12
INDIVIDUAL LESSONS

The Official Nutrition Education Association

HOME STUDY
COURSE IN
THE NEW
NUTRITION

RUTH YALE LONG, Ph.D.

Other Keats Titles of Related Interest

12 INDIVIDUAL LESSONS

The Official Nutrition Education Association

HOME STUDY COURSE IN THE NEW NUTRITION

RUTH YALE LONG, Ph.D.

Keats Publishing, Inc.　New Canaan, Connecticut

This information is made available as a public service by the Nutrition Education Association, Inc. It should not be used instead of medical advice or treatment by your physician. The Nutrition Education Association does not diagnose, treat, endorse, recommend or prescribe for any human disease or condition, nor does it dispense drugs or medicines of any kind. It is not commercially affiliated with any product, therapy or company, and neither the author, the Nutrition Education Association nor the publisher assumes any responsibility for use of the information herein.

RUTH YALE LONG, PH.D.
Houston, December 1988

**THE OFFICIAL NUTRITION EDUCATION ASSOCIATION
HOME STUDY COURSE IN THE NEW NUTRITION**

Copyright © 1989 by Ruth Yale Long

Library of Congress Cataloging-in-Publication Data

Long, Ruth Yale.
   The official Nutrition Education Association home study course in the new nutrition / by Ruth Yale Long.
      p.   cm.
   Includes index.
   ISBN 0-87983-381-5
   1. Nutrition—Study and teaching.   I. Nutrition Education Association.   II. Title.   III. Title: Home study course in the new nutrition.
TX364.L66 1989
613.2—dc19   88-12936
                                                           CIP

Printed in the United States of America

Keats Publishing, Inc.
27 Pine Street
New Canaan, Connecticut 06840

CONTENTS—HOME STUDY COURSE—ALL 12 LESSONS

Pages are numbered within lessons; *e.g.*, Lesson 1 runs from
page 1-1 to page 1-21. Index entries reflect this.

Lesson 1. A BASIC DIET PLAN AND USE OF FOOD SUPPLEMENTS

Getting started with Nutrition—Naturally. Philosophy of Nutrition. The Major Food Categories. Six Basic Rules for Good Nutrition. What Not to Eat. What to Eat for Meals and Snacks. Food Supplements for Adults. Accessory Food Factors. Food Supplement Program. If You're New to This Program. What's on the Chart. Marks, Notes and Abbreviations. The Chart of Supplements. Three High-Energy Drinks for You and Your Family.

Lesson 2. MENTAL PROBLEMS, STRESS, DEPRESSION, AND NUTRITION

New Brain Research. Mental Health and Nutrition. Brain Growth. Stress. Depression. Schizophrenia. Tranquilizers. Correcting the Incorrigible. Drug Addiction. Heavy Metal Poisoning. Diet. Suggested Additions to Food Supplements. Too Many Drugs—Time to Change.

Lesson 3. HEART DISEASE AND NUTRITION

Bypass Operations. Nutrition and Heart Health. Kinds of Heart Ailments. New Information "Trickles" In. Special Foods. Minerals. The Rinse Breakfast. Roundup. Food Supplements.

Lesson 4. ALLERGIES AND NUTRITION

Allergies and Nutrition. Allergens. Response to Allergens. The Liver. Pancreas. Adrenal Glands. Nutrients Needed. Results from My Program. Allergy Problems. Allergy Treatment. Allergy Symptoms. The Complete Allergy Program. Extra Nutrients for Allergies. Build Up Your Health.

Lesson 5. WHAT WE SHOULD AND SHOULD NOT EAT AND WHY

Is Our Food Good or Bad? Changes in Our Foods. What Shall We Drink? Nutrients Destroyed by Smoking. Fats and Oils. Carbohydrates. Calories. Imitation Foods. Additives. Automated Food Dispensing. Soil Determines the Health of Foods. The Future.

Lesson 6. VITAMINS FOR HEALTH AND ENERGY

Importance of Vitamins. Vitamin A. Vitamin B Complex. Vitamin B1 (Thiamine). Vitamin B2 (Riboflavin). Vitamin B3 (Niacin). Vitamin B6 (Pyridoxine). Pantothenic Acid. Folic Acid. Vitamin B12. Biotin. Choline. Inositol. Para-Aminobenzoic Acid. Vitamin C. Vitamin D. Vitamin E. Summary.

Lesson 7. MINERALS AND THEIR IMPORTANCE IN NUTRITION

Minerals Are Important. Chelated Minerals. Major Minerals. Trace Minerals. Dangerous Minerals. Hair Analysis. Food and Supplement Program.

Lesson 8. ARTHRITIS AND NUTRITION

The What and Why of Arthritis. Kinds of Arthritis. Stress Problems. Environmental Pollutants as a Cause of Arthritis. The Liver and its Influence on Arthritis. Arthritis of the Teeth. Diet Is of First Importance. Food Supplements. Suggestions for Nutritional Therapy. Arthritis as Allergy. Personal Experiences. Specifics of Arthritis/Nutrition Program.

Lesson 9. STAYING YOUNG WITH GOOD NUTRITION

How to Stay Young. Theories of Aging. Ailments of the Aging. Nutrients Needed. What We Don't Eat. What We Do Eat.

Lesson 10. BLOOD SUGAR LEVELS AND NUTRITION

New Diets for Blood Sugar Diseases. The Physiology of Blood Sugar. Hypoglycemia. Diabetes. Diet for Blood Sugar Problems. Food and Supplement Summary. Letters from Readers.

PREFACE

THE EXPLOSION of interest in nutrition that has occurred in the last few years has led to the publishing of this book as a guide for the general public. A natural food diet, plus moderate amounts of food supplements, as outlined in this book, will keep us well. You may ask, "What can I eat to stop the gas pains and the pains in my chest? How can I get more energy?" And the most important question of all: "How can I prevent cancer, multiple sclerosis, heart disease and other debilitating illnesses?" The partial answer is nutritious food. We eat to stay healthy, or we may become sick.

The general public is becoming more and more responsible for their own health. As an example, I received a letter from a woman who wanted to change her lifestyle now to keep from ending up in a wheelchair in a nursing home. The woman's mother was already undergoing that agony. We all hope to extend what Dr. Linus Pauling calls our "happy years," when we can move about and enjoy life.

More than 98 percent of Americans have filled, missing or decayed teeth; 3,000 of us die every day of cardiovascular disease, about 1,200 of cancer, and about 1,000 of diabetes. More than 50 percent of us have digestive problems, and one out of 10 will have such severe mental problems that they will have to be hospitalized. Presenile dementia (Alzheimer's disease) is now our fourth most prevalent killer disease; it is expected to be Number One in the 21st Century, which begins only 12 years from the time I am writing this. Good food and food supplements will help to improve most of our health problems.

Hundreds of people who have accepted this nutrition program have called or written to say how good they feel and how fast they are recovering. Some have muscular dystrophy, Crohn's disease, schizophrenia, chronic headaches, nerve diseases and allergies or arthritis that don't kill people but do make them miserable for 10, 20 or 30 years.

Nature's plan is that living creatures, including man, are provided with life-giving nutrients from natural foods. But these foods are perishable. Probably our three worst processed foods are white sugar, white flour and white rice. They last forever on the grocer's shelf, but they have so little food value they don't deserve space in our stomachs.

Occasionally, someone tells me that it is hard to eat well. What is really "hard" is being sick. Eating well is easy and pleasant. It may be different, but it is not difficult.

Many people are anxious to know what to eat so they can stay well. This *Home Study Course* will tell you what the body needs. The review questions at the end of each lesson will help you remember the most important points. My book, *Switchover! The Anti-Cancer Cooking Plan for Today's Parents and their Children* (Keats Publishing, Inc.) will help you to prepare nutritious food easily and quickly.

Our cells are made from the food we eat. If our cells are healthy, it's because we eat the food the cells need. If the cells are sick, it's because we senselessly feed our cells nonfoods or junk foods.

Won't you join me in eating good food that builds health with every bite? It will help us to be healthy, energetic and slim.

HOW TO USE THIS BOOK

Your new *Home Study Course in the New Nutrition* will be a pleasant, easy way to understand the importance of good nutrition.

Please read Lesson 1, "The Basic Diet Plan and Use of Food Supplements," first, because all the rest of the lessons are based on Lesson 1. For example, if you have allergies, you will want to go on the general diet in Lesson 1 to rid yourself of poisons and to build up your cells so you won't be allergic to anything. At the same time, you will want to add the special supplements and foods suggested in Lesson 4, "Allergies and Nutrition."

The same thing applies to arthritis, children's learning problems and the other disorders discussed in Lessons 2 through 12. If your ailments are more general—such as fatigue, indigestion or skin problems—Lesson 1 has all the information you need so that your body can heal itself.

Lesson 5, "What We Should and Should Not Eat and Why"; Lesson 6, "Vitamins for Health and Energy"; Lesson 7, "Minerals and Their Importance in Nutrition"; and (if you're over 30 years old), Lesson 9, "Staying Young with Good Nutrition," will tell you what good food and food supplements can do to *prevent* ailments, regardless of what they are.

Be sure to read the Chart of Supplements in Lesson 1 carefully. It has definitely stood the test of time. In the 18 years I have been "talking nutri-tion," I have received thousands of letters and phone calls from people as far away as Australia, islands in the Indian Ocean and from all 50 states, who have improved their health following the suggestions in the chart.

Many people tell me that they know they should be taking vitamin and mineral supplements, but they don't know what to take or how much to take. The chart tells in detail the supplements that you may need.

The companion book to this course is my cookbook, *Switchover! The Anti-Cancer Cooking Plan for Today's Parents and their Children*. It will help you prepare food that is good for you, tastes good and is quick and easy to prepare. You will never want to go back to your old diet of processed, refined nonfoods. Your new diet will build health with every bite.

A new feature in this course is the Review Questions, to reinforce the important points brought out in the text.

If you have any questions about the chart or other sections of this book, please write or call me.

Ruth Yale Long, Ph.D.
Houston, TX 77025

Lesson 1

THE BASIC DIET PLAN
AND
USE OF FOOD SUPPLEMENTS

LESSON 1—THE BASIC DIET PLAN AND USE OF FOOD SUPPLEMENTS

GETTING STARTED WITH NUTRITION—NATURALLY

NATURAL FOODS will help to keep us healthy, slim and peppy. They are the answer to many of our health problems. We should eat moderate amounts of fish, whole grains, legumes, fresh vegetables and whole fruits; small amounts of yogurt, natural cheese, nuts and seeds, chicken from health food stores and one or two eggs a day, also from health food stores. We can eat small amounts of red meat and milk, but these are not required.

To these natural foods, we add vitamins and min-erals in supplement form so that all the cells in our body will get the nutrients they need to prevent diseases—from dandruff to athlete's foot, and everything in between.

There are about 50 nutrients that we **must** have: about 20 vitamins, 20 minerals and 8 essential amino acids (building blocks of protein), plus carbohydrates, fats and water. "Essential" means we'll die without them.

Beginners' Questions

Every time I talk about my food program, invariably someone asks me the same four questions. Let me answer them now, in case you're wondering about these same subjects.

1. Nutrition and the Medical Profession. "If nutrition is as wonderful as you say it is, why don't doctors tell us more about it?"

I wondered about that myself, so in August 1973, I wrote to the American Medical Association and asked that question. The answer I received was, "Nutrition is wonderful, but doctors don't know about it because of a lack of nutrition training" (Moore, 1973). Recently, to bring myself up-to-date, I asked the same question, but the answer was the same: "Very little or no nutrition is part of a doctor's training."

So what can we do about this? We'll have to read and study on our own to learn how to be healthy. We can also ask our doctors to treat us with nutrition instead of drugs. I met a physician at a nutrition conference who said he didn't know anything about nutrition, but so many of his patients had asked about it that he realized he had to find out. Ask *your* doctor.

2. Heredity. Many balding men tell me, "My father and my grandfather were bald; I can't do anything about my thin hair because I inherited it." Many young women say, "My mother died of cancer; my aunt has cancer now. I know I'll die of it; I'm resigned to that, but I want to live as long as possible."

The answer to those people usually involves their genes and their environment. For a long time, geneticists knew that genes were very important, but now it is known that the environment has a lot to do with whether or not a bad gene develops. If a man gets every nutrient he needs, he probably won't lose his hair. If a woman keeps all the cells in her body healthy, they are not likely to change into cancer cells. We should be completely responsible for our own health; we can remain well if every cell in our body gets all the nutrients it needs.

Everyone has genetically different nutritional needs, and this *Home Study Course* will help you to find your specific requirements.

3. Mind and Body Stress. People tell me they are under a lot of stress: "It's not what I eat or don't eat," they say, "it's the awful stress at the office." Or maybe: "My son wants the car every night; my daughter stays out until three o'clock in the morning. The stress I'm under is killing me. Surely it's not what I eat. Isn't it just stress?"

About 50 years ago, Dr. Hans Selye discovered what happens in the body when we're under stress—it's the same for most of us. When we're confronted with a stress, the pituitary gland at the base of the brain sends a message to the adrenal glands, which sit on top of each kidney. The adrenal glands release their 32 hormones to prepare us to meet the

stress. Stored sugar pours into the blood to give us strength and energy in our arms and legs so we can move faster and do more muscular work if necessary. Also, more sugar in the brain allows us to think more clearly and quickly.

There are two ways to meet the stress—flight or fight. You run if you have to jump out of the way of a speeding car, but if your daughter stays out until three o'clock in the morning, you try to handle the problem by reasoning with her even though you are angry. Reasoning uses more blood sugar because the brain feeds on a sugar called glucose, and your brain gets a good workout trying to persuade your daughter to come home at a reasonable hour. You are actually fighting for your concern and possibly for your daughter's safety.

Whichever approach is called for—flight or fight—we hopefully make the right decision and conquer the stress. Then our bodies return to normal.

But the next hour or the next day we'll meet another stress, because that's the way life is. The pituitary sends its message and the adrenals try to pour out their hormones, but maybe all we had for breakfast was a cup of coffee, a doughnut and a cigarette. These nonfoods can't build up additional reserves of hormones, and the glands become exhausted. As time goes on, we try to meet the stresses of life with the help of our adrenal hormones, but we haven't fed the adrenals every nutrient they need. They become more and more exhausted until finally they begin to wither, damaged tissue builds up, the glands can't make hormones, the cells can't function and we're sick. We can't run and we can't reason.

Stress is perfectly normal. Healthy, well-fed adrenals handle stress well. But if the glands were unhealthy at birth because our mother lived on soft drinks and potato chips, or if they haven't been well fed since birth, they won't last long. And the day will come when the adrenals are so exhausted that they can't handle stress. Then one or more organs or tissues will be damaged. Weak adrenals are further weakened by the Standard American Diet (SAD), which is "bad enough to pull down even the strongest adrenals" (Tintera, 1958).

Stress is pleasant as well as unpleasant, so we don't want to eliminate stress from our lives. Hans Selye says even a passionate kiss is stress, so let's not try to live without stress. Let's feed every one of our cells so stress can't damage our minds or bodies.

4. Food Supplements. "If we eat a balanced diet, why do we have to take food supplements?"

The answer is easy—most of us don't get enough nutritious food. Most of it is so processed and refined, and so much of the food value has been destroyed, that we have to take vitamin and mineral supplements. The "protective nutrients," as Dr. Roger J. Williams (1973) calls them, have been lost from the food in the processing.

Many nutritionists also believe that the Recommended Dietary Allowances for vitamins and minerals are generally far too low to give us good health. Therefore, added supplements are often recommended.

PHILOSOPHY OF NUTRITION

Our philosophy of nutrition is that if every cell in our body gets every nutrient it needs, every tissue, every organ will be healthy, and we'll be healthy. We can't be healthy in any other way. All drugs have adverse reactions; all antibiotics damage the liver. Drugs can save our lives if we eat so poorly that we get sick, but, at the same time, they often cause more disease in the future. After years of such medications, our organs, especially the liver, can become so weak that a sudden infection or injury, even a mild one, can cause severe illness or even death.

Chronic Disease

Usually the first symptom of disease is fatigue. Next, we may get frequent infections, colds and flu ... then arthritis, diabetes, heart disease or cancer. Finally, after 15 or 20 miserable years of limping through life, we die. The reason is, usually, many years of nutritional deficiencies.

The sad thing is that most of our friends are limping also, with the same symptoms of disease, so we think that's normal. It isn't normal but it surely is average.

Statistics show that about 60 percent of us (that's more than every other person) have one or more chronic diseases. One million of these people are totally disabled, and 20 million have limited activity. At least three-fourths of us die of heart or vascular disease, and from other chronic diseases.

The difference between a chronic and an acute disease is that an acute disease either kills us or we get well, but a chronic disease is "incurable." A sick patient sees his doctor when he feels bad enough. Usually, drugs are prescribed. They work pretty well for a while. Then the patient feels worse again, and he takes another drug. For a time, he feels better again. The see-saw continues until drugs aren't enough. Then deterioration rapidly sets in.

One of my professors, an M.D., told his class that when he was in general practice, half the patients had nothing wrong that the physicians could determine. The patients felt bad, but there was no abnormal tissue, "nothing organically wrong." He and his colleagues gave their patients painkillers so the sick people could live with their symptoms, and that's all the physicians could do. My professor concluded, "Physicians can't tell the difference between someone who is okay and someone who is not okay."

A cancer investigator at a famous cancer institute says, "Doctors can cure 5 percent of human diseases; 95 percent of them we know nothing about."

Dr. Roger J. Williams (1973) notes that "doctors have to constantly make immediate decisions, and they must rely on what they've been taught. Physicians are not well trained to identify nutritional deficiencies except for gross under- and overweight, and that anyone can do."

Often our health problems begin in the womb. Our mothers didn't realize that poor nutrition before birth could stunt a child so he would never be as well, physically and mentally, as he might have been.

The illnesses that so many children have—the infections that strike about once a month all winter and are treated with antibiotics, make it more likely that another infection will strike—are usually caused by lack of vitamins and minerals. Another way of saying this is that they are caused by nonnutritious white sugar and white flour and fat, which make up 72 percent of the average American diet. Also, the hyperactivity, the behavior problems and the learning difficulties are virtually all nutritional deficiency diseases. Our children deserve to be well and to have good minds. We have to eat good food if we want to be mentally alert.

Some children seem well until they get to their teens. That's when they leave home to go to college or to get married; they are on their own. They don't have Mom to tell them, "At least drink your milk." From then on, it's more and more junk food, and their health eventually shows the strain.

Someone can die of a heart attack or stroke and his friends say, "Poor old Joe, he never had a sick day in his life." But Joe had really been sick for years. The fat had been building up in his coronary arteries or in the blood vessels in his brain. Finally a clot broke off a fatty deposit and floated through his bloodstream until it reached a spot that was too narrow to go through. The clot blocked the blood vessel, and the blood could not get through to take oxygen to the cells. Joe died.

It is surprising to learn that the first symptom of illness for one-fourth of the people in this country who die is death itself. Many people suddenly drop dead, and they didn't even know that their arteries were almost closed, their cells were dying, and death was coming soon.

Other chronic conditions can also cause such attacks. If the required minerals are not available in the heart muscle, the muscle gets weaker and weaker and finally stops beating. The person dies of a "heart attack," although his arteries are not blocked with fat as in the "usual" heart attack.

Let's Prevent Disease

We hear a lot about controlling disease with diet and food supplements, but the most important idea we can get across is how to *prevent* disease.

For prevention, we need a natural food diet. The proper food is primarily the same for allergies, arthritis, athlete's foot, dandruff, heart disease, cancer and all other diseases. If we eat all 50 nutrients, they will help us avoid disease, because our cells will be healthy. However, we can't just put those foods into our mouths and expect them to nourish our cells. We have to digest them, assimilate them into the blood and send them to every cell in the body. Every cell will take what it needs, and our bodies will heal themselves.

This food program is a way of life—not a crash diet to go on for only a week or a month or even a year. Good nutrition, which includes food and food supplements, must be continued forever.

You will recover from almost every ailment with this food program. Dr. Tom Spies, an early nutritionist, said, "If we just knew enough, we could cure all our ailments with food." Hippocrates said, "Food is our medicine; our medicine is food."

A tremendous amount of research shows that disease is related to poor diet. Dr. Ernst L. Wynder, president of the American Health Foundation, said in 1976 that "as much as 50 percent of all cancers in women and one-third in men relate to diet."

A natural food diet, he says, could also reduce the heart attack rate in this country by 25 percent, and infant mortality by 50 percent. Besides this, food bills would go down, since grains, fresh fruits and vegetables don't cost as much as convenience foods and highly processed junk food. Much more startling than that report is one which states that cancer is preventable, and gives guidelines for what we should eat to prevent it (*Diet, Nutrition and Cancer,* 1982). See my book *Switchover! The Anti-Cancer Cooking Plan for Today's Parents and Their Children* for more information about cancer and nutrition.

But if we eat better for a while and get to feeling better, then go back to the Standard American Diet, we'll get sick again, because it's the American diet of processed and refined foods that caused our illness in the first place.

A woman called me recently to talk about nutrition. She was going on vacation in three months and wanted to be "through" with the diet so she could eat anything she wanted from then on. It doesn't work that way.

Most people tell me that they would never go back to the old way of eating. They like what this food program does for them—it prevents disease and promotes good health.

Listen to Your Body

Our bodies will tell us when we're deficient in some nutrient if we'll just listen. We may know *now* that something is wrong. On our new diet, we will feel better. Then if we ever feel less than our best, we reread Lesson 1 very carefully, and we will almost always find that we've run out of one of our supplements, or we're not taking enough hydrochloric acid to digest protein, or we let our friends or relatives talk us into some food that wasn't right for us. It's usually very easy to find the reason we're fatigued or depressed.

When people tell me that they've changed their diets to improve their health, almost all of them stay on their new food and food supplement pro-

grams very carefully, and within a few days or weeks they write me: "I feel better physically and mentally than I ever have before. I would never go back to the old way of eating." However, during the years, a few people have gradually slipped back into their old habits of fast food and junk food, and they get sick again.

A fortyish woman called me recently and said that her allergies had returned. I knew that she wouldn't have developed allergies again if she had been following the food and food supplement program she had chosen before. She reviewed her program, and, sure enough, she was eating many junk foods. She was not eating six small meals a day, not taking balanced supplements, and she was missing so many of the nutrients she needed that she had developed the allergies. She realized what she should do, and said, "I really did feel good while I was on the program before. I won't get off of it again."

I'm sure she agrees with Dr. Roger J. Williams, who said in 1973, "The combination of good, natural food plus the correct nutritional supplements could eliminate most of the mental and physical problems, and is inexpensive compared to drugs and doctor bills."

Listen to your body; it will talk to you about food.

THE MAJOR FOOD CATEGORIES

Let's discuss proteins, carbohydrates and fats, our three major food categories.

Proteins

Although Americans are told that they eat too much protein, many of them aren't eating enough or not digesting what they eat. If they were, they wouldn't be sick.

When people come to me for counseling, they bring a list of everything they've eaten, drunk or snacked on for three typical days. Here's the list one woman brought in:

BREAKFAST
 1 toasted Danish
 1 cup coffee
SNACK
 diet cola
LUNCH
 pizza
 2 peppermints
 orange
 glass of water

SNACK
 handful of corn chips
 2 chocolate cookies
SUPPER
 1 Sloppy Joe sandwich
 handful of French fries
 ice tea
 vanilla ice cream

This is as bad a diet diary as I have seen. The only protein I could count was the Sloppy Joe sandwich, and that might be 10 grams if it were a big one. However, since it was on white bread, I guess we should take off a few points. She had just discovered that she had high blood pressure and that scared her. She also had frequent bladder infections, gas, bloating, too-full feeling after meals, fatigue and headaches. She was overweight and under severe stress. Ten grams of protein a day will never be enough to repair all her sick tissues. Women need from 44 to 46 grams of protein a day, men from 45 to 56. The sad thing about this woman's food intake is that she thought she was eating well.

Animal Proteins. What are our sources of protein? When we think of protein, we usually think of red meat (steaks, roasts, chops and hamburger), but many of us need to cut down on red meat. More and more research shows that people who eat a lot of red meat have more heart disease and cancer than people who don't. The suggested amount is no more than four ounces four times a week. Less is better, and none is all right; we can get our proteins from other foods more healthfully. Beef is said to be the most tainted red meat because of the growth hormones, antibiotics and pesticides the animals are fed. However, many nutritionists say that pork is just as bad.

Chicken from the supermarket is so tainted you probably will never want to eat another chicken. While I was working on my Master's in public health, I was taught that every fiftieth chicken that goes through the slaughterhouse line has cancer. The cancerous portion is cut off, thrown in a vat, cooked down a little and fed to the next batch of chickens. Thus, we're eating cancerous flesh, growth hormones, pesticides and antibiotics that the chickens were given in their feed. Obviously, none of these things is good for our cells. Chickens are often fed so much growth hormone that they can be brought to market in six weeks rather than 10 or 12. The farmer makes twice as much money, but the tainted chicken isn't really that good for us. Buy your chickens at the health food store. They cost more but they're worth it.

Although commercial chickens are often bad, commercial eggs are said to be acceptable. But once you've tasted an egg from the health food store, you'll never want to go back to supermarket eggs. We can eat one or two eggs a day and cook with extra eggs if we want to make muffins or custard. Eggs are an excellent example of complete protein—they have all of the amino acids in the amounts needed by our cells.

Don't worry about cholesterol in eggs; studies show that the cholesterol isn't what stacks up in our blood vessels. The average American eats 42 percent of his calories as fat, mostly in processed foods, and the tremendous amount of total fat (especially triglycerides) *does* cause fatty plaques in our arteries. On my program, we get all the nutrients needed to process the small amount of fat that we eat (10 to 20 percent of calories), so the fat serves as energy and doesn't stack up in blood vessel walls and form plaques. If lecithin is in the blood, it will emulsify the fatty plaques and send them into the blood as tiny globules that float along until they get to the liver, where they are made into bile. We can't live without bile, which is used to digest fat

and fat-soluble vitamins A, D, E, and K. So nature gave us a way to make cholesterol in every cell and to use lecithin to emulsify it. Egg yolks contain five to seven times more lecithin than cholesterol. So the medical journals are now saying we should eat more eggs since they are a good source of lecithin. Other good sources are soy, nuts, seeds and liver. So now, after 25 years or so, we're being told to eat more eggs, especially the yolks, which contain lecithin.

Fish is good animal protein; we can eat it several times a week. Man usually doesn't have anything to do with fish until he catches it, packages it and ships it. Fish may be soaked in a chemical during packaging, but that's probably not so bad when compared to what happens to some chickens and other animal protein.

Milk Proteins. If you can get raw milk, you're getting an excellent protein. Pasteurized, homogenized milk is heated and altered at the dairy and much of the food value is diminished. So we don't want to drink very much of it. One-half glass on cereal in the morning and one-half glass in a frozen fruit smoothie in the evening will be enough. But we must get calcium and other nutrients when we take our food supplements with yogurt during meals.

Cheese provides good protein if we eat natural, light-colored cheese and avoid the cheeses that are processed or colored with orange dyes.

Plant Proteins. The next protein category is probably more important than all the rest, especially for vegetarians. It is plant protein, which comes in two groups. Group A contains whole grains, nuts and seeds. Group B contains legumes, which are beans, peas and peanuts. When we combine these groups, we get complete proteins.

A complete protein is one that has the eight essential amino acids in maximum amounts for our cells, as in egg protein. There are 22 amino acids that we make our proteins from, just as there are 26 letters in the alphabet that we make our words from. The liver manufactures 14 of these amino acids if we eat the other 8 within 20 minutes of each other. If we have 21 amino acids ready to make hair or skin, we can't remain healthy if the liver doesn't have the raw materials to complete the 22nd amino acid.

In Figure 1, "A" represents the amino acid pattern of whole grains, nuts and seeds. Each of the eight spokes represents one of the essential amino acids. You'll notice that one of the spokes is very short. That's because one of the amino acids in these foods is in short supply. When we eat these foods alone, we get only the amount of protein represented by the small circle. The amino acids that extend beyond the circle are lost to us as protein. They are stored in the body as fat or are used as energy, but they have no protein value.

Now look at "B" in Figure 1. It represents the amino acid pattern of legumes (beans, peas and

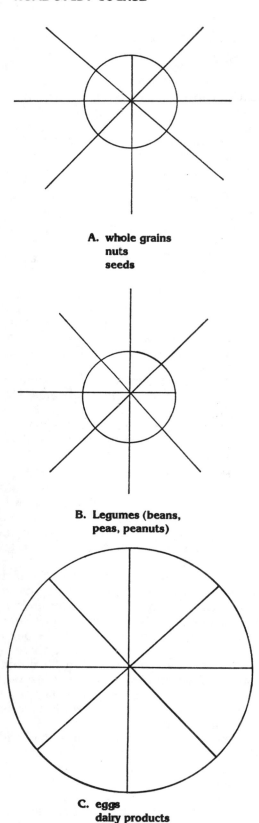

A. whole grains
nuts
seeds

B. Legumes (beans,
peas, peanuts)

C. eggs
dairy products
animal proteins

Figure 1. **The amino acid pattern of proteins.**

peanuts). One of the amino acids is in short supply. The small circle in "B" shows us that we're missing

a lot of good protein when we eat legumes by themselves.

Now look at "C" in Figure 1. We get this amino acid pattern when we combine group A (whole grains, nuts and seeds) with Group B (legumes—beans, peas and peanuts). They must be eaten in the same meal or snack. We can't eat the grains at breakfast and the beans at lunch and get complete proteins, because the amino acids will never get together in the digestive tract. By eating the groups together, we get all the amino acids needed for a complete protein—one group of foods complements the other.

The "C" pattern is complete protein as in eggs, dairy products and other animal proteins, so we aren't limited to combining groups A and B. We can also combine Groups A and C and Groups B and C. Thus, it is very simple to remember that when we eat Group A we must have either Group B or Group C. When we eat Group B we must have either Group A or Group C. We can always eat Group C by itself.

This chart is very simple. It's easy to think, "Here I have a dozen peanuts to eat. But I know that peanuts are not complete protein since they're legumes. So to complement them, I can eat a piece of whole-grain bread, a half glass of milk or yogurt, or a mixture of sesame and sunflower seeds." Those are a few of the many proteins to combine.

How much grain should we eat to balance the legumes? For a rule of thumb, we eat twice as much grain as beans. Therefore, if you eat one-half cup of millet, eat one-fourth cup of lentils; if you eat one cup of brown rice, eat one-half cup of red beans.

We have many choices of grains and beans, and you would be amazed at the various main dishes you can make with these excellent protein foods. Here are a few suggestions. Couscous—an Algerian dish made of cracked wheat and bits of meat and vegetables; cheese-grits soufflé; tamale pie made with cornmeal crust and spicy beans; No-Meat Loaf that looks and tastes like meat but has no meat in it—guaranteed to please the most red-meat-eating husband; patties made of garbanzo beans and millet; casseroles of grains, vegetables and cheese; omelets made with cracked wheat and steamed carrots or other vegetables; grain and bean burgers; crepes filled with anything from curried chicken to yogurt and crushed strawberries. The variety is endless. All the recipes I mentioned are in my cookbook, *Switchover!*

Protein Requirements. Some vegetarians eat plant proteins only, but they can get the amount of protein they need more easily if they eat eggs and drink milk. If they do, they're called lacto-ovo vegetarians. The main nutrient missing in plant foods is vitamin B12, but we can get it from meat, fish, milk and eggs. Vitamin B12 is not in brewer's yeast normally, but it has been added to some supplements. So read labels.

Think what we'll be saving when we eat proteins instead of so much beef. It takes about 20 tons of plant protein to feed animals, which returns to us one ton of animal protein. We can instead eat the plants and get a delightful variety of whole grain and legume combinations for good health, pep and energy.

Proteins are one of the most important items of diet. They are required to repair tissues; they are used for both growth and repair in children, so children need more for their size than adults do. Men need about 45 to 56 grams, women about 44 to 46, depending on their size. To get more exact figures for yourself, (according to the Food and Nutrition Board), divide your body weight in pounds by two. You'll get the approximate number of grams of protein you need. If you err, err on the high side. That is, it's all right to eat a little more than the minimum, but not so good to eat less.

Here's a short list of protein foods and their gram content.

egg 6
meat, fish, etc., 4 oz 25
yogurt, 1 cup 8
cottage cheese, ½ cup 15
tapioca pudding, ½ cup 5
desiccated liver, 2 tbsp 14
brewer's yeast, ½ cup 24
powdered milk, 1 tbsp 3
sardines, 3 oz 22
shrimp, 3 oz 20
beans, red kidney, ½ cup 8
lentils, ½ cup 8
soybeans, ½ cup 11
orange, 1, 3″ diameter 2
wheat germ cereal, ½ cup 10
millet, ½ cup 10

Let's review the do's and don'ts of protein. We eat animal protein including eggs, fish, poultry from health food stores, light-colored, natural cheese, whole milk (no skimmed or 2 percent) and small amounts of red meat (steaks, chops, roasts and hamburger). Let's add many plant proteins to our diet (whole grains and legumes). We'll feel much better for it, and we'll greatly enjoy the food.

Carbohydrates

Our next big food category is carbohydrates. We get energy from carbohydrates, which means that enzyme systems can't work and we can't work without carbohydrates.

The two protein categories we just talked about—whole grains and legumes—are also carbohydrates, because, as everyone knows, grains and beans have a lot of starch in them. Starch and sugar are carbohydrate foods. Starch is good; sugar is bad.

The two other big groups of carbohydrate foods are vegetables and whole fruits.

We eat more carbohydrates than either of the other food categories. You've heard for the last 25 or so years, "Eat a low-carbohydrate diet," and now I'm saying the opposite. We now know the importance of carbohydrates, but they must all be *complex* —not refined—not one ounce of white sugar, white flour or white rice.

Complex carbohydrates furnish energy for the cells' activities and save protein for repair. We won't get fat eating complex carbohydrates because grains, beans, vegetables and whole fruits are so filling and satisfying that we simply won't overeat.

Fats

The third major food category is fats. We should eat rather small amounts of both animal and vegetable fats.

The animal fat marbled through red meat is the worst kind because it contains poisons from the animal's food, air and water. The animal's liver detoxifies the poisons, but it doesn't store them; it sends them to the fat cells. Every day the cells furnish fat to the body for energy, and the poisons are eliminated when this fat is used. When we eat, we replace the fat. Our liver also sends a lot of the poison to be stored in the intestines, because those cells are replaced every one to six days, and the poison will be eliminated quickly. From 20 to 50 percent of our feces is sloughed cells, taking the poisons out of our bodies.

The three best animal fats are butter, cream and eggs. We should use only small amounts of butter—a natural fat—and we should never use margarine or hard, white shortening, both manufactured and so processed that they no longer fit the chemistry of our cells.

We should drink whole milk if we drink milk. As we've said, raw milk is best if we can get it. Cream contains five important trace elements, one of them chromium, which is required for glucose (sugar) tolerance. If we can't tolerate glucose, we'll have either low blood sugar (hypoglycemia) or high blood sugar (diabetes, our third largest killer disease). Fat in the cream also furnishes energy.

We drink milk to get calcium to feed our bones, teeth, nerves, muscles and other tissues. To assimilate the calcium, we must have fat; and the best kind of fat is the fat that comes in the cream. We're moderate about all fats, so we don't drink much cream, because too much is as bad as too little; we can't assimilate calcium if we overload our bodies with fat. I suggest no more than one glass of whole milk a day and one cup of yogurt.

The third good animal fat is egg yolk, which is almost all fat. It is now known that there are two kinds of cholesterol, one good, the other bad. The good cholesterol is mixed with lecithin, which emulsifies the cholesterol and keeps it flowing through the blood vessels. We cannot live without cholesterol. Every cell in the body can manufacture it, and the liver can make extra cholesterol in case some cells didn't produce enough to make bile. Cholesterol is part of our sex glands and adrenal glands, and it makes up from 5 to 10 percent of our brain tissue. On autopsy, the brains of Alzheimer's patients may be withered. Could that be because the patients did not get enough cholesterol?

Polyunsaturated vegetable fats are extremely important, but we get all we need from a small amount of nuts and seeds. They furnish linoleic and linolenic acids, the two essential fatty acids the body can't manufacture.

We don't want to eat vegetable oils from a bottle because they have been deodorized, depigmented, processed, refined, possibly hydrogenated and surely heated to a high temperature, even if the label says "cold pressed." The first few drops off the press can be cold, but the friction of pressing the oil heats it to a temperature that destroys food value. All of this processing changes the chemical structure of the oil molecule so it no longer fits the chemistry of our cells, and we can't use the abnormal molecule, called a "trans" fat (Hunter, 1971). But if we eat French fries, the trans fats are in our body. They get into the bloodstream and finally land in a cell where they can clog that cell so much that it can't function properly. If trans fats land in the liver, they can cause a liver problem; in the skin, a skin rash; in the kidneys, kidney damage; in the digestive tract, constipation.

What kind of salad dressing should we eat since we're not going to eat a lot of oil? Use a base of yogurt or buttermilk blended with part of the vegetables you're using in the salad. Or wash and dry Romaine, celery or any other raw vegetable, and serve with toasted nuts and seeds. Or butter a Romaine leaf with a thin film of peanut butter from the health food store or eat the leaf wrapped around a thin slice of white cheddar cheese, and you will join my new salad culture. I've appointed myself a committee of one to try to change American salad-eating habits, because we should cut down on so much oil with its trans fats.

We do need a small amount of linoleic acid from polyunsaturated vegetable oils. We should also eat three to six small amounts of nuts and seeds a day to get the linoleic acid we must have. What is a small amount? Two teaspoons of sunflower, sesame or pumpkin seeds, two walnut halves, four pecan halves, six almonds or 12 peanuts. You may need more if your skin is dry, if you're physically active, if you're a fast-growing child or if you need to gain weight.

If we eat three to six (depending on our size) small measures of nuts and seeds a day, we'll get the linoleic acid we need, but we won't get fat, because fat will burn fat. Remember, don't eat your entire quota of nuts at one time—spread them out through the day, one measure at each meal and snack. Combine nuts and seeds with other plant or animal proteins to make complete proteins as in the A/B/C groups.

Please note: peanuts (not really nuts, but legumes) must always be toasted. Raw legumes (beans, peas and peanuts) destroy trypsin, a digestive enzyme from the pancreas; they cause the villi in the small intestine to stick together and they can cause goiter.

Ratio of Protein to Carbohydrate and Fat

How much should we eat of each category—proteins, carbohydrates and fats? We need about 10 to 20 percent of our intake of calories as protein. Choose the higher level if you're ill and have a lot of tissue that needs repair. We need about 10 to 20 percent as fat. That leaves 60 to 80 percent of our intake of calories as *complex* carbohydrate—vegetables, whole fruits, grains and legumes. Actually, we don't count calories, we just estimate. A well-nourished hypothalamus region in the brain will tell us when to start and stop eating so that we won't eat too much or too little.

Let's put those percentages into small circles as in Figure 2.

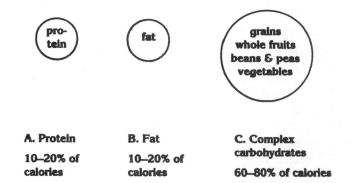

A. Protein
10–20% of calories

B. Fat
10–20% of calories

C. Complex carbohydrates
60–80% of calories

***Figure 2.** Amounts needed of proteins, carbohydrates and fats.*

Circle A represents the moderate amount of protein we will eat. Circle B indicates the small amount of fat. Although the percentage of fat and protein is the same, fat contains twice as many calories as protein, so the fat circle has to be half as big. Circle C represents the large amount of complex carbohydrates in our food program, but not one grain of white sugar or white flour. Whole grains, legumes, vegetables and whole fruits are excellent sources of vitamins, minerals and fiber.

When we eat lunch and supper, we should have a moderate serving of protein and a small amount of fat. The fat may be a thin film of butter on a muffin, plus nuts and seeds eaten out of hand or sprinkled on salad or on steamed vegetables. That means the largest amount of our food is vegetables (a big salad for lunch and a big serving of steamed vegetables for supper—or vice versa), plus fruits (for snacks), grains and legumes, which contain both carbohydrates and proteins (at any meal or snack, all through the day).

Often people ask me, "May I have snack food for breakfast and breakfast food at snack time?" Yes, that's fine, as long as you get everything on the list every day.

This diet may not seem magic to you, but so many people say they have greatly improved their health, it must have magic properties. The magic is that if we eat this way, we don't miss any of the 50 required nutrients. Our bodies will get what they need and they will heal themselves!

SIX BASIC RULES FOR GOOD NUTRITION

Here are six basic rules that we should live by. The first two are the most important. Both rules will help us digest our food better, and, since undigested food is poison to our bodies, good digestion is our number one priority.

Rule 1. Eat six times a day—three small meals at regular meal times, and three smaller snacks in between. I call this a nibble diet. If we eat small amounts of food at a time, we'll have enough enzymes—made from protein—to digest and assimilate our food, and enough carriers to take the food to our cells. There used to be a saying "We are what we eat." Now our saying is, "We are what we digest, absorb into our blood and assimilate into each cell," because, regardless of how good the food is, if we eat too much at one time, we can't assimilate it.

Almost everyone I talk to is pleased that they can nibble all day, but some people say they don't have time to eat six meals. Look around you. The average American eats six times a day, but he calls his mid-meal snacks "coffee breaks"; we call ours nutrition breaks.

In one study, laboratory rats were fed six small meals a day rather than three larger meals, as most people eat. Some of the rats started their nibble diet when they were two weeks old; others began when they were two years old (which is middle age for a rat). Both groups lived almost twice as long as the average. The food was the same, and they ate the same amount, but when they ate it in nibbles, they digested their food better and lived longer. Let's shout that from the housetops. Just think. One of the easiest ways to feel better and live longer is to eat less food at one time. It won't cost a cent extra, and we can start this procedure today.

Rule 2. I don't recommend drinking liquid with meals. And we should never drink coffee, tea, canned drinks, bottled drinks, cola, cocoa, alcohol or fruit juice.

Perhaps I should explain why we should not drink fruit juice. It is too sweet with natural sugar even if we don't add sugar. We can tolerate a medium-size whole apple or orange, but if we press or squeeze the fruit and make a glass of juice, it will have the equivalent of from four to seven teaspoons of sugar in it. The sugar goes to the liver quickly, where it should be stored. But the liver can't store that much sugar at one time. It releases the sugar to the

blood, and the heart pumps the blood all over the body. Since all that sugar goes through the pancreas, the pancreas secretes insulin, which takes the sugar out of the blood and puts it in the tissues so that we won't have diabetes. But we may have low blood sugar. It is estimated that 90 percent of Americans have low blood sugar, which often turns into diabetes if it isn't treated, and the only treatment is diet.

I know of many children who have continuous infections, sore throats, and some even lose their hair because of the large amounts of sugar they drink in fruit juice.

Since we shouldn't drink all those beverages, what does that leave us to drink? Milk and water, basically.

The important thing about water is to drink it 30 minutes before meals and snacks. The water goes from our stomachs into the small intestine about 30 minutes before the food gets to the stomach, where it must be digested in an acid medium. Water dilutes the strong hydrochloric acid needed to digest protein, which is why I do not recommend it with meals.

I receive more letters about immediate relief from gas and bloating when people stop drinking liquid with meals than on any other subject.

Rule 3. We should eat both raw and steamed vegetables every day. An easy way is to take raw vegetables to work or school and eat them with nuts and seeds. Steamed vegetables can be served at home with supper.

Rule 4. Vary your diet as much as possible. Every good, natural food adds something we need, but no one food gives us everything. For example, we should eat whole grains every day, but we should vary them so as to eat millet, bulgur, buckwheat, corn grits, etc.

Rule 5. Don't eat white sugar, white flour or white rice or anything made from these nonfoods. They are the worst empty-calorie foods. They deprive the body of B vitamins because it takes extra Bs to digest and assimilate those junk foods, and they don't contain enough of the vitamins and minerals needed for proper nutrition.

Rule 6. Eat almost no convenience foods—canned, frozen, bagged, packaged or "instant" foods. We can, of course, freeze our own garden produce, but otherwise we should buy fresh vegetables in season. We can eat moderate amounts of canned tuna, salmon and sardines.

WHAT NOT TO EAT

We should not eat processed meat such as ham, bacon, sausage or hot dogs. An occasional hot dog from the health food store will satisfy your children's desire for a weiner roast. Eat no processed cheese, cheese food or orange-dyed cheese; eat only natural, light-colored cheese such as Swiss, mozzarella, Monterey Jack and white cheddar. We should avoid margarine and hard white shortening; eat small amounts of real butter and nuts and seeds for the fats we must have. Eat no iceberg lettuce; instead eat dark green lettuce such as romaine, salad bowl, Boston, red tip and Bibb. Dark green lettuce has four times more food value than white, and we should not take up space in our stomachs with poor-quality food.

WHAT TO EAT FOR MEALS AND SNACKS

Let's go through the six meals of a day and see in detail what can be prepared from scratch.

On Arising

Drink water—six, eight or 10 ounces, whatever is right for your size and activity. I usually have about eight ounces the firsst thing in the morning and taper off to smaller amounts the rest of the day. I also put from one-fourth to one teaspoon of powdered vitamin C in the first glass because it's been six hours or more since my last dose. Many people use lemon juice. That's good too, but it doesn't have enough vitamin C, so we add powdered C.

Breakfast

Thirty minutes later, eat breakfast—one or two eggs; one for a little lady, two for a big man. Poached or soft-boiled are good. Hard-boiled eggs are acceptable if they're not overcooked but we don't have enzymes to break down overcooked protein. Scrambled or "over easy" eggs are fine if you "frizzle" them in butter in a moderately heated skillet. "Fry" means using a hot skillet with oil, and I don't recommend fried foods. If you have a good skillet that doesn't need grease, use that if you wish, but don't let it get too hot. If overheated, the finish on the skillet can send off toxic fumes.

With your egg, eat a small amount of whole-grain cereal. You can have a piece of toast, biscuit, muffin, pancake or waffle you've made yourself, or you can eat cereal hot (oatmeal, cracked wheat, four-grain or seven-grain) or cold (granola)—all from the health food store. There are so many delicious grains that we shouldn't limit ourselves to wheat, even though it's good. We can enjoy rye, triticale (a combination of wheat and rye), brown rice, corn, bulgur, buckwheat, oats, millet and barley. Dr. Josef Issels, a cancer specialist in Germany, says, "Whole grains are foods of incomparable perfection."

The important thing to remember about grains is not to get the supermarket kind. They have been processed and refined; the nutrients are so depleted that the grains don't have enough food value to justify taking up space in our stomachs. Degerminated grains are grains with the most healthful part removed. Don't buy them.

Health food store grains take longer to cook than supermarket varieties, but these hot cereals can be cooked with almost no effort. Try this method: The night before, place the grains in a wide-mouth thermos bottle with a plastic liner, not the glass kind. Add the right amount of boiling water needed for the grain. Put the top on, and swish the thermos around a little to mix the water and grain. Let it sit on the counter all night. In the morning, your breakfast will be waiting. The grains will be separate, cooked nicely and still slightly warm. The pint-size thermos makes enough for two or three servings.

Since we're going to eat six small meals a day, we don't overeat at any one meal. We always tell ourselves, "Stop eating, save space for your snack two and a half hours from now."

I once received a letter saying, "I had to get off your program because I can't eat that much." Since then, I've tried to emphasize that we need to eat *small* amounts—nibbles, really—especially at mid-meals.

Midmorning Snack

Thirty minutes before your midmorning snack, drink water. For the snack, eat a half or whole apple or any kind of fruit, with a nibble of protein. Good protein nibbles are a few nuts with a cracker you made, or peanut butter on a whole-wheat muffin. A square of natural hard cheese is healthful.

These few suggestions for nutritious snacks are by no means all. You'll find many more in my cookbook, *Switchover! The Anti-Cancer Cooking Plan for Today's Parents and Their Children.* Try some of the plant protein combinations. They're light and they digest well.

Lunch

Thirty minutes before lunch, drink water. For lunch, eat four ounces of a high-protein dish. This can be meat (occasionally), fish, poultry (from the health food store or from a farmer in the country); hard cheese, cottage cheese, yogurt, milk or a combination of the plant proteins: (A) whole grains, nuts and seeds, and (B) legumes (beans, peas and peanuts).

Choose millet soufflé, a casserole made with milk, eggs and cheese, plus tuna, potatoes, carrots, chickpeas (also known as garbanzo beans) or your choice of several lightly steamed vegetables mixed with a moderate amount of frizzled ground beef or other animal protein. The same combinations can also be made into meatless loaves or patties. These recipes are in *Switchover!*

With your protein dish you can have either a steamed green or yellow vegetable or a combination of several vegetables, including potatoes, if you wish. Once a day eat a raw vegetable salad. If you insist, you can have both salad and steamed vegetables for lunch and supper, but it's easier to prepare just one. If you work or go to school, pack a salad in a handbag-type cooler or in a small, wide-mouth thermos. Or, if your office has a fridge, stash it in there. It's easy to carry big chunks of vegetables, and they keep much better than if they're chopped fine. Eat small amounts of parsley often; it contains a lot of vitamin A and chlorophyll. Eat some nuts for their polyunsaturated oil content.

If you're still hungry, eat a whole-grain cracker or small piece of bread with a thin film of butter. You should be preparing all kinds of breads in advance and freezing them. Warm up just enough for one meal in the toaster-oven. You won't need bread if you've eaten potatoes, unless you want to gain weight.

Midafternoon Snack

Drink water 30 minutes before your midafternoon snack. This snack is the same as midmorning, with different fruits and different protein nibbles. You'll discover new and delightful snacks every time you leaf through a natural foods cookbook, and you'll probably make up some recipes of your own.

Supper

Thirty minutes before supper, drink water. Supper is the same as lunch—proteins, vegetables and maybe some grains. But make your choices different. Don't cook a roast and eat it at every meal until it's gone. Eat some at one meal and freeze the rest in meal-size portions. It's easy to double many recipes and to store a few dishes as you go along. Then you'll have a variety of protein dishes to warm in the steamer for future meals. Here are some protein choices your family might like:

LUNCH	SUPPER
egg salad	brown rice and red beans
chicken	millet burgers
poached fish	corn grits and cheese
cottage cheese	turkey breast
tamale/bean pie	lean roast beef

After five days or so, you can repeat some of the dishes as you try out new ones.

You also need variety in the grains and beans I suggest, the condiments served with them and the recipes for tuna, eggs, chicken, other animal protein and, of course, vegetables. Here are some choices of vegetables for lunch and supper:

LUNCH: steamed broccoli
tossed green salad
steamed mixed vegetables
carrot and raisin salad
avocado and grapefruit salad

SUPPER: coleslaw
steamed cauliflower
chopped green salad with toasted almonds
steamed green beans sprinkled with
sesame seeds
hearty vegetable soup

Evening Snack

Remember, don't eat too much at supper. You'll want to enjoy a small snack at 9:00 or so.

You'll be eating whole fruit in a smoothie or with nuts and seeds, plus custard, yogurt or a nibble of cheese. Thirty minutes before your evening snack, drink water.

In a Nutshell

Now that we've been over the day's meals in detail, let's summarize the program. But please re-read the detailed information occasionally.

On arising: Drink water at room temperature—the amount that is right for you. Don't drink too much, you won't be hungry for breakfast; don't drink too little, you'll be constipated the next day.

Breakfast: One or two eggs, whole-grain bread or cereal.

Drink water 30 minutes before snack.

Midmorning snack: Nibbles of protein and a small fresh fruit. An excellent protein is one-third to one-half cup of the Super Health Yeast Drink. (Recipe is in the chart at the end of this lesson.)

Drink water 30 minutes before lunch.

Lunch: Four ounces of a high-protein dish, plus steamed vegetables or raw green salad with nuts or seeds or oil-free dressing. One piece of whole-grain bread or half a muffin with a thin film of butter if you're still hungry—omit if on the weight-loss diet (see Lesson 12).

Drink water 30 minutes before snack.

Midafternoon snack: Same as midmorning. Drink water 30 minutes before supper.

Supper: Same as lunch.

Drink water 30 minutes before snack.

Evening snack: Same as midmorning.

Don't forget to eat from three to six small amounts of nuts and seeds a day, with some or all of your six small meals. Three servings are for little ladies; six for big men.

Different, Not Difficult

One of my counselees smiled sweetly when I told her she should make her bread. (It doesn't have to be raised bread; biscuits and muffins are fine.) She said, "I eat out every meal and I don't intend to change. I smoke and I don't intend to quit." I smiled too, and kept on talking about this food program.

I talked to her on the phone about two months later, and she said she was preparing all her meals from scratch, including bread. She didn't like to eat out any more, because the food was so much better at home, and she was enjoying the entire program and talking about it to her friends. She said she had smoked very few cigarettes because she just didn't think about lighting one. Then she added, "Besides, I'm saving a hundred dollars a month. This food is inexpensive compared to what I was paying for the food that was making me sick."

There's *nothing difficult* about this food plan, but it is probably very *different* to many people. When you get into the swing of things, you'll realize how easy it is.

FOOD SUPPLEMENTS FOR ADULTS

Linus Pauling believes that with the proper intake of vitamins and other nutrients, and by other healthful practices, we can live 25 to 35 years longer than otherwise. Also, more of us can live through the happy middle years, not confined to a bed or a wheelchair.

Our nutrition program must include food supplements. At nutrition conventions, I have heard many physicians say that, without supplements, they can't be as well as they like to be and that they can't keep their patients as well as *they* want to be. We need food supplements as insurance because our food is so processed and refined that much of the food value has been destroyed.

The Food Supplement Program on page 15 suggests amounts of nutrients for the average adult. If you're larger or smaller than the average, or if you're weak and ill, you might need more or less. If you're new to food supplements, begin with small amounts and work up gradually. Grind up the hard tablets and start with small amounts of the powder. Gradually work up to the amounts on the chart (see page 15). Stop short of those amounts if you're feeling like a million dollars.

We should take the supplements during meals for best assimilation, but since we don't drink water with meals, we can take our supplements with yogurt. We need yogurt every day anyway, to maintain the friendly bacteria in the intestines. Several supplement tablets slide down easily with a sip of yogurt (but start with one at a sip and build up).

When you are planning your own nutrition program with the help of this *Home Study Course*, start with small amounts of food supplements and build up gradually as suggested in the Food Supplement Program. Your body will let you know how much to take. When you feel better mentally and physically than you have felt before, you can take a little more and you'll probably feel even better. Later, you may want to decrease to a maintenance dose. If you don't feel up to par, go back to the original dosages. No one knows your body as well as you do.

ACCESSORY FOOD FACTORS

You'll find the vitamins discussed in Lesson 6 and the minerals in Lesson 7. This section will discuss some accessory food factors that will make your new food program even more helpful.

Yogurt. It helps to digest food and stimulates the kidneys; it's high in protein and vitamins. It helps to lower excess cholesterol, but sugar can cancel out its helpful effects. So eat the unflavored kind or make your yogurt at home.

Fiber. Miller's bran, available in health food stores, is an excellent source of fiber. Add it to all baked goods to help prevent constipation. It also helps to prevent heart disease, cancer of the colon, varicose veins, diverticulosis and obesity.

Lecithin. It helps to emulsify cholesterol and to remove it from blood vessel walls. It also helps to digest and absorb fats and prevent gallstones. And it helps to produce healthy nerves.

Blackstrap molasses. A good source of vitamins and minerals. (Brush your teeth after eating it.) Use sparingly in baked goods, since it has a very strong flavor.

Brewer's yeast. Excellent source of B vitamins, minerals and protein. Yeast is high in phosphorus, so check the label and buy yeast that has phosphorus balanced with calcium and magnesium. It helps to prevent heart trouble and constipation and to manufacture enzymes and cells in the immune system.

Wheat germ. It contains 24 grams of protein in one-half cup. It's high in phosphorus, so drink extra milk or add non-instant powdered milk to recipes to maintain calcium balance. Keep in freezer after opening. It's a rich source of vitamin E and fiber.

FOOD SUPPLEMENT PROGRAM

I receive many calls and letters about how easy it is to use this chart and figure out your own supplement program. Some call it "the best road map" they've ever seen. However, a few people have been overwhelmed by it. One young woman from Kentucky heard me speak there and bought some of my books. She glanced at the chart after she got home and thought she could never figure it out. She called me and said she wanted to come to Houston to talk with me in person. I told her I'd love to see her, but I wondered if she had really read this lesson. She said, "No, it just looks hard to me." I suggested that she read the lesson with a pencil in hand and mark in the margin every sentence she had a question about, then to call me and we could go over the lesson together.

She did that, and when she called she said she understood it very well, and there were only two questions she wanted to ask. She was impressed with how easy it was to figure out. I know you will be too.

Choose Your Own Diet

It is your prerogative to choose your own diet and to take food supplements. The products listed conform to the formulas suggested by outstanding researchers. The reader must construct the best possible nutritional program for himself. The author and Nutrition Education Association, Inc. are not responsible for the use or misuse of these products.

Health Food Stores

The products I discuss are available at health food stores. I don't list brand names; any brand at a reputable health food store will be all right if it has the same formula I have suggested. The relative amount of one vitamin or mineral to another is important.

If you cannot find the vitamins and minerals in the exact formulas I suggest, get the closest thing to them and fill in with individual formulas to equal the amounts listed in the chart.

Children's Vitamin Suggestions

The dosages in the chart are for adults. Children 13 and up take the adult dose, children six to 12 take one-half that amount and children from 1 to 6, take one-fourth. If your child is on the borderline, judge by his size which amount he should take or give him a fraction of the amount that fits his age. Don't overdo anything. For children under one year of age, get a liquid multi-vitamin-mineral for infants from the health food store, and give it according to instructions on the bottle.

IF YOU'RE NEW TO THIS PROGRAM

People who are new to this program may have been sick a long time, and their digestion isn't as good as it should be. At first their digestive systems just can't assimilate the added tablets and the different foods. Also, there may be large amounts of poisons in the system that the body needs to throw off. The poisons are usually released only in small amounts or not at all the first week or so. They will probably be released slowly the second and third week, until the poisons are gone. (It may take longer in some people.) By the fourth week, the poisons should all be gone, and you can increase to the amount your body needs. You will feel better than you've ever realized possible if you ease into this program, listen to your body and adjust the dosages according to what your body tells you.

Either poor digestion or stored poisons can cause gas, diarrhea, skin rash, nausea, dizziness, abdominal cramps, headache or other reactions. So grind up the hard tablets and take small amounts of the powder in order to assimilate them better or to slow down the release of poisons which are causing adverse reactions.

Grind Up the Tablets

If you have never taken supplements before or if you haven't taken a full program of supplements recently, you should grind all the hard tablets together and begin with small amounts of the powder at a time. The powder will have the correct ratio of one nutrient to another.

Grind up the amount of hard tablets suggested on the chart for one day. Don't grind the gelatin perles (usually A, D and E). Take them whole. Never grind the hydrochloric acid tablets or any enzymes. Take them whole also. They must dissolve in certain parts of the digestive tract.

The tablets can be ground dry in a blender or in a nut mill available at health food stores. Since the powder will be thrown all over the walls of the blender, scrape it down and dump it onto a paper.

Funnel the paper into a small jar. Keep the jar in a cool place.

How to Swallow the Tablets

How are you going to swallow the powdered tablets? Take them with yogurt or with any food soft enough to swallow without chewing, such as a mashed banana or apple sauce you have made in a blender with fresh apples. Put the amount of powder you're going to take in a small cup and mix in the soft food or yogurt. The B vitamins are bitter so swallow the powder quickly.

How Much Powdered Tablet to Take

Take about ⅛ teaspoon of the powdered tablets one to six times with meals the first day. (You won't use the entire amount of powder the first day; just save the rest for the next day.) If you have any reaction, stop for that day and start over after a day or two with a smaller amount. Continue to take small amounts until your system gets used to the supplements. When you can tolerate more, increase gradually at about three-day intervals until you are taking the entire amount suggested for one day. After you take the powder for two to four weeks, switch to the whole tablets and see if your system can tolerate them. Watch for undissolved tablets in your stool. If they're there, continue to take powdered tablets a while longer. It would be better to take the tablets ground, but you may be able to assimilate them whole after a few weeks. Sometimes strict vegetarians do not have sufficient hydrochloric acid in their stomachs to digest whole tablets and capsules.

Most people have no adverse reaction to taking the tablets whole, but if you do, come back to this section and review this information so you can slowly phase in your new food program.

Adjust Your Intake of Powdered Tablets

With this method of increasing the amount of food supplements, you will adjust your intake to what is right for your own body. Increase as fast as you can, because you won't get well until you get the nutrients your cells need. But don't increase so fast that you have adverse reactions. One of my friends told me she had gas and nausea after being on the program a few days. She said she had taken the full amount of tablets from the first day, although she knew she should take them in small amounts and build up. She said, "I just wanted to feel better faster." It's better to go slowly. Later, reduce the amounts of supplements to maintenance doses as shown on the chart. Your body will tell you if you need to increase again later.

Adjust Your Intake of Whole Tablets

If you start on whole tablets, go easy there too. Start with one or two of each kind and go up gradually to the total amount suggested.

If You've Been Taking Supplements All Along

You will probably be able to begin with small amounts of the tablets as noted on the chart, and work up to the full dosage in a few weeks.

WHAT'S ON THE CHART

The chart on the following pages gives the amount of nutrients suggested by nationally known nutritionists for the average adult. Also listed are deficiency conditions with suggestions for larger amounts of each vitamin and mineral if you suffer from that deficiency. Next is a suggested amount to be taken when you have recovered from the deficiency and you need a smaller amount for maintenance. We're all different, and we need different amounts based on our size, our activities and the condition of our health. We need supplements but there's no reason to take more than we need. Always remember, food is the most important part of this program, but we often also need food supplements.

MARKS, NOTES AND ABBREVIATIONS

(*) = essential	IU = international unit	t = teaspoon	Beg = Begin
(?) = special	mcg = microgram	T = tablespoon	Inc = Increase
(+) = accessory	mg = milligram	c = cup	Dec = Decrease

(x) = times to take a supplement; take the amount that's right for you

What Do the Marks Mean?
(*) (?) (+) (x)

Items marked (*) are essential and should be taken indefinitely because they are the basic vitamins and minerals that our bodies cannot manufacture. Most of them have been processed out of our food to a great extent.

Items marked (?) are for whoever needs them. Read the information in the paragraph and if the deficiency symptoms apply to you, take the items as needed.

Items marked (+) are called accessory food factors, and a healthy body can manufacture them if all nutrients needed to make them are circulating in the blood at all times. When people are sick, their cells may not be healthy enough to make these nutrients, so we help out by taking these food factors until the body can make its own. Some people might want to take them indefinitely; others might take them from time to time during the year. Taking them one month out of three will generally keep any ailment from sneaking up on us. Young people in good general health may take some of the items marked (+) one month out of six. Let your body tell you what you need. It's like cleaning out the carburetor of your car this month to avoid engine trouble next month. Take a moderate amount for three or four weeks, then stop taking them for a month or two and see how you feel. If you feel worse, take them again as long as needed. After all, they are just food. This way, we renew our cells even if we don't need all accessory food factors in supplement form all the time.

Occasionally I use an (x) under Brk, Lun or Sup. Some people will take liquid supplements; others, powder or tablets. So I couldn't say take "1" or "2." You'll need to take the correct amount by milligrams and take it at the times suggested: Brk, Lun and/or Sup.

Begin, Increase, Decrease
(Beg, Inc, Dec)

The chart suggests amounts for beginners, how to increase if needed and how to decrease to a maintenance dose. We're all different, and we need different amounts based on our size, our activities and the condition of our health. When the directions say "Increase," go up one tablet every three or four days until you get to the higher dosage. After your health problems have been solved, you may be able to decrease to a maintenance dose. That depends somewhat on your age and how well you stay on the food program.

Brk, Lun, Sup, Bed

Abbreviations to remind you to take your supplements at breakfast, lunch, supper or bedtime.

If Needed

I use "if needed" all the way through the chart. It means "if not noticeably better in one month, gradually go up." If you've never taken vitamins and minerals before, you should start with small amounts, but if your body needs more, go up gradually.

How Do We Use the Chart?

Let's go through the information on vitamin A and see how easy it is to use this chart. Vitamin A has an asterisk, which means that we take it every day from now on.

With your pencil, circle "Beta-carotene" and "25,000 IU." "Note" in the vertical column on the right side of the page says to begin with one at breakfast. That gives the dose needed by the average adult.

The next line in the right-hand column says "Increase if needed" to one at breakfast and one at supper. How do you know if you need to increase? Read the paragraph about vitamin A and you will see many signs of deficiency of vitamin A. If you have any of those signs, you may need to go up to two a day.

After you get over the deficiency, decrease to one 25,000 IU dose of beta-carotene with breakfast as a maintenance dose.

All the rest of the supplements are discussed in the same way.

THE CHART OF SUPPLEMENTS

VITAMIN A
(*) Vitamin A as beta-carotene—25,000 IU.

Relieves eye strain, infections, skin problems both inside and outside the body, liver and kidney damage, fatigue, loss of smell, inability to absorb calcium, respiratory problems, sinusitis (Kirschmann, 1975).

Helps prevent original cancers and recurrence of cancer; cancer patients may need much more (Nieper, 1983). See your nutrition-minded physician.

Note	Brk	Lun	Sup	Bed
Beg	1			
Inc if needed				
to	1		1	
Dec when able				
to	1			

Always take with butter or cream to stimulate enzyme activity.

VITAMIN B STRESS COMPLEX
(*) Vitamin B stress complex plus vitamin C. Choose any tablet with approximately this formula. Note that niacinamide and pantothenic acid are at five times the strength of B1, B2 and B6.
Each tablet contains:

30 mg B1	50 mcg B12
30 mg B2	150 mcg biotin
30 mg B6	100 mg choline
150 mg niacinamide	100 mg inositol
150 mg pantothenic acid	30 mg PABA
0.4 mg folic acid	500 mg Vitamin C

Note	Brk	Lun	Sup	Bed
Beg	1		1	
Inc gradually				
	3		2	
Dec when able				
(3 to 6 months)				
to	1		1	
Inc under stress				
to	2	2	2	2

Helps prevent mental conditions from poor concentration to stuporous depression, and others:

fatigue	arthritis	sullenness
pellagra	psoriasis	dizziness
headache	hypoglycemia	fat in arteries
neuritis	nerve problems	stress damage
diabetes	cirrhosis	aggressiveness
eczema	irritability	quarrelsomeness
stroke	hyperactivity	sensitivity to criticism
anxiety	loss of memory	pernicious anemia
insomnia	hostility	personality change
	tenseness	inability to concentrate

VITAMIN C
(*) Vitamin C. Suggested B complex has 500 mg of C in each tablet. After reaching 2,500 mg in B complex, increase C to bowel tolerance. Go up to 500 mg every three days or so until you get gas or diarrhea. Cut back about 1,000 mg and take that much every day.

Bowel tolerance increases with infections, stress and cold weather. Take ascorbic acid, calcium ascorbate or an ascorbate containing several minerals as buffers.

For colds, allergies, infections, pollution, smoke inhalation, toxic metals, stroke, heart disease, cancer and many more disease conditions.

Note	Brk	Lun	Sup	Bed
Beg	1			
Inc after a few days				
to	1	1		
Inc after a few days				
to	1	1	1	
Inc to bowel tolerance				

CITRUS BIOFLAVONOIDS
(*) Citrus Bioflavonoids—500 mg. Part of C complex.

For each bruising, miscarriage, nosebleeds, excessive menstrual bleeding, hemorrhoids, asthma, bleeding gums.

Note	Brk	Lun	Sup	Bed
Beg	1			
Inc if needed				
to	1		1	

VITAMIN D

(*) Vitamin D—400 IU for the average adult and child; 1,000 to 2,800 IU may be needed for a few months in pregnancy and lactation or for bone and dental disease. This vitamin can be toxic in very large amounts.

Note	Brk	Lun	Sup	Bed
1				

VITAMIN E

(*) Vitamin E—600 IU (young men), 400 IU (young women), 1,200 IU (70 year olds) (Passwater, 1976). Increase according to age. Choose d-alpha tocopheryl (or tocopherol) acetate or succinate, not the synthetic dl-alpha.

For many heart and blood vessel diseases, edema, burns. Dissolves scar tissue including acne scars, regulates menstrual flow. For arthritis, varicose veins, crossed eyes, nearsightedness, muscular dystrophy, headaches including migraines. Excellent for applying to skin lesions such as warts.

Note	Brk	Lun	Sup	Bed
	x			

MULTIMINERALS

(*) Multiminerals—tablets, amino acid chelated.

1,000 mg calcium	225 mcg iodine
20 mg iron	500 mg magnesium
1 mg copper	22.5 mg zinc
10 mg manganese	95 mg potassium
200 mcg chromium	200 mcg selenium
100 mcg molybdenum	

For physical, emotional and mental well-being. Helps cells use nutrients, activates enzyme systems. Don't take minerals in excess; they can become toxic more easily than vitamins.

Note	Brk	Lun	Sup	Bed
	x		x	

Take the amount needed to reach this potency.

TRACE MINERALS

(*) Trace Minerals—liquid or tablets. Of great importance, but only small amounts are required. Many trace minerals are included under multi-minerals.

Note	Brk	Lun	Sup	Bed

See label.

WHEAT GERM AND BRAN

(*) Wheat germ and bran. Add to baked goods and cereals. Adjust amount of bran needed to prevent constipation and diarrhea. Begin with 1 three times a day with meals. Go up as needed. Drink plenty of water at the right time: 30 minutes before meals and snacks.

Note	Brk	Lun	Sup	Bed
	x	x	x	

YOGURT

(*) Yogurt. Take supplement tablets with sips of yogurt during meals. Sugar cancels out the value of yogurt, so buy unflavored yogurt and add fruit if you wish. Or buy the starter at a health food store and make your own yogurt at home.

Note	Brk	Lun	Sup	Bed
	x	x	x	

LECITHIN GRANULES

(*) Lecithin granules. Take 1 to 1 T in Greek Drink, Yeast Drink or on cereal. For protection against fatty liver and fat in the blood vessels; for brain power and relief of depression. Ask for highest percentage of phosphatidyl choline.

Lecithin in gelatin capsules is not recommended; large amounts of gelatin are not easily digested by some people.

Note	Brk	Lun	Sup	Bed
See label.				
Beg	x			
Inc if needed				
to	x	x	x	

May double the amount for learning problems, senility, etc.

CALCIUM

(?) Calcium—500 to 1,000 mg more than in Multi-Minerals section and half that much more magnesium (both amino acid chelated). Vitamin D helps to absorb calcium to prevent or control arthritis or osteoporosis.

Note	Brk	Lun	Sup	Bed
If needed.				
	x		x	

PANTOTHENIC ACID

(?) Pantothenic acid (a B Vitamin)—100 to 200 mg in addition to B complex. For stress, allergies, arthritis, infections.

Note	Brk	Lun	Sup	Bed
Beg	1		1	
Inc if needed				
to	2	2	2	

TRYPTOPHAN

(?) Tryptophan—500 mg. For depression take these amino acid tablets in the mornings; for insomnia take tablets in the evenings.

Note	Brk	Lun	Sup	Bed
Beg	1			1
Inc				2
Phase out when able.				

OCTACOSANOL

(?) Octacosanol—1 mg. Dosage 1 mg for physical fitness (muscular strength, running time).

Note	Brk	Lun	Sup	Bed
	1			

(?) Octacosanol—for nerve-muscle diseases—from 2 to 5 mg daily. If no help, try 10 mg, but more than 10 would probably not help.

Multiple sclerosis, muscular dystrophy, amyotrophic lateral sclerosis, brain damage, myasthenia gravis and other conditions.

Note	Brk	Lun	Sup	Bed
Beg	1		1	
Inc gradually				
to	2	1	2	
Inc if needed				
to	4	3	3	

SUPPLEMENTS FOR CANDIDA ALBICANS

(?) Candida albicans supplements: garlic
taheebo tea (ask in health food store)
lactobacillus acidophilus
beta-carotene, 50,000 IU or more depending on severity. Vitamin A
thymus tablets, 3 to 6 a day (a raw glandular)
vitamin C to bowel tolerance
Plus natural food diet and moderate amounts of all other food supplements

Note	Brk	Lun	Sup	Bed
See specific entries in this chart.				

L-GLUTAMINE

(+) L-Glutamine—500 mg. Brain fuel for all ages. Helps in withdrawal from alcohol, cigarettes and sugar.

Note	Brk	Lun	Sup	Bed
Beg	1		1	
Inc if needed				
to	2		2	
Dec	1		1	

KELP

(+) Kelp—granular. Take ½ to 1 t daily. For weight control, sluggish thyroid, cold hands and feet, lethargy. Helps prevent radiation damage.

Note	Brk	Lun	Sup	Bed
Beg	¼t		¼t	
Inc if needed				
to	½t		½t	
Dec when able.				

PANGAMIC ACID (VITAMIN B15)

(+) Pangamic acid (including dimethyl-glycine (DMG), the active part of pangamic acid)—50 mg. Double or triple for emphysema, asthma or cancer. For listlessness, poor circulation, low mental levels, morning sluggishness. Supplies extra oxygen to tissues. Also for athletes.

Note	Brk	Lun	Sup	Bed
	1		1	

DESSICCATED LIVER POWDER

(+) Desiccated liver powder. Begin with 1 t a day; work up to 1 T. Ideal for afternoon snack so you won't have a five o'clock low. To mask the taste, take in canned vegetable juice. (The only time I advocate canned juice—to mask the terrible taste of desiccated liver.)

Note	Brk	Lun	Sup	Bed
Any time, but best as mid-meal snack.				

GARLIC

(+) Garlic—perles (some have no odor). Reduces high blood pressure; helps infections, asthma, diabetes, muscles, eliminates wastes including waste water. 15 mg of garlic oil a day (the equivalent of 3 or 9 cloves of garlic) lowers total cholesterol, increases HDL cholesterol and decreases LDL cholesterol.

Note	Brk	Lun	Sup	Bed
Beg	1	1	1	
Inc if needed				
to	3	3	3	

EPA

(+) EPA (eicosapentaenoic acid) with DHA (docosahexaenoic acid)—from fish body oils. 1,000 mg. Helps prevent heart attacks and strokes.

Note	Brk	Lun	Sup	Bed
Beg	1		1	
Inc if needed				
to	2		2	
Dec when able				
to	1		1	

CARNITINE

(+) Carnitine—250 mg. Helps to use fat and reduce triglycerides in the blood. Improves heart problems, muscular dystrophy and overweight. Our muscles can't move without carnitine.

Note	Brk	Lun	Sup	Bed
Beg	1		1	
Inc if needed				
to	2		2	
Dec when able				
to	1		1	

AMINO ACIDS

(+) Amino acids—powder, capsules or tablets. Continue taking all vitamins and minerals, especially B complex (5 a day) and C (bowel tolerance). This is *not* predigested protein or protein powder.

For physical benefit: high blood pressure, liver diseases, chemical poisoning including chemotherapy and radiation, bronchitis, emphysema, skin diseases, peptic and other ulcers, alcoholism, anemia, food and inhalant allergies, heart attacks, tumors, digestive problems, low and high blood sugar, cataracts.

Amino acids help to manufacture red and white blood cells, support the immune system and slow the aging process.

For mental and emotional benefit: mental retardation, nervousness, irritability, headaches, epilepsy, depression, schizophrenia.

Note	Brk	Lun	Sup	Bed
Beg	1,500 mg	1,500 mg	1,500 mg	
Inc if needed because of weight, size or severity of disease				
to	3,000 mg	3,000 mg	3,000 mg	
Phase out but continue from time to time.				

LACTOBACILLUS ACIDOPHILUS

(+) *Lactobacillus acidophilus*—tablets, liquid or powder (vary them). For healthy intestines and to achieve stools that are light colored, big around, soft (but don't disintegrate) and almost odorless, which means that 95 percent of the bacteria in the stools are "friendly" and almost none will be poisonous. *Bulgaricus* is not recommended because it is destroyed by the acid digestive juice in the stomach.

Note	Brk	Lun	Sup	Bed
See label.				
Inc if needed to double or triple that amount.				

RAW GLANDULARS

(+) Raw glandulars—tablets made from glands of young animals are available to help the corresponding gland in the human. Take according to the label.

Note	Brk	Lun	Sup	Bed
See label.				

BROMELAIN ENZYME

(+) Bromelain—protein-digesting enzyme that breaks down protein in acid or alkaline medium. 250 to 300 mg. Cancer, heart disease preventive.

Note	Brk	Lun	Sup	Bed
Beg	1		1	
Inc if needed				
to	2		2	

HCL and PANCREATIC ENZYMES

(+) Digestive enzymes—betaine hydrochloride with pepsin, glutamic acid hydrochloride, pancreatic enzymes.

For gas or bloating during or immediately following a meal, inability to taste meat or other proteins, belching and lower bowel gas one to two hours after eating, bursitis, arthritis, poor calcium and iron assimilation, anemia.

Symptoms of too much and too little acid are the same. By age 20, most people on the Standard American Diet (SAD) don't make as much acid as they need.

Note	Brk	Lun	Sup	Bed
Beg	1	1	1	
Inc	2	2	2	
or more if needed. Take from time to time or all the time, as needed.				

THREE HIGH-ENERGY DRINKS FOR YOU AND YOUR FAMILY

There are many health drinks on the market, but the best kinds are the ones we make ourselves. We should use whole food prepared fresh every day. This is an excellent way to take supplements. We never use these drinks to take the place of food, because food is still the most important. But we can include moderate amounts of special natural foods to improve our health pleasantly and quickly.

Here are recipes for three different drinks and suggestions about when to drink them. If you're new to these supplements, begin slowly and work up to the total amount suggested. If you become nauseated, you're increasing the amounts too fast. Poisons are being eliminated from the cells, and that might cause nausea or headaches, so go slowly at first.

Remember that if you phase out the drinks after you get to feeling good, continue to take the supplements marked "essential" (*) daily. Also, take the drinks from time to time to keep any ailment from sneaking up on you.

YEAST DRINK

(+) Brewer's yeast—super food, contains B vitamins, minerals, proteins.

Super Health Drink
Mix in blender: 1 c whole milk, yogurt, buttermilk or mixture or: 1 c nut milk (¼ c nuts powdered dry in blender, then add ½ to 1 c water)
add: 1 t to 1 T lecithin, according to the label. Add lecithin to either the Green Drink or the Yeast Drink, not necessarily both.
1 raw egg (leave out the egg if you'd rather have your egg cooked)
¼ t to 1 T brewer's yeast (begin with ¼ t and increase gradually)
add flavor with fruit, pure vanilla or almond extract

Take one-quarter to one-half cup as the protein for your midmorning and evening snacks, or with meals, with digestive enzymes if needed. Swallow the enzymes whole; do not dissolve. Or take 1 tablespoon every 30 minutes or so all day if you have trouble digesting food. This drink is excellent as a complete breakfast with a muffin.

GREEN DRINK

(+) This Green Drink will help to give you the power needed to maintain health and to help reverse the aging process. I like to drink it 30 minutes before breakfast. For faster recovery from any ailment, you can drink it 30 minutes before lunch and supper also if you're weak, depressed and tired. Since the Green Drink contains very little protein that must be digested in the stomach, it will quickly go through to the intestines and then to the blood and cells.

Green Drink
Into 6 or 8 oz of water, blend (or beat with egg beater):
1 t green barley powder
1 t (3 grams) free-form amino acids
1 t lecithin (or more, according to label).
Add lecithin to either Green Drink or Yeast Drink; not necessarily to both.
¼ t (1,000 mg) powdered vitamin C
¼ t granular kelp
¼ t L-glutamine powder
Add if you wish:
25,000 IU liquid beta-carotene (one day's usual dosage)
400 to 1,200 IU liquid vitamin E (see chart for potency)
liquid trace minerals (see label)
You will need only a light breakfast 30 minutes later, possibly one egg and one-half piece of whole-grain toast.

The above recipe makes one serving. If you drink more before lunch and supper, make another recipe for each drink. Don't make up more than enough for one day.

LIVER DRINK

(+) I may have saved the best for last, but the Liver Drink doesn't taste the best. It's not bad when mixed with vegetable juice. The liver drink will increase your energy and furnish many vitamins and minerals for your cells.

Liver Drink
1 t to 1 T dessicated liver, blended well with
6 oz of mixed vegetable or tomato juice

I have talked to many people about this drink, and they say it helps them feel better than any other recommendations. You will probably want to begin with 1 t of the liver and increase to 1 T as your midafternoon snack. You'll be peppy right through the afternoon, and you'll have plenty of energy to prepare the evening meal of steamed vegetables and protein.

Please Note:
The way this program is designed, the nutrients in the tablets and in the drinks are divided through the day so that they will maintain your energy and good health all day every day.

As you begin to feel better than you've ever felt before, you will become more energetic, your ailments will begin to leave your body, and you will get to your correct weight without being on a strict diet. You will be healthy, energetic and slim.

QUESTIONS

TRUE/FALSE

1. It is imperative that we get all 50 nutrients (proteins, carbohydrates, fats, vitamins, minerals and water) in order to be well.

2. Some diseases are inherited, but usually, if a certain disease runs in families, it's because the family members ate the same kind of food with the same deficiencies.

3. Stress is an abnormal condition, and our bodies have no way to handle it.

4. The first symptom of illness for one-fourth of the people in this country who die is death itself.

5. Dr. Roger J. Williams says, "The combination of good, natural food plus the correct nutritional supplements could eliminate most of the mental and physical problems, and is inexpensive compared to drugs and doctor bills."

6. Red meat is required in a natural food diet.

7. It is possible but difficult to be a strict vegetarian.

8. We should not drink skimmed or 2-percent milk because the cream has important nutrients needed to help digest calcium.

9. As a general rule, we should eat 10 to 20 percent of our calories as protein, 10 to 20 percent as fat, and 60 to 80 percent as complex carbohydrates, but not one gram of white sugar or white flour.

10. Rule 1 of good nutrition is to eat three small meals at regular meal times, and three smaller snacks in between.

11. Rule 2 of good nutrition is never to drink liquids with meals because we don't want to dilute the hydrochloric acid needed to digest protein in our stomachs.

12. Recent research suggests that the average adult should eat one or two eggs a day.

13. B-complex vitamins are used in large amounts by the brain.

14. Vitamin D is manufactured by sunlight shining on our skin.

15. Studies show that vitamin E helps lower high blood pressure.

16. Chelated minerals are better absorbed in the body than some other minerals.

17. Nutritionists advise large doses of phosphorus as supplements.

18. Our muscles don't coordinate well without manganese.

19. Wounds may not heal well without zinc.

20. Potassium deficiency can cause paralyzed muscles.

MULTIPLE CHOICE

1. Nutritional deficiency diseases include: (a) hyperactivity, (b) behavior problems, (c) learning disabilities.

2. To be well, we must: (a) eat at least 25 of the 50 nutrients, (b) digest our food well, (c) assimilate the food into the blood and (d) send digested food to each cell.

3. Excellent proteins include: (a) chickens from a farmer who raises them without pesticides, antibiotics and growth hormone, (b) eggs, (c) fish, (d) certified raw milk.

4. Which of the following combinations are complete proteins: (a) brown rice and red beans, (b) nuts and seeds, (c) soufflé made with cheese, eggs and milk, (d) black-eyed peas and corn bread.

5. The three best animal fats are: (a) lard, (b) butter, (c) cream, (d) eggs.

6. Which of the following are healthful salad dressings: (a) yogurt-based dressings, (b) mayonnaise made with safflower oil, (c) fresh nut butter or ground nuts, (d) Swiss cheese, grated or sliced and mixed with vegetables.

7. We should not eat raw beans, peas and peanuts because they: (a) destroy trypsin, a digestive enzyme from the pancreas, (b) cause the villi in the small intestines to stick together, (c) make us fat, (d) cause goiter.

8. Other rules of good nutrition include: (a) eating steamed and raw vegetables daily, (b) varying our diets, (c) not eating highly refined foods, (d) eating almost no convenience foods—canned, frozen, instant.

9. We should not eat: (a) processed meat, (b) processed cheese, (c) margarine, (d) hard white shortening.

10. Some of the best foods for freezing are: (a) whole grains, (b) dried beans, (c) watery vegetables, (d) all kinds of bread.

11. Vitamin A has the following effects on the body: (a) as a cancer treatment, it destroys the shield that the cancer builds around itself to repulse the body's immune system, (b) it helps heal wounds, (c) it helps heal bed sores, (d) it can be used as a gargle for sore throat.

12. Vitamin C helps against: (a) pollutants, (b) smoking, (c) arteriosclerosis, (d) petechiae.

13. Calcium truths include: (a) deficiency of calcium can cause the heart to beat irregularly, (b) nutritionists suggest taking hydrochloric acid to help dissolve the calcium we eat, (c) the large amounts of phosphorus in the tissues can pull calcium out of the bones, (d) undissolved calcium can build up in the tissues and joints and cause hardening of the arteries or arthritis.

14. Symptoms of deficiency of magnesium include: (a) blood clots in the heart and brain, (b) twitching muscles, (c) softened tooth enamel, (d) epileptic seizures.

15. Sodium deficiences are unlikely, but they can

cause: (a) intestinal gas, (b) weight loss, (c) nerve pain.

16. Helpful accessory food factors include: (a) wheat germ, (b) garlic, (c) dessicated liver, (d) lecithin.

ANSWERS

True/False

1. T 2. T 3. F 4. T 5. T 6. F 7. T 8. T
9. T 10. T 11 T 12. T 13. T 14. T 15. T
16. T 17. F 18. T 19. T 20. T

Multiple Choice

1. a,b,c 2. b,c,d 3. a,b,c,d 4. a,c,d 5. b,c,d
6. a,c,d 7. a,b,d 8. a,b,c,d 9. a,b,c,d 10. a,b,d
11. a,b,c,d 12. a,b,c,d 13. a,b,c,d 14. a,b,c,d
15. a,b,c 16. a,b,c,d

REFERENCES

Ballentine, R. *Diet and Nutrition, A Holistic Approach.* Honesdale, PA: The Himalayan International Institute, 1978.

Bland, J. Carnitine. *Health News and Review*, March-April 1986.

Cheraskin, E. and Ringsdorf, W.M. *Psychodietetics.* New York: Bantam, 1976.

Diet, Nutrition, and Cancer. Washington, DC: National Academy Press, 1982.

Downs, R. W. New Products for Enhanced Health. *Bestways*, May 1986, p. 38–39.

Garrison, R. H. Jr. and Somer, E. *The Nutrition Desk Reference.* New Canaan, CT: Keats, 1985.

Hunter, B. T. *Consumer Beware.* New York: Bantam, 1971.

Kirschmann, J.D. *Nutrition Almanac.* New York: McGraw-Hill, 1975.

Levinson and Bigler, 1960.

Moore, M.E. Personal Letter from Nutrition Education Section, American Medical Association, 1973.

Nieper, Hans. Tape of talk at Atlanta, Southeast Conference of Clinical Nutrition, P.O. Box 592, Colony Square Station, Atlanta, GA 30361. May 13–15, 1983.

Passwater, R. *Supernutrition.* New York: Pocket Books, 1976.

Pauling, L. *How To Live Longer and Feel Better.* New York: W. H. Freeman, 1986.

Pfeiffer, Carl C. *Mental and Elemental Nutrients.* New Canaan, CT: Keats, 1975.

Select Committee on Nutrition and Human Needs of the United States Senate. (In) Diet Related to Killer Diseases V, *Nutrition and Mental Health.* Washington, DC: U.S. Govt. Printing Ofc., 1977.

Selye, H. On Just Being Sick. *Nutr. Today*, 5(1):2–10, 1970.

Tintera, J. What You Should Know About Your Glands and Allergies. *Woman's Day*, Feb. 1958.

Williams, R. J. *Nutrition Against Disease.* New York: Bantam, 1973.

Wynder, E.L. Nutrition and Cancer. *Federation Proc.* 35:1309–1315, 1976.

Lesson 2

MENTAL PROBLEMS, STRESS, DEPRESSION AND NUTRITION

LESSON 2—MENTAL PROBLEMS, STRESS, DEPRESSION AND NUTRITION

NEW BRAIN RESEARCH

ALL MENTAL problems are physical problems. That statement might surprise you, but it is true because our brains are made of cells that determine whether or not our minds work well. If they do, we are intelligent; if they do not, we are stupid. Our brain cells also determine our emotions. Sometimes we are pleasant, sometimes we are vicious and aggressive.

Obviously, we want our brain cells to make us intelligent and pleasant. How can we bring this about? With good food, which will supply every cell in the brain with every nutrient it needs. Which of the approximately 50 nutrients are needed for brain food? All of them. We need all of the vitamins, minerals, proteins, carbohydrates, fats and water to have healthy brains that can develop to their best potential. We all *deserve* good brains; now it is known that the health of the brain depends on the food we eat.

The food needed by the brain is the same that we talk about in this entire series of lessons—natural food, unprocessed and unrefined, which contains all the essential nutrients in sufficient amounts so that our brains will never lack even a microgram of any nutrient. A lack of such an infinitesimal amount as that may cause a needed cell to be manufactured incorrectly, to become sick or to die. Such deficiencies lead to mental retardation, schizophrenia, mood swings and mental abnormalities ranging from poor concentration to stuporous depression.

Much of this information has been discovered within the last 10 or 15 years. It was formerly thought that the brain was completely separate from the rest of the body, and that the blood brain barrier determined which substances could cross that barrier. Now it is known that if the brain cells do not get the nutrients they need from the food we eat, the cells cannot control what crosses the barrier. It is also known that natural, whole, unprocessed foods containing all vitamins and minerals allow our brains to work well, and that one meal of junk food can keep us from thinking well; one meal can cause our emotions to get out of control. Uncontrolled emotions may cause divorce, migraines or hostile behavior. We may see a gun and pick it up and shoot someone.

PRECURSORS AND NEUROTRANSMITTERS

More information about nutrition and the brain is available now than has ever been known before. The brain has been called the last great frontier, and now that frontier is being explored. Since all the cells in our body are connected to a nerve cell, it is clear that what we eat affects our intelligence, our moods, our desire to eat and what to eat, and even the way our muscles work.

Our nerves are directed to do what they do by neurotransmitters, which are messengers that travel from one nerve cell (neuron) to another to activate cells anywhere in the body. Neurotransmitters are made from the food we eat—enzymes, coenzymes, vitamins and minerals. A special ingredient called a precursor, also made from the food we eat, is required. If the nutrients and the precursors are plentifully supplied, our neurotransmitters will function and our nervous systems will run our bodies so well that we will have no mental or physical disease.

Let's make a list of the precursors and neurotransmitters we'll be talking about. We need to know these new terms.

Precursors	Neurotransmitters
tryptophan	serotonin
tyrosine	dopamine
choline	acetylcholine

Each precursor, usually an amino acid from the protein we eat, furnishes part of the nutrients needed to make a specific neurotransmitter.

Each neurotransmitter manufactured in a nerve cell must leave that cell and go to a receptor in another nerve cell. There the receptor activates a nerve and changes a mood or causes sleepiness or keeps us from feeling pain or alters the composition of the blood plasma in the brain so that other changes occur (Wurtman, 1983). A neurotransmitter in a hyperactive child may reach a receptor that will inhibit the child's activity. Or it may reach a receptor that will say "eat" so that we won't become anorexic, or "stop eating, you've had enough" so we won't get fat.

Neurotransmitters and precursors of neurotransmitters also activate nerves that increase our learning ability, our behavior, our memory and even the movement of our muscles. Our nerve-muscle diseases include multiple sclerosis and muscular dystrophy. In fact, neurotransmitters can influence any activity pertaining to nerve cells.

Tryptophan—Serotonin. If rats, and probably humans, are given a high complex carbohydrate-low protein meal, brain tryptophan (a precursor) is increased, and more serotonin (a neurotransmitter) is manufactured. The reactions may be better memory, easier learning or less insomnia. However, if rats and humans are given a high-protein meal, less serotonin is available. That's because tryptophan is the least abundant amino acid, and it isn't able to get a carrier to take it across the blood-brain barrier to help make the serotonin if a lot of other amino acids are competing for carriers. Thus, if you took tryptophan to help you go to sleep and ate a hamburger at the same time, you probably would have put so many other amino acids into your blood that they would crowd out the tryptophan, and it wouldn't get "a seat on the bus."

Instead, if you had eaten a banana, which contains almost no protein, the tryptophan would probably find a carrier into the brain, since there were so few amino acids competing, and you would go right to sleep.

Tyrosine—Dopamine. Parkinson's disease is marked by a deficiency of the neurotransmitter dopamine. Neurons (brain cells) work better when we eat tyrosine, an amino acid precursor of dopamine, which is manufactured in our bodies. Dopamine is also activated by drugs such as L-dopa and by tranquilizers, both of which are hard to regulate. They may cross the blood-brain barrier too easily if the barrier cells are not healthy. Both these drugs have severe side effects. We can avoid them by making our own neurotransmitters if we eat good food. Then the neurotransmitter dopamine can combine with vitamin C to help stop or prevent the tremors of a Parkinson's disease patient.

We can increase the brain output of the neurotransmitter dopamine by eating more protein, which contains tyrosine, or we can buy tyrosine in powder or tablet form at health food stores. Tyrosine often helps Parkinson's patients and patients with depression as well.

Another vitamin, B3, is considered the natural anti-anxiety substance. It is attracted to receptors which inhibit anxiety. Tranquilizers such as Valium, Librium and Serax also do the same thing, but they have severe side effects. B3 is like vitamin C in that a large percentage of the vitamin will not cross the barrier. But when large doses are given, more of the nutrients get across. Once B3 gets into the brain, it is a powerful anti-anxiety agent, and it has no bad side effects.

Choline—Acetylcholine. Another food team to help our brains is choline (precursor) and acetylcholine (neurotransmitter). Probably most of us have been eating lecithin as part of our natural food program. It is an excellent source of phosphatidyl choline, the preferred form of lecithin. Choline (or lecithin) from the health food store has been used successfully to treat tardive dyskinesia, (a disease in which muscles fire out of control), mania (hyperactivity and talkativeness) and ataxia (lack of muscular coordination). Alzheimer's disease (presenility) may respond to long-term usage of lecithin combined with a natural food diet and food supplements (Wurtman, 1983). Therefore, the time to start preventing Alzheimer's is now.

Future of Neurotransmitters. These precursors— tryptophan, tyrosine and choline—will be used a great deal in the future to treat mental problems. Until now, the treatment has not been allowed because there was controversy about whether the compounds were foods or drugs, and it had not been decided which government agency should regulate the products.

It is imperative that all vitamins and minerals and a natural food diet should be used with any neurotransmitter or precursor in order to furnish all nutrients that may possibly be needed. It would be no good to take only the precursors or neurotransmitters or both. There are no magic bullets, but there is magic in feeding our cells all needed nutrients.

MENTAL HEALTH AND NUTRITION

To understand the effects of nutrition on the brain, let's review E. Shneour's book, *The Malnourished Mind.*

The Malnourished Mind

The entire course of human existence is largely determined by the nutrition received during gestation and to the age of two years. The growth of the brain during that time is one of the earliest, fastest and largest developments of the body.

After birth, the brain continues to grow at a much faster rate than the rest of the body. At four years, the brain is at 90 percent of its adult weight; the rest of the body is at 20 percent. The structure of the brain undergoes many changes, but nutritional deficiencies can never be made up later.

Direct evidence is lacking, but indirect evidence and many studies show that intelligence can be impaired by poor nutrition. We can improve our diets now; it will be too late to wait for direct evidence. Like radiation, bad effects of malnutrition don't show up until years later, when it's too late to do anything about them.

In the world, 350 million children, 7 out of 10 under age six (20 million in the United States alone), suffer from malnourishment or starvation. Of the 200,000 children born every day, more than half suffer from malnourishment, which leads to crippled brains and/or bodies.

Many Americans, addicted to quick, irregular meals and reinforced by the money-grabbers in the food industry, may be affected by brain-damaging malnutrition. Mild, sustained malnutrition may cause brain damage just as much as starvation, but results will be harder to identify.

Rats can find their way through simple mazes even if half their brains have been cut away. But in complex mazes, slight damage caused by brain surgery shows up very clearly. Malnourished brain cells usually don't show up until people have to use advanced mental skills to survive.

If we don't feed babies well before and after birth, all other efforts to solve mental deficiency problems are likely to be futile.

Human Brain Size

The brain of the human baby increases at the following rate:

Newborn	340 grams
6 months	750 "
1 year	970 "
2 years	1,150 "
3 years	1,200 "
6 years	1,250 "
9 years	1,300 "
12 years	1,350 "
20 years	1,400 " (3 pounds)

The greatest growth is soon after birth. The infant triples in size during the first year. This rate is not shared by any other animal. An infant with a full-size brain could not be delivered through the female pelvic canal, and yet, without a full-size brain, man could probably not have survived. So the major part of the brain develops after birth. This created a new problem: to develop, the brain must have adequate nutrients. No other organism shares this problem to the same degree.

Prenatal Growth

Prenatal growth is even more remarkable. Plenty of raw materials must be available to develop the brain. If one nutrient is missing, the brain will never be properly completed. Resources will be used somewhere else. There is some overlapping of nutrients, but a mild, chronic deficiency such as malnutrition cannot always be reversed, and a defective brain will result.

Pregnant women often do not eat well enough so that their babies can develop completely. Sometimes poor women eat a lot of starch, which makes them fat but does not furnish the protective nutrients they need. Doctors may put them on weight-reducing diets and they're deprived of even more nutrients.

Winick (1976) says that chronic, borderline malnutrition is common in the United States because of the large amounts of refined sugar and flour that so many people eat. Obviously this affects brain development in human babies. He says that changes in the brain tissues of starved animals are the same as changes in the nonbrain tissues of malnourished children. Of course, there is no direct way to study human brain tissue.

Brain Cells

The human brain contains 11 billion nerve cells (neurons). These are needed for acquiring, transferring, processing and analyzing information. In other words, for thinking. Throughout the entire period of prenatal life, 20,000 neurons have to be produced every minute. Billions of glial cells ("glial" means "glue") manufacture an essential fatty substance, myelin, which surrounds the neurons and holds them together.

Glial cells are replaced by new cells; neurons are not. After birth, the brain continues to grow by making more glial cells to produce myelin. The neurons that die are never replaced. Thus prenatal malnutrition can seriously affect a person's entire life by limiting the number of neurons produced before birth.

The brain is 2 percent of the total weight of the body and uses up to 20 percent of the total oxygen and 20 percent of the total nutrients. It uses 500 calories of a 2,500-calorie diet. A rich blood supply of one and one-half pints flows through the brain every minute.

The brain has no margin of safety and no reserves. A five-second interruption of blood flow brings unconsciousness; a few-minutes interruption brings irreversible damage or death. The brain can withstand a great deal of abuse (as far as nutrition is concerned) in an adult. But not in children.

As the fetus receives nourishment from the mother, it begins to grow. When the placenta forms to give the fetus nutrients and oxygen, blood flows through— as much as 30 quarts per day, flowing at the rate of four miles per hour. The placenta, as the afterbirth, weighs about a pound. Children who have a defective placenta cannot receive adequate nutrition. This results in permanently smaller children, physically and mentally, even if they receive adequate nutrition in later life.

There are periods of "growth spurt," and if nutritional deficiencies occur during such a time, an organ may be permanently stunted. Early-life malnutrition results in a decreased number of cells in the brain and in other organs. The organs most affected are the ones that had nutritional deficiencies during their growth spurts.

Defects

X-rays and gamma rays decrease cell growth. Diagnostic X-rays cause stunted development of offspring, especially in the brain. The child may suffer from mental retardation that cannot be reversed. This is called microcephalic idiocy.

Other factors cause defects. German measles (rubella) during the first three months causes eye and ear defects. Thalidomide during the first seven weeks caused babies to be born with flipperlike stumps instead of arms and legs. It is during the first seven weeks that the "growth spurt" in human limbs takes place. Other investigators say that deficiencies of B vitamins were caused by the thalidomide.

The growth spurt of the brain occurs between the fifteenth and twentieth weeks of pregnancy and between the twenty-fifth week of pregnancy and the end of the second year after birth. Thus brain stunting depends on when the malnutrition occurs and how long it lasts. There is a decrease in the size and number of neurons, which multiply only during pregnancy.

Some brain cells perform only one function, but others can pinch-hit in different ways. Without adequate nutrition, however, the cells that are supposed to pinch-hit may not be available.

Protein Malnutrition

Protein malnutrition is one of the most serious deficiencies. Studies show that pregnant women who eat 50 grams or less of protein per day have babies who weigh less and have smaller skulls than women who eat 70 grams per day. More babies of low birth weight are mentally retarded. This has been known since 1919. Small-for-date children and prematures do not reach their potential, mentally or physically, no matter how well they are fed in later years. They have a much higher incidence of physical and mental handicaps.

Until recently, it was an accepted fact that dietary deficiencies resulted in stunting of the body. Now, it is realized that the brain is particularly vulnerable. It was formerly thought that IQ was 80 percent heredity. It is now thought by many researchers that IQ is only 30 percent heredity and 70 percent environment, including nutrition.

Hospital Records

Most hospitals do not keep records or perform tests to identify malnutrition. A government survey asked the 50 state boards of health to find out how many cases of malnutrition or deficiency disease were diagnosed in their hospitals in a given year. Ten states ignored the request, and 35 of the remaining 40 said they didn't keep such records. Many explained that they assigned the reason for being in the hospital or the primary cause of death to some other factor, even though this factor was caused by malnutrition.

Fasting and Crash Diets

When we go on a crash diet or fast, the brain loses little weight, but water is substituted for some tissues. A mature adult will usually recover, but a young child will not, and his brain suffers more than any other organ because the brain requires all nutrients at all times.

Brain Fats

Brain membranes are formed early in life. If the membranes don't develop because of nutritional deficiency, mental retardation may result. Fats form part of the structure of the membranes. Most fats can be manufactured by the body (if all nutrients are present), but a few cannot. These are called essential fatty acids (EFA) because we must eat the fats we cannot make.

An unusual study was made of South African children. Their growth was stunted by poor diet. When they were given more protein, they began to grow, but they became deficient in EFA. The reason was that when children grow fast they need more EFA. Deficiencies can cause growth retardation, skin damage and partial malfunction of many organs, including the brain (Shneour, 1974).

Winick and his colleagues (1976) tell us that the adult brain contains 10.7 percent cholesterol. Phospholipids, which are fats combined with phosphorus, such as lecithin, are 12 percent of gray matter and 17 percent of white matter. If we eliminate too much fat from our diet, we might be eliminating brain power.

BRAIN GROWTH

Early brain growth is mainly due to cell division and to an increase in the number of cells. Later growth is an increase in the size of cells (Winick, 1976).

If animals are undernourished during cell division, the number of cells is reduced. This change is permanent and can't be reversed after the cells stop dividing. If malnutrition is present when cells are enlarging, they won't enlarge, but they will enlarge again when nutrients are increased. Rats undernourished during the first 21 days of life had total number of brain cells reduced, and no amount of nutrition could build new cells (Winick, 1972).

Malnourishment during the first three weeks also interferes with fat assimilation. There is a substantial loss of brain cholesterol and phospholipids up to one year of age. In the rat, the fatty sheaths (myelin) around the nerves are decreased and become shorter and thinner. The part of the brain called the cerebellum has the fastest cell division, and this part is damaged first in the rat.

Cell migration is also slowed down. In the rat, neurons move into the hippocampus on the fifteenth day after birth. Neurons are thinking cells. Without good nutrition, it appears that these cells cannot migrate. It may be that cells aren't dividing.

In animals, neurons and glial cells in the spinal cord and the brain degenerate without good nutrition. In pigs, there are not as many neurons in the gray matter, and the ones that are there are swollen. In rats, enzyme production is delayed, and the number of enzymes in the brain and cord is reduced. If malnutrition in a human infant's brain continues after eight months of age, the brain has fewer and smaller cells. Brain growth depends on nutrition during cell division. All cell types are affected. If a child is malnourished into the second year, brain cell size is reduced, but cell size in other organs is not (Winick, 1976).

Brain in Jeopardy

Lesser (1977) agrees that nutrition of Americans is "so poor that human brain development is in jeopardy." Sometimes the poor nutrition is because the expectant mother wants to lose weight. Felig (1973) says, "Crash starvation diets in pregnant women are to be absolutely condemned."

It appears that the quantity and quality of the food fed early in life decide the final makeup of the adult. If rats are weaned early, they have a poor memory and can't learn well. But these effects can be cancelled out if the animals are fed a high-fat diet from age 18 to 30 days. Evidently the fat in the diet is important for development of the brain. Something similar happens when male rats are weaned early. If they are given a refined-carbohydrate diet, their testes degenerate. But fat in the diet corrects this.

Dieting

Lack of sufficient food can affect the brain. Ancel Keys conducted an experiment on 32 healthy men. He gave them a diet of only 1,570 calories—about the percentage of food that someone on a crash diet would be getting compared to what he needed. The men ate only two meals a day, at 8:30 A.M. and 5 P.M. They became psychologically disturbed, irritable, depressed and had masklike faces (Shneour, 1974).

Survival of the Brain

In the early 1950s, Aldous Huxley wrote, "The nervous system is more vulnerable than any other tissue of the body; therefore, vitamin deficiencies affect the mind and behavior before they affect the skin, bones, mucous membranes, muscles and viscera." If anyone isn't getting an adequate diet, his brain will not be as efficient as it should be. It may not survive as a brain.

The substances needed for health of the brain are not found in adequate amounts in schizophrenics, alcoholics, older people who have somewhat lost their memory or who have become depressed or senile, or in children with learning disabilities. Often when the diet is improved, the first symptoms of relief are less fatigue, more alertness and less depression; the recovery depends on how long the symptoms have been present. Finally, let us quote Cheraskin and Ringsdorf (1968), who say, "It is not possible to find a mental patient who does not have something organically wrong."

STRESS

Most of the people I talk with at nutrition meetings tell me they aren't really sick and they don't really have poor diets. They claim that all of their ailments are caused by stress—just stress. However, we can all generally handle stress without any ill effects if we eat well. So let's find out what to eat in order to handle the stress and not have it damage our cells.

Stress is a condition that harms the body and causes cells to die. Stress can be pleasant or un-

pleasant. It can originate from many causes: anxiety; overwork; too little sleep; poor diet; not enough exercise; use of drugs, antibiotics, even aspirin; going to too many parties or going out in cold weather.

Every nutrient is needed in larger than usual amounts to withstand the stress. People often say, "I'm just too tired to eat." But food and nourishment for all the cells is essential if we are to stay healthy.

Everyone suffers from stress, but many of us just complain and rely on tranquilizers. The only way we can get real relief from stress is to feed our cells the nutrients they need. In this way, we can handle the stress without getting sick. We don't eliminate the stress; if we did, we'd live like vegetables. If we roll with the punches, stress won't harm us, providing we eat a nutritious diet to keep our cells healthy.

Here's what happens when we're under mental or physical stress. A world-renowned expert, the late Hans Selye, figured this out 40 years ago, and it has been corroborated in thousands of studies since then (Selye, 1970).

The Stress Reaction

When we're confronted with stress, the pituitary gland at the base of the brain sends a message to the adrenal glands, which sit one on top of each kidney. The adrenal glands release their 32 hormones into the blood to prepare the body to meet the stress. The heart beats faster, consequently the blood flows through the blood vessels with more force. Proteins are withdrawn from the thymus and lymph glands and are broken down into sugar; part of the sugar goes to the blood to furnish energy; the rest goes to the liver to be stored until needed. The lungs take in more air more quickly. And, even if we've just eaten, we stop digesting our food. We use the blood to withstand stress and, while digestion is delayed. So blood rushes to our arms, legs and brains so that we can run fast if necessary, use our arms forcefully and think clearly and quickly. All of this exaggerated activity prepares us to handle stressful situations.

Let's pretend that we've met a man with a gun in a dark alley and we don't have a weapon. Our logical response is to run—fast. And we will be able to run faster than we ever ran before because of the additional blood sugar in our muscles. But if our teenage son wants the car every night and our daughter stays out until three o'clock in the morning, we need extra blood in our brains so we can persuade our teenagers to be more considerate. Sometimes we have to fight for our reasons, which can be very stressful.

These two reactions represent the flight or fight

syndrome—the two major reactions to stress. With the extra power from increased blood sugar, we respond to the stress more easily. Sometimes people can perform miraculous feats of strength during stress. A magazine article several years ago told of a 12-year-old boy who lifted the wheel of a car off his father, who had been pinned underneath when the car rolled.

Repair

After we have handled the stress, our bodies repair themselves with needed raw materials, which are nutrients from the food we've eaten. But if we have eaten only doughnuts, potato chips and candy, which contain almost no nutrients, there aren't enough raw materials to repair tissue and the exhaustion stage sets in. We get sick. We may get stomach ulcers because of not enough proteins in the stomach to protect it against the very strong digestive juices. So the acids eat a hole in the lining of the stomach. The urinary loss of protein is equal to the protein from four quarts of milk. But if sufficient protein is supplied, stress will not cause ulcers or other damage. Stress caused by accidents, burns or drastic surgery can destroy so much protein that the body can progress to severe illness within one day (Selye, 1970).

But let's say we have no drastic stress, just the usual daily problems. Maybe the car wouldn't start, maybe the boss suddenly thought of a report he wanted at the last minute or maybe your spouse brought a friend home for dinner when you planned to have leftovers. Your adrenal glands are still working well enough to help you meet all those emergencies.

But the next morning something happens to cause additional stress. Your adrenal glands try to release their 32 hormones to prepare you to meet this stress. But all you had for breakfast was coffee, a cigarette and a croissant made with white flour. The hormones have not been replaced because they require something like whole-grain muffins, real butter and fresh yard eggs. We need 50 nutrients from proteins, fats, carbohydrates, vitamins, minerals and water to repair the damage and we haven't eaten enough nutritious foods to make new hormones.

Another Stress

If we meet another stress, we go to pieces because our glands can't function. We're tired, we never seem to get anything done, our personalities change. We're irritable, crabby. We can't tell what's real and what isn't. Some pepole have nervous and emotional upsets, high blood pressure or gastric and duodenal ulcers. Certain types of rheumatic, allergic, cardiovascular and renal diseases appear to be essentially stress diseases (Selye, 1970).

Cold weather is a severe stress. When the weather is cold, we have to manufacture 300 percent more heat so we won't get colds, flu or pneumonia. This takes extra nurients, especially vitamin C, which is destroyed within seconds when we're under stress, and vitamin A, which is depleted within minutes. If we don't have extra vitamin C, we get a "cold," because vitamin C is used in large amounts by white blood cells to destroy the bacteria and viruses that caused the cold. Thus we can't fight an infection without vitamin C (Mount, 1976).

Many people who have lived with stress for years become so ill that they are given cortisone, an adrenal hormone. They improve, usually, but everyone knows the severe side effects of cortisone given as a drug. When our bodies make it in the adrenal glands, we get the exact amount needed for our cells. But it is impossible for synthetic, man-made cortisone to work the same way our natural cortisone works.

"All people with nutritional deficiencies have trouble coping with problems," says J. D. Moriarty in the *Journal of Applied Nutrition* (1974). Often we just eat more sugar and drink more coffee. That's like whipping a tired horse. Our pancreas can't handle the sugar, and our adrenals are withering away from exhaustion and lack of nutrients.

Thus our bodies suffer, usually from fatigue, then ulcers, colds and headaches. We can have digestive upsets, low- and high-blood sugar, heart disease, cancer and many diseases of the immune system.

Adrenal Diseases

When our adrenals are so poorly fed that they get exhausted and can't produce any more hormones, the glands enlarge. Then the damaged, malnourished cells develop sores and begin to bleed. The sores finally heal and produce scar tissue. But scar tissue can't make hormones. If this condition gets bad enough, it's called Addison's disease. The patient gets weaker and weaker, his skin gets darker, his blood pressure falls, and he vomits and has diarrhea. Thus, we must keep our adrenal glands healthy so they will always make enough hormones, especially if we have stressful jobs or are in other stress-related situations.

Hydrochloric Acid

When we're under stress long enough, we quit making hydrochloric acid (HCl) in the stomach. Then the proteins we eat can't be converted into amino acids to repair tissue. Undigested protein causes allergies and diseased cells all through the body. We also have gas, bloating and a too-full feeling after meals. Many people take antacids, which destroy even more hydrochloric acid and make their digestion worse. The gas leads to such ailments as diverticulosis and cancer of the colon, the second most common location of cancer. Without HCl, our food putrefies; poisonous bacteria move into the intestines and then travel all over the body. This causes a variety of diseases and may even affect the brain. We can be depressed, not able to think well and have persistent worry and strain. Some brain ailments are called cerebral allergies, but the ailments are caused by the fast food and junk food we eat. Undigested protein also causes gas, which leads to such ailments as diarrhea or constipation. If our bowels are sluggish, minerals and vitamins can't be digested and absorbed. (Selye, 1970).

Some people at my nutrition seminars argue that they must already have too much acid in their stomachs because they sometimes can taste acid in their throats when they belch. They do have too much acid, but it's the wrong kind of acid. Here's what has happened. All metabolic processes involving foods result in waste acid being formed. When we eat eggs, which contain sulfur, we make sulfuric acid. Most foods have phosphorus in them, so we make phosphoric acid. Many people are familiar with the term uric acid; it is said to cause gout. We must get rid of the waste acid or we will have acidosis, a serious disease. Nature arranged to have it excreted in the urine or breathed out in carbon dioxide. But if anything goes wrong with either of those methods, the waste acid collects in the stomach. That's the acid people taste in their throats. We have to get rid of it. The easiest way is to take hydrochloric acid, which seems like the opposite of what we need. But the hydrochloric acid will eliminate the waste acid and help us digest protein.

When we eat junk foods, we don't make enough HCl, and, as we age, we make less and less. At age 40, we make 12 percent less than we did at 30, and at 60, 30 percent of us don't make any. Those people are often in wheelchairs, nursing homes or hospitals. The other 70 percent of the 60 year olds are struggling through life able to manufacture only 15 percent of the HCl they made at age 25. No wonder people are sick.

Other people argue that they surely don't need HCl because they don't have gas, bloating or a too-full feeling. They don't realize how many symptoms can be caused by HCl deficiency.

One young man, very much into nutrition, said he had finally solved a problem he had had for a long time. He said he sometimes felt "mean and ornery," but when he took HCl, his meanness left; he was cheerful and he felt good. Obviously he was then able to assimilate the vitamins and minerals he needed.

Other people ask me, "Why don't I feel better? I'm taking all the vitamins and minerals and watching my diet carefully, but I just don't feel good." I always ask, "Are you taking HCl and pancreatic enzymes?" They reply, "No, I ran out and I forgot to buy more," or some other excuse. Young people probably won't need to take these enzymes indefinitely, just long enough for their cells to start producing the enzymes. This would probably take from two to four weeks. Older people may want to take them from now on.

Other Causes of Stress

It is difficult to realize how many varied circumstances cause stress or result in stress. Illness is a severe stress to the body, especially fever. Vitamin A is excreted and a deficiency of A can cause blindness. Maybe that's why children who have measles have to stay in darkened rooms to protect their eyesight. A disease like measles uses a lot of vitamin A to fight the infection. A positive calcium balance is impossible to maintain with a high fever. That means more calcium is leaving the body than is being taken in. This deficiency can result in weak bones and teeth and a weakend heart as well, because the heart must have calcium in order to beat. B vitamins are also used up fast during illnesses, and deficiencies can lead to severe infections and beriberi, with symptoms of paralysis, fatigue, heart failure and wasting of the limbs. A folic acid deficiency can be caused by an infection, and this leads to severe illness because, without this B vitamin, the body cannot manufacture new cells to replace old, worn-out cells.

The release of amino acids to make more sugar, which we've already mentioned, causes more protein to be excreted in the urine. This causes a negative protein (nitrogen) balance, which means that we're losing more protein than we're eating. Then muscles must be broken down to make protein for tissues that we need the most, especially the brain and lungs. Muscles in arms and legs are depleted first, but if the deficiency continues the muscles of the heart may be broken down to feed the brain.

In diarrhea, much protein is lost in the urine and less is obviously absorbed. Tonsilitis and acne, broken bones and burns also cause loss of protein, as do pain, anxiety, fear and migraine headaches (Scrimshaw, 1969).

The negative protein balance continues after the stress is over, until the cells are built up again, which usually takes a long time. Normal growth in children can't take place until cells are restored, so nutrition should be as good as possible for early recovery.

Why is it so important that we get plenty of protein? Because all of our body tissue is made and repaired with protein. If a certain hormone made in the adrenal glands requires 20 amino acids for its manufacture, and there are just 19 available, we can't make nineteen-twentieths of a hormone; we can't make any. So if we can't make the 32 adrenal hormones, we can't handle stress. This can result in any physical illness and/or any mental and emotional problem you can name.

Noise—A Stress. Noise can cause stress reactions. Studies show that most adults can tolerate the mild noise of office typewriters, but a few people become upset. Also, tests show that adolescents are apparently not harmed by moderate noise.

I'm sure everybody is glad to know that, but if you've ever chaperoned a high-school prom, you know that the "noise" there is far from moderate. We've been told for years that such loud music can cause hearing loss.

Television—A Stress. Ten medical students were shown film clips of murders, fights, torturing and executions. These are the very scenes that children often watch on television. The medical students excreted 70 percent more adrenaline than usual. Adrenaline is one of the adrenal hormones released when the body is under stress. It increases blood pressure, stimulates the heart muscle, makes the heart beat faster and increases the output of blood from the heart. Thus, these typical stress reactions can be caused by watching violence on television.

Large amounts of adrenaline paralyze the muscles that keep the anus closed, so stress can cause people to defecate without wanting to. Terrified animals are also known to do this (Ballentine, 1978). This reaction pulls sugar out of the muscles and results in the destruction of muscles and excretion of protein.

Sleep Loss—A Stress. Going without sleep causes stress and protein loss, but usually on the second day rather than the first day after sleep loss. Most people have noticed this. When we miss sleep, we usually get along surprisingly well the next day, but the day after fatigue hits us.

School—A Stress. Many adolescents are borderline deficient in nutrients, yet they are often under great stress because of their emotional states and school pressures. Final exams and social events increase the secretion of adrenaline. Young children, too, undergo stress because of peer pressure at school. They are also less immune to infection than are adults. These stresses can have an important effect on their health (Scrimshaw, 1969).

Surgery—A Stress. Surgery is a severe stress on the body. R. J. Peshek, D.D.S. (1974), prescribes special nutrients for his dental surgery patients to avoid damage from stress. He says he obtains "remark-able results." Nutrients include vitamins E and C, zinc, digestive enzymes and fat-soluble chlorophyll, a good scource of vitamins A, E, F and K and of the minerals magnesium and potassium. Potassium helps the blood clot. The chlorophyll helps to heal wounds and regenerate tissues. Dr. Peshek says that if he had only one product to use it would be fat-soluble chlorophyll.

Weight Loss—A Stress. Sometimes dieting to lose weight causes stress. If we eat less than 900 calories, protein from the diet is used for energy rather than for growth or repair of tissues. Adding protein doesn't help. We need complex carbohydrates for energy.

During stress, the body loses large amounts of vitamin C, protein, carbohydrates, fats and many vitamins and minerals. All of these nutrients must be replaced in order to withstand the stress.

Don't Eliminate Stress

We've talked about avoiding stress, but we can't really eliminate stress from our lives. We wouldn't want to if we could. Stress can be pleasant. It's anything, good or bad, that puts a greater than usual demand on the body. We can be playing hard and loving every minute of it and still be stressed. The other day a friend of mine said, "Maybe that's why I get sick every Christmas—stress. Too many sweets, late hours and booze. My adrenals may be exhausted."

Hans Selye says that even a passionate kiss is stress! So let's not try to get rid of all stress. Let's eat well so our adrenal glands won't be damaged. Those glands regulate our disposition, our efficiency and even our personalities. If the glands do a good job or a poor one, it's because of what we've been eating.

Foods and Stress

We should eliminate the processed foods, the refined carbohydrates, white sugar and white flour from our diet. We need proteins and fats in moderation, with plenty of complex carbohydrates—whole grains, vegetables, whole fruits, nuts, seeds and legumes (beans, peas and peanuts).

Selye says that physicians and dieticians usually don't realize what an important role nutrition plays in stress. They are the very people who decide what sick people in hospitals get to eat. Selye says, "Poor food certainly induces stress that can delay recovery" (Selye, 1970).

Foods to Avoid. To prevent damage from stress, Page (1972) suggests foods to avoid.

1. Eliminate sucrose. This would eliminate 90 percent of our ills.

2. Give up all packaged, frozen, boxed, canned and dried foods.

3. Avoid everything with white flour or white sugar in it.

4. Eliminate anything (almost) in jars and bottles such as soft drinks, jam, jelly (make your own).

5. Avoid processed meats and cheese—anything with nitrites, nitrates and dyes.

Foods to Emphasize. Page also suggests foods to emphasize:

1. Yogurt, kefir or acidophilus products.

2. Seeds—sesame, sunflower, pumpkin.

3. Nuts of all kinds, especially almonds, walnuts, peanuts.

4. A blender drink with lecithin, yeast and bran.

Most nutritionists suggest a natural food diet that is said to greatly improve the health of the vast majority of people.

Protein. Protein makes up about 15 percent of the calories in the diet.

- small amounts of muscle meat (4 ounces four times a week or less).
- dairy products, including one or two eggs a day.
- poultry (from the health food store) and fish.
- combinations of legumes (beans, peas and peanuts) and whole grains, nuts and seeds—amounts suggested are about 20 percent to 50 percent as much legumes as whole grains.

Fats. Next are fats, some animal (best are butter, cream and eggs), and some vegetable (best are nuts and seeds). We should not use bottled vegetable oil; we should eat small measures of nuts and seeds per day in divided amounts. Small measures are two teaspoons of sesame, sunflower or pumpkin seeds, or two walnut halves, four pecan halves, six almonds or 12 peanuts. Peanuts must always be cooked; other seeds and nuts can be eaten raw.

Carbohydrates. The third category is complex carbohydrates—whole grains; vegetables, both cooked and raw; and whole fruits. This should be about 75 percent of our calories. Most people don't differentiate between the good and bad carbohydrates, but just lump all carbohydrates together and try to avoid them.

The truth is that complex carbohydrates are excellent foods and we need to eat the bulk of our calories from this category. "Bulk" is the right word, because complex carbohydrates furnish bulk. They have a lot of fiber that keeps food moving through the alimentary canal. Thus, undigested food can't

stack up in the colon and cause constipation, which can lead to cancer.

When we emphasize the importance of whole fruits, we are de-emphasizing the importance of fruit juice. Don't drink it; it's too sweet. One medium orange or apple has one teaspoon of natural sugar in it. But by the time we squeeze or press fruit to make a glass of juice, we drink from four to seven teaspoons of sugar. One would never eat four to seven apples or oranges. Fruit juice increases our blood sugar level so much that insulin is overproduced in the pancreas, and it takes too much sugar out of the blood. Then we have low blood sugar.

DEPRESSION

The most common symptom of mental illness is depression.

Depression is not just sadness; it is also hopelessness. Kline (1974) says depression is the most undertreated of all major diseases. It has been estimated that as many as 20 percent of the population suffer from depression at any one time. Other emotional problems affect another 25 percent of the people at any one time. These figures were quoted in the report of the President's Commission on Mental Health.

That makes depression one of the most frequent mental disorders, and also one of the most common of all serious medical conditions (*Medical Tribune*, 1976). Twice as many women as men suffer from depression.

Depression and the Liver

A healthy liver can help us avoid depression by maintaining constant blood sugar levels. Our brains use glucose, a form of sugar, for energy. The brain needs a tremendous amount of energy to keep our 12 billion brain cells working every minute of every hour of every 24 hours. In fact, the brain weighs only 2 percent of our body weight, but it uses the first 20 percent of the food we eat as energy for its own cells.

The liver does much more than maintain blood sugar levels. It filters the blood and removes the wastes, contaminants and toxins that might damage cells all over the body. It removes pesticides, insecticides and poisons created by the breakdown of foods.

If the liver doesn't work well, these poisons circulate through the body. They are especially harmful in the brain, where they can cause "don't-carish" feelings, laziness and depression.

Some authors say that a damaged liver is the main cause of depression. Actually, the main cause is poor diet, because the liver has to have all nutrients brought to it in the blood so it can work well and prevent depression.

We must first determine how much to eat. If we overeat, the enzymes in the liver are overworked and they can't change the food into nutrients the liver needs. The undigested food enters the bloodstream, where it is a foreign invader that can cause allergies. Between meals, we are deficient in nutrients because so much food was passed along in the overload that the liver doesn't have enough nutrients stored. Thus, when the liver works poorly, we can't get an even flow of nutrients and depression develops.

Internal signals should tell us when we have eaten enough or when we need to eat more. If the liver doesn't work well, these signals may not work, partly because of liver problems, and partly because of a hypothalamus weakness. That's the region in the brain that regulates the appetite.

If there are large amounts of refined foods in the diet, either the food can be absorbed too quickly or it can't be used by the body. Then the liver has to detoxify the foods that are causing the trouble. But the liver is so overloaded that it can't detoxify the poisons. The same thing happens when we eat food loaded with chemicals. The body can't use chemicals that the liver couldn't detoxify, and the chemicals become allergens that can attack us anywhere, even in the brain, and lead to diseases such as depression.

Some of the side effects of drugs that supposedly combat depression are inability to urinate, fast pulse, dry mouth and frequent low blood pressure. Sometimes the drugs cause heart blockage, jaundice and seizures such as epilepsy. Even with these side effects, one of every 10 prescriptions written in this country is for antidepressant drugs (Kline, 1974). Natural foods and supplements of vitamins and minerals do no damage, yet they furnish nutrients needed by a sick brain.

Depression and the Brain

Depression is really one of the easiest problems to solve. The needed vitamins, minerals and foods will act quickly if we just take advantage of the new knowledge that has been discovered.

Tryptophan. Tryptophan is being used to treat depression. This is an amino acid found in all complete proteins, such as meat, eggs and milk.

Tryptophan is a precursor of the neurotransmitter serotonin, a messenger that helps impulses move along nerves. When we need to eat, to stop eating, to remember something, to think well on examinations and especially to not be hyperactive or depressed, impulses must travel along our nerves to accelerate or inhibit these activities.

Many nutrients are required for the manufacture of serotonin, especially tryptophan, an amino acid that we can't make and must eat. All minerals and vitamins are required as coenzymes, especially B complex and C. For energy, we need carbohydrates and fats. All of these nutrients must be available in large amounts, flowing through the capillaries in the brain at all times. If one is missing, the message will be garbled, and depression may result. Since so many vitamins and minerals are not available in adequate amounts in the average American diet, it is easy to see why so many people suffer from depression and other mental problems.

The neurotransmitters were discovered recently, and a tremendous amount of research has been published in medical and nutrition journals that tells of their importance in relieving depression. What is so different about recent scientific thinking is that, if enough of the nurients needed to make the precursors and the neurotransmitters are floating in the blood, the sheer force of the large amounts of both substances will allow enough of the needed nutrients to get into the brain cells so the messages will be received, and the nerves will be activated to relieve depression.

Without the precursors and other nutrients, it's like a telephone switchboard operator trying to complete a call without plugging in the cord. The message can't get through.

A study in *Lancet* (1975) reported on 42 people who received either tryptophan or a drug. Nine doctors agreed that there were highly significant improvements with fewer side effects in the tryptophan group.

A fringe benefit of tryptophan treatment is that insomnia may be relieved. Investigators believe that insomniacs are really suffering from depression (*Medical World News*, 1976). As little as one gram (1,000 mg) of tryptophan was helpful.

Drugs to help people sleep often leave them feeling groggy in the morning. Most of the drugs for insomnia sold over-the-counter are either worthless or unsafe (special report of the FDA advisory review panel, Dec. 1975). Since tryptophan is a nutrient required by the body, it does not cause side effects when taken as directed.

It isn't possible to just eat more protein to get more tryptophan. The blood levels of serotonin do go up, but they also go up for 5 other amino acids that compete for transport. It is suggested that, in depression, 1,000 mg of tryptophan be given in addition to what is eaten (Wagman and Brown, 1975). The tryptophan should be given with the mid-morning snack of whole fruit, and no protein should be given at the same time. Usually we eat protein and whole fruit together for snacks, but tryptophan has to compete with other amino acids for carriers to take it where it needs to go in the body, and if we eat protein, the competition would be too great. Because there is less tryptophan in protein than any other amino acid, it hardly has a chance to find a carrier if it is eaten with other protein.

Choline. Another precursor that helps prevent and relieve depression is a fat named choline. Its neurotransmitter is acetylcholine, which helps us remember, helps us think and relieves depression.

Everyone who eats natural foods knows about choline because it is one of the major ingredients in lecithin, available at health food stores and recommended for much more than preventing depression. It helps us keep fats from stacking up in the blood vessels and in the liver, and it is recommended for gallstones.

There are many studies using choline in medical and nutrition journals. One woman was kept in a hospital and given every drug ever used against depression. She became more and more depressed. Then the researchers gave her lecithin with its high content of choline, and after a few weeks she said she felt better than she ever had before. Then the investigators put her back on medication and she became depressed again. Finally, she was given lecithin again and she became well.

Hydrochloric acid. As we have stated, if we have too little hydrochloric acid, we can experience hopelessness, depression and feelings of inadequacy. A deficiency of HCl allows bacteria to overgrow in the intestine, causing gas, indigestion and an overloaded liver.

SCHIZOPHRENIA

Schizophrenia is a broad term for many mental diseases. It is an illness of perception (Cott, 1973). The senses of sight, hearing, taste, touch and smell can become distorted. Also, a person's thinking changes. People become paranoid, they mistrust their closest relatives, their loved ones, their motives and everything that is said and done for them.

Profound depression is part of schizophrenia. The suicide rate is very high. Early symptoms in childhood are withdrawal and depression, but symptoms are not as clear as in an adult.

Watch for Signs

If you're on a natural food diet, don't be worried about the possibility of getting schizophrenia, but you might like to know some of the warning signs of the illness. They include insomnia, headaches, an offensive body odor, irrational crying fits, devastating fatigue, severe depression, inner tension, changes in personality, a constant feeling of being watched, a feeling of terror and a fear that you will lose your self-control (Cheraskin et al., 1971). Some of these signs are found in other illnesses, but if you notice several at once, see your nutrition-oriented physician and begin the food and food supplement program immediately.

Nutrients Needed

The most important vitamins to prevent or control schizophrenia are B3, B6 and C. Pantothenic acid has a calming effect, so it's also important. Minerals are required. For example, magnesium activates about 120 enzyme systems in every cell. Also when we take extra B6, we need extra magnesium. Zinc activates about 60 enzyme systems. Zinc and magnesium together keep copper from accumulating. If it does accumulate, and if there's not enough zinc, copper can cause schizophrenia (Pfeiffer, 1975).

Copper is in our plumbing, and soft water picks it up. Birth control pills add copper, as do intrauterine devices and copper bracelets.

Megavitamin Therapists

More and more physicians and other health professionals are becoming interested in megavitamin therapy.

Pauling. Linus Pauling (Hawkins and Pauling, 1973) says that vitamins, especially B and C, are inexpensive, almost entirely nontoxic, and free of side effects when compared with ordinary drugs. "Increased intake has small probability of doing harm and large probability of doing good."

Pfeiffer. The Brain Bio Center in Princeton, New Jersey, has treated more than 400 patients with schizophrenia. The treatment with vitamin B6, zinc and magnesium, plus a good diet, has been 95 percent successful (Pfeiffer, 1975).

Dr. Carl C. Pfeiffer, director of the center, says the most important aspect of schizophrenia is that, if people had had adequate nutrition, they might have prevented their illnesses (Pfeiffer, 1975).

Lesser. Dr. Michael Lesser, a psychiatrist from Berkley, California, is president of the Orthomolecular Medical Society. He says that about twice as many people recover from mental illness if they're treated with orthomolecular therapy—extra vitamins and minerals but no drugs—as recover without nutritional therapy. This treatment also helps "ordinary people" reach their potential in life, that is, they have health and energy to do what they want to do.

Dr. Lesser reported that 67 percent of his psychiatric patients suffer from low blood sugar because they eat large amounts of refined sugar and flour. Much investigation shows that low blood sugar is associated with violent behavior.

Low blood sugar, if untreated, develops into diabetes (high blood sugar) and the accepted treatment is generally diet. Diabetes often leads to other serious diseases such as hardening of the arteries and other circulatory problems, resulting in blindness, heart attacks and amputation of feet (Lesser, 1977).

Hoffer and Osmond. Studies of nutrition and schizophrenia have been going on for over 30 years. The original work was done by two Canadian psychiatrists, Abram Hoffer and Humphry Osmond. They began using vitamins, minerals and amino acids to balance the chemistry of the brain cells.

They first used niacin and vitamin C to treat schizophrenia, plus a high-protein diet, with very few refined carbohydrates. Let's differentiate between complex and refined carbohydrates. Complex carbohydrates are whole grains of all kinds—wheat, corn, brown rice, buckwheat, millet, bulgur and oats—that have not been refined and depleted of their nutrients. Refined carbohydrates are white flour, white sugar and all products made from them. They have lost so much food value—vitamins and minerals—in the processing that they deprive the body of nutrients. Even enriched bread, which we hear so much about, is detrimental to health. About 20 nutrients have been removed from whole wheat, and only 4 have been put back in, really not much enrichment.

Self-Test for Schizophrenics

These questions are from a shortened version of the Hoffer-Osmond Diagnostic Test for schizophrenia (HOD) from *New Hope for Incurable Diseases* by Cheraskin and Ringsdorf (1971).

You can take the test by yourself. It will let you know what's happening in your head and remind you that something can be done about it, if needed.

Sight
People's faces seem to change in size as I watch them.
My hands and feet sometimes feel far away.
People watch me a lot more than they used to.
Sometimes the world seems unreal.
Pictures appear to be alive and to breathe.
I sometimes feel that I have left my body.

Sound
I often hear my thoughts inside my head.
I often have singing noises in my ears.

Touch
I sometimes feel I am being pinched by something I can't see.
I sometimes feel that there are crawly things under my skin.
I sometimes feel strange vibrations shivering through me.

Taste
Some foods I used to like now taste funny.
Water tastes funny.

Smell
Things smell very funny now.
I sweat much more than I used to.
I can no longer smell perfume.

Time
I can no longer tell how much time has gone by.
The days seem to go by very slowly.
I find that past, present and future seem all muddled up.
I have much more trouble keeping appointments.

Thought
There are some people trying to harm me.
I can read other people's minds.
Most people hate me.
I am not sure who I am.
There is some plot against me.
I now become easily confused.
I can't make up my mind as well as I used to.

Feelings and Emotions
I usually feel alone and sad at a party.
Life seems entirely hopeless.
I am constantly keyed up and jittery.

There's the list. If any of the comments describe you, it's time to begin your new food program that will nourish your brain cells. Your thoughts, feelings, hearing, sight and touch will probably improve as well.

Schizophrenia therapists watch for three possible minor problems that may arise.

1. If you have a stomach ulcer, stay on your ulcer medicine, and see if your physician will phase it out for you. Or use buffered niacin, which should relieve any pain.

2. High blood pressure patients using reserpine-type medications may have nausea or a drop in blood pressure. This might not be dangerous, but could be uncomfortable.

3. Patients who schedule liver or glucose-tolerance tests should stop taking niacin a week before the test.

These two researchers have had phenomenal success with the test and their therapy, and have added most other essential nutrients to their patients' food and food supplement programs.

Megavitamin Therapy. Hoffer and Osmond found that 82 percent of schizophrenics can be helped with vitamin therapy, which is cheaper than drugs, has no side effects and is safer because nutrients are natural substances normally present in the body and are absolutely essential to life.

Schizophrenics are often treated by diet alone.

They formerly lived on junk food; they ate candy bars and drank coffee and colas by the gallon. By giving them moderate amounts of protein, and complex carbohydrates and by removing junk foods, there is often a dramatic improvement in schizophrenics. Some patients need high doses of some of the nutrients.

The usual person can get along well with 20 mg of niacin, but some investigators suggest that a schizophrenic may need much more, plus 3,000 mg/day of vitamin C, 200 to 1,000 mg/day of B6, and moderate amounts of all other nutrients, especially zinc and magnesium. Some patients respond better than others.

See your nutrition-minded physician.

Large doses of niacinamide (B3)—1,000 to 3,000 mg/day—sometimes reverse early senile dementia, delirium tremens and other alcohol psychoses (Moriarty, 1974). More than 3,000 mg a day may cause depression.

Pauling and other researchers studied the number of schziophrenics who had to be hospitalized for their disease and found that schizophrenics were low in all three vitamins—ascorbic acid, B3 and B6—and were 40 times as likely to be in the hospital for schizophrenia as people who weren't low in those vitamins. Only 6 percent of schizophrenics were not deficient in any of the three vitamins. That means that 94 percent of the schizophrenics studied were low in one or more.

TRANQUILIZERS

About the time Drs. Hoffer and Osmond began using nutrients to help schizophrenics, tranquilizers were discovered, and physicians in the United States used them a great deal. Tranquilizers do not cure schizophrenia and other mental illnesses, they just keep the patient quiet while he's suffering from his mental disease. They are patentable, though, and drug companies spend money to test and advertise them. Drug companies cannot patent vitamins and minerals, so they cannot make as much money on them. But many doctors continue to prescribe drugs for treatment of mental illness (Lesser, 1977).

Although patients aren't hospitalized so long when they take tranquilizers, there have been more patients admitted to mental hospitals since tranquilizers have been available. There are so many side effects from tranquilizers that patients quit taking them and have to be hospitalized again. Side effects include shaking, tremors, visual disturbances and sudden death. One ailment that pertains to the muscles is called tardive dyskinesia, which means that muscles fire at any and all times. Muscles all over the body can flutter, but much of the problem is that muscles in the face are affected and uncontrollable. There can be a quick fall in blood pressure, and the patient dies. Some people use tranquilizers to commit suicide.

CORRECTING THE INCORRIGIBLE

For years, nutrition investigators have been saying that deficiencies of nutrients contribute to juvenile deliquency.

American Laboratory (September 1977) published a report of 11 years of study of juvenile delinquents, their treatment by nutritional means and the outstanding success from that treatment.

The report is called "Correcting the Incorrigible."

One thousand difficult youngsters in a correctional institution were seen from 1963 through 1974. A total of 86 percent of those young people treated with nutrition have not returned to an institution or been arrested again. The 5-year follow-up rate for the highest-funded federal center for incorrigible young people is only 5 percent success.

These young people were physically, not mentally sick but they are still sick in the strictest sense. They had all been through psychotherapy for several years, but they had never been examined for physical health. Many had diabetes, hypothyroidism and complete lack of hydrochloric acid in the stomach.

The youngsters were about 16 years old and had been in and out of correctional programs for years. Some were in special education classes in elementary schools, some in reform schools, some in jail.

Some of the stresses these young people endured were poor health in general and frank malnutrition. Many had fast, irregular heartbeats. Half of them did not show any response when given a mild electric shock. Fully half did not have normal eye blinks. One-fourth did not blink at all at a ball falling against a clear plastic shield in front of their eyes or to a jet of air or water into their eyes. The investigator said, "This is difficult to comprehend and is a startling finding."

Half the delinquents had malabsorption syndrome. That is, the nutrients that should be absorbed through the walls of the small intestine were not absorbed. Deficiencies were pronounced for pantothenic acid, B6, vitamin C, sodium, potassium and manganese.

Lead, a dangerous poison, was especially high in most of those entering the school. Lead interferes with the use of zinc, a required mineral, which helps to control hyperactivity and mental illness.

Nearly every adolescent had either high or low blood sugar. All of them were put on a diabetic diet—no refined sugar or flour, no soft drinks or other junk food. They had supplements of vitamins and minerals, including one gram of ascorbic acid at each meal and hydrochloric acid tablets. All these helped lower the lead content of the tissues. To help relieve their hyperactivity, the students took vitamin C, which probably helped by making their adrenal glands work better.

Many children diagnosed as autistic became normal when given 400 mg of B6 daily and a good diet. Any psychiatric therapy is useless unless excellent nutrition is provided first.

Other symptoms these delinquents had were low thresholds for fatigue and confusion, allergies to foods and actual breakdown of central nervous system tissue. Treatment emphasized support of the adrenal glands. That means all vitamins and minerals were given, but no white sugar or flour was allowed.

DRUG ADDICTION

Drug addicts take drugs to change their moods or emotions—to get a high. We've mentioned that neurotransmitters can activate brain cells, causing acceleration or inhibition of a mood or emotion. Street drugs and doctors' drugs change the amounts of the neurotransmitters present in the brain cells, thus they cause greater acceleration or inhibition and lead to addiction. Megavitamin therapy has been found to reverse the addiction (Wurtman, 1983).

Investigators Alfred Libby and Irwin Stone have used such therapy with their drug-addicted patients. They reported in the *Journal of Orthomolecular Psychiatry* in 1982 on a pilot study with hard-drug addicts. They were given sodium ascorbate, a buffered vitamin C that does not cause gas or diarrhea when taken in large amounts. The investigators said that the sodium would not cause a problem with blood pressure because the sodium is not absorbed into the tissues. Ascorbic acid is also available as calcium ascorbate, which means that the buffering agent is calcium, and as an ascorbate buffered with several minerals. Also given were multivitamins and minerals and liquid amino acids for a few days, along with a good diet.

Megadoses of Vitamin C

The amount of ascorbate given depends on the amount of drugs the patients usually took. As a rule of thumb, a $50-a-day habit requires 25 to 40 grams of ascorbate; $150- to $200-a-day habit, about 60 to 75 grams. Errors should be on the high dosage side because of ascorbate's extremely low toxicity and lack of side effects. These megadoses are continued for four to six days. During this time, there should be no withdrawal symptoms. If there are, the dosage should be increased.

Early Improvement

Generally, in two or three days, appetite returns, and patients begin to eat well and sleep restfully for the first time since they became addicts. One of the first things noticed is that the patients feel good. After a few days, the megadoses are gradually reduced to doses of about 10 grams of ascorbate a day. The liquid amino acids are stopped, and the patient is eating well and feeling good. The case histories of these patients show that they return to happy, healthy, worthwhile lives after years of drug addiction.

HEAVY METAL POISONING

Our brains are easily damaged by poisonous metals—more so than any other parts of our bodies. Tons of the metals have been dug up and spread all over the earth, and it is impossible to avoid them. Besides that, many of the foods that would protect us from the poisons have been refined, and the helpful nutrients have been processed out.

Lead

Lead is the major toxic mineral we're exposed to, and we suffer from headaches, restlessness, agitation, irritability and depression. Our memories are not as good as they used to be, and we can't concentrate well. We can't sleep, we have nightmares and we may even hallucinate. Also, we are bothered by muscle aches and pains, nausea and indigestion.

In ancient Rome, wines were stored in lead containers, and water pipes were made of lead. The fall of Rome has been blamed on the low birth rate of the upper classes caused by lead poisoning.

Lead from air, food and water is stored in our bodies. Only a few years ago, lead was used in baby food cans. Now it has been banned. Only about two years ago, lead was banned from canned foods for the rest of the population. The FDA ruled recently that tuna, salmon, vegetable, fruit and all other food cans must be made without lead in the seams. Until that time, canned food was the largest source of lead intake in the country. We absorb lead through our skin when we hold the newspaper, when we clean engines, work with putty or dye our hair with certain dyes.

Although we excrete much of the lead we absorb (in the urine), we take in more than we excrete. Children absorb, and retain in the soft tissues, 35 percent of the lead they take in. Any hyperactive child may be affected by lead. It can cause learning disorders, autism, epilepsy and mental retardation. Many adults who have severe reactions to lead are criminals or live in slums. Their major items of diet are white sugar and white flour products, which furnish little protection against the poisons. We can partially protect ourselves against lead because the good minerals in our food will help our cells repulse the bad. Of course, coffee, tea, alcohol and diuretics allow our good minerals to be excreted. We should take supplement tablets of minerals to add to a good, natural food program to save our health.

Dolomite and bone meal, formerly popular supplements, may be contaminated with lead from the bones of the animals that were exposed to lead as they grazed, usually near highways or chemical plants.

Aluminum Is Dangerous

Aluminum will probably be the most dangerous of the metals in the future. It is 8 percent of the earth's crust, and investigators say it will cause more deaths in the future than even heart disease and cancer. Many researchers say aluminum cooking utensils are not dangerous, and that antacids and antidepressants are our major source of aluminum. The metal is also in many processed foods.

Much of the aluminum finds its way to the brain, and an ailment we hear a lot about these days—Alzheimer's disease—often develops. It is presenility, and it is now our fourth killer disease. It is estimated that during the twenty-first century, it will be our first killer disease. Many people begin to lose their short-term memory around age 30. Many of those same people are diagnosed as Alzheimer's patients in their forties. At autopsy, their brains show cell degeneration, with excess aluminum in the brain and spinal fluid. When aluminum salts are injected into the fluid surrounding the brain in laboratory animals, the animals' brains degenerate just the way senile human brains do.

Aluminum is used to purify drinking water; it is added to most salt to keep it from caking. Toothpaste contains aluminum, as do many baking powders. Health food stores sell baking powder without aluminum. We can easily get rid of the major sources of aluminum and keep our brains in better condition.

DIET

Food

The basic diet needed for mental problems of all kinds is the one given in Lesson 1 of this course.

1. 10–20 percent of calories as protein from grains and beans combined. These are our best protein foods, as they furnish the fiber we need for good digestion. We can eat moderate amounts of fish, poultry from the health food store, milk, eggs, light-colored, natural cheese—but very little red meat. Use meat as a condiment to give flavor.

2. 10–20 percent of calories as fat. Butter can be used to cook with and to spread on bread. Nuts and seeds furnish polyunsaturated fat, which contains linoleic acid.

3. Near zero refined carbohydrates (white sugar and white flour).

4. 60–80 percent of calories as carbohydrate from whole fruits, vegetables, whole grains and legumes.

5. Appropriate vitamin-mineral supplements, especially vitamin C and the whole complex.

Food Supplements

Food supplements will greatly help to pep up a tired brain. Their major advantage is that they will work more quickly than food by itself.

B Complex, Especially. Supplements of all nutrients are needed for people with mental problems, but emphasis is on B-complex vitamins because tissues that suffer most from B deficiencies are those that use a lot of energy, such as the nerves and the brain.

Other brain problems result from swelling of the inside of the blood vessels in the brain and blocking the capillaries. The cells that these capillaries are supposed to feed can't get food, so they die. This is a small stroke. If a person has a number of small strokes he becomes senile because his brain is dying little by little. The earliest symptom of nerve damage is in the brain and spinal cord and results in a nerve disease that causes feelings of inadequacy, insomnia, lack of attention, failure to concentrate and irritability.

Other symptoms of B deficiencies are vague fears, emotional disturbances and inflammation of the nerves, which causes paralysis, wasting, disappearance of the nerve reflexes, pain and tenderness over the nerves, a feeling of small insects crawling over the skin or abnormal sensations such as burning and prickling. Mental symptoms are common: apathy, confusion, emotional instability, irritability, depression, fear of impending disaster and defective memory. Sometimes mental symptoms are seen after only a few days of deficiency. Some people suffer from apprehension, loss of ability to use the hands efficiently and inattention to detail. Early brain damage is irreversible, so early improvement of the diet is important. A sudden severe deficiency can cause profound mental changes.

Behavior problems include poor manual speed and coordination, poor eye-hand coordination, unsteadiness of hands and body sway. Persons on pep pills, those who fast and those who go on crash diets may have these symptoms.

Two diseases formerly thought to be caused by alcohol poisoning are now known to be due to a B-vitamin deficiency. Wernicke's syndrome, which causes mental changes, and Korsakoff's syndrome, which is loss of memory of the recent past, respond to B-vitamin therapy.

L-glutamine. An amino acid called L-glutamic acid is especially important. It is present in rather high concentrations in brain and nerves, and it helps them function. The average intake in protein foods is 5 to 10 grams a day. Tremendous amounts can cause increased activity and nausea. But epileptics and persons with other mental problems may need more than they get. The form recommended is L-glutamine, which is a derivative of the amino acid, because the amino acid itself can't cross the blood-brain barrier. L-glutamine crosses the barrier, then when it gets to the other side it changes into glutamic acid (Williams, 1971). Many patients with mild or moderate mental deficiencies have improved their personalities and increased their intelligence, as shown by 5 to 20 additional IQ points (Pauling, 1968). This amino acid can be used as brain food in addition to glucose (Williams, 1971).

Vitamin B1 (Thiamine). A deficiency in thiamine causes mental depression, irritability, confusion, loss of memory, inability to concentrate and sensitivity to noise (Williams, 1971).

Vitamin B3 (Niacin). A deficiency of B3 causes mental diseases. The vitamin is absolutely essential for the metabolism of brain cells, and unless the cells have been damaged beyond repair, they begin to function again when malnutrition is corrected (Williams, 1971).

Some people take niacin best if it is dissolved in warm water and swallowed while the stomach is empty. Most gastric burning occurs when the vitamin is absorbed low in the intestinal tract. The flush may still appear.

The flush is well known. The reddening appears first on the head and face and it feels hot. The sensation of needles pricking the skin follows. Usually the flush lasts only 30 or 40 minutes. It is slightly uncomfortable but is not dangerous. Niacin should be taken in small amounts at first, and built up gradually. Ascorbic acid should be given with niacin (Newbold, 1970). Niacinamide, another form of niacin, does not cause flushing, but may cause nausea or depression in large doses, over 3,000 mg a day.

Vitamin B6 (Pyridoxine). Sixteen autistic children were given or denied vitamin B6 in a double-blind crossover study. The children lived in widely scattered areas, from California to Florida. They were given their usual vitamins, minerals and prescription drugs, plus megadoses of ascorbic acid and niacin, and either B6 or a placebo. It has been shown that large doses of B6 will elevate serotonin levels. Serotonin is a substance that allows nerve impulses to flow along the nerves.

The children were found to need extra folic acid (a B vitamin) and extra magnesium when taking large amounts of B6 for a long time. The children's behavior improved significantly while taking the B6, and deteriorated significantly when it was withdrawn (Rimland, 1978). In another study, a deficiency of B6 caused convulsions. In a sample of 800 psychiatric patients, the needs ranged from 5 to 400 mg daily (Williams, 1971).

Pantothenic Acid. Deficiency of pantothenic acid causes degeneration of nerves in animals. Prisoners on a diet deficient in pantothenic acid were severely depressed mentally. People stand stress better when they receive large doses of this B vitamin (Williams, 1971).

Biotin. Biotin is made by friendly bacteria in the intestines, if this is not prevented by an excess of poisonous bacteria. A deficiency of biotin leads to depression. Persons with severe depression improved on IV injections of 150 or more mg a day. The usual dosage is 150 to 300 mcg a day (Kirschmann, 1975).

Choline. A study at Massachusetts Institute for Technology by Dr. John H. Growdon and his colleagues found that oral doses of choline, one of the B-vitamin cousins, apparently improve memory and "virtually any brain disease due to too little choline." Manic depression may be one of the treatable diseases using choline (Davis, 1978). Choline is the basic ingredient in lecithin, and it prevents the depositing of fat in the liver (*Dorland's*, 1974).

Inositol. Inositol, another B-vitamin cousin, may be of special value in brain nutrition. Hoffer uses a compound of niacin and inositol to treat mental illness (Williams, 1971). Sometimes all nutrients are fed but aren't assimilated. Extra vitamins may be needed for best absorption (Williams, 1971).

Folic Acid. A deficiency of folic acid, a B vitamin, was found in 48 of 59 elderly patients admitted to a psychiatric hospital. Patients with mental disease have low levels of folic acid. Anticonvulsants and other drugs contribute to disturbances and personality changes. Suggested supplements are vitamin C (2,000 mg) and zinc gluconate (30 mg) morning and evening. Folic acid can't be made into folacin, its active form, without vitamin C (Williams, 1971).

Vitamin B12. Poisonous bacteria in the intestine feed on B12, so there is not enough left for the patient. The deficiency leads to mental illness that is often more severe than physical illness, and to pernicious anemia. In anemia, the intrinsic factor is missing rather than B12, but mental symptoms can often be seen for years in patients before physical symptoms show up (Pauling, 1968).

A B12 deficiency causes symptoms ranging from

poor concentration to stuporous depression, similar to schizophrenia. Patients with psychiatric symptoms and deficiency states were given B12 and folic acid. All improved (Williams, 1971). Since B12 is found only in animal foods, vegetarians might not get the amount they need without a supplement.

Other Vitamins. The B complex, of course, isn't all that is needed for mental health. The body's vitamin C stores can be exhausted in only a few seconds of stress. If the stress continues, the adrenal glands grab all the C, and the other tissues of the body suffer from a deficiency.

Linus Pauling says that if everybody took adequate amounts of vitamin C, world leaders as well as the people of the world would be able to think 10 percent more clearly. Think how much better off everyone would be. Patients with mental disease have high demands for vitamin C and have body levels below normal. Also, they use up vitamin C 10 times faster than those who are not ill. Some patients given 36 to 48 grams of ascorbic acid a day became definitely better (Stone, 1974). Many schizophrenics soak up huge amounts of vitamin C—up to 70,000 mg (Moriarty, 1974).

SUGGESTED ADDITIONS TO FOOD SUPPLEMENTS

To simplify the information about additional nutrients for mental health, here is a chart of supplements to add to those suggested by the references listed in this lesson and in Lesson 1 of this series.

Nutrient	Total amount suggested	Number of doses	Comment
B complex	150 mg or more	3	Bs are not dangerous in large amounts (they are excreted in the urine). However, B2 and B6 should usually be taken in equal amounts. (B12 and biotin and folic acid are listed in micrograms.)
Niacinamide (B3)	100 mg to 3,000 mg	3	Dr. Richard Passwater (in Supernutrition) says to begin with 100 mg and increase until you have a sense of well-being. Large doses or doses over extended periods may cause depression or nausea. Always take the entire B complex with niacinamide.
Niacin (B3)	75 mg to 750 mg	3	25 mg after each meal for one week. Increase 25 mg every week to a feeling of well-being—usually not over 250 mg three times a day

Nutrient	Total amount suggested	Number of doses	Comment
Pantothenic acid	600 mg to 800 mg	3	Helpful in any stress situation.
L-Glutamine	2 to 20 grams	2	Begin with a small amount. Increase gradually to a feeling of well-being. Some researchers suggest 10 to 20 grams a day.
Pyridoxine (B6)	200 to 1,000 mg	3	Behavior may improve dramatically. Take all food supplements together. Decrease B6 when able. Intake varies greatly.
Vitamin C	3,000 mg to 6,000 mg or more	3–6	"Bowel tolerance" is suggested by many nutritionists. This means take 500 mg six times a day. If this causes gas, cut down below that level until you get relief. If it doesn't cause gas, go up until you get gas and cut down below that level. (Bowel tolerance means to take C until diarrhea develops.)

We are all different, not only from each other, but also within ourselves from day to day and from hour to hour, depending primarily on the stress we are under. Stress affects our adrenal glands and thus the way we use food.

Whenever you take nutritional supplements, it is a good idea to start slowly and build up to the large amounts. Also, remember to listen to your body. Since we are all different, we must adjust all nutrients to our own individual needs.

TOO MANY DRUGS—TIME TO CHANGE

In this country, we have spent almost all our money and energy in the past trying to find drugs to treat stress and mental illness. "The drugs we use to treat mental illness are not very good. They are not very specific and they have terrible side effects," said Dr. Fridolin Sulser in the Houston Chronicle.

It is time we used natural foods, needed by every cell to build and repair tissue. I have heard from many people who have suffered cruelly for up to 40 years on a drug program, then have found nutrition, and, gradually, almost like a miracle, they improve. How tragic to remember the 40 years they wasted limping through life, suffering from physical or mental ailments that should have been treated naturally so many years ago.

QUESTIONS

TRUE/FALSE

1. All mental problems are physical problems.

2. Neurotransmitters are messengers that travel from one nerve cell to another to activate any cell in the body.

3. Researchers suggest that Alzheimer's disease may respond to long-term usage of lecithin.

4. The brain grows faster before and soon after birth than any other part of the body.

5. The brain weighs 2 percent of the total body weight, but it uses up to 20 percent of the total oxygen and 20 percent of the total nutrients.

6. We become unconscious if our blood stops flowing for five seconds; we suffer irreversible damage or death if our blood stops flowing for a few minutes.

7. Pregnant women who eat 50 grams or less of protein per day have babies who weigh less and have smaller skulls than women who eat 70 grams per day.

8. Aldous Huxley stated in the early 1950s: "The nervous system is more vulnerable than any other tissue of the body, therefore, vitamin deficiencies affect the mind and behavior before they affect other tissues."

9. We can all handle stress without ill effects if we eat well.

10. Our adrenal glands manufacture 32 hormones that protect us from stress if we eat good food needed to make the hormones.

11. In cold weather, the stress of producing extra heat for our bodies uses up vitamin C much faster than usual.

12. Page says that if we eliminate white sugar from our lives, we would eliminate 90 percent of our ills.

13. Depression is one of our most frequent mental disorders.

14. Drugs given to patients with depression often cause severe side effects, but even so, one of every 10 prescription drugs written in this country is for antidepressant drugs.

15. Hoffer and Osmond found that 82 percent of schizophrenics can be helped with vitamin therapy.

16. Linus Pauling stated that patients low in vitamins C, B3 and B6 were 40 times more likely to be in the hospital for schizophrenia than people who weren't low in those vitamins.

17. The aluminum that gets into our blood from foods and antiperspirants is attracted to the brain, and it is said to be partly the cause of Alzheimer's disease.

18. Researchers emphasize B complex to help prevent nervousness, insomnia and poor memory.

MULTIPLE CHOICE

1. We should eat well so we won't have the following ailments: (a) mental retardation, (b) schizophrenia, (c) mood swings, (d) stuporous depression.

2. Neurotransmitters are made from the following nutrients: (a) vitamins, (b) minerals, (c) precursors, (d) all of the above.

3. Neurotransmitters and their precursors are made from the food we eat, and they activate nerves that impact on one or more of the following conditions: (a) moods, (b) learning, (c) memory, (d) movement of muscles.

4. List the statements about the brain that are true: (a) During prenatal life, 20,000 neurons have to be produced every minute, (b) The body does not furnish nourishment for the brain, (c) glial cells hold the neurons together, (d) prenatal malnutrition can seriously affect a person's entire life by limiting the number of neurons produced before birth.

5. Deficiencies of essential fatty acids can cause: (a) growth retardation, (b) skin damage, (c) partial malfunction of the brain and other organs, (d) all of the above.

6. Often when the diet is improved, the first symptoms of relief are: (a) less fatigue, (b) more alertness, (c) less depression.

7. Stress is anything that taxes the body, such as: (a) anxiety, (b) overwork, (c) poor diet, (d) going out in cold weather.

8. Which of the following conditions cause stress on our bodies: (a) noise, (b) violence on TV, (c) sleep loss, (d) poor food.

9. Nutrients needed to combat depression include: (a) aspartic acid, (b) tryptophan, (c) vitamin B complex, (d) carbohydrates, (e) fats.

10. Warning signs of schizophrenia include: (a) insomnia, (b) headaches, (c) crying fits, (d) changes in personality.

11. Side effects of tranquilizers, often given to schizophrenics, include: (a) shaking, (b) visual problems, (c) sudden death.

12. Brain damage can be caused by heavy metal poisoning which causes: (a) lack of concentration, (b) nightmares, (c) hyperactivity.

ANSWERS

True/False

1. T   2. T   3. T   4. T   5. T   6. T   7. T   8. T   9. T
10. T   11. T   12. T   13. T   14. T   15. T   16. T
17. T   18. T

Multiple Choice

1. a,b,c,d   2. a,b,c, or d   3. a,b,c,d   4. a,c,d   5. d
6. a,b,c   7. a,b,c,d   8. a,b,c,d   9. b,c,d,e   10. a,b,c,d
11. a,b,c   12. a,b,c

REFERENCES

Ballentine, R. *Diet and Nutrition, A Holistic Approach.* Honesdale, PA: The Himalayan International Institute, 1978.

Cheraskin, E. et al. *Diet and Disease.* New Canaan, CT: Keats, 1987.

——— et al. *Psychodietetics.* New York: Bantam, 1974.

——— et al. *New Hope for Incurable Diseases.* New York: Exposition, 1971.

Cott, A. *J. App. Nutr.* 25(1,2):15–24, 1973.

Dorland's Illustrated Medical Dictionary, 25th Edition. Philadelphia: W. B. Saunders, 1974.

Fineberg, S. K. The Realities of Obesity and Fad Diets. *Nutr. Today*, July/Aug. 1972.

Garrow, J. S. Diet and Obesity. *Proc. R. Soc. Med.*, 66:642–44. July 1973.

Goodhart and Shils. *Modern Nutrition in Health and Disease.* Philadelphia: Lea and Febiger, 1973.

Guyton, A. C. *Textbook of Medical Physiology.* Philadelphia: W. B. Saunders, 1976.

Hall, Ross Hume. Overweight: Clue to Decline in Quality of Nourishment. Entrophy Institute, Vol. 1(5), July/Aug. 1978.

Hawkins, D. and Pauling, L., eds. *Orthomolecular Psychiatry: Treatment of Schizophrenics.* San Francisco: W. H. Freeman, 1973.

Hoffer, A. Nutrition and Behavior. In: *Medical Applications of Clinical Nutrition* (Ed. J. Bland). New Canaan, CT: Keats, 1983.

Horrobin, D. F. *An Introduction to Human Physiology.* Davis, 1973.

Houston Chronicle, page 9, section 4; Monday, May, 29, 1978.

Jensen, K. et al. *Lancet*, ii(7941):920, 1975.

Kirshmann, J. D. *Nutrition Almanac.* New York: McGraw-Hill, 1975.

Kline, N. S. Antidepressant Medication: A More Effective Use by General Practitioners, Family Physicians, Internists and Others. *JAMA*, 227(10):1158, 1974.

Lesser, M. *Nutrition and Vitamin Therapy.* New York: Grove Press, 1980.

———. *Select Committee Report.* Washington, DC: U.S. Govt. Printing Ofc., 1977.

Mann, G. V. The Influence of Obesity on Health, Part II. *N. E. J. Med.*, 291(5):226–31, 1974.

Medical Tribune, February 11, 1976.

Moriarty, J. D. *J. Appl. Nutr.*, 26(3):27–35, 1974.

Mount, L. E. Energy Expenditure During the Growing Period. (in) *Early Nutrition and Later Development.* Chicago: Yearbook Med. Pub., Inc., 1976, pp. 156–163.

Page, M. E. and Abrams, H. L., Jr. *Your Body Is Your Best Doctor!* New Canaan, CT: Keats Publishing, 1972.

Passwater, R. A. *Supernutrition.* New York: Pocket, 1975.

Pauling, L. *Science*, 160:265–271, 1968.

———. Sugar: Sweet and Dangerous. *Executive Health* 9(1):1–4, 1972.

———. *How to Live Longer and Feel Better.* New York: W. H. Freeman, 1986.

Peshek, R. J. Surgery—a Stress. *J. Appl. Nutr.*, 26:6–20, 1974.

Pfeiffer, Carl C. *Mental and Elemental Nutrients.* New Canaan, CT: Keats, 1975.

Schauf, G. E. *JIAPM*, 3(2):33–41, December, 1976.

Scrimshaw, N. The Effect of Stress on Nutrition in Young Adults. (in) *Adolescents, Nutrition and Growth*, ed. F. P. Heald.New York: Appleton-Century-Crofts, 1969, pp. 101–117.

Seddon, G. and Burrow, J. *The Natural Food Book.* New York: Rand McNally, 1977.

Selye, H. On Just Being Sick. *Nutr. Today*, 5(1):2–10, 1970.

Sherman, W. C. Obesity. *Food and Nutrition News.* National Livestock and Meat Board, 45(1):3, November, 1973.

Shneour, E. *The Malnourished Mind.* New York: Anchor, 1974.

Stone, Irwin. *The Healing Factor: Vitamin C Against Disease.* New York: Grosset & Dunlap, 1972.

Williams, R. J. *Nutrition Against Disease.* New York: Pitman, 1971.

Winick, M., ed. *Nutrition and Aging.* New York: John Wiley and Sons, 1976.

Wurtman, R. J. Behavioral Effects of Nutrients. *Lancet*, 1 (8334): 1145–1147, May 21, 1983.

Lesson 3

HEART DISEASE AND NUTRITION

LESSON 3—HEART DISEASE AND NUTRITION

WILL YOU be one of the one million people who die of heart disease this year? Death due to heart disease is equal to 10 jumbo jet airline disasters every day (Whitaker, 1982). More than 600,000 of the deaths occur outside of a hospital, and for many victims, the first symptom that a person has a life-threatening disease is death itself. You don't have to be one of those victims.

So much exciting information has been published to help us prevent heart attacks and strokes that we don't have to worry about this number one killer. If you'd like to avoid pain from angina pectoris, avoid a stroke that cripples your mind or body, avoid dropping dead from a coronary occlusion, avoid a blood clot in your leg that causes agony (or that breaks off and travels to your lung and blocks *those* blood vessels) and avoid the popular and sometimes tragic "heart bypass" operation, there is a way.

BYPASS OPERATIONS

Before we discuss the easy way to prevent and control heart disease, let's talk about what's wrong with the bypass operation so often used, overused and abused.

In 1981, 159,000 bypass operations were performed, up 22,000 from 1980. The number of oper-ations has been going up at the rate of 15 to 25 percent a year since 1971. What is the cost of the operations? At least $20,000 for one operation, and $3.2 billion a year for all operations.

A bypass operation never prevented a heart attack, and, worse than that, the *New England Journal of Medicine* reports that only 15 percent of the patients who live through the attack are likely to live longer if they have surgery. Five percent of the patients who have surgery continue to have angina pains. That's because 20 percent of the new veins clog up within the first year after surgery, and more and more clog up as the years go by. In fact, a higher percentage of people who have the surgery have heart attacks in the future than people who have not had surgery.

Only about 35 percent of the patients return to work after they have the bypass operation; more patients return to work after some types of heart attack than after bypass surgery. *Lancet*, a prestigious British medical journal, says that there is "no conclusive medical evidence that bypass surgery is better than other therapies," and the operations seem to be performed "to financially maintain the current crop of cardiopulmonary surgeons." Two experts in the field have said, "Generally, the bypass operation is just one in a series of fads, and if the patient doesn't change his lifestyle" (give up junk foods, quit smoking, etc.), "the benefits of the operation will be only temporary."

The Journal of the American Medical Association (JAMA) published a food program recommended for heart patients that consisted of low-fat foods, plus fresh fruits and vegetables. No unusual exercise was suggested. In just 24 days, patients could work harder and longer. Those with high cholesterol reduced their levels more than 20 percent; they had a 91 percent drop in angina attacks, and 18 of them either reduced their medication or went off it completely. The article concludes with the information that bypass surgery may be needed at times to save lives, but the improvement may last only a short time. Many of those who have surgery get worse and even require another operation. The power of the AMA is obvious by its advertising and promotion of this money-making operation, but a preventive medicine program should be publicized to emphasize its value for vibrant health of the heart.

NUTRITION AND HEART HEALTH

The new excitement about heart disease and all other related ailments, lumped together as atherosclerotic cardiovascular disease (ASCVD), comes in four parts:

1. Cholesterol and animal fats aren't the villains that most investigators have thought.

2. Vegetable oil (polyunsaturated fat), although an essential food, not only won't cure ASCVD, but too much may be dangerous.

3. The vitamins and minerals in unprocessed, unrefined whole foods are the new "treatment" that cuts down on atherosclerotic cardiovascular disease.

4. Supplements of vitamins are usually needed, mostly because it's difficult to get unprocessed food with the nutrients left in, and because pollutants in the environment use up or cancel out some of the nutrients we do get. Drugs have been used to lower the cholesterol content of the blood, but Clofibrate, one of the drugs most prescribed, has been found to cause an across-the-board increase in death. Also, Clofibrate causes an up to 45 percent increase in damage to the gall bladder.

What's the answer? Our natural food program, with moderate amounts of all food supplements and large amounts of some. This food plan will reduce the fatty plaques and allow the consistency of the blood to be not too thick and not too thin. Thus one of the major causes of heart attack and stroke will be eliminated. The program also provides all nutrients needed for the heart muscle to beat. It is well known that minerals are required for muscles to

contract, and if the heart muscle can no longer contract, the heart cannot beat. About 20 percent of so-called heart attacks, on autopsy, show that the blood vessels were not blocked by fat; the muscle just stopped contracting, and the heart failed to beat. Death followed.

All this new knowledge is ours for the taking. We may have to change what we eat, but think of the freedom of not worrying about having a heart attack any minute. Have you lost a close friend or relative that way? We can't be certain it won't happen to us unless we eat properly to prevent heart problems. If you're already taking medication for your heart, whole foods and food supplements will improve your condition, and soon you'll probably be able to take fewer and fewer drugs. Your doctor will probably be able to take you off drugs before long, but *don't* take yourself off. If you stop some drugs suddenly, you may bring on a heart attack. So don't take any chances.

We should eat moderate amounts of fresh fruits and vegetables, whole-grain cereals, legumes (beans, peas and peanuts), fish and small amounts of lean meat, natural, light-colored cheese, the wonderful seeds and nuts, and one or two eggs a day. All these foods must be unprocessed and unrefined. Nuts and seeds that have been roasted either with or without oil have been damaged by heat. Raw legumes contain a substance that inhibits trypsin, one of the pancreatic enzymes that help to assimilate protein.) Rancid nuts can be processed to mask the rancidity, but the danger remains. Also, many whole-grain flours have been sprayed with chemicals to keep them from spoiling. Cottage cheese often has so many additives that it is damaging to the cells. We'll be buying almost no foods that have confusing labels because we will be buying natural, unprocessed foods.

You're probably already saying, "My doctor lets me eat only one egg a week." You won't have a high cholesterol level on my program because it contains all vitamins and minerals, which adjust the amount of cholesterol in your blood vessels. Many people have excess cholesterol in their blood, but it is because vitamin C or one or more of the other nutrients required for healthy cells is missing. Let's enjoy one or two eggs a day, along with as perfect a diet as we can get, plus moderate amounts of all vitamins and minerals in supplement form.

Let's also enjoy eating six small meals a day rather than three larger meals. This plan helps to reduce the number of heart attacks, which often follow a heavy meal. When food is being digested, blood is drawn to the stomach and intestines to help with digestion. The heart may not get enough blood to furnish oxygen and nutrients, especially if its arteries are full of fatty plaques or if the artery walls are damaged because they don't get the nutrients needed to make healthy cells.

I told a friend of mine that I was writing a book about heart disease, and he said, "You're too late for me; I've had my heart attack." Then he quickly added, "But mine was caused by stress. I'm healthy. I seldom even have a cold. It was just stress." He obviously hadn't heard that we can handle stress if our bodies have all the nutrients they need. Physical and emotional stress use up nutrients so rapidly that the body often can't replace them fast enough. That sounds simple—and it is. As simple as the cure for scurvy, which stumped the medical world for hundreds of years. Finally someone said, "Eat limes." He was ridiculed for suggesting that simple remedy. And yet that's what saved the world from scurvy—eating limes and other foods high in vitamin C.

KINDS OF HEART AILMENTS

High blood pressure and atherosclerosis are the two major causes of heart deaths.

High Blood Pressure

High blood pressure contributes greatly to many illnesses and deaths related to heart disease. With a natural food program, as eaten by primitive populations and by modern nutrition-minded people, high blood pressure is practically nonexistent (Ershoff, 1981). These people eat a ratio of about 10 times more potassium than sodium. But in the United States, the ratio is reversed, with people eating from 1¼ to 5 times more sodium than potassium.

The average adult probably needs no more than 500 mg of sodium a day, but he eats from 5,000 to 17,500 mg. Populations that eat the largest amounts of sodium have the highest rates of high blood pressure. However, all people who eat large amounts of salt do not have high blood pressure. About 17 percent of adult Americans develop high blood pressure on a daily sodium intake of about 3,000 to 6,000 mg per day. The Food and Nutrition Board of the National Academy of Sciences, National Research Council, suggests that ½ to 1 teaspoon of salt a day would be safe. That's 1,100 to 3,300 mg. But the average American eats 2 to 4 teaspoons of salt a day. This amount causes half the people over age 65 to develop high blood pressure.

If everybody, including the 17 percent who are especially sensitive to salt, ate no more than 1,380 mg of sodium a day for life, they would probably not get high blood pressure. But if high blood pressure has been present for a number of years, restricting sodium will lower the blood pressure somewhat, but not enough. The salt intake for those people may have to be as low as 230 mg a day or less. Many people take diuretics that get rid of the sodium, but a low-sodium diet will often reduce the blood pressure without a diuretic. Some doctors, however, believe that patients should be given diuretics if their kidneys are healthy enough to filter the sodium.

This recommendation is not best for the patients, but it is aimed at allowing them to eat more salt so that their food will be palatable. Of course, on a natural food diet they would lose their need for salt. It is well known that we can't taste food without needed amounts of zinc and the B vitamins, nutrients often refined out of processed food and severely missing in the average American diet.

Natural foods are low in sodium and high in potassium. They provide only about 500 mg of sodium and 7,800 mg of potassium per day. When food is processed, canned or frozen, salt is added in such large amounts that the average American consumes from 5,000 to 10,000 mg of sodium a day. Although the sodium content goes up in the processing, the potassium content stays the same. Thus, 20 percent of American adults have high blood pressure, and 40 percent of older Americans have a blood pressure problem. The best solution for these people seems to be a diet of natural foods plus a moderate amount of potassium as a supplement. This is exactly what my food program offers. If patients have a kidney problem, it would be dangerous to increase the potassium just by giving potassium tablets. If there were no problem already, one might develop.

Some of the highest sources of sodium are restaurant foods and fast foods. Thus people who regularly eat those foods may develop high blood pressure. If large amounts of potassium tablets are given, the following side effects are common: poor taste, abdominal cramps, nausea, diarrhea, vomiting and others. However, if people take the same amount of potassium in natural foods, such reactions rarely occur. Low-sodium high-potassium foods include almost all raw fruits and vegetables, plus almonds, Brazil nuts, peanuts and walnuts. As an example, fresh raw peas contain two mg of sodium; frozen, 116 mg; and canned, 236 mg in 100 grams of peas—about three-eighths of a cup.

Atherosclerosis

Atherosclerotic cardiovascular disease includes several other heart and blood vessel ailments, but atherosclerosis is the most common disease of the blood vessels. It involves the depositing of fatty plaques on the lining of the vessel walls. Arteriosclerosis is the hardening of those plaques caused by calcium deposits. They can be brittle like glass. Why is calcium deposited in the arteries rather than going to the bones and teeth where it belongs? Because we don't have enough hydrochloric acid in the stomach to dissolve the calcium. Undissolved calcium can't go to the bones and teeth; it collects in the joints and causes arthritis, or in the blood vessels and causes hardening of the arteries.

Most of the trouble is caused by the fatty plaques, because they narrow the blood vessels so much that only a trickle of blood gets through to feed the heart. We feel as if we're suffocating because the heart can't get enough oxygen. That's angina pectoris. If the plaques get so thick they close up the vessel, we have a heart attack. Doctors call it cardiac insufficiency.

Sometimes there's so much fat that it forms a clot in a branch of a coronary artery and plugs up the artery. That also causes a heart attack. This condition is called coronary thrombosis, coronary occlusion and cardiac infarction. Part of the heart actually dies. If a large part dies, we die; but sometimes new blood vessels open up and send blood around the blocked artery. If the artery is small, there's little damage done; but if the artery is large, and the clot grows fast, new blood vessels haven't had time to form; then cells in that part of the heart die because they don't get enough blood.

Often a clot breaks off somewhere in the body and floats along in the blood until it gets to a smaller vessel or a narrow place with lots of thick plaques. The clot plugs up the vessel and causes a heart attack (coronary embolism). Many young people have this kind of heart attack. Almost every year we read about a football player who dies of a coronary embolism.

Infarcts. Infarcts (death of tissue because of blood clots) can happen anywhere in the body. An infarct in the brain is called a stroke (apoplexy) and in the lung, a pulmonary embolism. We might even say you'd be lucky to have angina pains. Then you'd be warned of a possible heart attack and you'd have time to do something about it before anything happened. Kannel (1970) says that only 20 percent of those who have a myocardial infarction have angina beforehand.

Many of those other 80 percent have infarctions and don't recognize them. Dr. Kannel found that 23 percent of the people who had an infarction didn't know they had one. They probably had pain but they didn't think it was serious, or they wanted to avoid doctors, or they just ignored their own discomfort. Probably many men think it's unmasculine to complain; so they probably took an aspirin and forgot about it. Men with high blood pressure or diabetes have twice as many unrecognized infarctions as others do. Ten percent of the people have a silent or painless infarction, and they won't know it until they have an electrocardiogram later on during a routine checkup, which shows that some time in the past they had a mild heart attack or stroke. Even if the first infarction is so mild that you don't notice it, it won't make the second one any lighter. It doesn't seem to matter about age either. Many people from 30 to 79 have had mild heart attacks or strokes and didn't know it.

Dr. Henry A. Schroeder, in his book, *The Trace Elements and Man*, says that mild strokes cause ringing in the ears, loss of speech, loss of vision, numbness in certain places, maybe even just dizziness. We're dying by inches, or maybe just becoming senile. Recently a friend of my husband's died of a heart attack early one Sunday morning. He hadn't missed a day's work; he had even played golf the day before. I asked my husband if there had been any indication of anything unusual, and he said, "Yes. He had had indigestion for several weeks." It is well known that indigestion pains may not be indigestion but angina. It seems strange that anyone with this discomfort wouldn't see a doctor.

Some doctors tell me that the medical profession is not doing enough to help cut down the one million deaths from heart and blood vessel disease every year. At a meeting of physicians, Dr. Ancel Keys, one of the most prominent heart disease researchers, spoke about this dilemma in *Atherosclerosis Proceedings*. Let me quote him exactly. "What about meeting the big challenge, the need for primary prevention of coronary heart disease (CHD). Nothing now is being done or is even seriously proposed to reduce in any important way the incidence and mortality rate of CHD." He goes on to say that although doctors have been trying for a third of a century to find the answer to heart disease, nothing has really been accomplished.

Fortunately there is now slightly less artherosclerosis, but it is still our biggest health problem. The medical community and nutritionists don't agree on why there is less of it. The medicos say it's because more people are eating margarine, but the nutritionists say it's partly because 30 million Americans are taking vitamin E (Passwater, 1975) and other vitamins and minerals.

Here's a good way to get atherosclerosis, according to Dr. Schroeder. Drink a lot of coffee all day with plenty of sugar and cream, eat white toast for breakfast with lots of jelly, eat a bologna sandwich on white bread for lunch with a piece of pie, and for supper, eat fried potatoes, pork with rich gravy and more pie for dessert. That diet will surely lead to high cholesterol, low chromium and—worst of all—atherosclerosis.

NEW INFORMATION "TRICKLES" IN

The exciting information in the medical and nutrition journals about heart attacks has actually been trickling in for quite a few years. A lot of it is about fats—animal, vegetable and cholesterol.

What About Fats?

I will make three points about fats. There are two kinds of cholesterol; good (high-density lipoprotein—HDL) and bad (low-density lipoprotein—LDL). HDL contains lecithin, which reams the cholesterol out of the blood vessels and sends it to the liver to make bile. LDL is the kind that stacks up in the arteries. Almost every journal I read these days tells us how to get rid of the LDL and how to *increase the HDL.* So if your doctor tells you your cholesterol count is high, tell him if it is HDL, that's just the way you want it.

Let me emphasize three points about fats.

1. The cholesterol we eat doesn't increase the amount of cholesterol in the blood.
2. Polyunsaturated (vegetable) fats in large amounts do not help prevent coronary heart disease (CHD). In fact, they can cause more heart, cancer and other disease problems, mostly by increasing our need for vitamin E.
3. Triglycerides (fats made in the body from sugar, starch and alcohol) are really the major villains.

And there are two significant points to make about eggs, high-protein foods and complex carbohydrates—the whole foods.

1. Eggs and dairy products and other high-protein foods with moderate amounts of animal fat and cholesterol are such good foods, with lots of vitamins and minerals to keep our blood and tissue cells healthy, that we should include them generously in our diets.
2. Refined carbohydrates (white sugar and white flour) cause more damage than anything else. We must replace them with complex carbohydrates—unprocessed, unrefined fruits, vegetables, whole grains and legumes.

What About Cholesterol?

Let's look first at cholesterol. There never has been general agreement among the investigators that the cholesterol we eat is such a menace. One investigator wrote in the *South African Medical Journal* in 1973: "One distinguished American research physician has written that blood cholesterol is a biochemical measurement in search of clinical significance." Cholesterol *must* circulate in the blood. We need it in every cell. It puts a strong, smooth lining in the blood vessels so the blood that rushes through so fast won't wear away the lining. It helps make sex and adrenal hormones, bile acids and vitamin D. Dr. Schroeder says that the brain and pancreas contain from 5 to 10 percent cholesterol, and the liver more than 1 percent. Without cholesterol, the skin would become dry. The average American diet contains from 200 to 800 mg of cholesterol a day, but we make it in the liver, small intestine and in every cell in the body—a total of 2,000 to 3,000 mg a day. Even with a high-cholesterol diet, the body makes 60 to 80 percent of the total cholesterol it needs every day. In a no-cholesterol diet—all vegetarian—the body makes all the cholesterol it needs. (There is no cholesterol in plant food.)

A friend of mine at a Saturday night party said, "I'm so glad tomorrow is Sunday. I can eat an egg." I asked her what eating an egg on Sunday was all about. She said that her doctor let her eat only one egg a week because her cholesterol count was high, and she was a person who manufactured too much cholesterol. She liked eggs so much that she saved them for Sundays. I tried to explain that a lot of new research shows that cholesterol isn't dangerous, and that everybody manufactures it. I suggested that she talk it over with her doctor. She said, "Oh, I can't. He died of a heart attack."

Almost everyone appears to have enough fat in his blood to produce atherosclerosis, says Dr. Kannel (1969). We all have at least a moderate amount of atherosclerosis by the time we're 20, but the disease doesn't usually bother us until we're 40. Also, practically everybody who has a moderately bad case of atherosclerosis has a mild form of diabetes. People who have serious cases of diabetes have serious atherosclerosis, says Dr. Schroeder, and it usually eventually kills them.

Many people are trying to lower their cholesterol the "easy" way, with drugs. But that may backfire because desmosterol, which is the last step in the chain before cholesterol is formed, can't change to cholesterol. So there is a buildup of desmosterol. That causes cataracts.

There was a study in Massachusetts called the Framingham Study, which went on for about 20 years with 912 men and women. It is called "one of the nation's most respected heart studies." This report says that a person's cholesterol level "does not largely depend on the amount of cholesterol in his diet. But we shouldn't believe that there is no relationship between heart disease and food intake." (We'll get to that later.) The *Medical World News* of September 1970, which published this article, says this news "may prove shocking to many doctors, and certainly to the public."

The Framingham report is shocking because we've been programmed to avoid high-cholesterol foods. It's generally accepted that a diet of 42 percent of calories in fat, most of it from animals, which is the average American intake, is too much for a well-balanced diet. And investigators agree that we need some vegetable fats. But one or two tablespoons a day are recommended—not more.

What About Vegetable Fats?

For years we've been eaing more and more vegetable fats. In fact, the ratio of vegetable fats to animal fats has gone up 37 percent. Studies show that if animals eat polyunsaturated fats, tumors develop faster than if the animals eat saturated fats. (National Research Council, 1982.) A report by Dr. Broda O. Barnes in his book, *Heart Attack Rareness in Thyroid-Treated Patients*, also suggests that patients on high polyunsaturated fat diets may be more susceptible to cancer. Dr. Barnes says, "It is apparent that previous suggestions of dietary alterations to prevent heart disease (those diets which say cut way down on animal fats and up your intake of vegetable fats) were premature and should be abandoned immediately until such alterations can be clearly demonstrated as safe and effective."

A report on the prevention of cancer, put out by the Committee on Diet, Nutrition, and Cancer (1982), suggests reducing total fats, not just saturated but polyunsaturated fat as well.

What has happened to heart disease during the low-animal-fat, high-vegetable-fat era? It strikes a higher percentage of us every year. And it hits more and more young people. Figures for this chart are from the National Center for Health Statistics.

HEART DISEASE RANK AS CAUSE OF DEATH

Age	Sex	Rank
1 to 4	Both	7th from top
5 to 24	Both	5th
25 to 44	White males	2nd
45 up	White males	1st
Women get a bit of a break.		
15 to 24	Females	3rd
45 to 64	Females	2nd
65 up	Females	1st

So, by age 65, the women catch up with the men, and heart disease is their first cause of death also.

After all these years of propaganda in favor of vegetable oils, Karvonen (1972) says, "As the cholesterol-lowering effect of polyunsaturated fatty acids became known, it was hoped that their use might prevent coronary heart disease. The incidence of CHD has not been reduced, nor has the disease already evident been retarded." Polyunsaturated fatty acids don't keep the blood from clotting, either. Shank (1973) says that even though the diet has changed in the last 25 years—a much higher amount of polyunsaturated fat is being eaten—there are more people every year getting atherosclerosis.

The Really Dangerous Fats

Fats that are always dangerous are hydrogenated fats. They're the hard margarines and also the shortenings that are hard at room temperature and keep forever on the shelf. Even soft margarine is marked on the label as "partially hydrogenated" or sometimes "partially hardened." The reason hydrogenated fats are bad is that hydrogen is bubbled through the liquid oils until the oils are saturated. Fats in the body are in chains, and if the chain has blank spaces, nutrients needed to metabolize that fat can get in to do it. But if the links in the chain are filled up with hydrogen, the nutrients can't get in.

Heated fat is particularly bad (*Journal of Atherosclerosis Research*, 1967). When oils are heated to 200 degrees centigrade and fed to rabbits on an average cholesterol diet, atheroslcerosis was much worse than when cholesterol was given by itself. The serum cholesterol levels didn't go up, but a lot more fat was deposited on the vessel walls.

Some of the worst foods, says Dr. Henry G. Bieler in his book *Food Is Your Best Medicine*, are those that combine heated fat and starches, such as French fried potatoes, doughnuts, potato chips and buttered popcorn. Popcorn cooked in a hot air popper is all right. The *Encyclopedia of Chemical Technology* (1965) states that commercial oils are refined by being heat-treated to extract oil from the vegetable seed, then bleached, and, worst of all, deodorized by being heated above 215 degrees C. for several hours.

Dr. Roger J. Williams in *Nutrition Against Disease* concludes that most commercial polyunsaturated oils possibly produce atherosclerosis and should not be used.

Too Much Triglyceride?

Recently we've heard a lot about triglycerides. Many investigators say that triglycerides are the worst fats of all. They are made in the liver from the refined sugar and starches we eat and the alcohol we drink.

As long ago as 1964, investigators were saying in the *American Journal of Clinical Nutrition* that the major cause of coronary heart disease must be that people are eating so much simple sugar and syrup. After all, the average person eats about 128 pounds of sugar a year. As you read this book, you're probably thinking that you eat very little sugar, so think of the person who is eating yours and his both. At 256 pounds a year, he is likely to have a lot of triglycerides in his blood. If he's eating that much sugar, he can't possibly have room for much else. He may not know he's eating it either. Sugar is the substance that is added in highest quantity to prepared, processed foods.

The government requires all manufacturers to list ingredients on labels in order of greatest amount by weight to the least amount. So if you see a can of stewed tomatoes with sugar listed second, you know that sugar is the second largest ingredient by weight in that product. However, the manufacturers try to fool us by listing sugar as "dextrose," "corn sweetener" or another name, so we won't realize how much sugar is in the product. When we add up all those different sugars, we often find there's more sugar than anything else. That's another good reason *not* to eat canned, frozen or otherwise processed food.

Dr. John Yudkin (1973) says that the only test investigators used to use for blood fats was a test for cholesterol. Recently, they've been testing for triglycerides and finding them, obviously because we consume so much more sugar and alcohol than we used to. He says sugar is related to coronary heart disease more than any other foodstuff. Yudkin also says that if we all gave up refined carbohydrates and reduced "the diet to the evolutionary level" (which means natural, unrefined whole foods) the incidence of CHD would be almost nil."

In his investigations, Dr. Yudkin has found that "myocardial infarction occurs in men who usually eat about twice as much sugar as men eat who have no history of infarction." That's often the person who is eating your 128 pounds of sugar and his too.

What About Butter and Eggs?

I said we were going to enjoy dairy products again. Let's start with butter. Investigators now have found that butter is an excellent natural food. Naimi (1965) fed rats a diet containing 40 percent butter, which was 65 percent of the total calories. The rats got fat, but their blood fat or fatty plaques did not get worse. The nutrients in the butter and in the other 35 percent of their diet counteracted any adverse effects of the high-fat diet.

When cream is taken off milk, almost all of the chromium, manganese, cobalt, copper and molybdenum in raw milk appears in the butter. Magnesium and zinc remain in the skim milk (*American Journal of Clinical Nutrition*, 1971). We can't afford to lose all those minerals; we should drink whole milk.

The new research on eggs shows that egg yolk is an excellent source of lecithin, which emulsifies the cholesterol and reams it out of the blood vessel walls. The tiny little globules of cholesterol then float through the blood until they get to the liver, where the liver uses the cholesterol to make bile, required to digest fats and fat-soluble vitamins. We were told in the past to restrict eggs, but now we know that eggs are one of our best foods.

Years ago, Dr. Roger J. Williams said that although eggs have been condemned on the grounds of high cholesterol, they're one of the most perfect foods, rich in vitamins, minerals and essential amino acids. Eggs help keep the cholesterol-lecithin ratio in the blood normal, which means that the lecithin in the egg will keep the cholesterol in the egg moving through the blood and won't let it stack up in the walls of the vessels. We don't want to overdo anything, so let's eat no more than one or two eggs a day, but we can cook with extra eggs if we want to make muffins or custard.

Dr. Gladys Sperling and her colleagues (1955) fed rats a stock diet with 10 percent whole egg, and the life span of males seemed substantially increased. Raw eggs are considered more nutritious than cooked eggs, says Dr. Allan Nittler (1974). But they can deplete our biotin if we eat too many.

Two pediatricians tested the egg substitute Egg Beaters to find out if it would be good to feed infants and small children a low-cholesterol substitute rather than whole eggs or egg yolks. Navidi and Kummerow (1974) of the University of Illinois first list the ingredients in Egg Beaters: egg white, corn oil, nonfat dry milk, emulsifiers (vegetable lecithin, mono- and diglycerides and propylene glycol monostearate), cellulose and xanthine gums, trisodium and triethyl citrate, artificial flavor, aluminum sulfate, iron phospate, artificial color, thiamin, riboflavin and vitamin D.

These researchers added calcium lactate to both eggs and Egg Beaters fed to weanling rats and chow-fed rats used as controls. The pups fed Egg Beaters averaged 31.6 grams in weight at three weeks; those on eggs, 66.5 grams; and those on chow, 70 grams. The pups fed Egg Beaters developed diarrhea in one week; those on eggs had no diarrhea.

Both sets were weaned at five weeks. All the Egg Beaters pups died within three to four weeks after weaning. The animals became coated with the Egg Beaters and were washed gently with a mild detergent solution and dried with paper towels. The washing removed some of the hair along with the foodstuff. The investigators concluded that Egg Beaters lack essential nutrients and that they are not good food for infants.

Refined Carbohydrates Are Dangerous

Other dangerous foods that are ruining our hearts are canned and frozen fruits and vegetables, refined grains, processed meats and cheeses, and almost anything in a can, box or package. Dr. Schroeder (1971) says that he tested 723 foods to find out how much nutrient value of two B vitamins is lost when foods are canned and processed. This is what he found.

B6 losses from:

canned vegetables	57 to 77 percent
frozen vegetables	37 to 56

Pantothenic acid losses from:

canned vegetables	46 to 78 percent
frozen vegetables	37 to 57
frozen animal products	21 to 70

Flour milling losses of:

7 vitamins	50 to 86.3 percent
5 bulk minerals	60 to 84
7 trace minerals	40 to 88

To avoid so many processed foods, we'll have to change our diets, but here's what one heart expert says about that. Ancel Keys (1970) says, "There are those of us who try to change people's diets, but it is not worth considering in middle-aged men, and is impossible in younger people." Probably many of us have had trouble trying to get a middle-aged man or a young person, say a teenager, to change his diet, but think of the advantages if he will change. I have many letters from people who *have* changed. They say they would never go back to the old way of eating, and they enjoy eating whole grains and vegetables they never ate before such as broccoli, greens, cauliflower and many others.

One thing we should do, says Linus Pauling (1986), is to eat less fructose than many people are now eating. They obviously think that, since it comes from fruit, it won't harm them. But many studies show that animals fed fructose had more heart attacks than the controls. Our rule is to be moderate in everything. That includes the sugar called fructose.

Our rule of moderation also applies to saturated fat and cholesterol. Just because they aren't such villains doesn't mean that we can go overboard on them. It stands to reason that if the blood cholesterol is high, we want to get it down. We're just going to find a better way to do it than by not eating eggs, since we now know that won't work.

We can add good food a little at a time. For every bite of poor-quality food we give up, let's eat a bite of healthful food, and little by little we'll improve

our health. Moderation is the key. And moderation is the way to try anything new—usually. When I changed my diet, I did it all at once, and it worked for me. But sometimes the body reacts adversely to a great change. The best thing to do is to begin cautiously and observe the reactions.

The Great Complex Carbohydrates

Now let's find out more about the other group of whole foods—the complex carbohydrates. They are unprocessed, unrefined fruits, vegetables, legumes (beans, peas and peanuts) nuts, seeds and whole grains.

The W. E. Conners research team (1972) recommended 60 to 65 percent complex carbohydrates, 20 to 25 percent fats (animal and vegetable about half and half) and 15 to 20 percent protein. Other investigators (among them Pritikin, in his book *Live Longer Now*) suggest 10 percent protein, 10 percent fats and 80 percent complex carbohydrates. Between these extremes will probably be where we want to set our intake. That would give us an intake of calories from:

Protein:	10 to 20 percent
Fats:	10 to 20 percent
(both saturated and unsaturated)	
Complex carbohydrates: 60 to 80 percent.	

Heart disease in Peru, where the natives live more than 16,000 feet above sea level in the Andes mountains, is almost nonexistent, says Dr. Herbert Hultgren, director of Stanford's cardiovascular laboratory. Dr. Hultgren studied natives in the Andes for 15 years. When these people move to sea level, they get sick with heart disease and high blood pressure, which he says may be caused by a change in diet. The diet of the natives at 16,000 feet is about 85 percent complex carbohydrate, mostly from whole-grain wheat and bananas.

Blood pressure usually goes up with age in Americans, but these Peruvians keep their same low level all their lives. Even Americans who move to the Andes and eat the native diet have lower blood pressure within five years—equal to that of the natives.

SPECIAL FOODS

Many special foods are known to help prevent and control heart attacks and strokes.

Alfalfa

Alfalfa has many nutrients that we need, it's an excellent food and it's easy to grow. In a study financed by a U.S. Public Health grant, calves were fed an excessively high cholesterol diet. They survived no more than four months, but after only two months they had severe plaques. Their cholesterol count was 1,000 mg. When they were given alfalfa, their cholesterol count dropped with "no waiting period." When they were taken off alfalfa, their count went up again (Cookson, 1967).

We can easily grow alfalfa sprouts, even in a one-room apartment. My favorite way—because it's so easy—is to put into a quart jar a tablespoon of alfalfa seeds (from the health food store, so you won't get any that have been sprayed for planting). Cover the seeds with water. Put a piece of nylon net over the top, held in place with a rubber band. Put the jar in a dark place. The next day pour off the water and put it in soup if you like. It has vitamins and minerals in it. Every day for three or four days, rinse the sprouts with water, and then drain them by standing the jar upside down in a bowl. The jar must be slightly tipped so the water won't collect and cause the seeds to become sour. When the sprouts get about an inch-and-a-half tall and have two little leaves, bring them into the light, and the leaves will get bright green. Now's the time to harvest your crop and put them in the refrigerator. They will keep several days.

These sprouts are delicious in salads, in omelets and on sandwiches instead of lettuce. Make your own egg foo yung. A friend of mine grinds sprouts and an apple in her baby food mill and gives them to her year-old daughter. The baby doesn't like sprouts by themselves, but she likes the combination.

Vitamin C

Some investigators say that the earliest lesions (sores) on the walls of the blood vessels are caused by a deficiency of vitamin C. Sokoloff (1966) said that if enough C is given quickly enough, the lesions will go away, but without C, lesions that have been building up for a long time are much harder to get rid of. Lesions make rough, uneven spots in the tough lining of the blood vessels. Globules of fat floating along in the blood stick to the rough spot. More globules stick to the first one, and soon a clot is built up. Several investigators in different experiments reduced excessive blood cholesterol levels by giving only half a gram of C three times a day by mouth. The count dropped 35 to 40 percent. Dr. Sokoloff also lowered the triglyceride rate from 195 to 85 with ascorbic acid (vitamin C).

When two top-ranking investigators get together to review atherosclerosis and try to find new ways of preventing the killer, something good is bound to happen. Carlos Krumdieck, M.D., Ph.D. and C.E. Butterworth, Jr., M.D. base their investigation on these concepts:

1. Atherosclerosis in the early stages is reversible.

2. It should not be thought of as inevitable when we get old.

3. It is not just a result of high blood fat content, but also of injuries to the blood vessels caused by deficiencies of vitamins and minerals.

These doctors found a great amount of literature that says that vitamin C helps keep the blood vessels from being injured. They also found evidence that C and lecithin help excrete blood fat in the feces and also keep it flowing so it can't stack up in the vessels.

Many researchers, say Krumdieck and Butterworth, relate atherosclerosis to scurvy, and scurvy is definitely caused by a lack of vitamin C. In scurvy and in atherosclerosis, sores on the lining of the blood vessels are the same. Lesions appear in the lining long before the fatty deposits form. Even back in 1757, Lind wrote that people with light cases of scurvy "drop down dead upon an exertion of their strength." Thus, although there are very few cases of scurvy today, there are millions of cases of the forerunner of scurvy—atherosclerosis.

When an investigator fed guinea pigs several diets, the diet that caused the most atherosclerosis was one without ascorbic acid, and with cholesterol supplements. The investigator, Fujunami (1971), fed one group of guinea pigs a diet supplemented with both ascorbic acid and coconut oil. After only two weeks, the pigs fed coconut oil, had high levels of cholesterol, but those fed the same oil with ascorbic acid had very low levels.

Drugs—over-the-counter and prescription alike—lower the ascorbic acid level. They include aspirin, barbiturates, ether and many cancer-causing substances found in the atmosphere and in cigarette smoke. When rats are exposed to these pollutants and drugs, they manufacture much more ascorbic acid to offset the danger. Drugs and cigarette smoking in polluted cities contribute greatly to the deficiencies of vitamin C in humans. Also, convenience foods, which have much of the vitamin C processed out, deprive the body of vitamin C. A study by Willis and his co-workers (1954) reported that in half of his patients (those on ascorbic acid therapy) the fatty plaques cleared, but in the other half (the untreated patients) the plaques remained.

How much vitamin C should anyone take in a day? Let's first consider how much an animal should have. Monkeys and guinea pigs are the most common animals besides man that do not make their own vitamin C. Other animals manufacture the vitamin in their bodies. The Committee on Animal Nutrition recommends 10 mg/kg of body weight for monkeys in the laboratory, and from 20 to 50 mg/kg of body weight for guinea pigs. These amounts keep the animals in optimal health, maintain growth and resist infection. The amount recommended in the Recommended Dietary Allowance, set by the Food and Nutrition Board of the National Academy of Sciences, National Research Council, for a healthy, resting young man is 0.7 mg/kg. That's only one-tenth to one-fiftieth as much as recommended to keep an animal healthy. The total intake recommended by Linus Pauling in his book *Vitamin C and the Common Cold* was 2,300 mg a day, or about 40 times the RDA. Dr. Pauling's new book, published in 1986, suggests from 6,000 to 18,000 mg a day.

Dr. Pauling says that all hospital patients, no matter what illness they have, should be getting more vitamin C than provided in hospital diets. He believes that there are no significant differences between the natural and synthetic varieties, and that more expensive brands are not necessarily superior to less expensive ones.

Bioflavonoids

Also beneficial in preventing or controlling heart disease are the bioflavonoids. They're also called vitamin P, and are part of the vitamin C complex, found mostly in the white rind of citrus fruits and in buckwheat. Rutin is one of the bioflavonoids you'll find on supplement labels. Robbins (1967) fed 260 albino rats bioflavanoids in four experiments. Every experiment cut down on the plaques. The bioflavonoids "deaggregate" blood cells, which means they don't form clots, and the blood flows more freely.

B6 and Its Associates

Vitamin B6 (pyridoxine) seem to be a key nutrient, but whenever we take B6 we should take all the rest of the Bs, because they work together. The best sources are liver, yeast and wheat germ; whole grains are also an excellent source. We should probably all take supplements of B6 in tablet form.

Monkeys fed diets deficient in B6 developed atherosclerosis rapidly, but when they were given supplements of B6, their atherosclerosis improved even if they were eating more saturated fat (Rinehart, 1951). B6 is destroyed by heat; thus canned, evaporated, powdered and pasteurized milks that have been heat sterilized have had most of the B6 destroyed.

Dr. Schroeder, in his book, *The Trace Elements and Man*, agrees with many investigators who say that B6 is one of the important assists in helping us avoid heart diseases. Experimental monkeys that don't get enough B6 develop lesions in the walls of their arteries. These lesions fill up with fat; thus Dr. Schroeder says a deficiency of B6 probably starts

the whole process of fatty buildup. Remember that person who is eating your sugar and his too? He's obviously eating so much refined food that he uses up the little B6 he gets and doesn't have enough to keep his heart and blood vessels healthy.

Here's a study that puzzled the investigator. Mann (1974) studied a group of 24 young Masai men in Africa. The Masai have been confounding the experts for years because they eat mostly meat and milk. Those are two things that experts say make our Western diet cause CHD, but the Masai don't have the disease. These young men were put on a diet of all the milk they could drink. But the milk was soured beforehand with lactobacillus. That's one of the ingredients that keep our intestinal flora healthy. It is one of the bacteria used to make yogurt.

The men drank an average of four liters a day, with 120 to 150 mg of cholesterol per liter. The investigators didn't want the men to get fat, so they organized soccer games for exercise. The Masai usually don't compete among themselves, but finally they decided to play soccer. Some of them got tired playing and sat around and drank milk all day—up to eight liters.

When the experiment was over, the investigators announced the "unexpected results." The men who had gained six pounds or more had lowered their cholesterol count 28 mg; those who had gained less than six pounds had lowered their count only 8 mg.

Dr. Williams explained what happened in his book, *Nutrition Against Disease* (1971). He said that if people eat enough yogurt to have good intestinal bacteria, the bacteria manufacture enough B vitamins, including B6, to keep the cholesterol count down. In treatment of humans, Samsonov and his associates (1973) found that their heart patients were below normal in vitamin C, P and B6. When the patients were given supplements of these vitamins, their cholesterol count fell to normal within two weeks.

Wonderful Vitamin E

Vitamin E, or tocopherol, is one of our best bets to avoid CHD, but there are four cautions with vitamin E. If you've ever had rheumatic fever, you may never be able to take more than 150 IU a day. If you have congestive heart failure, don't take E without advice from your nutrition-minded physician. If you have high blood pressure or diabetes, take 30 mg a day and increase 30 mg a day every month (Passwater, 1975). You'll be taking 360 mg a day at the end of the year. Passwater says if anyone has diabetes and is not taking vitamin E, he's virtually committing suicide.

It's extremely difficult to analyze the vitamin E content of food because most tables are not reliable. Also, tocopherols lose much of their potency when they're stored or processed. The highest sources of vitamin E in our diet, according to Harris and Embree (1963), are vegetable oils, grains, fruits and vegetables. I wrote to five vegetable oil companies about the content of tocopherol in their oils, and two of them answered. One said 0.1 percent; the other said, "very low, but people don't take vegetable oil for its vitamin content." The more oil we eat, the more E we need, which we're evidently not getting in the oil.

Cereals lose large amounts of E when the bran and germ are removed, and bleaching removes nearly all of what's left (*British Medical Bulletin*, 1956). Freshly ground whole-grain cereal gives us a good supply, and we can grind our own. A little mill made to grind small amounts of grains and seeds is available at health food stores, mail-order houses and maybe some hardware stores. Here is a list of 14 seeds, nuts and grains chosen for their vitamin E and linoleic acid content. (More about linoleic acid later.) I grind one tablespoon of the mixture—it takes less than 15 seconds—and mix it with milk, bran and wheat germ for breakfast. The seeds I use are wheat berries, buckwheat groats, oat groats, rye, millet, sesame, flax, alfalfa, almonds, pumpkin seeds, sunflower seeds, chia seeds, walnuts and pecans—equal parts by weight. You might like to check the food value in *Composition of Foods*, Agriculture Handbook No. 8, put out by the U.S. Department of Agriculture. Green, leafy vegetables are an excellent source of vitamin E and they can be eaten raw so the E isn't destroyed by processing. Raw greens furnish us with much of our E.

Bunnell and his associates (1965) tested sample menus that showed that the average intake of vitamin E in our diet is 7.4 mg. The RDA is 10 to 30 mg. (We'll see in a minute what the Drs. Shute from Canada recommended.) Yet many doctors and dieticians are still saying that we get enough E in a varied diet.

Karvonen (1972) fed 25 dogs a diet that made them die of kidney disease. On autopsy, they had severe plaques in the arteries. Then he fed the same diet to four other dogs, plus 2.5 to 4 mg vitamin E per kilogram of body weight. None of the four dogs had any plaques.

Toone, in a letter to the editor of the *New England Journal of Medicine* (1973), wrote that he put 11 heart patients on vitamin E supplements and 11 on placebos. All had been taking from 110 to 240 nitroglycerin tablets a month. The men on vitamin E were able to reduce their nitroglycerin doses to only one or two tablets a month, and they also "had a sense of well-being." In the placebo group, not one of the men was able to reduce his intake of nitroglcyerin to that low level.

Another reason why vitamin E helps our hearts so much is that it is an antioxidant. Since we can't live without oxygen, it sounds funny to say that we need something "against" oxygen, but oxygen is toxic under certain conditions (Tappel, 1973). Sometimes it reacts on polyunsaturated fats to form free radicals. Free radicals are compounds that affect proteins and enzymes and make them link up with other substances in the cell incorrectly.

One of the writers explained the free radical activity by comparing such a substance to a man attending a convention without his wife. He's ready to join up with anybody who is not attached to somebody else.

When these cross-linkages happen, two other things happen: (1) the proteins and enzymes can't get into the systems they belong in, so the metabolic process goes haywire, and (2) the waste matter of the damaged cell membrane collects in the cells like garbage. Some of the damaged membranes are turned into pigments that accumulate in the heart, brain and muscle. This pigment—sometimes called age pigment—builds up at the rate of about 0.6 percent of the heart muscle volume each decade. Thus, some polyunsaturated fats wind up as pigments that damage our hearts, doing more harm than good. Food that has been oxidized has had its minerals and vitamins destroyed. Ground meat, for example, has many surfaces exposed to air with more chance for the nutrients to be destroyed. A copper plate that is exposed to air has a dark film on it like the dark pigment in our tissues.

But there is something we can do about this whole oxidation process. Vitamin E is the most important antioxidant. Also, vitamin C and the mineral selenium increase the power of E. We can get E from some foods, as I mentioned, or as supplements. We get C from whole citrus fruits, from sprouts and from other fresh foods. Sometimes C is processed out of frozen fruit juices. Supplements of C combined with bioflavonoids are helpful. We also need special sulfur-containing amino acids—especially methionine. Methionine comes along as a scavenger and helps clean out the debris in the cell before the pigment can be formed. Eggs are one of the best sources of methionine.

Two friends of mine rubbed the brown age spots of the backs of their hands with vitamin E squeezed from a capsule. Gradually the brown spots became lighter. Many people have brown spots on their foreheads. You can prick a capsule, squeeze out a drop and keep the rest of the capsule in the fridge until used up.

Vitamin E and the Doctors Shute

Two brothers, Dr. Wilfrid and Dr. Evan Shute, in Canada, were famous for using vitamin E for heart patients.

Dr. Evan Shute spoke at a meeting of doctors and lay people in Illinois in December 1970 (Shute, 1973). He gave these answers to questions about vitamin E.

1. When vitamin E is given, the body can get 12 percent more oxygen from the air. That means a lot to someone with blocked arteries.

2. The average dose for a young woman should be about 400 units a day; for a young man, about 600 units, unless they're under stress—then more. (Remember the cautions.) The amount needed depends on the intake of vegetable oils—the more oil, the more E. Dr. Shute says he's asked about dosages all the time, but there's no exact answer. If a man has a low sperm count, 100 extra units a day might increase the count, but if he has arteriosclerotic legs, Dr. Shute would start him on 1,600 units a day. That much might be too painful, because new capillaries would grow into the area and it would feel like thawing out a frozen foot. If too painful, the patient can start with smaller doses and work up. Also, if anyone is taking inorganic iron or cereals enriched with iron, he should take the iron at breakfast and the E at night, because the iron destroys the E. Iron should be taken as an amino acid chelate, which is an organic form.

3. There's no reason to take divided doses; vitamin E takes hours to be absorbed.

4. Vitamin E ointment penetrates through the skin.

5. An expectant mother should take vitamin E; some infants, even prematures, have been born with ateriosclerosis. The infant should have E with the first breath.

6. One of the best uses of vitamin E is to avoid a series of small strokes.

7. Vitamin E can kill chronic rheumatic heart patients. They can't take more than 150 units. Once in a great while, high blood pressure patients can't take large doses. They should start with 30 units. Diabetics may suddenly need less insulin if they start on vitamin E. They should carry candy for the first few days.

8. You can cure any acute phlebitis with vitamin E.

9. If a person is taking digitalis, he will almost certainly need less if he starts taking vitamin E.

Dr. Roger J. Williams said (1971) that possibly one of the reasons why the Drs. Shute had such good luck with vitamin E therapy is that people have been eating so much polyunsaturated fat in the last 30 years that they've given themselves a deifiency of vitamin E. At least, the one million people who die and the many others who have heart attacks or other problems probably have such a deficiency.

How About Lecithin?

Lecithin is also a major help in preventing and controlling atherosclerosis. It is an emulsifying agent. Ahrens and Unkel, back in 1949, said that the ratio of lecithin to cholesterol in our bodies should be 1.2 to 1. Even if people have high blood fat, if that ratio is kept, they don't have atherosclerosis. To test this, Ahrens used an enzyme that removed the lecithin, and the blood got milky-looking, with large particles of fat—the kind that stick to the walls of blood vessels.

If we are healthy, our livers make lecithin and cholesterol in the ratio of 1.2 to 1. Morrison (1958) says that lecithin was the most effective cholesterol-lowering agent he ever used. Fifteen patients had been on low-fat diets from one to 10 years, but their cholesterol levels hadn't been reduced enough. Then they took two tablespoons of lecithin, three times a day. After three months, their average cholesterol reduction was 41 percent; total fat, 129 mg. Then they went on a maintenance dosage of one to two tablespoons a day. Investigators reported that when they injected cholesterol by itself into experimental animals, the animals developed lesions; then cholesterol and lecithin were injected together. No lesions formed.

Medical World News (November 22, 1974) discussed research on lecithin by doctors at the Simon Stevin Research Institute in Bruges, Belgium. They agreed that polyunsaturates in moderate amounts are needed by the body. Lecithin from soybeans, a vegetable source, contains from 65 to 75 percent polyunsaturates. These Belgian doctors gave intravenous doses of lecithin to 100 patients, and their blood fats were lowered, especially excess cholesterol, which was lowered by 40 percent. Soybean lecithin is a "nontoxic, natural product with no local reactions and no side effects observed in the organs," they say.

The lecithin molecule found in the body, according to the Belgian doctors, is one of the main fat carriers. The injected lecithin is also a fat carrier, and activates the enzyme that starts the breakdown of cholesterol in the body so it can be used as needed by every cell. Lecithin removes the cholesterol from the blood and changes it to the form used by the cells.

The Belgian doctors have tried oral doses, but did

not get quite such good results. As most investigators agree, although unintravenous injection is faster acting, oral feeding is much easier since we can feed ourselves. While the doctors are studying ways to administer the drug, we can take our own oral doses of lecithin and prevent cholesterol buildup and can probably dissolve any buildup that has already taken place. Later in this lesson, Dr. Jacobus Rinse suggests how to take lecithin orally. Also, new forms of lecithin have been developed that give better results in getting rid of fatty plaques.

Foods containing lecithin are eggs, liver, nuts, wheat (whole grain) and soybeans. We can take supplements of lecithin in powdered, granular and liquid form, and in capsules. Granular lecithin is suggested, with as high a potency of phosphatidyl choline as can be found. The percentage should be at least 30, and a higher potency is available. Be sure that the percentage given is phosphatidyl choline.

Since lecithin is a phospholipid (that means it is a fat with a lot of phosphorus in it), we need to make sure we get enough calcium to balance the phosphorus. Milk, cheese, yogurt and green leafy vegetables are the answer.

Fiber

You've heard how valuable fiber is in providing roughage—especially unrefined bran from the health food store. Now there is a lot of information in the medical journals about how fiber helps us to avoid atherosclerosis.

Burkitt (1974) tells about several investigators from England and South Africa who have been writing a great deal about unrefined bran. They advise taking two teaspoons of bran with each meal. Dr. Fredrick Stare said that as we eat more fiber, the fat in the feces increases. Thus not so much goes to the blood.

Rabbits were fed all essential nutrients, except for natural fiber. They ate only chemical cellulose. They developed fatty deposits and clots in their arteries. If the diet was high in bran, a natural fiber, none of the experimental animals got atherosclerosis (Kritchevsky et al., 1968).

The fringe benefits of eating bran are many. It controls or prevents diverticulosis, varicose veins, deep vein thrombosis, hemorrhoids, acne and cancer of the colon (the second most common location of cancer), as well as coronary heart disease.

You might want to start with only two teaspoons of bran at breakfast. If you need more, take it at the other meals too. It will help if you're constipated or if you have diarrhea. Cellulose is the most common plant ingredient. It's found in vegetables and fruits as well as in whole grains.

That apple-a-day adage is still good advice also.

Pectin, found in apples, reduces serum cholesterol. Investigators think it increases the excretion of cholesterol in the feces (Atherosclerosis, 1969).

Keys (1960) concluded that fruits, leafy vegetables and legumes (all high-fiber foods) produce lower cholesterol counts than sucrose and milk sugar.

MINERALS

Many nutritionists are now saying that minerals are often more important than vitamins. You may agree when you find out how they are needed to prevent heart problems.

Calcium

A study which lasted for five years, 1964 to 1969, was made by Knox (1973). He studied the effect of calcium on the incidence of heart disease. He found that if the calcium intake is high, the deaths from heart disease are low. He said that this implies "the possibility of achieving very substantial alterations of ischemic-heart-disease mortality through relatively simple dietary manipulations." And it certainly is relatively simple to add calcium and all other nutrients to our diets rather than have heart disease.

We get calcium in dark green leafy vegetables, almonds, sardines, salmon and blackstrap molasses. (Be sure to brush your teeth after taking blackstrap.) The only problem with dark green leafy vegetables is that some of them are high in oxalic acid and they "bind" calcium and excrete it in the feces. The vegetables highest in that acid are spinach, beet greens and swiss chard. If we go by Rule 4—Vary Your Diet—we won't eat a lot of any one thing; therefore, we won't eat enough of those vegetables to cause a problem.

We shouldn't depend heavily on pasteurized, homogenized milk and cheese because so much of the food value is destroyed in the processing, and it is hard for many people to digest. Also we should drink whole milk, because the calcium we eat can't be absorbed without fat. The best fat to help absorb the calcium is the fat that comes in milk, cream or butter (*Journal of the American Dietetic Association*, 1967).

Another reason for eating butter or drinking whole milk is that it helps keep the correct calcium-phosphorus balance better than fats with high melting points, such as hydrogenated fats—margarine and hard white shortening (Chanda, 1949). Also the correct calcium-magnesium ratio is twice as much calcium as magnesium.

In the past, many nutritionists recommended raw bone meal, which supplies calcium, phosphorus and trace minerals. But now there is controversy about this supplement because some animals that furnish bones for the bone meal take in lead with their food, which can cause lead poisoning in humans.

Marvelous Magnesium

Magnesium may help as much as calcium to avoid heart attack. Of 64 patients with myocardial infarction treated with magnesium by Seelig and her colleagues (1974), only one died. Researchers in many foriegn countries, especially Germany and France, report success in treating angina with magnesium.

If cholesterol is high, magnesium is especially needed to help manufacture lecithin, which, in turn, will help dissolve the cholesterol. Too much calcium may cause a magnesium deficiency, which would cause the blood vessels of the heart to constrict. More magnesium makes the coronary vessels dilate.

If you're on digitalis now, you might like to know that a deficiency of magnesium might cause digitalis toxicity. Also, magnesium helps counteract unnatural rhythms of the heart (Seelig, 1974). Other drugs (adrenergic catecholamines) may cause death of part of the heart muscle because they throw the calcium-magnesium ratio out of balance.

Whole foods are the best sources of magnesium: whole grains, blackstrap molasses, legumes, nuts, seeds and yeast. The correct mineral balance is built into these foods.

And we can help with supplements. The best form is said to be amino acid chelated, which means that the mineral is combined with an amino acid in the laboratory the way it must be combined in the body so it can be absorbed into the tissues correctly. Magnesium and all other minerals need acid to help assimilate them into the system. If they are taken with calcium, which is also alkaline, we especially need acid. Many nutritionists suggest betaine hydrochloride with pepsin, the acid that should be secreted in the stomach to digest our food, but which is often partly missing, especially after age 40. If you have pains after eating, the television ads say you need antacids. But symptoms of too much and too little acid are the same. To find out which you have, take one of the hydrochloride tablets. If you feel better, which you probably will, you'll know you need them. If you feel worse (one in a million), take two glasses of water to dilute the acid and don't take any more acid.

One easy way to get magnesium is to take about ¼ teaspoon of Epsom salts every day in a large glass of water. (That won't be enough for a laxative). My heart used to beat hard and fast, especially when I was quiet, just before going to sleep. After taking the Epsom salts for a few days, I suddenly realized that my heart had calmed down. Now it gently purrs along.

Fringe benefits of magnesium are that it helps keep kids from being irritable and it also keeps all of us from having muscle twitchings and cramps (Goodhart and Shils, 1973).

Fabulous Chromium

There is a lot of information in the medical journals about the value of chromium. It works with insulin to metabolize (use) sugar, and a deficiency leads to fatty plaques in the aorta. When rats are fed a lifetime chromium deficiency, they have all the symptoms of coronary heart disease. A 150-pound man needs about 500 micrograms per day, but when hospital food was analyzed for two days, only 100 micrograms a day were found.

Dr. Schroeder and his associates gave rats a diet of half white sugar, torula yeast (which is low in chromium) and lard. Cholesterol and blood sugar were both high. But when they gave chromium or dark brown sugar, which has six times as much chromium as white sugar, their cholesterol count was low.

With the typical American diet of about 70 percent of calories from refined sugar, refined flour and fat, we get very little chromium. Not enough to help us use all that refined food or to replace what we lose in the urine. In white sugar, there are only two micrograms of chromium to 100 calories; in purified honey, there are 10; but in blackstrap molasses, there are 37 micrograms. Whole-wheat flour is a good source—175 micrograms in 100 grams, but refined white flour has only 23 micrograms in 100 grams.

Butter is a good source of chromium, as are wheat germ and bran. Rye has very little. Buckwheat and millet, carrots, beets and beef are good sources.

If we don't eat enough chromium, we have to use our body stores (if we have any) to metabolize the carbohydrates and fats; thus we might end up with a net loss.

We could easily get chromium if we ate the cattle. Refined white flour that people eat has only 0.23 ppm. chromium, but cattle eat the "shorts" and bran with 2.22 and 2.18 ppm. Of course, we can buy stone-ground whole wheat flour or grind our own. Then we'll get all that's there. We also get a good amount from fish, shellfish and chicken. Meats have several times as much chromium as vegetables, grains and fruits. That means fresh meats, organically raised, not proceced cold cuts.

Here's another fringe benefit of adding chromium to your diet. Since there should be large amounts of chromium in the cornea of the eye, as there are in the skin, a deficiency of chromium can cause cataracts and those little blood vessels which show up right under the skin (vascularization). Enough chromium will help to do away with the cataracts and with the ugly little blood vessels, which always mean that something unpleasant is going on inside where we can't see it. The large blood vessels are getting lined with fat so that the blood has to open up new, smaller vessels near the skin.

Chromium is available in supplement form at health food stores. It is also found in some brewer's yeasts—check the label.

Zinc vs. Cadmium

Cadmium is a trace mineral that's dangerous. The worst thing about it is that the body accepts it in some systems, thinking it is zinc. The systems can't use it, but by the time the body finds out it has the wrong substance, it's too late, and it can't drop the cadmium and pick up zinc.

Dr. Schroeder says that zinc is especially important in helping us avoid high blood pressure, which makes our hardened arteries get hard faster, and increases our chances of having artherosclerosis. It also causes two other changes in the body: an enlarged heart and diseases of the arteries in the kidneys.

Dr. Schroeder experimented with rats during their lifetimes, giving them 5 ppm of cadmium in their drinking water. He also gave them the same amounts of many other trace elements in different experiments, without any signs of high blood pressure. But with the cadmium, the rats had every symptom of human high blood pressure. The cadmium permeated the kidneys and knocked out the zinc.

Human kidneys in modern industrialized countries generally have a ratio of zinc to cadmium of about 1.5:1. In kidneys of tribal Africans, the ratio is about 6:1; in beef, 40:1; and in pork, 72:1. In laboratory rats with hypertension, the ratio averaged about 1.3:1. In people dying of hypertension, the ratio was about 1.2:1.

After hundreds of thousands of analyses, Dr. Schroeder has concluded that too much cadmium and too little zinc in kidneys "is a contributing, if not the whole cause, of high blood pressure."

Some of the foods with the highest ratios of zinc to cadmium are our old friends, the complex carbohydrates. Whole grains and cereals have a ratio of 111:1; legumes, 357:1; root vegetables, 49:1; and nuts, a whopping 684:1. Meats are good too, with a ratio of 35:1; oysters, have 379:1. But when these same foods are processed, instead of the ratio of 35:1 in whole-wheat bread, white bread has only 5:1.

Many drinks, both alcoholic and nonalcoholic, have too little zinc for the amount of cadmium. Coffee and tea have low ratios of zinc to cadmium, and so do wine, vermouth, gin, brandy and whiskey (both Scotch and bourbon). Soft drinks don't escape. One cola drink, widely advertised, tested high in cadmium.

Selenium

Selenium, a mineral found in many foods—if the foods are grown on soil rich in selenium—is related to the health of the heart. Pigs deficient in selenium have hearts that collapse into a flat sheet almost completely without fiber and muscle. Hearts from normal pigs will retain their shape. Because of this reaction, it is thought that heart disease in humans may be related to a deficiency of selenium. Rats and lambs were deprived of selenium, and the blood vessels in their hearts hemorrhaged. Pigs without enough selenium develop a disease called "mulberry heart disease," because the cardiac blood vessels hemorrhage and give the heart a reddish-purple color like that of a mulberry.

In general, selenium in the diet appears to keep the heart muscles from breaking down. Thus, when people get enough selenium, there aren't so many heart disease deaths (Shamberger, 1979).

Carnitine

Carnitine will help reduce triglycerides and clear the blood of fats. It is made from the amino acids lysine and methionine, if we digest and assimilate the protein we eat. It is not found in large amounts in any one plant protein, thus vegetarians might not eat enough to reduce the blood fats. Also, if we don't have adequate amounts of vitamin C, the carnitine can't be manufactured (Leibovitz, 1984).

How About Water?

Even water can lead to heart disease if it's the wrong kind. In the past 10 years, many investigators have found that in areas where the drinking water is soft, heart disease death rates are high, possibly because there's not much calcium, magnesium and other trace minerals in soft water. Also, we may retain more sodium when we don't get enough calcium (Crawford, 1972). Artificial water softeners make the water high in sodium.

Schroeder explains that hard water contains calcium and magnesium bicarbonates that collect on the insides of metal pipes and coat them with such a hard substance that they don't easily corrode. They will corrode if the water is acid, but hard water is very seldom acid. You can test your own water for hardness; if soap doesn't lather easily, the water is hard; if it is hard to wash soap off your hands, the water is soft.

On the other hand, soft water is usually acid. Schroeder worked with a Japanese investigator who found that the more acid in the water in an area, the more strokes the people have. Strokes are the leading cause of death in Japan.

We know that there is more cadmium in soft water areas to account for the extra atherosclerosis, strokes and heart attacks. Schroeder stresses that the hypertension is not caused by the soft water directly, but by the cadmium pulled from the pipes by the acid soft water. To test the acidity of water, use nitrazine paper from the drugstore.

When people are short of zinc because of processed, refined foods, and a lot of cadmium is added from water, Schroeder believes that the difference in the cadmium-zinc ratio is the difference in having high or normal blood pressure.

Animal products, especially shellfish, are the best sources of zinc. Also we can use zinc supplements.

If you have an annoying, even frightening, irregular heartbeat, many nutritionists say that you may need the minerals we've been talking about: calcium and magnesium as well as potassium and folic acid (one of the B vitamins).

THE RINSE BREAKFAST

I've saved one of the best recommendations for last. One of my favorite heart disease writers is Dr. Jacobus Rinse, whose well-documented article appeared in *American Laboratory*, July 1973. Scientifically inclined readers will enjoy Dr. Rinse's article, but nonscientifically-inclined readers can understand it too.

Dr. Rinse had angina at age 51 in 1951. He took the drugs his mother advised for several years, but he didn't improve much. Then, since he is a chemist, he scientifically analyzed what he should do for himself. First, he took garlic and he could work harder without feeling chest pains. (Garlic is highly recommended as a treatment for high blood pressure.) Dr. Rinse also took 1,000 mg of vitamin C daily and a multivitamin pill.

For breakfast every day, Dr. Rinse ate the following:

cereal with milk
1 tablespoon wheat germ
1 tablespoon food yeast
1 tablespoon lecithin
1 tablespoon safflower oil

After every meal he took 100 mg vitamin E. That complete breakfast brought about his "cure." Since then, he has had no angina pains or any other ailment. He eats no processed or refined foods, because he thinks that the vitamins and minerals removed from them cause so many of us to have heart disease. One year after he began this program, he was able to do heavy outdoor work and even run.

He said, "The results seemed too good to be true."

Here's Dr. Rinse's interesting explanation of why the lecithin and safflower oil work so well.

"Hard fats in the body melt at high temperature. What we need is to have those fats melt at body temperatures. Then they will be flushed out of the blood vessels. Lecithin and any vegetable oil high in linoleic acid (safflower, soy, sunflower, sesame) dissolve the hard fats. Neither one by itself will do as well. It's as simple as that."

Later research shows that we should eat whole foods, not what Donald Davis (1983) calls "dismembered foods." These foods include "unrefined" and "cold-pressed" oils, which supply "calories in abundance, but very little else. Corn, soybeans, sunflower seeds, etc. are fine whole foods, but this is not true of any oils which can be separated from them." Thus, our food intake should include little or no oil, and instead, we should get our linoleic acid, one of the polyunsaturated fats, from nuts and seeds.

Dr. Rinse says, "Our working hypothesis is that food deficiencies are the main cause of atherosclerosis, and therefore all other known influences, such as tension, smoking, obesity and maybe also heredity are only contributory."

Dr. Rinse goes on to say that physicians often assume that those four villains are the principal causes of heart disease. These factors probably contribute to the disease, he says, after it has started because of deficiencies in the diet.

Obesity will probably not be a problem on a whole-food diet, because your food will satisfy your appetite, and you won't want to eat so much. Exercise helps because it flushes the blood vessels, improves circulation and speeds more nutrients to every cell.

Several thousand people in Holland and the U.S.A. and some in England and Belgium use the Rinse supplements, he says, "although most physicians ignore the method."

Many of my friends don't ignore it. One, who had a heart bypass operation in August, was scheduled for another one the following October. He started the Rinse Breakfast, and at his next physical, his doctor said he wouldn't have to have another bypass. Needless to say, my friend spread the word about his new treatment to all his family and friends.

Another friend had angina so badly that he couldn't walk across the room. He changed his diet completely, to one that included every nutrient in maximum amounts, and almost overnight he began to improve. A year later he dug up half his backyard and planted a garden.

ROUNDUP

Let's see in a nutshell what we can do for our hearts. First, go by the diet and food supplement program in Lesson 1.

Eat moderate amounts of animal proteins such as dairy products and organically grown muscle meat (steak, roasts, chops and hamburger). Eat one or two eggs a day and cook with extra eggs if you want muffins and custards. Eat additional protein from whole grains and legumes (beans, peas and peanuts).

Eat a small amount of fats, both animal (best are butter, cream and eggs) and vegetable (best are nuts and seeds).

That leaves the bulk of our diet as complex carbohydrates. These are legumes; whole grains of all kinds; vegetables, both cooked and raw; and whole fruits, fresh, raw and ripe.

It is dangerous to suddenly stop taking some drugs recommended for high blood pressure. See your physician; let him take you off when the right time comes.

FOOD SUPPLEMENTS

The food supplements will be those mentioned in Lesson 1. They are all available at health food stores.

Supplements especially important for the heart are listed here.

Vitamin E. Remember the cautions mentioned in the section on vitamin E. If necessary, begin with 30 IU of vitamin E and increase gradually. If the cautions don't apply to you, begin with 100 IU and go up about 100 a month until you get to 600, which is the lower amount recommended by Dr. Evan Shute. If you're nearing 70, Dr. Shute suggests 1,200 IU.

EPA stands for eicosapentaenoic acid. It is a new product to ward off heart attacks and strokes. It is a fish body oil, not fish liver oil, which might contain so much vitamin D that it could be toxic. Take the EPA according to the label.

Pangamic acid, also called dimethyl-glycine, helps the tissues use oxygen more efficiently. The recommended amount is 50 mg twice a day.

Selenium is another definite help (Shamberger, 1979). The suggested amount of selenium is 100 mcg (micrograms) twice a day.

Garlic perles may help you reduce high blood pressure. Studies show that they help 40 percent or more of patients. Suggested amount is three perles, three times a day.

The suggested dose of carnitine, to help cleanse the blood of fat, is 500 to 1,000 mg a day, in divided doses (Leibovitz, 1984).

In heart disease or any other disease, it is extremely important not to ever overload the digestive system. Here's where much of our trouble begins, because we eat too much at one time, and we can't digest the proteins down to amino acids to repair tissue. By the time you've been on this program for a while, your hypothalamus will be working, and you won't feel hungry all the time. The hypothalamus sets our appetite, and tells us when to start and stop eating. In fact, one of my counselees wrote, "One remarkable result of the nutrition program is that I am no longer constantly hungry. This is really remarkable to me. I am satisfied with less food, and feeling satisfied is a new situation for me."

It would probably help almost everybody to take hydrochloric acid (HCl) with each main meal, for a while at least. If you're young, stop taking it after two to four weeks. One counselee wrote, "With HC1, I no longer have the horrible feeling that my heart will give out." This person, a physician, had been rushed to the hospital several times with severe angina pains before he got on a good diet.

But first and last, eat the Rinse Breakfast. You may portion it out any way, just so you get all the nutrients Dr. Rinse suggests. I use a raw egg, one teaspoon to one tablespoon lecithin, depending on the brand, and from one-fourth to one tablespoon brewer's yeast in about one cup of milk, nut milk or soy milk (vary these, too) almost every morning for breakfast. I also eat a small piece of whole-grain bread or muffin. If you're a beginner with brewer's yeast, start with the smaller amount and work up to one tablespoon a day—or more.

I get the polyunsaturated fat I need in nibbles of nuts and seeds during the day, and the rest of the vitamin and mineral tablets as part of my meals. This "insurance" makes me confident that I am feeding my body as well as possible. It isn't a hardship—it's a pleasure to be responsible for my own good health. My husband took a dim view of the drink because of the taste of the yeast. When I showed him an article about yeast being good for the hair, he "joined the club."

Maybe some of these ideas are so new that you're a little leery of them. Just start moderately, as we mentioned before, and see how much better you feel. You'll be hearing more and more about whole food and food supplements, because more and more people will be relieved of their heart pains and be alive to tell about their good health.

These suggestions are designed to furnish all nutrients needed so that the body can heal itself.

QUESTIONS

TRUE/FALSE

1. Often the first symptom that a person has a disease he'll die from is death itself.

2. Heart bypass operations always prevent heart attacks.

3. If you stop taking some medicines suddenly, you might have a heart attack.

4. We should eat three small meals and three smaller snacks a day to help prevent heart attacks.

5. Physical and emotional stress use up nutrients so fast that the body suffers.

6. High blood pressure and atherosclerosis are the two major causes of heart deaths.

7. The best defense against high blood pressure is to eat about 10 times more sodium than potassium.

8. When both fat and unwanted calcium stack up in the arteries, the condition is called "hardening of the arteries."

9. Some researchers say that only 50 percent of the people who have heart attacks have chest pain beforehand.

10. Nutritionists say that fewer people have heart disease now than formerly because more people are taking vitamin E.

11. Triglycerides are made in the body from the refined sugar and starch we eat and the alcohol we drink.

12. Dairy products can be eaten in moderate amounts without the fear of heart disease.

13. Vitamin C and lecithin keep blood fat flowing so it won't stack up in the blood vessels.

14. One of the best reasons for taking vitamin E is to avoid a series of small strokes.

MULTIPLE CHOICE

1. If a person has a heart bypass operation, he should: (a) stop eating junk food, (b) quit smoking, (c) cut down on fats.

2. New research shows: (a) that some cholesterol is not dangerous, (b) vitamins and minerals in food help prevent heart disease, (c) we should eat unprocessed food.

3. A natural food program will: (a) help reduce fatty plaques in blood vessels, (b) keep the blood too thick, (c) help keep the heart muscle beating.

4. Processed foods contain a higher ratio of sodium to potassium than natural foods because: (a) natural foods are low in sodium and high in potassium, (b) when foods are processed, canned or frozen, salt is added in large amounts.

5. List information about high blood pressure in Americans: (a) 20 percent of American adults have high blood pressure, (b) 40 percent of older Americans have the disease.

6. Side effects of taking excess potassium tablets include: (a) nausea, (b) diarrhea, (c) vomiting.

7. We should not eat poor foods, such as: (a) vegetable oils in large amounts, (b) eggs and dairy products, (c) refined carbohydrates.

8. Cholesterol: (a) is needed in every cell, (b) helps to make vitamin B, (c) causes dry skin.

9. Vegetable fats: (a) may make people susceptible to cancer, (b) do not keep the blood from clotting, (c) eaten in large amounts can cause heart problems.

10. The worst fats are hydrogenated: (a) and they keep forever on the shelf, (b) and they cause more atherosclerosis than cholesterol causes, (c) and they are heated to such a high temperature that they lose food value.

11. Refined carbohydrates that are ruining our hearts include: (a) canned fruits, (b) whole grains, (c) processed meats, (d) processed cheese.

12. Complex carbohydrates include: (a) whole grains, (b) vegetables, (c) legumes.

ANSWERS

True/False

1. T 2. F. 3. T 4. T 5. T 6. T 7. F 8. T
9. F 10. T 11. T 12. T 13. T 14. T

Multiple Choice

1. a,b,c 2. a,b,c 3. a,c 4. a,b 5. a,b 6. a,b,c
7. a,c 8. a 9. a,b,c 10. a,b,c 11. a,c,d 12. a,b,c

REFERENCES

Ahrens, E. H. and Kunkel, H. G. *J. Exp. Med.*, 90, 409, 1949.

Am. J. Clin. Nutr., 14:169, 1961.

———, 24:562, 1971.

Atherosclerosis. Second Symposium, 1969.

Barnes, B. O. *Hypothyroidism, The Unsuspected Illness*. New York: Crowell, 1976.

Bland, J. *J. Appl. Nutr.*, 34(2): 91–102, Fall 1982.

British Med. Bull. 12:14, 1956.

Bunnell, R. H. et al. *J. Clin. Nutr.*, 17:1, 1965.

Burkitt, D. P. *British Med. J.*, Feb. 3, 1974.

Chanda, R. *British J. Nutr.*, 3:5, 1949.

Composition of Foods. Agriculture Handbook #8, U.S. Dept. of Agriculture (Revised) 1963.

Conners, W. E. *Preven. Med.*, 1:49, 1972.

Cookson, F. B. *J. of Athero. Research*, 7:69, 1967.

Crawford, M.D. *Proceedings of the Nutrition Society*, 31:347, 1972.

Davis, Donald R. *J. of Appl. Nutr.*, Spring 1983.

Encyclopedia of Chemical Technology, 8:805, 1965.

Ershoff, B. H. *J. Appl. Nutr.*, 33(2):160–166, Fall 1981.

Goodhart and Shils. *Modern Nutrition in Health and Disease*, p. 292, 1973.

Harris and Embree. *Am. J. Clin. Nutr.*, 13, 385, 1963.

JADA, 51:57, 1967.

J. Athero. Research, 7:647, 1967.

Kannel, W. B. *Minnesota Medi.*, 52:1225, 1969.

———. *Geriatrics*, 25:75, 1970.

Karvonen, M. J. *Proceedings of the Nutrition Society*, 31:355; 1972.

Keys, Ancel. *J. of Nutr.*, 70:257, 1960.

———. *Circulation*, 41:1970, #1.

Knox, E. G. *Lancet*, June 30, 1973.

Kritchevsky, D. P. et al. *J. Athero. Research*, 8:697; 1968.

Langer, S. E. *Solved: The Riddle of Illness*. New Canaan, Conn.: Keats, 1984.

Leibovitz, B. *Carnitine*. New York: Dell, 1984.

Mann, G. *Am. J. Clin. Nutr.*, 27:464, 1974.

Medical World News, Sept. 1970.

———. November 22, 1974.

Morrison, L. M. *Geriatrics* 13:12, 1958.

Naimi, S. *J. of Nutr.*, 86:325, 1965.

Navidi, N. K. and Kummerow, F. A. *Pediatrics*, 53:565, April 1974.

Nittler, A. *Let's Live*, Feb. 1974.

Passwater, R. A. *Supernutrition*. New York: Pocket Books, 1975.

Pauling, L. *Vitamin C, the Common Cold and the Flu*. San Francisco: W. H. Freeman, 1970.

———. *How To Live Longer and Feel Better*. New York: W. H. Freeman, 1986.

———. *Institute of Science and Medicine Newsletter*, 1(6):4, Spring 1979.

People's Medical Society Newsletter, June 1983.

Pritikin, N. *Live Longer Now*.

Rinehart, J. F. *Proceedings of the Society of Experimental Biological Medicine*. 76:580, 1951.

Rinse, J. *The Rinse Formula*. New Canaan, Conn.: Keats, 1988.

Robbins, R. C. *J. Athero. Research*, 7:3, 1967.

Samsonov, M. A., et al. *Nutrition Abstracts and Reviews*, 43:69, 1973

Schroeder, H. A. *J. of Chron. Diseases*, 23:123, 1970.

———. *Am. Clin. Nutr.*, 24:562, 1971.

Seelig, M. *Am. J. Clin. Nutr.*, 27:59, 1974.

Shamberger, R. J. *Executive Health*, March 1979.

Shank, R. E. *JADA*, 62:611, 1973.

Shute, E. *J. Appl. Nutr.*, 25:25, 1973.

Sokoloff, M. *J. Am. Ger. Soc.*, 14:1239, 1966.

Sperling, G. *J. of Nutr.*, 55:399, 1955.

Stare, F. *Modern Nutrition in Health and Disease*, p. 902.

Tappel, A. L. *Geriatrics*, 20:415, 1973.

Toone, W. M. *N. E. J. Med.*, 289 #18:979 1973.

Tujunami. *Circulation Journal*, 35:1559, 1971.

Whitaker, J. M. *J. Appl. Nutr.*, 34(2):103–110, Fall 1982.

Williams, R. J. *Nutrition Against Disease*. New York: Pitman, 1971.

Willis, G. C. et al. *Canadian Med. Assn. J.*, 71:562, 1954.

Yudkin, J. *South African Med. J.*, 47:44, 1973.

Lesson 4

ALLERGIES AND NUTRITION

LESSON 4—ALLERGIES AND NUTRITION

ALLERGIES AND NUTRITION

DO YOU have allergies? Does your nose run, your skin itch or do your lungs wheeze when you breathe? Do you sneeze constantly at certain times of the year? Do you have headaches or depression—now often called "cerebral allergies"? Does food make you hyperactive or not active at all?

All of these complaints are related to allergies, and millions of people are afflicted with one or more of these reactions.

It is easy to get over your allergies. You need a new food program that includes all natural foods and moderate amounts of all food supplements, with large amounts (for a while) of some. When you think how easy and inexpensive it is to conquer allergy, you'll be glad that you finally found the way to do it, especially if you've been suffering for many years.

You're wondering why I can say it's easy. I say it

because all allergy is caused by food that doesn't nourish the cells. Even inhalant allergies are caused by the poor food we eat. So when we eat good food, we build up our sick cells, and we won't have allergies.

ALLERGENS

When pollen we inhale hits the moist, healthy cells in the sinus cavity, the pollen slides on into the digestive tract and is excreted. We never knew the pollen was there because the body got rid of it quickly. Thus, we don't have an allergy to pollen or other inhalants. Other healthy cells all over our bodies also protect us from food allergies.

Many food allergies are caused by undigested food, because we can't use food unless it is digested and broken down to its simplest parts with the help of enzymes. Thus proteins have to be changed to amino acids before they can repair our tissue. *Undigested* proteins, therefore, are foreign invaders. When we eat an egg or an apple, we can't make cells out of those foods. At that time, they are allergens— something foreign to our bodies that should not go into our cells. After the proteins are broken down to amino acids, the amino acids are converted into hair, eyes, skin and all other body tissues.

Sometimes the undigested proteins get into our blood. Healthy cells are so strong that they don't allow the wastes and cell debris to squeeze in, but when our cells are sick from not getting the nutrients they need, they become permeable to anything that comes along, including the egg and apple we ate but didn't digest.

Undigested foods can go all over the body and clog up cells. The clogged cells cause skin rashes, diarrhea and all types of allergies. *Digested* proteins nourish cells. We are not allergic to foods that nourish our bodies.

Our cells must get all 50 nutrients to be healthy and protect us from allergies. If every cell in our bodies gets the nutrients it needs, every cell, every tissue, every organ will be healthy, and *we* will be healthy.

Let's trace an allergen and see why we have skin rash, asthma, hay fever, itchy skin, even shock from penicillin and other drugs.

The first thing that goes on in the body, as we've already mentioned, is that something gets into our tissues that doesn't belong there. It can be pollen, dust or chemicals that we breathe in, food we eat that we don't digest or bacteria or viruses that enter the tissues. These are allergens (anything we're allergic to).

What Are Allergies?

Allergies are not small local spots that cause sniffles, a rash, headache or leg ache. They actually start with adrenal gland failure caused by a deficiency of nutrients poorly processed by a sick liver. Strong adrenal glands and liver defend us against invading allergens; weak adrenals and liver can't protect us.

Tintera (1959) said that in 20 years of a busy practice he relieved all his allergic patients of their allergies, whether they were suffering from asthma, hay fever, sensitivity to pollen, house dust, tomatoes, parsnips—or whatever the allergen happened to be—by building up their adrenal glands. He also emphasizes the importance of a healthy liver and pancreas. We need to build up all the organs the same way at the same time—with good food and food supplements.

The cells of our immune systems patrol our blood vessels and our body cells constantly, searching for some substance that doesn't belong there. When they find pieces of egg, for example, the pieces have to be changed into something the body can use, such as amino acids, vitamins, minerals, fatty acids and simple sugars.

But if a substance that doesn't belong in our body gets into the tissues, such as dust, pollen, dog dandruff, undigested proteins or chemical additives in food, it must be surrounded by other cells of the immune system and disposed of. Bacteria and viruses have to be killed or they cause infection.

Ragweed Pollen

Let's use ragweed pollen as an example. Pollen gets into the body through the mouth or nose and burrows into nasal membranes. If the allergen enters the alimentary canal and goes all the way through, it won't hurt us. But if it burrows into our tissues, it causes allergic reactions.

As we've said, when pollen is breathed in and lands on the membranes in our sinus cavities, healthy membranes that secrete mucus will be moist, and the pollen will be washed out of the sinus cavity and down our throats and will be excreted through the digestive tract. We won't have any allergic reaction to the pollen.

But if the membranes aren't healthy, they don't secrete mucus, and the cells get dry. Dry cells can't wash off the pollen. The pollen penetrates the tissues and becomes imbedded in the walls of the sinus cavity.

The body has to get rid of the pollen, so its defense system gets into action. A message goes to the adrenal glands. They pour out hormones that make antibodies to surround the pollen. Then the white blood cells come through the bloodstream, slip through the capillary walls into the tissues and surround the antibody and pollen. All this happens in a flash. We don't even know that this process is going on. This reaction is called the inflammatory response, and if this response works, the person is not allergic (Tintera, 1959).

The words "inflammatory response" sound bad, but the response will get rid of an allergen; therefore, the response is good. When the response works, we don't have allergies. We can stand in a hay field and not have hay fever.

RESPONSE TO ALLERGENS

Cortisone, made in the adrenal glands, is one of the hormones that are called out in the inflammatory response. It is well known that cortisone will relieve allergies, but we all know that cortisone given as a drug causes serious side effects, even death. This is partly because it is impossible for anyone to know how much cortisone is needed. But if our adrenal glands make our cortisone, they make and release exactly the amount needed at all times (if the nutrients are present to make the hormone out of), so there won't be an excess. If there are foreign proteins in the liver or if the liver doesn't have enough amino acids to make hormones and enzymes, or if the adrenals aren't working well enough to make the antibodies, the defense fails.

Any allergic reaction can take place in the sinuses, bronchials, stomach or skin. More and more allergens accumulate in the sinuses causing sinusitis; those in the bronchials cause respiratory problems; in the stomach, digestive problems; in the skin, a rash or itch; and particles of proteins go to the brain, lodge there, and cause cerebral allergies which lead to learning and behavior problems.

The antibodies can't be made until the allergen gets into the tissues, because the body doesn't know what kind to make. If the adrenals are weak, they can't make antibodies, and allergens can't be destroyed. Tintera says that weak adrenal glands are the basic cause of allergies and infections.

The adrenal glands must be healthy if we are to avoid or control allergies. Thus we suffer from allergies because we have poor livers and adrenal glands. It doesn't matter what the substance is that we're allergic to, we need to build up those glands.

Chemicals

It isn't just pollen or other pollutants in the air that cause allergies. We have many other invaders that can get into our bodies and cause allergic reactions.

We've mentioned undigested foods, especially proteins. We must have a very strong acid medium in our stomachs to digest protein. It is called hydrochloric acid (HCl). Without HCl, the proteins cannot be changed into amino acids.

Then the proteins go into the small intestine. Some of them get through the walls of the intestine and into the blood vessels; then they go on to the liver. If the liver isn't healthy enough to detoxify undigested proteins, they go into the blood. The undigested protein molecules may travel through the blood to the skin, the brain or to any other tissue, where they cause allergic reactions.

Histamine

Weak adrenals cannot make enough antibodies, and allergens build up in the tissues. That buildup leads to damaged cells which then release histamine. When histamine is in the blood, the blood vessels dilate, the capillary walls weaken and the plasma oozes out of the blood vessels and collects in the tissues. Our noses run or our skin breaks out in a rash from the plasma. When penicillin is injected, it can cause an even more serious reaction. So much plasma may leave the blood that people can die of shock within a few minutes.

When the histamine goes through the liver, it should be destroyed by an enzyme called histaminase. (The ending "ase" denotes an enzyme.) But if the liver isn't in good condition, liver cells can't make histaminase. Choline, magnesium and vitamin E must be present for the liver to make the enzyme. Without the enzyme, histamine piles up in the blood and tissues and irritates the cells. You probably know someone who has to go to the drugstore to get antihistamines. His liver doesn't work well or he could make his own histamines. Antihistamine drugs are often toxic and cause stomach ulcers and bleeding. The drugs may damage the liver so that it can't produce histaminase.

Adrenal Hormones

Let's review this inflammatory response. The adrenal glands react to the allergens by secreting hormones that call out antibodies which go to the invaders and surround them. White blood cells digest the antibody-allergen combination, and the body recovers from its allergic attack. If all the cells in the body work right, this inflammatory response keeps us from having allergies.

A junk-food diet can cause the adrenals and the liver to fail, as can emotional upsets, lack of sleep, infections, use of drugs or other stress. Any of these conditions can bring on an allergic attack. We can't avoid stress or allergens. We just need to feed our bodies so our cells won't be damaged. Tintera (1959) says, "The average American diet is bad enough to exhaust even the strongest adrenals." Kasper Blond (1960) adds that toxic proteins released to the blood by a damaged liver can cause irritation of all tissues.

THE LIVER

Let's continue our discussion of allergies by learning more about the liver, the adrenal glands and the pancreas. That may seem like a roundabout way of getting to the subject, but allergies aren't just on the skin, in the sinuses or in the digestive tract. Allergies are caused by damaged glands. So in order to eliminate the allergies, we have to build up these glands. They and the rest of the body will be well if we eat plenty of good, natural food, and take enough vitamins and minerals to make healthy cells.

Let's find out how the liver helps us use the food we eat. A small amount of the carbohydrate (starch and sugar) is digested in the mouth. When the food reaches the stomach, carbohydrate digestion stops and protein digestion begins. Protein is only partially digested in the stomach, then it is sent to the small intestine, which finishes converting the protein to amino acids, the carbohydrates to simple sugars and the fats to fatty acids. No food can be used by our bodies for energy or repair of tissue unless it has been broken down by enzymes.

The breakdown products then go through the walls of the intestine into the capillaries. All the capillaries of the entire 20 feet of the small intestine converge into larger and larger blood vessels until they all flow into one large vein that leads into the liver. This is called the portal vein.

The portal vein then spreads out into thousands of capillaries as the blood goes through the liver. On the top side of the liver, the blood converges into one vein again, called the hepatic (liver) vein, which then goes into larger veins until it gets to the heart. There it empties into the general circulation where the food we've eaten—which has been changed to nutrients and is now in our blood—is pumped all over our bodies to feed all our cells.

Let's go back to the liver and find out what happens to the blood there. The blood going into the liver contains breakdown products of almost all the food we've just eaten. It has all the amino acids (building blocks of protein), all the carbohydrates and 10 to 20 percent of the fats. The rest of the fats go into the lymph system from the intestines and join the blood circulation near the heart.

When the liver receives all these nutrients, it must change them to enzymes, hormones, hair, eyes, muscles and even to emotions. It has been estimated that more than 500 different activities take place within the liver cells.

The Liver and Proteins

First of all, the liver makes proteins such as hormones and enzymes from the amino acids it gets. If the liver could not make proteins, we would not live more than a few days. The liver may change some of the amino acids into carbohydrates and fats for energy. This process releases ammonia. If ammonia accumulates in the blood, it becomes a poison, especially to the brain. It must be changed to urea by the liver so it can be excreted. But if the liver doesn't have enough cells working to make the change, the brain may be affected, and coma can occur, which can cause death (Guyton, 1976, p. 943).

The liver also forms 85 percent of the plasma proteins, all except the gamma globulins, which are part of the immune system. The plasma proteins circulate in the blood plasma and are used in the cells.

Also, the liver makes what are called the nonessential amino acids. This doesn't mean we don't need them; it means that since the liver can make them, we don't have to get them in food. But we do have to have the eight essential amino acids, plus energy from the carbohydrates and fats.

The liver makes bile, some from the cholesterol made by our own cells and the rest from the food we eat. Bile is sent to the blood, then to the small intestine to help digest and assimilate fats and fat-soluble vitamins. Besides this, the liver has to detoxify all the foreign substances and poisons that get in the blood in the small intestine. Remember that label on the box of cookie mix you read at the supermarket? It has many chemicals foreign to the body, which the liver must get rid of. If the liver ever gets so weak that it can't detoxify poison, death follows (Blond, 1960).

The Liver and Carbohydrates

The liver also has to handle all the carbohydrates it gets from the intestines. These are already broken down to simple sugars. The liver immediately releases as much glucose (sugar) as the body needs to keep the blood level of sugar high enough so we won't have hypoglycemia, low enough so we won't have diabetes and just right to give us plenty of energy. Then the liver stores the rest of the glucose as glycogen. This is starch, very much like the starch you see when you cut a potato in two, but in animals and humans it is called glycogen. This glycogen can be picked up out of storage and turned into glucose immediately when the blood sugar starts to drop (Robbins, 1974). Glucose furnishes energy for our cells, especially to the brain. However, if the liver cells aren't healthy, the liver can't store glycogen. The sugar is then released into the blood. When the sugar goes through the pancreas, the pancreas overreacts and pours out too much insulin, which takes sugar out of the blood and puts it in the tissues. This makes the sugar in the blood low. This is a typical case of hypoglycemia, which often turns into diabetes if it isn't treated, and the only treatment is proper nutrition.

The Liver and Fats

The liver also processes the major part of the fats we eat. Although only 10 to 20 percent of the fats go into the liver from the small intestine, the rest of the fats go into the general circulation and eventually come back to the liver, where they are processed into substances that go into the energy cycle. Most of our energy, except for that of the brain, comes from fats.

Other Work of the Liver

Another thing the liver does is to store nutrients from our food, especially vitamins and minerals. These are sent into the blood circulation until we need them. Literally hundreds of enzymes are used by the liver for all of these activities.

When we have healthy livers, we know that all these activities are going on continuously to keep us healthy and to help us absorb the nutritious foods we eat.

But what if we haven't been eating nutritious foods? If we eat the average American diet of fast foods and junk foods, we might expect our livers to deteriorate—to lose cells.

One of the amazing things about the liver is that many of its cells can die but it can still function for a while. This is because the liver has tremendous reserves. You've probably heard that a large part of the liver can be cut away and it will grow back. In animals in the laboratory, 90 percent of the liver can be removed and the liver can still do its work. A report in a medical textbook tells of a man who had 90 percent of his liver cut away to remove many small benign tumors. The patient recovered, and the liver was completely regenerated within a few months (*Annals of Surgery*, 1964).

Since a great amount of damage can be done to liver cells and we can still function, we must always eat well, because we never know when we are living on the last 10 to 20 percent of our liver cells.

A Sand Castle Analogy

We can lose many liver cells without knowing it, because we don't feel sick. The liver can be compared to a sand castle on the beach (Robbins, 1974). A little ripple of water comes from the sea and laps at the castle, washing away a few grains of sand at a time. Soon, a larger wave rushes in and maybe a big chunk of sand flows out to sea. Finally, a big wave flows over the castle and it is *all* washed out to sea.

For a while, the liver can stand small waves of injury such as infections, too much coffee or booze,

a hemorrhage, a deficiency of small amounts of nutrients or too much white sugar, white flour and fat. But little by little, the liver cells die without causing symptoms or signs of disease. The liver is losing its reserves.

The absence of some enzymes the liver should make keeps us from assimilating the nutrients. If we don't have vitamins and minerals, if we take in a lot of chemical toxins, if we're malnourished or addicted to drink or drugs, then we can have liver failure and disease anywhere in the body.

We often have food products in our livers that have not been broken down to their simplest forms. If they haven't been, they are poisons in our cells.

Poisonous Proteins

Proteins that come to the liver through the portal vein, for example, can cause a disturbance anywhere in the body—even in the brain. Toxic proteins that cause mental disorders including behavior problems can accumulate in the brain. Two of the most common symptoms are irritability and never being pleased with what's going on.

The sad thing about the people with such problems is that they don't want to have behavior problems any more than their friends and loved ones want them to. People whose behavior problems are caused by glands weakened by poor food could become cheerful, cooperative human beings if they ate good food. Instead of being fed well, they are usually told to "get your head on straight." Nobody can get his head on straight unless he has eaten and digested all the nutrients needed by the brain. Nobody! Many criminals, drug addicts and miserable people whose brains are loaded with poisonous proteins should be fed well so that they can solve their behavior problems.

Several mental disorders can cause death. If a person dies early, he usually dies of liver damage; if he lives longer, a brain tumor may develop (Blond, 1960). Toxic proteins can be found in the placenta of a pregnant woman with a damaged liver. The infant can be born with allergies, asthma or convulsions.

Have you ever heard of a young mother who couldn't nurse her baby because the baby was allergic to her milk? The mother may have liver damage, which causes her milk to be toxic, and the baby's liver may not be mature enough to cope with the toxic milk (Blond, 1960).

These poisonous proteins can irritate a lot of different kinds of body cells. Sometimes red blood cells break down. At other times, the lymph glands and the white blood cells don't work right (Blond, 1960).

Doctors' Drugs

Drugs prescribed by doctors can cause severe side effects, and many of them cause the death of liver cells. The most notorious ones are those that cause hypersensitivity or allergies (Robbins, 1974). Some of these drugs are thiouracil, mercaptopurine and tolbutamide. Others are sulfonamides. All antibiotics (especially tetracycline) damage the liver.

Tetracycline keeps proteins from being manufactured in the body. That's why it works against bacteria, which are proteins. Tetracycline shouldn't be used during tooth development—the last half of pregnancy to the age of eight years. These drugs also go into the mother's milk during lactation. There are many other warnings against their use. They are especially dangerous for people with kidney trouble. Fungi such as Candida albicans, known widely as a yeast infection, can overgrow. Blood may not clot. The liver, the blood and the kidneys should be examined regularly for damage. Many adverse reactions are listed in the standard reference in this field, the *Physicians' Desk Reference*, as usual with most drugs, because many tissues are damaged when proteins can't be manufactured.

Everyone who takes these drugs doesn't have adverse effects. It seems obvious that people with good nutrition may avoid problems if the drugs aren't continued too long. Of course, if nutrition was good enough, people probably wouldn't need to take drugs in the first place. When the drugs are stopped, the adverse effects stop if the liver hasn't been too damaged (Robbins, 1974).

Another category of drugs is far more dangerous and may cause massive cell death. It contains halothane, isoniazid, iproniazid, para-aminosalicylic acid, phenylbutazone, urethane and 6-mercaptopurine. It is suspected that these drugs cause a sensitivity reaction, which is another way of saying they cause allergies.

Too Much Food

One of the worst things that can happen to the liver is that we eat too much at one time. First, the stomach gets overloaded and there aren't enough enzymes to break down the proteins. The mass of food goes into the small intestine, but there's too much to get digested there too. When the food enters the liver, there are many foreign proteins—toxins that should have been changed into amino acids but a weak liver fed with junk food couldn't change them.

Many people have a habit of eating 12-ounce steaks, big baked potatoes, and a little bit of white head lettuce that doesn't contain enough nutrients to pay for its space in the stomach. (We should eat dark green-leaf lettuce—it has more vitamins and minerals than light green lettuce.) Most people can't digest that much food at one time. They may someday find that their liver cells have been so damaged by all this flood of poorly digested food that something goes wrong in their bodies. Wherever there is a weak place in the system—adrenal glands, heart muscle, the skin or other tissues—anything from allergies to cancer may develop (Blond, 1960).

Liver Cells Die

It is frightening that all this can happen without our knowing that liver cells are dying. There may be no forewarning of serious trouble. Suddenly the big wave comes along and washes the sand castle out to sea.

When the liver doesn't get enough nutrients from the intestine, it can't make the hormones, enzymes and energy the body needs. It may not be able to detoxify the poisons from food. Jaundice is a sign of liver damage, but long before that ailment shows up, there can be allergies, personality changes, confusion, nervous symptoms and mental problems.

Liver Disease Symptoms

The first symptom of severe liver disease may be hypoglycemia. It threatens the patient's life. The first sign of something wrong may be excitement, then in extreme cases the muscles become uncoordinated; then stupor, convulsions, coma and death may follow (Davidson, 1970).

In other symptoms and signs of liver damage, men develop female-like breasts, both sexes can have redness of the palms, the body can develop a sweet-sour odor, and the urine can become rather pungent. The kidenys can even become damaged. The changes in the kidneys may not seem to be severe, but kidney failure can be serious enough to cause death (Robbins, 1974).

Veins can show up as red, spidery forms under the skin. There may be a high fever. A condition called Caput Medusae may appear. This is enlarged veins around the naval, given its name because the veins look like the snakes on the head of Medusa in mythology.

When the liver has too few working cells, it can't make enough protein. There may not be enough albumin, globulin or prothrombin in the blood. If not, wastes can't be picked up, so water collects in the tissues. Maybe you know people who wake up with puffy eyelids or who have swollen hands and their rings get tight, or swollen feet when they stand. Also, without enough globulin, there may not be enough proteins to make enzymes or hormones. Without prothrombin, the blood can't clot sufficiently, and people may have hemorrhages.

Such toxic proteins can cause lesions of the bones, abnormal protrusions of the eyeballs, loose teeth and irritability. Allergies are usually found where tissues are damaged.

Now for the happy part. Although all these problems may sound severe—and they are—they can possibly all be reversed if the final big wave hasn't come along to sweep the entire sand castle out to sea. The liver can be regenerated by good food and food supplements (Blond, 1960).

It is important to remember that there may be no signs of illness until the liver has suffered "extensive damage" (Robbins, 1974, p. 988).

An investigator at one of the world's outstanding medical research institutions once told me that the medical profession "can treat successfully about 5 percent of the diseases of mankind; 95 percent of them we know nothing about." It seems obvious that physicians who don't know much about nutrition know very little about how to treat diseases—most of which are caused by nutritional deficiencies that lead to sick and dying liver cells that can affect every tissue in the body. A healthy liver will help make all needed nutrients so that we won't be allergic to anything.

PANCREAS

The main work the pancreas does to prevent allergies is to make enzymes that help digest our three major foods: proteins, carbohydrates and fats. In addition, the pancreas manufactures sodium bicarbonate, which helps produce the rather high alkaline medium needed to digest food in the small intestine. If the pancreas is not healthy, it cannot do this work. Many acute and chronic diseases may be caused by an inability to digest food because of a lack of enzymes and bicarbonate.

Undigested Proteins

Some investigators think the most common problem of the pancreas is that it doesn't make enough bicarbonate, not that it doesn't make enough insulin. Proteins are digested in the small intestine in an alkaline medium, from pH 8 to 9, and they can't be broken down to amino acids unless there is plenty of bicarbonate. A deficiency causes toxic proteins to circulate in the blood and results in allergies. Philpott (1977) says that amino acids in tablets or capsules, plus pancreatic enzymes, can reduce or eliminate allergies in severe degenerative diseases.

This will keep undigested proteins (those that can't be used by the body) from getting into the bloodstream and setting up an allergic reaction.

Injury to the Pancreas

The pancreas can be injured in two ways. In addition to making enzymes to digest proteins in the small intestine, the pancreas makes hormones such as insulin from foods it gets from the blood. If it is overworked because it gets too much food at one time, it can't work well. Also, the pancreas can be injured by the enzymes it makes. The enzymes are supposed to go to the small intestine to digest all foods, but if we haven't been eating enough zinc, the pancreatic duct will clog, and the enzymes can't get out of the pancreas. This can happen when there is a deficiency of vitamin A, because without A, the cells that line the duct swell up and completely close it. So many enzymes accumulate there that they may begin to eat the pancreas itself. This is called pancreatitis. Many people have mild attacks of pancreatitis but they don't know it—they think they are having mild stomach pains.

ADRENAL GLANDS

We've already talked about the liver and pancreas. Let's see how these organs relate to the adrenal glands and to allergies.

The adrenal glands sit one on top of each kidney. They help us avoid damage from stress, but they have other important functions pertaining to allergies. When the body's response to allergies begins, the adrenal glands pour out their hormones to make antibodies. The antibodies get into the bloodstream and float along, determined to find any foreign invader—any allergen—and destroy it. They surround the pollen, undigested protein or foreign chemical and keep it from irritating the tissues. At the same time, the white blood cells, fortified by vitamin C, have received a message to contact the antibody that has surrounded the antigen and destroy both. They will then be sent to the nearest opening that allows waste to flow into the excretory system and be eliminated from the body.

NUTRIENTS NEEDED

How can we stop the allergies that seem to never end? We can build up our cells so that they will resist foreign invaders. As we've said, the invaders are far too large to enter healthy tissue. But when nutrients are missing, the cells become permeable, and the large molecules can get in to start their allergic reactions.

Hoffer (1983) says, "I am convinced that were we still eating foods to which we had adapted over geological time, in the same seasonal pattern, we would have few allergic people." Thus, he agrees that the foods now available are a major cause of illnesses of the American people. The average American diet can never build health because man has processed the food so that it has almost no food value.

Vitamin A

There are many nutrients that help protect us from allergens. One is vitamin A, which is partly responsible for the health of the skin inside and outside the body. If there is enough A, the cells in the sinuses make mucus to wash away invaders. Vitamin A also helps keep the membranes healthy so the allergens can't enter the cells—whether they are in the sinuses, skin or digestive tract.

Vitamin A must be guarded by vitamin E, which protects the fat in cell membranes from becoming rancid. Oil-soluble vitamins are made rancid by oxygen, just as butter is when it sits out in a warm kitchen. Rancid fat will cause holes in cell membranes through which allergens enter the cells. Vitamins A and E can't be absorbed well unless the fat-digesting enzymes in the intestine are activated by the presence of fatty food, which allows the fat-soluble vitamins to be digested along with the food. If we drink whole milk with the fat (cream) left in, we have a better chance of digesting the fats than if we drink skimmed milk.

Vitamin C

Vitamin C is extremely important. It has an anti-histamine action, it makes our own cortisone work better, cells aren't so permeable with plenty of C and C even detoxifies foreign substances entering the body. The amount of vitamin C needed depends on how many allergens reach the tissues.

Vitamin C as ascorbic acid may cause gas and diarrhea in large doses. It is suggested that we take calcium ascorbate, which is ascorbic acid buffered with calcium, or an ascorbate containing several minerals as buffers. These can also cause gas and diarrhea if taken in excess, but for those who are susceptible the system can usually tolerate more buffered C than straight ascorbic acid.

Nutrition-minded physicians suggest that people take their bowel tolerance of vitamin C. Adults begin with about 500 mg four times a day, then increase by about 500 mg daily until they get gas or diarrhea. This means that the cells are saturated with vitamin C, and when more is taken, the cells can't accept it, so it spills over into the intestines, which causes the discomfort. We don't want that, so the dose should then be reduced by about 500 to 1,000 mg and that much should be taken every day. When you're under extra stress you will need even more. Vitamin C is destroyed within seconds when we're under stress. Many people have told me that

vitamin C helps prevent allergies better than anything they have ever tried.

Linus Pauling, one of whose specialties is vitamin C, suggests 6,000 to 18,000 mg every day, and adds, "Don't miss a day." The more severe the infection, the more vitamin C we can take without getting gas or diarrhea and the more the body needs to prevent allergies and other ailments (Pauling, 1986).

Vitamin C makes the allergens that reach the blood harmless if we take enough of it. Linoleic acid from raw seeds and nuts (toasted peanuts—don't eat peanuts raw) and vitamin C help keep our cell walls and connective tissue strong so allergens can't get in. Connective tissue is what holds the organs in place.

Vitamin C is especially helpful to avoid asthma, hay fever, insect bites, poison oak and ivy, yellow jacket stings and other such problems. Yellow jackets kill up to 100 children and adults a year. Reactions imitate a heart attack. Always carry a large amount of vitamin C when you're on a camping trip or hike in the woods.

B Complex

The vitamin B complex will help. The entire B complex should be taken, but B6 and pantothenic acid are of special importance. Cortisone can't be produced without pantothenic acid, and, as we've said, we need to manufacture cortisone and all other adrenal hormones to make antibodies to knock out allergens.

Some of us need much more pantothenic acid than others. If allergies seem to run in families, there may be a higher need in that particular family for pantothenic acid then in other families. Adrenal glands of animals deficient in pantothenic acid are filled with scars. Recovery may take weeks after the animals start taking the vitamin before the scar tissues can be repaired. If there is no scar tissue, recovery may be very rapid.

Any time we're under stress, we need more pantothenic acid because it is destroyed quickly by stress. Panto is nontoxic in high amounts. Adults have taken 10,000 mg a day for weeks safely (Davis, 1972). Vitamin C helps panto work, and less is needed.

If the diet is deficient in any of the B vitamins, not enough digestive enzymes can be made. When liver, rich in B vitamins, has been given daily, allergies have disappeared,

Babies don't have enzymes to digest solid food, so if solids are given before six months, babies may develop allergies.

RESULTS FROM MY PROGRAM

No vitamin or mineral supplements alone can take the place of an excellent diet. Often, allergic persons are taken off many good foods. They gradually become allergic to whatever foods are left in the diet because their diets become so limited that they don't have enough nutrients to keep their livers and adrenal glands working well. Soon they're left with so few foods that cells all over their bodies become damaged by lack of nutrients, and many ailments set in. We have to have good nutrition to repair cells, and the sooner we eat good food, the sooner we can feel better.

A Lovely Lady

I counseled an older woman once who said she ate nothing but chicken and cornbread for lunch and fish and cornbread for supper because skin tests showed she was allergic to everything else. She also had arthritis and digestive problems. Sometimes my counselees are rather overwhelmed by the diet and food program I plan because it's all so new to them. This lady said it would probably take time before she could work it all out. I said, Yes, she should work into it gradually, but to please get digestive enzymes on her way home and start taking one tablet with each meal, and work up to the amount needed to avoid allergies.

I called her in a week or two, and she said she had bought the enzymes that day, taken some with supper that night, and felt much better. She hadn't told her husband because she thought it was just a coincidence that she felt better. After two more days of digestive enzymes, she realized it wasn't just a coincidence, so she told her husband, and he started taking them too.

Then she said with a tear in her voice, "You don't know how wonderful it is to be able to sleep at night. Many a night I've walked the floor because I was in such pain I could not even lie down comfortably, much less sleep."

Isn't it a shame that somewhere in all those years of struggle with poor digestion that caused pain and allergies, someone hadn't told her about digestive enzymes that break down proteins into substances the liver can handle, thus eliminating allergy-causing, toxic undigested proteins from the body.

A Young Mother

Another thrilling story concerns a young woman who walked into my house for counseling. When she was seated, she said, "I feel as if I ought to hug your neck. You've done so much for me these last five weeks." I had never seen her before so I asked how I had helped.

She said, "Five weeks ago, I took my children to a doctor. He had no help for us, and suggested we go to an allergist. But I had already tried that route for years." She said, "I actually sat in that doctor's office and cried." She almost cried just telling about it.

"That same day," she went on, "I called you for an appointment for nutrition counseling. You said you were booked up for five weeks, and you suggested that I read Lesson 1 and 4 of your *Home Study Course in the New Nutrition*. The book recommended a natural food diet, moderate amounts of all food supplements and large amounts of the complete B complex, vitamin C and plenty of pantothenic acid. Also, no junk food, especially white sugar and white flour. You made an appointment for me, but if my family got well, I was to call back and cancel the appointment.

"We ate exactly that way and took all the supplements. It's been like a miracle. My three children are almost completely free of allergies. One of the boys has had asthma for years. He is greatly improved. Another one was hyperactive and had behavior problems in school. Those problems are practically over. It is almost unbelievable. I've been telling all my friends about nutrition—all their children are sick. But they just look at me as if I were crazy. They don't believe it. I keep telling them to just try nutritious food and food supplements. They think that sounds too easy. But I know it works.

"I thought about calling you to cancel the appointment since we are all doing so well, but I wanted to come to tell you about it in person."

So just by reading a book and being open-minded enough to try a new idea, her health problems and those of her children were virtually solved. Such a small price to pay—giving up junk food—to really feel well.

I'm not always successful with allergic people. One of our oldest friends has been snorting around with hay fever for about 40 years. Last fall I asked him if he'd like to get rid of his allergies. He said, "No, I've had them so long I'm kind of used to them."

Others Are Helped

Other people I've counseled about nutrition to prevent or eliminate allergies have written to me. I am quoting excerpts from their letters with their permission.

"I have never felt so well physically and mentally in my entire life after changing my diet to natural foods. My daughter's allergies cleared up within two weeks, and my husband's health problems are leaving."

A young woman had both severe allergies and severe colitis. As usual, we talked about the foods and food supplements needed, because her only chance to renew her cells and heal both ailments was to get plenty of nutrients. Every food I suggested, she said, "I'm allergic to that," or, "That upsets my colon."

We decided that she should feed herself just as a six-month-old baby is fed when he first takes solid food—¼ teaspoon of a new food at a time. She ate mostly the few foods she was not allergic to, but every day she ate a small amount of a food she had not been able to tolerate. If she had no reaction to that amount, she ate more several times a day. Little by little, she could eat more different foods.

I knew that she could get well faster if she could get more nutrients from food supplements. Since her digestive system was so irritated, we thought tablets as food supplements would irritate her intestines even more. So she ground up all the hard pills in the blender with a little water and took just a few drops several times a day. She swallowed the gelatin perles (oil-soluble vitamins) and could tolerate those. She didn't grind up any kind of enzyme tablets—hydrochloric acid or pancreatic enzymes.

Gradually she absorbed enough nutrients so that both her conditions improved. About three weeks after she started on the program, she called me and said she could already eat many more foods than before, although still in small amounts.

It is important to know your body and know your surroundings. When you go into a situation that might upset you, such as a hayfield or a house where there are dogs, prepare for it by taking extra vitamins, especially B and C. Your cells will appreciate having plenty of nutrients to work with to throw off the allergens.

Closed Minds

When I'm speaking to a group I like to watch their faces. If they're clued in to nutrition, they nod and smile in agreement with what I say.

If they're kind of a captive audience and didn't come because the program was on nutrition, many faces look antagonistic. These people won't listen to new ideas. They've heard the opposite of what I'm saying, because their knowledge of nutrition is mostly from television, with its ads for sugar, cola drinks and potato chips. Those ads are preceded or followed by ads for antacids, which weaken the hydrochloric acid in the stomach, making it impossible to digest protein to amino acids. Thus, we can't make antibodies and other cells needed for a healthy immune system.

That's not all. Calcium and other minerals won't go into solution so they will be taken up by the bones unless we have a very strong acid in the stomach. A lack of minerals leads to arthritis, osteoporosis and many other ailments.

The antagonistic people don't believe me because they think if what I'm saying is true, they would surely have heard about it before. But the truth about natural foods has been tragically ignored. The big food companies plan their advertising campaigns so people will buy processed foods. There's more money in selling potato chips than potatoes.

ALLERGY PROBLEMS

Many people take skin tests for allergies. Many of the people I talk to who take the tests tell me, "I'm allergic to 79 of the 89 foods I was tested for." They seem rather proud to say that. When I ask them how their allergies show up—as hay fever, rash or headaches—they say they haven't noticed any reactions, the allergies just showed up on the skin tests. Many also tell me they can't tell much difference when they don't eat the foods they're supposed to be allergic to—they never really feel good anyway!

Individuals who are ill, tired or emotionally upset don't digest their food well, and they have allergies at times. These allergies don't show up on skin tests because the people are not ill, tired or emotionally upset all the time.

Food

Babies taken off milk because of allergies seldom improve. Usually babies are given solid foods when they're too young, and they often lack enzymes to digest such foods. As we've mentioned, undigested foods cause allergies.

The allergies usually get worse, and the babies are taken off one solid food after another until the diet is so limited they're not getting all the nutrients. They shouldn't have been put on solid foods in the first place.

Pediatricians who know about nutrition say babies should have only breast milk for six months. If that is not possible, then formula. But no solid foods for six months. Then no purchased "baby food"—it should be prepared from the family table in the blender or in a baby-food mill. After all, if the food isn't good enough for baby, it isn't good enough for the rest of the family either. Set aside for baby family food that does not have extra salt or sugar.

If a woman's adrenal glands are exhausted when she is pregnant, her baby's adrenals will not be able to make cortisone. The baby will have allergies.

When the adrenals are not making their hormones, blood sugar drops and people crave sweets. They are tired, irritable and nervous. Allergies are most severe when the blood sugar is lowest. After no food all night, the blood sugar is low, and asthma attacks often occur in the morning.

Adelle Davis (1965) gives general suggestions for allergies:

1. Give yogurt if milk is not tolerated.
2. Give a diet high in protein, calcium, magnesium and B vitamins.
3. Eat small meals.
4. Eat no refined foods (white sugar, white flour) in any form.
5. Goats' milk may be substituted for a short while.
6. Use no soy.
7. The most common allergy is to wheat; any other whole grain can be used until the glands are built up.
8. Hard-boiled eggs may be tolerated better than soft or raw.
9. Eat no chocolate. Carob is preferred.

Anyone who is allergic to sugar will get sick when he eats sugary food. He may develop hives, rash, itching, swelling, skin tautness and pain. The urinary bladder may shrink. Children with this condition may wet the bed. The central nervous system may react and cause tension, anxiety, depression, thought disorders and changes in behavior. Mood may be changed or may swing from pleasant to unpleasant.

Eating dairy products may cause these ailments if people are allergic to them. Remember our rules for allergy:

1. Overeating any food may cause allergy because our digestive enzymes are overworked and they can't digest food. People are usually allergic to undigested food and junk food rather than whole, natural food.
2. Often people are allergic to foods they like, probably because they eat too much of them. Thus, if we eat too much of anything, we may not have enough enzymes to digest it, and obviously, we won't have enough variety in our limited diets to get *all* nutrients needed.

Some people are allergic to one food, others to another. Some people get relief from certain vitamins that others are sensitive to. The only way to solve this problem is to eliminate for a while any food or vitamin that you think might be causing a problem. Then, slowly start eating it again; as your cells and glands improve, you will be able to adjust

to it gradually. You may be allergic to the fillers in a particular brand of vitamins. So try other brands.

Pollutants in the Environment

Many children are allergic to pollutants in schools. Janitor supplies, bleaches, powders, furniture polish and window cleaners have labels that read: "Do not breathe—keep away from children." Other products too, such as insecticides, paint, enamel, spray snow, plastic, rubber cement, pen markers and fixatives all carry warning labels, but are used constantly.

No-pest strips are especially dangerous. The label says, "Do not use in rooms where food is prepared or served." I've seen them in people's homes hanging over dining room tables!

Levine (1983) is concerned with the chemical pollutants in the environment which can be present in such massive amounts that no bodily defense can overcome the damage.

These chemicals are literally poison—they are completely foreign to our cells. If we swallow arsenic, we probably will not live, depending on the dosage. There are many chemicals that poison us slightly, but we can often overcome their damage if our defenses are strong enough.

Pollutants in Foods

One time I phoned a young woman, and I could tell she was chewing something. She said, "Oh, I just took a bite of a candy bar. You would call just now!" When we got around to her problem, it turned out to be allergies. I said the candy bar was making her allergies worse, and she said, "Do you really believe that?"

Yes. Because it's true.

The *Wall Street Journal* of December 27, 1976, reported that an allergy doctor and his wife were allergic to foods grown or treated with chemicals. They ate only chemical-free, organically grown foods that cost them $6,000 a year. That was about $3,000 more than food from a supermarket would have cost. They deducted the $3,000 from their income tax as a medical expense, but the IRS didn't allow the deduction. When the case was brought to the tax court, the court sided with the couple, saying, "Their special diet is the only method of effectively treating chemical allergies."

Cerebral Allergies

A new slant on allergies was published in *Lancet* (Pearson, Keith and Bentley, 1983). A study was done to determine whether or not the many people who claim to have allergies actually have them. The researchers said that when people are told they are allergic to certain foods, they might leave so many good foods out of their programs that they would be worse off than if they ate *all* nutritious foods even if they thought they shouldn't. Also, sometimes people are put on such limited diets by their physicians that the diets can cause allergies, and the patient is worse off than before.

ALLERGY TREATMENT

Most allergists treat their patients by telling them not to eat foods that cause allergies and by warning them to avoid inhalants.

This treatment just leads to more allergies. When good foods such as wheat, milk, corn, etc. are given up, the diets become so limited that the liver, pancreas and adrenal glands don't receive enough food nutrients to build health. Soon the victim is left with so few foods that cells all over the body become damaged and many ailments set in.

The Usual Treatment

The "in" thing with allergists these days is an elimination diet, which begins with a four-day fast with return of foods one at a time to determine which foods can be tolerated. These allergists never suggest building up the body. These methods that eliminate good foods further damage organs starved for vitamins and minerals, and lead to more and more allergies, until the poor victim becomes isolated.

Some allergists suggest a house with no rugs, drapes or wallpaper. The walls, ceiling and floor are covered with glazed tile to eliminate dust, and the victim lives out the rest of his miserable existence in this box.

Imagine what happens if he ever sticks his nose out of his antiseptic environment into the real world. He has no reserves in the liver to fight the pollution.

A Better Allergy Treatment

The only sensible way to treat allergies is to build up the body so the immune system can work. When it does, we don't have allergies. If this seems too good to be true, try it. There are many letters in my files from people who got rid of their allergies. The two words they use the most to describe their response are "miracle" and "unbelievable." To me, the one word that applies to these cases is "natural." Nature put us on this earth and gave us everything we need to be well, but man changes the food so much that the nutrients we need are no longer available for our use.

Isn't it unreal to suggest that mankind had to wait until 1954 (or thereabouts) for tetracycline to be invented so that we could be healthy? That doesn't make any sense.

The allergy diet contains moderate amounts of all nutrients, varied daily, with no more than four 4-ounce portions of red meat (steaks, roasts, chops and hamburger) a week. Most people past 20 or so should take hydrochloric acid to digest protein, because undigested protein is poisonous to our cells and causes allergies. If we eat a diet high in refined foods, we won't get enough nutrients to make the hydrochloric acid we need.

Young people may take hydrochloric acid from time to time, about one month out of three or six, so that no ailments will slip up on them. That's like cleaning out the carburetor this month to avoid engine trouble next month. Anyone who has allergies should take HCl until he is no longer allergic, and from time to time after that. Usually, the older a person gets, the more HCl he needs, and the oftener he should take it—up to 3 or 4 tablets during each meal, every day. I often get a phone call or a letter from someone who says, "HCl has helped change my life." It is a simple remedy, and the sicker a person is, the more he needs, because he has more cells that need repair. Won't it be nice when everyone knows that all diseases from allergies to cancer are primarily caused by inability to convert proteins into amino acids used to repair tissue?

Allergy Clinics

A friend spent several weeks in a famous clinic for elimination-allergy treatment. When she came home, she gave a talk about her experiences at a health meeting. She tried to play a cassette tape during her talk. She had a lot of trouble because she said she was bothered by the fumes arising from the tape.

I asked her later if her allergist had ever suggested improving her diet and taking food supplements to build up her organs, especially her immune system. She said, "No. In fact, I can't take vitamins. I'm allergic to them." Thus she eliminated her best chance for recovery. Researchers tell us that we can't be allergic to something the body requires for life.

Actually, if anyone were allergic to vitamins and didn't get any he would die. Often a binding agent causes the allergy, not the vitamin.

I finally met that woman again several years later. She told me that she had never really improved after being on the program in the famous allergy clinic. She told me I had been right all along, and finally after suffering many more months, she had given up on that clinic and taken on the responsibility for her own health by eating nutritious foods and taking moderate amounts of most food supplements and large amounts of vitamin C and B complex. She had improved amazingly, and was rightly upset because she had wasted so many years trying to recover her health without benefit of nutrients.

ALLERGY SYMPTOMS

Let's investigate the causes and symptoms of allergy as discussed by most allergists who do not treat nutritionally. It seems now that almost any ailment can be called "allergy." We'll start with the two main groups: mental and physical.

One Basic Reason for All Disease

There is one basic reason for all disease—lack of nutrients needed to build healthy cells and repair tissue. There are two ways our nutritional deficiencies react on our tissues.

1. Signs—Changes in the structure and function of the tissues, such as wounds, tumors, blockages of blood vessels, kidney tubules or other tubes, and other such physical problems. Signs of these diseases are easily recognized; for example, pneumonia, heart disease, kidney problems and infections. "Signs" refers to evidence of disease that a physician can determine by tests or by examination.

2. Symptoms—Changes in the cells or tissues that may not be obvious at first. The patient feels bad mentally, physically or emotionally, but there are no outward signs of illness. "Symptoms" refers to the way a patient feels—the evidence of disease as perceived by the patient. Symptoms cannot be determined by a physician.

Mental Problems: Tension

This disorder affects the nervous system. A person suffering from tension can have physical symptoms as well, such as asthma, hay fever and skin rash.

Some manifestations of tensions are:

overactivity
clumsiness
inability to relax
oversensitivity
adverse reactions to light
restlessness
poor use of hands
irritability
insomnia
extreme sensitivity to pain and noise

Mental Problems: Fatigue

The fatigue symptoms may be one or more of the following:

tiredness
sluggishness
mental depression
feeling of unreality
inability to concentrate

burning or prickling sensations
achiness
lack of response to ordinary stimuli
irrational behavior
nervous tics

Almost always present with these signs and symptoms are:

pallor
dark circles under the eyes
stuffy nose

And common signs, but not present in all patients, are:

watery eyes
increased salivation
headache
increased sweating
abdominal pain
bed wetting

Mental Problems: Behavior

Cerebral (brain) allergies affect behavior and cause poor perception, feeling and thinking. This has been known for 80 years, according to information in recent medical journals. But for thousands of years, it has been known that certain foods cause tension, irritability and depression. Have you ever seen someone with asthma who isn't tense, irritable or depressed to some degree when having an attack?

Some psychiatrists years ago said that patients had a psychological upset that caused the tenseness and other symptoms. Thus, they were treated by psychiatrists who thought the problem was in their subconscious minds. Now it is known that the brain cells are physically damaged by lack of nutrients, and *that* is what causes the tenseness or other brain allergies.

Good digestion of food in the stomach and small intestine is crucial for the health of the brain. If we take wheat, corn, milk and other good foods out of the diet, allergies extend to still more foods because there are fewer and fewer vitamins and minerals available to make healthy cells, and our glands become weaker and weaker.

People with allergies are unpleasant to be around. But just think what it must be like to *be* one of those people. They have behavior problems, but they don't realize that they were caused by pizza with a white flour crust, imitation cheese and tomato extender, washed down with a 12-ounce bottle of cola. The cola not only weakened the acid needed to digest the food, but also flooded the body with so much phosphorus that it upset the calcium-phosphorus balance and caused arthritis. That's why, when people discover natural food and overcome all those problems, they use the words "miracle" and "unbelievable."

Many practitioners call almost anything that affects our mental ability a cerebral allergy. An allergist notes that when children suffer from mental problems, they don't want to learn, they may be hyperactive or sleepy, and they may have physical problems as well. Some of the children are clumsy and awkward, they may dart from one object to another and seemingly need to touch everything they see, especially if they're in a new place. They don't conform to school, society or family. They are irritable and aggressive. Their attention span is short.

In a medical library, you can find that every one of those conditions has been studied and written up in a medical or nutrition journal. Subjects in the studies proved the value of food, because after their diets were improved they had no more mental problems. The answer: Build up the body.

Adults may suffer from the same symptoms, and they sustain their allergies by chain-smoking or by drinking one cup of coffee after another. It is known that schizophrenics are allergic to foods and inhalants, and are low in blood histamine, needed as part of the body's immune response that fights the allergens. Ninety-two percent of schizophrenics are said to have allergies. Chain-smokers, coffeeholics and 100 percent of schizophrenics will be better off if they build up their bodies.

When a person is allergic, he craves the food he is allergic to. You've noticed that people who crave sweets usually feel good after they eat a lot of sweets. People who smoke feel better when they're smoking, and they seem to be nervous when they haven't had a smoke for a while. It's the same with drugs and alcohol. These patients will become normal when they build up their bodies.

Physical Problems

It isn't just mental problems—tension and fatigue—but physical problems as well that result from malfunctioning, malnourished organs and glands.

There can be pains in the abdomen (we've mentioned that these may be mild attacks of pancreatitis). Headaches are common (we've mentioned that big molecules of protein can get into the tissues and cause the tissues to swell because of irritation from histamine). Legs ache, and there are aches and pains in other joints and muscles. These complaints are similar to arthritis or rheumatism.

Children may wet the bed. This complaint and others connected with the urinary tract can cause

inflammation, which can be aggravated by soaps or other irritants.

The respiratory tract reacts to lack of nutrients in the glands by sneezing and itching of the nose. Patients may have coughs that hang on for days or weeks. Attacks of bronchitis or pneumonia are frequent.

Also one of the physical problems that some people call allergies is poor function of the liver. It simply doesn't receive enough amino acids, vitamins and minerals. Our adrenal glands can't make the hormones we need because we can't make hormones out of soft drinks, doughnuts and candy bars.

Other physical problems include a pancreas that cannot make enough enzymes or bicarbonate to adjust alkalinity of the small intestine to the proper pH so we can digest our food. What do we make enzymes out of? Amino acids. But the Standard American Diet (SAD) can't change enough of our proteins to amino acids.

Some patients who are allergic have a fast pulse rate. Normal is 70 beats a minute. A smoker's pulse rate is usually 80; a nervous person's, 80 to 110; and a well-trained runner's usually 50. The pulse rate rises when we exercise, but it returns to normal quickly. It rises after a meal if a person is allergic to the food he ate. A simple test for allergy is to count the pulse both before and after meals. If the rate goes up after eating—build up the body.

Fasting Is Dangerous

The new treatment provides nutrients so all the brain cells will be healthy. Some allergists suggest that patients fast for four days, then add one food at a time to determine what food was causing the allergic reaction. The four-day fast is helpful in getting the person off junk food. Anyone who doesn't eat at all is better off (for a while) than anyone on the average American diet of processed food. Fasting is not usually good for people except that it eliminates food that is making them sick.

Fasting stops the food supply to the three pounds of microorganisms in our intestines which can then change from friendly to poisonous. If we eat and digest food well and feed the microorganisms plenty of fiber, 95 percent of them will be friendly and will manufacture B vitamins for us. Also, they will overpower the bad bacteria.

Tests for Allergies?

Tests are usually given by allergists. Some physicians use sublingual food tests, which are probably the best. The intradermal tests are usually the least accurate, because food seldom interacts with skin outside the body as it does with the skin inside the mouth, stomach and intestines. The intradermal tests, however, can be used to test contact allergens.

Usually, most people can eat a food they test positive to, if they eat very little of it and don't eat it very often. Allergy tests are frustrating to some patients because there are different kinds of allergies (Pilar, 1983). Allergens that are not in the bloodstream can be found by a scratch test. These include allergies to eggs, peanuts, nuts, fish, shellfish and strawberries. It is much harder to detect allergens in the bloodstream. They include milk, wheat, chocolate and coffee. Pilar says that allergy sufferers should not become frustrated, because there are new therapies and explanations being developed every day; soon someone will discover how to get rid of allergies. We've already discovered how—build up the body.

My approach to these expensive and aggravating tests is not to submit to them. Everyone should be on a good, natural food diet, and take moderate amounts of all food supplements, which will almost always clear up the allergies. It isn't really critical that you know what you used to be allergic to, because in a few weeks or months you won't be allergic to anything.

A good nutritionist or a nutrition-minded physician can discover cerebral problems by taking a medical history and analyzing the diet. Any child who feels worse after eating or who has stomachaches or colic obviously may need different foods. Many people realize they feel bad after they eat, but very few connect their depression, anxiety or fatigue with food.

If you really want to get rid of allergies, it is easy. Much easier than living with them. Relief is so pleasant that many people won't believe their allergies are caused by the junk food they eat. In fact, most people claim that they eat well-balanced meals. Here's an example of a list one counselee brought as her intake of food for one day.

Breakfast—nothing
Lunch—nothing
3:50 P.M.—processed cheese and coffee
5:00 P.M.—coffee
Supper—after the nutrition meeting

This girl is trying to lose weight, and she is obviously on a dangerous food program. She will be so sick that the 10 pounds she was trying to lose will be the least thing she has to worry about.

She may try to make up at the evening meal for her poor food all the rest of the day. If she eats a lot it will put more weight on since it will be at 11:00 P.M., when she gets home from the group counseling session. But if she eats a big meal, as much as her 70 trillion cells need, she will be so stuffed that she won't have enough enzymes to break down the food, and she will add to the undigested food already poisoning her cells. So she must eat a small meal to be able to digest at least some of it, if her cells can make at least some HCl, which is doubtful. A large meal would cause so much gas and bloating that the food wouldn't do her any good, and, besides that, she'd feel miserable.

Here's another person's food list for one day:

Breakfast—Diet soft drink with 1 tablespoon protein powder
Lunch—White crackers and processed cheese
3:30 P.M.—Diet soft drink with 1 tablespoon protein powder
5:30 P.M.—Two pieces commercial fried chicken, white flour biscuit with apricot preserves, one medium-size orange

Anything wrong with that? Yes. Diet soft drinks can cause osteoporosis (porous bones) because the phosphates in the drinks pull calcium out of the bones. If they are sweetened with Nutra-Sweet, they can cause many health problems because for every molecule of Nutra-Sweet that goes into our bodies, one molecule of wood alcohol is produced. The wood alcohol can cause blindness if enough is taken, and when it is concentrated, it turns into formaldehyde, a known cancer-causing agent. Also, extra phenylalanine, which is combined with aspartic acid (Nutra-Sweet), has been shown to cause brain damage in animals. Protein powder is a man-made processed food. We need complete proteins from natural foods, as in the Super Health Drink in Lesson 1 of this course.

Keep a list of your food intake for a few days or a week. You may be startled by what you write down. Many of my counselees tell me they didn't realize they ate so much junk food until they had to write it down to bring in for counseling.

Problems of All Ages

Learning problems in children are common, as is fuzzy thinking in older people, especially in senior citizens. After years of deterioration of the organs and glands because of poor diet, people lose their brain power. This is easy to understand in children who eat mostly junk food; in middle-aged men, who often overload on thick steaks (called the "motorcycle" of the middle-aged); and in oldsters who make up much of the "tea and toast" group. It is well known that the older we get, the slower our bodily reactions become; thus, we need *more* good food and food supplements, not less (Kugler, 1977).

Solving More Problems

As I have stated, children under six months of

age should not be given solid foods. Their digestive tracts cannot handle solids, and they might develop allergies that last for many years.

Some of the problems with proteins as allergens are solved when proteins are cooked. Some people cannot tolerate raw or pasteurized milk but can handle boiled milk. It is known that skin tests have little value in finding allergies to food. Mayer (1970) says that scratch and skin tests may show up allergies to so many different substances that it is almost impossible to interpret the results.

Learning-Disabled Children

One of the most interesting groups of young mothers I've ever worked with all had children with learning disabilities (LD). I was asked by the director of the school for LD children to teach nutrition to their mothers.

All the mothers had either allergies or hypoglycemia or both. After four to five weeks of classes, the mothers reported that their allergies and blood sugar levels were improving on their new diets and food supplement programs. They said that, as far back as they could remember, they had never really felt good. Even as teenagers, they had suffered from fatigue, depression, headaches and, of course, allergies. These women were typical victims of poor nutrition that caused weakened organs, especially adrenals, pancreas and liver. They often had acute infections, but mostly they limped through life suffering from headaches, digestive problems, lack of energy and depression. What a waste to spend 15 or 20 years like that when food and food supplements will relieve all those ailments.

But the most exciting result of their new knowledge of nutrition was the impact it had on their children. Their health improved, they got over their hyperactivity, behavior problems, allergies and learning disabilities. Studies show that LD children, including those with Down's syndrome, can bring up their IQs as much as 10 to 50 points.

One woman had an eleven-year-old daughter who had been on Ritalin (speed) for five years. With the food and food supplements, she got off Ritalin and maintained good conduct and good health. It is really thrilling to see a group of people improve this way, and no one is happier than those who have suffered the longest and seen their children suffer.

My Two-Year-Old Friend

Many people are pale and have dark circles under their eyes. I have talked to and read about many pediatricians who see these signs and immediately say, "Get them off milk." The parents of one two-year-old child that I know were told to take her off milk after the child had a series of infections.

Without the major source of protein in her diet, her infections were almost continuous. She would take cold and be put on antibiotics. (All antibiotics damage the liver.) It would take two weeks to recover from the effects of the drug. She would be fairly well for a week, then get another infection because the liver was too weak to throw it off, and the cycle would start over.

She was so run down after three months of this that the flesh on her little arms and legs was like mush instead of the firm flesh of a healthy child. Finally, her parents gave up all medication. They put her back on milk and on the diet and food supplements suggested in Lesson 1 and at the end of this lesson.

Within three days she had improved noticeably. Her mother remarked, "She even plays around the house more happily." Her cough, which bothered her mostly in the morning before she got out of bed, was the last sign to leave. That took 10 days. But long before that, her improvement was like a miracle, especially when we realize she had been drugged and deprived of good nutrients for three months, going downhill all the time. Her recovery was exciting and rapid, as is usual with natural foods.

THE COMPLETE ALLERGY PROGRAM

I don't want to imply that all cases of allergy will be healed "miraculously" or "unbelievably." It may take time—weeks or months in some cases. But improvement will begin soon, and healing will come when the body gets enough of the nutrients needed. Obviously, it will help to stay away from large amounts of foods that cause adverse reactions.

Gradually add small amounts of new food. Avoid inhalants that cause problems. This is only common sense. The time will come when the body heals itself, and all healthful foods can be enjoyed.

EXTRA NUTRIENTS FOR ALLERGIES

(Use with Supplement Chart in Lesson 1)

You should work with your nutrition-minded physician on this program.

Of first importance is to change your diet and food supplement program to the suggestions in Lesson 1. There is no "magic bullet" for allergies or any other ailment. Each cell must get its full quota of all nutrients so it will be healthy. When all cells are healthy, the body is well.

Suggested amounts of vitamins and minerals are for adults. Children age six to 12 take one-half this amount; ages one to six take one-fourth this amount. If your child is on the borderline, allow about one-third the amount. Totals are given, not amounts to add to what you're already taking.

Beta-carotene

Beta-carotene is changed to vitamin A in the body only when it is needed, so there can be no toxic amount of vitamin A.

25,000 IU at breakfast
25,000 IU at dinner
Double each amount if allergies are severe.

Vitamin B Complex

Take as suggested in Lesson 1: Begin with two tablets a day and gradually increase to five, in divided doses. In times of stress or flare-ups of allergies, increase to eight tablets a day in divided doses (two tablets, four times a day) with food.

Pantothenic Acid

In addition to the amount in the B complex (there are 750 mg daily in 5 B-complex tablets as suggested in Lesson 1), take 100 mg panto at each meal and midmeal, if and when allergies are severe. If needed, go up to 200 mg several times a day with and between meals. Phase out the extra panto when possible, but continue with the amount in the B complex.

Vitamin C

Vitamin C is the only vitamin that tells us how much to take. We begin with 500 mg three times a day with main meals. Increase every other day or so to the amount that causes gas or diarrhea. When your cells are saturated, they can't hold more vitamin C. If you take more, your cells can't accept it, and it spills into the intestines and causes gas or diarrhea. Cut back 500 or 1,000 mg and take that much every day. That is called "bowel tolerance" —all you can tolerate without gas or diarrhea. Your bowel tolerance goes up when allergies are severe and/or when you're under stress. Take more at those times. Vitamin C will be of great benefit to everyone who has allergies to anything. Use it.

Linus Pauling (1986) suggests from 6,000 to 18,000 mg a day for everyone. He says, "If you take cold when you're taking that much vitamin C, you're not taking enough."

Don't forget, if you're new to this program:

1. Grind all of a day's *dry* tablets together (don't grind hydrochloric acid or digestive enzymes). Take small portions of the ground mixture at meals and midmeals with a sip of yogurt. We don't drink water with meals. Increase gradually to the amount suggested on the chart, or to the amount your body says is right for you.

2. Hydrochloric acid and digestive enzyme tab-

lets and gelatin perles *must* be taken whole with meals so they won't irritate the mouth, throat or empty stomach. Swallow quickly with yogurt or buttermilk.

See Lesson 1 for details of the entire food supplement program.

Let's always remember that food supplements won't keep us well by themselves. We have to get off junk food and on to a good diet for the whole program to work.

BUILD UP YOUR HEALTH

What all allergic people should do is build up their general health, especially the liver, pancreas and adrenal glands. I have many letters in my files from people who are no longer allergic to anything and are enjoying the delicious foods that their cells were formerly too sick to accept.

If you have been on a restricted diet because of allergies, you will have to build back slowly. First, you should gradually take the food supplements suggested (all of those in Lesson 1 and the extras listed in this lesson). Your adrenal glands will begin to improve.

You should gradually add good foods even if you haven't tolerated them for a while. Start the way you would start a baby on solid foods—small amounts of one food you haven't eaten recently. If there is an adverse reaction, it's because your tissues and/or your immune system are not working perfectly. Don't eat any more of that food for a week or so. However, the next day, you can try a bite of another food you hadn't been able to eat. Little by little, your system will improve so you will not be allergic to anything.

While I was writing this, a young mother called me and said, "Your food and food supplement program completely eliminated all my four-year-old daughter's allergies."

Today's mail brought this message: "I have read your lesson on nutrition and allergies and am extremely impressed with your clear and easy-to-understand descriptions and recommendations. My 14-year-old son and I have suffered with allergies all our lives, and have been taking two injections a week for a number of years. I have a stack of books on allergies—you wouldn't believe—but yours is the first I felt we could follow.

Those are messages that nutritionists like to hear! Maybe I'll be hearing you call and tell me that *your* allergies are gone!

QUESTIONS

TRUE/FALSE

1. Allergies can be caused by food that doesn't nourish the cells.

2. Allergies are related to failure of the adrenal glands caused by nutritional deficiencies.

3. Cortisone can relieve allergies, but it may cause severe adverse reactions.

4. Sometimes when a young mother can't nurse her baby because the milk doesn't agree, it's because the mother has liver damage.

5. All antibiotics, especially tetracycline, damage the liver.

6. When we eat too much at one time, we can't digest food, and the undigested food causes allergies.

7. An early sign of liver disease is swollen tissues with water retention.

8. The pancreas makes hormones such as insulin and enzymes to digest proteins.

9. The adrenal glands pour out their 32 hormones to help make antibodies to destroy allergens.

10. Vitamin A, the skin vitamin, protects the cells in the sinuses from allergens.

11. Pantothenic acid is a B vitamin that helps produce our natural cortisone.

12. Antacids cause poor digestion of protein, which leads to gas, bloating and a too-full feeling after meals.

13. Calcium and other minerals must be dissolved in hydrochloric acid so they will be taken up by bones and teeth.

14. Studies show that often people think they have allergies, but instead they have symptoms of depression and anxiety.

15. Fasting is usually not good for people except that it eliminates junk food that is making them sick.

MULTIPLE CHOICE

1. Allergens can cause: (a) skin problems, (b) sinus inflammation, (c) upset stomach, (d) behavior problems.

2. To get rid of allergies, we must have healthy: (a) pancreas, (b) adrenals, (c) liver, (d) all of the above.

3. Histaminase is: (a) an enzyme, (b) made inside the liver, (c) made with the help of choline, magnesium and vitamin E, (d) needed to destroy histamine, a troublesome body chemical.

4. The liver: (a) changes starches to sugars, (b) does not process fats, (c) stores vitamins and minerals for later use, (d) will deteriorate unless the diet is good.

5. The liver: (a) makes enzymes, (b) makes hormones, (c) makes energy, (d) detoxifies poisons in food.

6. Signs and symptoms of liver damage include: (a) personality changes, (b) confusion, (c) nervous symptoms (d) coma and death.

7. Foods available for Americans are: (a) a major cause of the illnesses of the American people, (b) unrefined and healthful, (c) often filled with damaging chemicals, (d) processed until they have almost no food value.

8. Vitamin C does the following: (a) it acts like an antihistamine, (b) it makes our own cortisone work better, (c) it helps keep foreign invaders out of our cells, (d) detoxifies foreign invaders.

9. Suggestions to prevent allergies: (a) give yogurt if milk is not tolerated, (b) give a diet high in protein, calcium, magnesium and B vitamins, (c) eat large meals, (d) eat no white sugar.

10. Many people don't relate their ailments to the poor food they eat, which causes: (a) depression, (b) anxiety, (c) fatigue, (d) tension.

ANSWERS

True/False

1. T 2. T 3. T 4. T 5. T 6. T 7. T 8. T
9. T 10. T 11. T 12. T 13. T 14. T 15. T

Multiple Choice

1. a,b,c,d 2. d or a,b,c,d 3. a,b,c,d 4. a,c,d
5. a,b,c,d 6. a,b,c,d 7. a,c,d 8. a,b,c,d 9. a,b,d
10. a,b,c,d

REFERENCES

Annals of Surgery 159:513–519, 1964.
Blond, K. *The Liver and Cancer.* 1960.
Davidson, C.S. *Liver Pathophysiology.* 1970.
Davis, A. *Let's Get Well.* New York: Signet, 1965.

———. *Let's Have Healthy Children.* New York: Signet, 1972.
Guyton, A. C. *Textbook of Medical Physiology.* Philadelphia: Saunders, 1976.

Hoffer, A. Nutrition and Behavior. In: *Medical Applications of Clinical Nutrition* (Ed.) J. Bland. New Canaan, CT: Keats, 1983.

————. What To Do About Your Allergies. Huxley Institute, *CSF Institute Newsletter* 10(3), July 1983.

————, and Walker, M. *Orthomolecular Nutrition*. New Canaan, CT: Keats, 1978.

Kugler, H. Slowing Down the Aging Process. In: *New Dynamics of Preventive Medicine*, Vol. 4, *Tomorrow's Medicine Today*. Overland Park, KS: IAPM, 1977.

Levine, S.A. Allergy Research Review, *Newsletter*, 2(1), 1983.

Mayer, J. *Postgr. Med.*, 47:230–233, 1970.

Passwater, R. Prevention of Aging and Cancer by Application of Antioxidant Therapy. (in) New Dynamics of Preventive Medicine, Vol. 4, *Tomorrow's Medicine Today*. Overland Park, KS: IAPM, 1977.

Pauling, L. *How to Live Longer and Feel Better*. New York: W. H. Freeman, 1986.

Pearson, D. J., Keith, J.B.R. and Bentley, S.J. Food Allergy: How Much In the Mind? *Lancet*, June 4, 1983.

————. Letter to the Editor. *Lancet*, July 16, 1983.

Pfeiffer, C. C. *Mental and Elemental Nutrients*. New Canaan, CT: Keats, 1975.

Philpott, W. H. Proteolytic Enzymes and Amino Acid Therapy in Degenerative Disease. In: *A Physician's Handbook on Orthomolecular Medicine*, New Canaan, CT: Keats, 1977.

Pilar, S. Food Allergies, Huxley Institute, *CSF Institute Newsletter* 10(3), July 1983.

Robbins. *Pathologic Basis of Disease*. 1974.

Tintera, J. *Woman's Day*. Feb. 1959.

Lesson 5

WHAT WE SHOULD AND SHOULD NOT EAT AND WHY

LESSON 5—WHAT WE SHOULD AND SHOULD NOT EAT AND WHY

IS OUR FOOD GOOD OR BAD?

"THE FOOD in the United States is so poor that it is hazardous to your health." "Americans are the best-fed people in the world." We hear both of those statements over and over. Which is right?

Nutritionists know that much of the food that Americans eat is so processed and refined that the average American should not eat the Average American Diet.

We'll find out in this lesson what we should and should not eat and why. Also we'll find out what has happened to our food that makes it so poor, and how we can get food that is fit to eat.

What We Should Eat

Although we talk a lot about food supplements, food itself is the most important part of this health program. Our food should be as natural as possible. We eat moderate amounts of red meat, but it isn't required. If you wish, you can eliminate it from your diet, but most nutritionists say that a little

will be helpful if it isn't contaminated. We are now able to get more organically raised beef, so hopefully we can eat and enjoy moderate amounts of red meat. We should eat more fish than meat, one or two eggs a day and cook with extra eggs. Don't worry about the cholesterol. (See Lesson 3 for cholesterol information.) We can drink a small amount of milk—no more than one or two glasses a day, half of that yogurt or kefir. You don't have to drink milk if you don't want to, but if you do drink it, drink whole milk, not 2 percent and not skimmed. We don't fractionate foods because the fraction we don't eat may have special food value. This is the case with milk. The cream contains five important trace elements, one of them chromium, which is part of the glucose tolerance factor that helps us to avoid low and high blood sugar. If it is available, raw milk is more healthful than pasteurized or homogenized milk. We can eat moderate amounts of cheese if it is natural and light colored. Check the label. Other excellent protein foods are beans and grains, which should be combined to furnish amino acids missing in each.

We should eat butter on our bread rather than margarine, and we can cook with butter if the recipe calls for oil or shortening. Another excellent fat that is required for life itself is linoleic acid, a polyunsaturated fat. The best source is nuts and seeds. Eat some nuts and seeds raw, others toasted for flavor. Always eat peanuts toasted.

The next big category of food is carbohydrate. We obtain most of our calories from this category. The big carbohydrate groups are grains, legumes (beans, peas and peanuts), vegetables and whole fruits. These foods furnish energy and they provide the protein we eat so it can be used to repair tissue.

These are the natural foods that will keep us well. This program is easy, different (not difficult) and the food tastes so good that you will never want to go back to the old way of eating fast foods and junk foods.

The reason this program works for everybody is that if every cell in our bodies gets every nutrient it needs, every cell will be healthy; every tissue, every organ and *we* will be healthy. That is obvious, but it seems too simple for some people to accept. They often find it hard to believe that anything as simple as natural food can keep us healthy. Then they try the program and call me. They are ecstatic about their new health. You can be too.

CHANGES IN OUR FOODS

Food is a 200-billion-dollar-a-year industry, and the food companies spend about 6 billion dollars a year (3 percent of the total) persuading us to buy what they make the most money out of.

We also pay 26 billion dollars a year (13 percent of the total) to wrap up the foods we take home (Brewster and Jacobson, 1978).

Most of the ads are for processed foods. For instance, have you seen a TV commercial lately that advertises fresh, raw potatoes? No, not often, but there are plenty of ads for potato chips, sugared cereals, candy bars, snack cakes and sugared drinks, whether you add the sugar or it comes in the drink. Nutra-Sweet has almost taken over the sweetener market. We'll talk more about that later.

Vending machines are fairly new sources of a quick snack, and 100 years ago there were very few of the machines. Now the machines collect 10 billion dollars a year for snack foods with very little nutritional value.

The biggest change has been in the restaurant business. One out of three of our food dollars is spent "eating out," mostly in restaurants. That figure is expected to rise to one dollar out of two by 1990.

Many of those dollars are spent at fast-food chains. McDonald's is the largest chain. The sales went up from 129 million dollars in 1964 to 10 billion 576 million dollars in 1986. Some of the biggest changes may surprise you. We're eating 70 percent fewer fresh apples, 876 percent less butter, 75 percent less fresh potatoes and 65 percent less fresh cabbage. On the other side, we're eating 90 percent more beef, 179 percent more chicken, 224 percent more corn syrup, 681 percent more margarine, 465 percent more frozen potatoes, 995 percent more food colors and a whopping 1,300 percent more canned tuna.

It's easy to see that we're eating less natural food and more animal protein and processed, packaged, man-made foods. Such foods contain fewer vitamins and minerals—and there goes our good health, lost to the food processors.

WHAT SHALL WE DRINK?

Since we're talking about what we should and should not eat and drink—and why—we'd better start with water. We all need plenty of it.

Water

Water is the most important substance in the body (Horrobin, 1971). If you are a slim man, 60 percent of your body weight is water. If you're fat (or a woman), it's a little less.

Most everything in our cells is dissolved in water. The blood is mostly water and the urine contains wastes dissolved in water. Although we can live for days if we don't eat, we die in a few days if we have no water.

Acid Water Erodes Tissue

Certain elements in man's drinking water may cause mental illnesses or death. These are heavy metals such as lead, mercury and cadmium—poisons that accumulate through the years and cause damage to the body in the same way barnacles damage ships (Pfeiffer, 1975).

The poisonous metals take the place of zinc, manganese and copper required to make enzymes in the brain and other cells. Deposits of the minerals can cause hyperactivity. Even good minerals such as iron—if we eat too much of it—can take the place of the same three minerals, and the excess shows up as insomnia, high blood pressure and restless activity.

Acid soft water erodes plumbing, which produces toxic amounts of heavy metals. In some areas of New Jersey, soft well water produces pinholes in copper piping in only 10 years. The lead and copper go into the drinking water. Studies show that rats that drank water with a lot of cadmium in it died 10 to 15 percent sooner than those that drank water without cadmium. They developed hardening of the arteries, enlarged hearts and high blood pressure. Cadmium seems to be part of the cause of high blood pressure and stroke. Soft, acidic water corrodes galvanized pipe and releases cadmium into drinking water.

Also, since the water is soft, there is very little calcium in it, which means that more lead will be absorbed into the cells, because the cells accept lead if they can't get calcium. Soft water is also related to heart disease and deaths. Other studies show that people who live in soft water areas have more poisonous lead in their bones than those living where the water is hard.

Schizophrenia is also related to excess copper and iron, with low levels of zinc and manganese. Copper and iron are both required by the body, but like all minerals, can be toxic in excess. Copper pipes can allow toxic levels of copper in drinking water if the water is soft and acid.

Milk

Our next big beverage category is milk, but cow's milk is a very controversial food, and many nutritionists say we shouldn't drink milk after we're weaned. We shouldn't drink cow's milk before we're weaned, either, because we should drink breast milk. Cow's milk is not made for babies, and they often respond to a cow's milk formula with many problems (Frazier, 1979).

The first problem is often colic, with diarrhea, vomiting and abdominal pain. Other reactions include bleeding from the stomach and intestines, which usually starts in the first month of life. The infant may tolerate the milk when he gets a little older. Iron deficiency can also cause anemia, usually when the baby is from four months to one year of age. Allergies are common, and they cause asthma and runny noses.

The infant's digestive system is so immature that he can't digest proteins well. Cow's milk has three times more protein than breast milk, and the baby on cow's milk usually has allergies to protein. Many children are given soy milk, but a quarter to a fifth of the children who are allergic to cow's milk are also allergic to soy.

Some infants lack the enzyme lactase, which is needed to digest lactose (milk sugar). This deficiency occurs worldwide. Symptoms of lactase deficiency include acidic diarrhea, vomiting, bloating and abdominal pain. Usually the highest amount of lactase is available just after birth, and by age 3, a child may not make as much as he needs. About 70 percent of North Americans and northern Europeans continue to make lactase after age 3, but other people in the world often cannot drink milk as adults.

Anyone, even if he has a lactase deficiency, can probably eat soured milks such as yogurt, buttermilk and cottage cheese. Possibly it will be found in the future that taurine, an essential nutrient found in high levels in breast milk and low levels in cow's milk, plays an important role in brain development.

Alcohol

There surely is no controversy about whether or not we should drink alcohol. Obviously, everyone agrees that excess alcohol is bad. Many nutritionists and biochemists say it should be eliminated from our diet.

Roger J. Williams (1981), one of the world's outstanding nutritional biochemists, suggests that people with an alcohol problem take L-glutamine as a special supplement to help them kick the habit. L-glutamine is needed, not glutamic acid, which is an amino acid. It can't cross the blood-brain barrier, but the derivative, glutamine, can, and when it gets across, it changes to the acid form and nourishes the brain. L-glutamine is a natural substance manufactured in the body, but all of us do not make as much as we need, thus we should take it as a supplement. Many alcoholics respond well to a daily dose of two grams, divided through the day, which is about half a teaspoon of the powder. The product is also available in tablet form. Williams suggests taking 500 mg of L-glutamine one-half hour after meals and before bed, dissolved in a little water if powdered, or taken with a swallow of water if in tablet form. Heat destroys L-glutamine. It is available at health food stores.

Everyone who drinks is not an alcoholic, but those who are often follow their addiction to insanity and death. Alcoholism, associated with physical, emotional and mental damage, is one of our greatest killers. Also, it upsets its victims' ability to work or to live well socially (Cheraskin, Ringsdorf and Medford, 1971).

Sometimes people drift into alcoholism without realizing they have the disease. Some of the signs that alcoholism is sneaking up include:

1. Guilt over drinking.
2. Sneaking drinks.
3. Loss of memory after drinking.
4. Drinking in the daytime.
5. Low self-esteem.
6. Deceiving family.
7. Aggressive outbursts.
8. Self-pity.

9. Reduction of sex drive.
10. Hiding bottles of liquor.
11. Neglecting eating.
12. Prolonged confused thinking.
13. Serious physical diseases.

That is also a list of symptoms of nutritional deficiency. If there were no deficiencies, there would probably be no alcoholism. A companion disease to alcoholism is low blood sugar, according to many nutritionists, who say that every alcoholic suffers from hypoglycemia, which, of course, is caused by nutritional deficiencies.

Some people cannot remove the toxic products in alcohol from their systems. The toxicity results in tension, anxiety, irritability and thirst. These symptoms disappear if the alcoholic takes another drink. At first, alcohol is a sedative, but if the body can't remove the toxins, it becomes an irritant. A missing enzyme causes the addiction and the adverse effects.

Rats in a laboratory were given alcohol, but they didn't develop a taste for it until they also ate sugar. Then they became heavy drinkers. Half of the rats were then given a natural food diet, and they immediately began to eat less sugar.

Many nutritionists recommend a natural food program with all food supplements, like the program in Lesson 1. Special supplements are recommended by certain therapists for alcoholism. Cheraskin, Ringsdorf and Medford (1971) emphasize a natural food diet with moderate amounts of all food supplements and massive amounts of vitamin B3, approximately 3,000 mg a day, divided, at three meals and at bedtime. By itself, B3 will not give the results desired, so the whole program must be followed carefully.

Vitamin B3 can be taken as niacin, which is preferred by many nutritionists, but it causes in susceptible people a flush that lasts from 45 minutes to an hour or more, and is uncomfortable to many people. If the niacin is too uncomfortable, buffered niacin or niacinamide or nicotinic acid may be used. Begin with 50 mg each time and work up. If it is too uncomfortable, take niacinamide instead of niacin. About five people out of 100 get headaches. If severe, any painkiller can be used. Some people become nauseated or vomit, have a skin rash or a reaction that causes a drop in blood pressure. Often, these reactions can be stopped by switching from niacin to niacinamide or vice versa.

Three problems appear over and over in alcoholics (D.R. Hawkins, quoted in Cheraskin, Ringsdorf and Medford, 1971). The first is the use of tranquilizers, which have been noticeably damaging in every case.

Second is low blood sugar, and third is disorders of sight, sound, touch, taste and smell.

Every alcoholic patient in Hawkins's practice is now screened with the HOD test for schizophrenia, which is closely related to both low blood sugar and alcoholism. See Lesson 2 for a sample of the HOD test.

Alcohol consumption goes up every year, and the age of the consumers goes down. In 1973, the drinking population (15 years old and older) drank 2.69 gallons per person. After 1973, the drinking age population included 14-year-olds (Brewster and Jacobson, 1978).

Alcohol is probably the worst threat to health of all the substances that we put in our mouths. It leads to cirrhosis of the liver with 30,000 deaths annually, 40 percent of which are said to be caused by alcohol consumption. Alcohol causes birth defects, and the FDA suggested that labels on liquor bottles should warn pregnant women to drink no more than two drinks a day. The limit should be *no* drinks a day.

Alcoholics consume many more calories than nonalcoholics—about 210 more calories a day on the average.

Coffee

If you drink coffee, you get a lift, and you can work harder and think more clearly. Later, you'll become tired; you'll think how good a cup of coffee would taste. You drink coffee off and on all day, and you may not admit it, but you're addicted. You may think you can get off coffee with no withdrawal headaches, but often you can't.

Caffeine is found in coffee beans, tea leaves, cola nuts and the *maté* plant. *Maté* is a South American caffeine drink, and it can be found wherever herbs are sold. But you should avoid it; people may drink it without knowing it has caffeine in it.

Caffeine is a powerful stimulant that acts on the central nervous system. The constant stimulation can adversely affect our health, and eventually the effects can be disastrous (Abrams, 1976).

Degenerative diseases that relate to coffee consumption include heart disease, cataracts, diabetes and senility. Caffeine upsets the body chemistry, but it can also stimulate the liver to send glucose—energy fuel—to the blood. Coffee is a drug that is so acceptable that people who do not drink coffee are looked on as rather strange.

Coffee and tea contain the same amounts of caffeine—100 to 150 mg a serving. Tea also contains tannin, which may cause constipation. Cola drinks contain from 35 to 50 mg of caffeine. Coffee contains specific oils which may cause irritation of the stomach and the intestines, and lead to diarrhea.

Caffeine is such a powerful stimulant that, if taken in large amounts, it can cause death. A medical report tells of one suicide using coffee. Smaller regular doses can cause stress—which may be due to dehydration—and many other degenerative diseases. One report from a Harvard School of Public Health researcher says that coffee drinking is related to cancer of the lower urinary tract and bladder.

A disease called caffeinism was described in the *Journal of the American Medical Association* for December 1967. Symptoms are insomnia, loss of weight, loss of appetite, irritability, feelings of chilliness and sometimes low fever and conjunctivitis (irritation of the delicate membrane that lines the eyelids). These symptoms are common among people who drink a lot of coffee. A woman who drank 18 cups of coffee a day had painful swelling in her feet for 10 years. She gave up coffee and the swelling stopped. After drinking tea, her symptoms returned, then left again when she finally stopped drinking caffeine.

Caffeine increases fatty substances in the blood and can cause irregular heartbeats. It relates to diabetes and low blood sugar. Researchers say that many patients can stabilize their blood sugar levels by giving up coffee and eating a natural food diet with moderate amounts of food supplements.

In a study using 25,000 former college students, it was found that those who drank two or more cups of coffee a day had a 72 percent higher incidence of ulcers than those who didn't drink coffee, and those who drank cola had a 48 percent higher incidence.

Patients who had formerly had heart attacks and who drink up to five cups of coffee a day were shown to have a 50 percent greater risk of heart attack than those who did not drink coffee. If patients drank six or more cups a day, the risk was increased to 100 percent.

Some investigators think that caffeine will someday be recognized as one of the major health hazards of our society. It will upset the body chemistry and cause health problems if people continue to drink it. The damaging effects may be described as noncognizant, subliminal drug addiction.

If you've cut down on coffee since the prices went up so much, you're not alone. In 1946, people drank an average of 1,005 cups a year (20 pounds per person), but by 1976 they were down to 560 cups. More people are reaching for a soft drink rather than coffee. The intake of soft drinks was about four times more during the time that people were drinking less coffee.

The use of tea is more stable, and people through the years have been drinking about 160 cups a year. Caffeine in coffee and tea has caused fertility problems, miscarriages and stillbirths in pregnant women.

Cocoa is not a very popular beverage. It seems that people who eat chocolate candy are about the only ones who drink cocoa. The price of cocoa beans is so high that manufacturers are using substitutes for cocoa. I heard the president of one of the big candy companies interviewed on television recently, and he said he really didn't know what was being used in the candy his company made to get the chocolate flavor.

NUTRIENTS DESTROYED BY SMOKING

Everyone knows that cigarette smoking is hazardous to our health, but possibly everyone doesn't know why. One reason is that smoking destroys nutrients our bodies need.

The more you smoke, the more vitamin C you need. Cheraskin and Ringsdorf (1975) studied about 700 members of the health professions and arrived at the following statistics about cigarette smoking.

1. Nonsmokers tend to consume more vitamin C than do smokers.
2. Nonsmokers take in more vitamin K, B1, pantothenic acid, B6, total protein, B2, valine (an amino acid) and vitamin E than do smokers.
3. Nonsmokers eat fewer refined carbohydrates (white sugar and white flour) than do smokers.

This tells us that people who smoke and eat junk food have an addiction or at least a craving that perhaps they would not have if they had eaten satisfying food that feeds all cells all the nutrients they need all the time.

Obviously, smokers and nonsmokers eat differently. Nonsmokers are possibly more health conscious and eat more healthful foods. It may be that smokers are trying to correct a condition, possibly hypoglycemia. When the condition is not present, there is no need to smoke.

One point that seems completely clear is that people who eat poorly and smoke have more disease. People who eat well, take their vitamin C and do not smoke have more resistance to disease; thus they have better health.

I have counseled many smokers who had been trying for years to give up smoking, but the craving was so severe they couldn't give it up, and they always began to smoke again. When many of the smokers went on my natural food diet, they had no craving for cigarettes.

I'll never forget one young woman in her 20s who said she smoked and was not going to stop. We kept on talking and smiling, and when we parted, she still had not said she would stop smoking. I called her in about a month, and she said she was enjoying the new natural food. It satisfied her appetite and she had smoked only three cigarettes that whole month. Obviously, when smokers begin to eat well, they no longer have the desire to smoke.

PROTEINS

Americans have generally eaten plenty of protein, but statistics about how much is actually eaten can be confusing. Many of us do get too much, especially red meat, but in my 18 years of studying nutrition, I have talked with hundreds of people who don't eat enough protein. Many of those people are over 50. They are widows or widowers who eat alone, and they don't prepare nutritious foods. They tell me, "It's too much trouble to cook just for me." They grab a junk food snack, maybe a cup of tea and a piece of white flour toast. Those nonfoods keep them from being hungry, but they do not build or repair the millions of cells that they wear out every day. This "tea and toast" group is heading for disaster.

Also, as we age, we produce less hydrochloric acid in our stomachs, and therefore, we can't digest and assimilate the proteins we eat, especially red meat. Undigested protein is not only of no benefit to our cells, it is absolutely poisonous. Some of the poisons get out of the intestines and travel all over the body in the bloodstream. Then they go into cells anywhere and cause adverse reactions such as skin rash, diarrhea, sinusitis, shortness of breath and many more. Reactions in the brain include depression, inability to concentrate, violent and aggressive behavior and even schizophrenia.

Also, undigested protein goes through the 20 feet of small intestine and 5 feet of large intestine and collects in the sigmoid colon. By that time, the protein is rotten and putrefied, and is causing tremendous gas pressure, which explodes into a bubble or grape-shaped pouch that extends into the body cavity. The pouch is filled with rotten fecal matter, and the thin membrane surrounding the pouch has no muscles, so the fecal matter can't be pushed back into the colon to be excreted. The pouches are called diverticula, the disease is diverticulosis and when the pouches get inflamed, it is called diverticulitis. We can never get rid of the pouches except by surgery, even if we go on my excellent diet. But the diet will keep the disease from getting worse, and it should never turn into cancer. Diverticulosis is a precursor of cancer, and the colon is the second most common location of cancer in both men and women. (The most common cancer in men and women is cancer of the lung.) The average length of life after diagnosis of cancer of the colon is 2.2 years.

Thus, the most important information about protein is to get a varied intake of plant and animal protein and to eat small amounts at a time so it can be well digested. We can then break the proteins down to amino acids that will build and repair tissue rather than having them foul the body because we ate so much that we can't digest the proteins.

Anything we consume in amounts larger than needed leads to disease, whether it is red meat, whole-grain bread, nuts and seeds (all of which nourish the body) or oxygen or water (both of which we can't live without). "Too much" leads to obesity, which leads to diabetes, heart disease, even cancer, because we can't digest "too much" of anything, whatever it is.

Restructured Meat

You may have forgotten the good taste of fresh cooked roast beef. Many restaurants serve "roast beef" made of chunks of beef mixed with fat, salt and soy vegetable protein and stuffed into a sausage casing. When served, usually at fast-food chains, it looks like the real thing, with fat marbled through it. It can be listed on the menu as "steak" (Hunter, 1978).

These products are also found at supermarkets and are made to look like veal "steaks" or lamb "chops" that have been grilled, barbecued or baked. Vegetable protein (soy) can replace up to 20 percent of the meat in packaged products. Fat solids, which cost less than one-fifth as much as beef, can replace from 20 to 26 percent of ground beef without changing the taste. Hot dogs and cooked sausage can contain 15 percent fat solids. They are also found in stews, soups, canned meats and spaghetti sauce.

Reconstructed Protein

Let's say you are determined to buy old-fashioned beef for your family. At dinner, you realize there is little flavor in the meat. Animals are often fed so much growth hormone that they go to market much earlier than they should, and they don't have time to develop tasty tissues.

Cattle may be fed with Masonex, a waste product of the Masonite industry (Hightower, 1976). The cattle eat more in a day when fed Masonex, probably because chemicals in Masonex stimulate the appetite. That the beef tastes like cardboard doesn't seem to matter.

Supermarket ham is no better. Ham used to be slow-cured so it developed a good flavor. The ham now is quick-cured with nitrite. The label can say "country ham" when it is aged no longer than four days. Old-fashioned country ham was aged at least four months, sometimes a year.

Hamburger

Fast-food hamburger chains often serve synthetic foods, because their products don't have to follow labeling codes other meats follow, and because the people who eat hamburgers don't expect high quality (Hightower, 1976).

Schools aren't far behind in using synthetics. The Department of Agriculture allows the school breakfast and lunch programs to use up to 30 percent soy protein in meats. When the kids start young on such tastes and textures, they will never remember any other kind of food, and their early programming becomes their lifestyle.

They may never know that their allergies, frequent colds and possibly stomachaches or worse were caused by nutritional deficiencies in the artificial food they ate in school. However, the nonfood can certainly be flavorful. The chemical companies will see to that. They make every flavor from "bacon" to "strawberry," either in liquid or spray-dried form. Another flavor is cooked tomato, completely synthetic, no tomatoes in it, and used for soup, sauce and ketchup.

An interesting expression was used in an ad for one of the synthetic flavors that was touted as "natural." It was called one of a series of "scientifically reconstituted, artificial oils" (Hightower, 1976).

Antibiotics in Animal Feed

Antibiotics have been called miracle drugs, and very few humans have escaped being treated with them. The first antibiotic used was chlortetracycline. It had been developed as a medicine for humans, but when it was fed to chickens, the chickens grew faster. The antibiotics were later used for animal feed to make the animals mature faster so the farmer could sell them sooner and make more money (Hall, 1976).

In 1971, after about 20 years of using antibiotics, the FDA estimated that 78 percent of the meat and eggs eaten in this country comes from animals fed medicated feeds (Hall, 1976). This is happening all over the world, and, in Italy, a physician realized that the children he saw were maturing at younger ages than normal. After much research, he realized that veal caused the problem. Many Italian parents fed their children veal because they thought it was more healthful for children than older beef. The physician went to the government and asked that antibiotics not be allowed in the animal feed, so the government banned them in veal. Later the physician realized that the children were still maturing early because of the antibiotics in chicken and beef feed. He went to the government again and asked for a ban on those antibiotics. The government refused this request saying that if farmers couldn't force early maturity and fast growth of the animals, there would not be enough protein for the people to eat.

What else do all these antibiotics do to the humans who eat the animal flesh? No one knows the answer. Everyone is guessing, but only one study has been reported. As the animals grow, they gain weight, but with antibiotics, 16 percent more pig can be produced with the same amount of feed. Their bones break more easily because bones don't grow as fast as the soft tissue, and the bones can't support the added weight. Thus, many of the animals suffer from broken bones in the feedlots and while awaiting slaughter. Chances are that other side effects are found, but agriculture experts are not eager to find out for sure. Hall (1976) says, "Ignorance seems to be preferred."

One of the most obvious problems is that the microbes are becoming resistant to the antibiotics. When the weak bugs die, the powerful bugs are found in larger numbers because the antibiotics formerly used do not kill off the resistant bacteria. Also, all the antibiotics that are used in human diseases are used in animal diseases and vice versa.

Before 1955, resistant bacteria were rare, but only 10 years later, 60 to 70 percent of all common bacteria in the intestine were somewhat resistant. As more and more antibiotics are used, more bacteria become resistant, until humans must often take larger doses than were previously needed (Hall, 1976). The best way to prevent both animal and human diseases is to eat to build a healthy immune system to fight off disease.

Fresh Eggs Are Good Food Again

When the American public thinks of eggs, they usually think of cholesterol. Eggs are good food, and we can eat one or two a day; the cholesterol will not harm us unless we get too much, and anything that we eat too much of, including water, harms us. Cholesterol is required in every cell, and every cell is able to manufacture it; if our cells are healthy, they make just the right amount, and we never get too much.

Now nutritionists suggest that we eat one or two eggs a day and cook with extra eggs if we want muffins or custard. Although many people eat very few eggs because they're still afraid of cholesterol, other people are eating as many eggs per year as their parents and grandparents ate in 1935—about 280 per person (Brewster and Jacobson, 1978).

Restructured Eggs

Have you seen the eight-inch egg? It isn't fresh, it isn't natural, but it's called "egg." You've probably eaten slices of it at restaurants without knowing it.

When a hard-boiled egg is sliced, some of the slices will be all or nearly all white. The eight-inch egg is made by machine from mashed egg whites and mashed yolks, molded into shape. They are kept frozen for up to two years, then sold to restaurants for salads, sandwiches and garnishes.

Substitute eggs have been manufactured in factories for years. The product, made from fish, was used in mayonnaise, in ice cream and in baked products (Hunter, 1978).

Another product, Egg Beaters, was tested on young rats, but the rats didn't grow as fast as they should. They had gained only 31.6 grams of weight at three weeks of age. Rats fed shell eggs averaged 66.5 grams during the same time period. The rats got some of the mix from the Egg Beaters on their fur when they were feeding, and the investigators tried to gently wipe it off with tissues. The rats' fur came off with the mix. The Egg Beaters rats died within three to four weeks after being weaned.

Some people have described Egg Beaters as tasting like soft, hot cotton. Others say they taste like wet cardboard with mayonnaise.

Milk and Milk Products

Have you been longing for a piece of real strawberry shortcake with real, heavy whipped cream? You may not be able to find the old-fashioned kind of cream. Almost everything now is nondairy. But those products may be higher in calories and fat than the old-fashioned kind and highly saturated at that.

Nondairy whipped toppings may look good, but they're made of about 30 percent saturated fat, 10 percent sugar and 2 percent protein, with a lot of water, flavors, colors and stabilizers. Nondairy coffee creamers are similar.

Milk has picked up a few more labels—"filled" and "imitation" are two. Imitation milk is made from soy and other materials; it costs less to make, but the consumer pays the same amount. Filled milk is any milk that has fat other than milk fat added. These milks are not equal to cow's milk, and they differ from each other. Some have no vitamin A, and others have too much; some are low in total protein and in both calcium and phosphorus. They have been judged unsuitable for infants and children and potentially harmful for pregnant and lactating women and older people.

Vegetable Proteins

When soy is added to beef to make patties, the soy absorbs up to four times its weight in water, and the customers pay a high price for the water. Some states do not allow the use of the word "burger" or "hamburger." The patties must be called "imitation hamburger" or any term that tells the customers what they're getting. Some areas have very little control, and some "pure beef" hamburgers from fast-food outlets contain soy, starch and more fat than is allowed.

In institutions, soy is used in codfish cakes, sardine salads, oatmeal cookies and even in scrambled eggs. Maybe that was what I had recently on an airplane. The yellow mass on my plate looked something like eggs, but it tasted more like cotton than anything else. I really meant to write to the president of that airline. That's the only way airlines and others will ever know what the public thinks about such foods.

Soy is acceptable as an extender in protein dishes; in fact, I add small amounts of soy flour to cookie recipes. But I never advocate adding soy to the many dishes we've mentioned.

The most interesting, varied and different vegetable proteins are whole grains and legumes (beans, peas and peanuts). Try some whole wheat, rye and triticale (a combination of wheat and rye that the botanists put together). The combined foods are complete proteins, but one of the most important things about these proteins is that they are delicious and healthful. Try red beans seasoned with pizza flavoring and spread on a crust of whole wheat, corn bread or oat flour. Add mounds (or less, to your taste) of grated light-colored natural cheese, and enjoy a new, natural pizza that tastes even better than the old kind and is healthful as well. Sprinkle some frizzled, organically raised ground beef over the top if you're still eating meat. You'll never crave the white-flour-crust-and-canned-tomato pizzas you used to like.

Here's another super vegetable protein dish: chickpeas, also called garbanzo beans, blended with millet plus eggs and seasonings—all patted into a pan and frizzled until golden and crusty. One day my son, who is a meat-and-potatoes man, came by while we were eating supper. He ate some of our frizzled millet and garbanzos and said, "Mom, these sure are good patties." I told him what they were made of, and he said again, "Mom, these sure are good patties." ("Frizzled" means cooked in a moderate skillet with butter. I don't use hot oil; we should never fry anything.)

I cook grains and legumes ahead and freeze them. That's the way we get convenience foods, and we easily and quickly prepare super dishes from these excellent protein foods.

Trying new recipes is fun, and you'll probably be making up some of your own before long. Many more recipes are in my cookbook, *Switchover! The Anti-Cancer Cooking Plan for Today's Parents and Their Children.*

Should You Be Vegetarian?

Man should eat meat and other animal proteins. That is the position taken by Abrams (1980), who begins his argument by noting the possible dangers in eating raw plant foods. Many such foods are poisonous and must be cooked to neutralize unwanted substances, as in, for example, raw potatoes and raw brussels sprouts. When these vegetables are cooked they are much more easily digested than when they are eaten raw. Other common foods such as grains and beans must also be cooked.

When man discovered fire, he could eat more plants because he could digest cooked food more easily, but man has used fire only during the last 2 percent of the several million years he has lived on earth. Before that, man gathered fruits, nuts and other plants he could eat raw.

Thus, man evolved eating animal proteins, but when the supply of game began to dwindle, he turned to agriculture. He had not planted vegetable foods before because he preferred animal foods, and he lived better using buffalo and other animals as a source of food and also as clothing and housing.

The American Indians seemed to be very healthy on this diet. Since it takes about eight square miles to feed one person on a hunter-gatherer's diet, early man had to turn to agriculture and domesticated animals when the population increased. Six thousand people could be fed on eight square miles of land.

Actually, no culture has been entirely vegetarian. Man learned to combine grains and beans for complete protein, but he always added at least small amounts of animal proteins: fish, domesticated guinea pigs, turkeys, ducks and even native dogs. He also ate worms and mosquito larvae. (My family moved to Mexico City in 1953 and marveled at the taco stands on the street where natives sold tacos in their version of a smorgasbord. One of the choices on a taco was maguey worms—animal protein.)

Some societies domesticate animals and use milk for protein. Most present-day cultures reject milk as food, and it has never been widely used. However, a tribe in Africa called the Masai live very well on a high intake of blood and soured milk.

The health of the people of the world has degenerated because of the high-carbohydrate diet of refined and processed foods. Refined carbohydrates are much less satisfying than whole grains, and man becomes obese when trying to eat enough of the refined foods to satisfy his appetite day after day. Obesity itself is a health problem. Meat is filling and satisfying, so we don't have to eat it in large amounts. If we eat no animal protein, we'll spend a lot of time eating large amounts of vegetables, grains and whole fruit to get the calories we need.

The answer lies in the natural food diet as set forth in these lessons. We may eat moderate amounts of red meat, fish several times a week, one or two eggs a day (and cook with extra eggs), chickens from the health food store, natural light-colored cheese in small amounts, one or two glasses of milk a day if you wish (half of it yogurt), combinations of grains and legumes for plant proteins and for excellent complex carbohydrates, vegetables cooked and raw, whole fruits, butter to cook with and to spread on bread and nuts and seeds in small amounts several times a day.

This food program provides all nutrients, which go to the blood and then to all cells to build and repair tissues and to furnish energy to make it all work.

FATS AND OILS

Since 1957, Americans have been eating about 17 pounds of fats and oils per person per year. But they used to eat half butter and half margarine, and now they're eating about 5 pounds of butter and 12 pounds of margarine for the same total—17 pounds! The FDA has ruled that both products must contain 80 percent fat. Butter can contain only milk, cream, salt and coloring. Margarine may contain fats, oils, milk solids, salt, flavoring and vitamins A and D. As much as 20 percent of the fats and oils in shortenings can be from beef fat and lard (Brewster and Jacobson, 1978).

Vegetable Oils

Vegetable oil, praised and prescribed as the answer to heart disease, has become a disaster because of the way it's processed. We must have oil from plants as a source of linoleic acid, the one essential fatty acid the body can't manufacture and we have to eat. But oil becomes damaging to our cells when it is extracted from the seeds and nuts, processed and put into bottles.

The oil is extracted in two ways. In mechanical extraction, the seeds (corn, sunflower, soy and others) are crushed, water is added and the slurry is then heated for 30 minutes at 230 degrees F, then cooked again to extract more oil. Then the crushed seeds are pressed at 10 to 20 tons per square inch (Hall, 1976).

In the solvent method, the crushed seeds are treated with gasoline or other chemicals that release more oil than pressing. Up to 100 ppm of solvent remains in the oil. Some countries allow only 10 ppm of solvent to remain.

The oils then must have undesirable free fatty acids removed with lye at 160 degrees F. Then the oil is bleached and deodorized at 330 to 380 degrees

F for about 12 hours. Finally a preservative, usually BHA, is added.

Such high temperatures cause the oil to be carcinogenic. Many oils are used to deep-fry potatoes and chicken, and they are heated over and over, which makes the oil molecules even more damaging to our health.

Vegetable oils are not allowed on my food program, because many natural food nutritionists report that all processed, bottled oil is detrimental to our health. No one seems to consider the food value of such additives. So we eat fresh nuts and seeds to get the excellent oil we need.

Hardened Fats

After the oils are prepared, they are hardened to be used as margarine and shortening. The melting point is raised by adding hydrogen to the oil. The oil is heated to about 380 degrees F. Since the fatty acids in the oil are saturated by the processing, the oil is no longer polyunsaturated. It is a saturated fat. These new fats are unnatural.

When we eat nuts and seeds, we are getting unsaturated fats designed by nature, called *cis* fatty acids. But the manmade saturated fats are changed to *trans* fats. The change is caused by higher heat and pressure when the oils are hydrogenated. Trans fats melt at temperatures of up to 111 degrees F; cis fats only up to 55 degrees F (Hall, 1976). Since cis fats melt at 55, they are obviously liquid at 98.6, the normal body temperature, and they will flow in the blood instead of stacking up in the arteries and causing heart attacks and strokes. Obviously, the trans fats remain hard at 111 degrees F. Thus, they don't melt and flow through the blood vessels; they stack up in the arteries, causing atherosclerosis.

Rancidity

Exposure to oxygen causes unsaturated fats to become rancid. BHA added to margarine and salad oils keeps those foods from spoiling, but the preservatives may be as damaging as the rancid oils.

The fatty acids combine with each other to form unnatural structures, especially when they are used for deep-fat frying. The longer they stay in the cooker, the more unnatural they are. Trade journals for fast-food places advertise products that will "renew" the overheated rancid oils so they can be used as much as one month longer. Cancer-causing agents are more likely to be in the oils that have been reheated many times.

Margarine or Butter?

Have you ever heard of butterine? That's an early name for oleomargarine. The name was not so hard to change as the color. In the early days, margarine was white, and the butter industry wanted it to stay that way, because sales of margarine were not very high because people didn't want to eat white margarine that looked like lard.

Later, laws were passed to allow colored margarine to be sold in all states except two strong dairy states, Wisconsin and Minnesota, and those states too finally legalized colored margarine. Then margarine sales skyrocketed, and margarine outsold butter by 100 million pounds a year.

When the cholesterol scare developed, the margarine manufacturers exploited the fear of heart disease into a bonanza for themselves. They aimed their advertising at physicians, and since the physicians didn't know the dangers of hydrogenation—hardening vegetable oils so they would not become rancid so easily—they recommended margarine.

Hardened fat no longer fits the chemistry of our cells. It was known as early as the mid 1950s that hardened vegetable oil was dangerous. Studies with animals and humans showed that it contributed to the incidence of nerve diseases, heart disease, hardening of the arteries, cataracts, arthritis and cancer.

Thus these abnormal fatty acids damage our cells and cause the very diseases they are supposed to prevent. It is illegal for advertisers to say that polyunsaturated fats will prevent or control heart disease, but every time a TV announcer says, "rich in polyunsaturates," most viewers relate "polyunsaturates" to preventing or controlling heart disease, and they subconsciously get the message to buy the product when they go to the supermarket. They still believe that hydrogenated oils are healthful, 30 years after the first adverse reactions were reported.

The American public must be educated to the danger of hardened fats—that more atherosclerosis (fatty deposits in the arteries) is caused by margarine than by butter and eggs.

Almost everywhere I speak, people are surprised by these statements. They almost always are pleased as well, and they say they're glad to go back to butter; they never really liked margarine anyway!

Butter Is "In"

Salted butter isn't good for us, and many people have changed to unsalted butter because it has such a fresh taste. If you like salted butter, you've probably been eating too much salt, and your taste buds don't work well enough for you to taste subtle flavors. Your system may need zinc and B vitamins; both of these nutrients help our sense of taste work better.

Salted butter doesn't spoil easily because the growth of yeasts and molds is slowed down. Unsalted butter has fewer additives, so it's better for us, but it must be used quickly. If you like salted butter, buy unsalted and salt it lightly at the table (Hunter, 1978).

CARBOHYDRATES

People like most carbohydrates; they'll eat them, good or bad, even though some of them are made with substances you'd never want to put into your mouth. What are the unpleasant carbohydrates? They're called microcrystalline cellulose, which is a bulking agent in food. What does that mean? Cellulose is the structural component of cotton, paper waste, rayon and cellophane. It can be purified to a white powder that flows freely, is odorless, tasteless and has no calories. It can be substituted for flour in baked goods and is used in potato flakes, salad toppings, puddings, soups and desserts. It is used in candies and pretzels; the more cellulose in a food, the fewer calories it has, and no one can even tell it's there (Hunter, 1978).

Wood and Paper Cellulose

Another additive that devitalizes our food is cellulose from wood, which has been used instead of bran in bread. It holds a lot of water, so the main ingredient of these breads is water. They are advertised as having 400 percent more fiber than wholewheat bread, but if humans eat too much fiber, it can bind fats, cholesterol and minerals, which means that the nutritive value of the bound substances is not available to the body. Nutritional deficiencies can result.

Researchers were asked if the high-fiber bread would cause nutritional deficiencies, and the answer was, "It depends on how much bread a person eats, and on what else he eats." They also said that it might be all right for adults to eat the bread, but the situation would be quite different for growing children. They admitted that "20 years later, we'll look back and find that something has gone wrong."

This fiber is used to coat fried fish and chicken and to make thin potato chips strong and breakresistant. Added to hot dogs, sausage and ground meat, it swells the quantity and also absorbs fat to make the products juicier. It makes salad dressings and mashed vegetables smooth and thick. It can be added to yogurt, fish cakes and soft drinks. Anything it is used in is less appetizing and less healthful (Hunter, 1978). Of course, fiber is needed in the diet, but the best way to get it is from natural foods such as whole grains, legumes, vegetables and whole fruits.

As strange as it seems, the average American eats less carbohydrate than he did in 1910. But the carbohydrate is refined and processed and has less food value than it used to have.

Our two main sources of carbohydrates are cereal grains and sugars. "Whole grains are foods of incomparable perfection" is one of my favorite quotations. It is from Dr. Josef Issels, a cancer specialist in Germany. Whole grains contain starch, which is digested slowly and changed to sugar for energy. Such unrefined carbohydrates contain vitamins, minerals and excellent protein. Fiber from whole grains cannot be digested, so it cannot be taken into our cells. It provides bulk to make our bowels move. As the wastes are flushed out of our bodies, they leave a pleasant home for the friendly bacteria that live in our intestines. The bacteria manufacture B vitamins to help us stay well. These complex carboydrates should furnish from 60 to 80 percent of our calories, so they will be a very important part of our intake of food.

Sugars contain almost nothing but calories, but Americans eat 30 percent of their calories as white sugar (sucrose) and white-flour foods. We should reduce this amount to zero.

Glucose is the kind of sugar that our brains feed on. It is required, and starch is broken down to glucose to feed our cells. Humans have been using about 300 grams of glucose, mostly from starch foods, every day for millions of years (Pauling, 1986).

Pauling says that the intake of sucrose (white table sugar) should be kept low. It includes white sugar, brown sugar, raw sugar, honey, candy and refined, commercial desserts. We can eat the excellent desserts we make ourselves from natural ingredients.

Pauling also says that we shouldn't eat much fructose. Through the years, humans have eaten only about eight grams of fructose from fruits and honey. But in the last century, they have eaten large amounts of sucrose, which is half glucose and half fructose, and our intake of fructose jumped to about 74 grams a day. Pauling quotes studies that show that the tremendous number of deaths from heart disease is related to the amount of sugar, especially fructose, in the diet. When fructose is digested, acetate is formed, which is partially changed to cholesterol.

Many studies show that the fat, and especially the cholesterol, in our diet is not causing the high incidence of heart disease. What causes it? The tremendous amount of sugar we eat. It is not a good source of energy for our cells.

Corn syrup, which is glucose, also called dextrose, is an acceptable sweetener in moderation (Pauling, 1986). Health food stores carry powdered dextrose. If you want to try corn syrup, check the label, because some corn syrup has sucrose or refined sugar added. We don't want that.

Candy

It's rather surprising to hear that people don't eat as much candy as they used to. In 1968, they ate about 20 pounds per person, but in 1976, they ate only a little over 16 pounds per person. That was probably because the candy bars are so much smaller and more expensive than they used to be. Also, children eat most of the candy, and there is a smaller percentage of children in the population. From 1970 to 1976, the number of people under 13 years of age fell 10 percent.

During World War II, the intake of candy sky-rocketed, probably because sugar was severely rationed to individuals, but the candy industry had a large allotment of sugar, and servicemen were allowed candy in their rations.

Carbohydrates and Triglycerides

Sugar and starch are both carbohydrates. Starch is an excellent food for energy, but sugar increases the blood levels of triglycerides (TGs)—fats that clog up our arteries and cause heart attacks and strokes.

Studies show that human beings who eat white table sugar have high levels of triglycerides in their blood regardless of what else is eaten. However, humans who eat high levels of starch have lower levels of TGs (Reiser, 1983). TGs also go up when the food is consumed by gorging rather than by nibbling.

Recently I talked with a young woman who is a manic-depressive. She said she had been sick for 15 years and had become much worse during the last year. I asked her what she had for breakfast, and she said she hadn't eaten anything. She did have a morning snack—a cola drink and some cookies. She skipped lunch and had a rather large meal for dinner, but the food was processed and refined and had lost much of its nutritional value. She started on the natural food program with moderate amounts of all food supplements, and she began to improve as soon as she ate food that would supply her brain cells with all 50 or so of the essential nutrients. It is thrilling to hear from the people who have been so sick for so long and who improve on this program and live normal lives. They are determined to be well and eager to stay on the program.

Carbohydrates and Cholesterol

In studies with animals, Reiser (1983) says that if the animals were fed high levels of fructose, the cholesterol level of the blood increased significantly, but if they were fed identical diets containing high levels of starch or glucose, the blood levels of cholesterol did not increase. Thus, when we eat white table sugar or white flour, the cholesterol count will probably go up.

Human studies show that white sugar causes higher blood cholesterol than starch even if the humans eat a lot of cholesterol and saturated fat and little or no fiber. Thus, we see again the importance of whole grains, with their natural content of fiber. All of these studies back up our natural food diet.

Also, it seems that men and older women may be more susceptible to white sugar than younger women. This is borne out by the death rate figures that report heart disease as the major cause of death among men in their forties, but not among younger women. However, for women past menopause, heart disease is the biggest killer.

Several other studies were reported (Reiser, 1983) of humans fed either sugar or starch from natural foods, such as cereals, vegetables, beans and potatoes, all high-fiber foods. In all cases, carbohydrate from white table sugar raised cholesterol blood levels, but carbohydrates from natural foods lowered the levels. One of the most common fallacies is that fruit juice is healthful. As we've seen in Reiser's report and in Pauling's book, fructose is partly responsible for the disease that kills more Americans than any other. The first and easiest new habit we can adopt is to stop drinking fruit juice. That is probably the most concentrated amount of fructose the average American consumes.

Let's remember, however, that we do eat whole, fresh, raw, ripe fruit. Our bodies can profit by the amount of sugar in whole fruit. We get too much only when we press or squeeze fruit to make a glass of juice that contains four to seven teaspoons of sugar. We would never eat four to seven whole apples or oranges in one setting.

Let me condense Reiser's concluding statements to three sentences that from now on should be a part of everyone's knowledge about living and eating to avoid disease.

1. Our natural food program includes whole foods, especially complex carbohydrates (whole grains, beans, vegetables and fruits).
2. They will furnish needed fiber and excellent carbohydrates that will almost wholly eliminate the desire for white table sugar and fruit juice.
3. This food program will help build health so we will not be subject to the many environmental factors that produce the high level of degenerative diseases in our society.

CALORIES

In the old days, people ate more calories than they do now, but the calories were distributed differently. In 1910, the average intake was about 3,500 because people were more active then and needed more energy. Later, around 1960, people averaged about 3,200. Now the intake is up to about 3,400 a day. Since our activity level is no higher, on the average, there are more people who are overweight. And since we eat so much white sugar and white flour, which contain almost nothing but empty calories, we overeat because we never feel satisfied. A food program like this one contains all nutrients needed by every cell, thus the appetite is satisfied and we don't overeat.

Also, we eat more fat than we used to, and more than we need. Our intake averages 42 percent of calories, most of it in junk food. The suggested amount for good health is 10 to 20 percent of calories. Our major sources of fats are butter and nuts and seeds. In 1970, the average man weighed 10 pounds more than he did in 1960, and the average woman, seven pounds more.

IMITATION FOODS

All through our inspection of what we should not eat, we find man-made, synthetic foods (Hightower, 1976). This didn't just happen; it was planned. In an article urging people to eat synthetic foods, an executive with a large food company says: "This is not an intriguing prospect for most people, so the soy-protein foods should look like foods we are familiar with." An executive of a major food manufacturing chain said, "Eventually we'll have to depend on artificial foods to feed the world's population. By using artificial ingredients now, we're helping in their development."

Much of our food is labeled "imitation," but what exactly does that mean? Sausage was formerly called imitation if it had more than a little cereal or water; cheese, if it didn't have enough fat; and jelly, if it didn't have the standard amount of fruit (Hunter, 1978).

People don't like to buy imitation foods, so the labeling rules were changed to allow labels that weren't so negative. Imitation maple syrup can be labeled "pancake" syrup, and imitation bacon can be called "breakfast strips." These foods, if not imitation, would have to have labeling information, but imitation foods do not have to, nor do they have to be equal nutritionally to their real counterparts.

Doesn't it seem to you that the big food companies are going out of their way to turn the food industry to synthetic foods? Why not just try to do what's been done since man evolved, which is furnish real food that nourishes our bodies.

With fake foods, food companies can buy raw materials cheaply when the market is stable. Then they can patent their new discoveries and discourage competition. The executives keep their jobs, and the company will have raw materials regardless of the weather or anything else. They can control the market and be sure of profits. In other words, nothing ever spoils, and the shareholders are happy.

Imitation Foods Lack Variety

A variety of nutrients is seldom available in imitation foods. People who buy ready-to-eat imitation chicken, ham, tuna and turkey made from soybeans are getting only the nutrients in soybeans. The foods are called "textured vegetable proteins." This way of eating breaks Rule Four of my *Home Study Course*, which says "vary your diet." If we eat the chicken and turkey from the health food store, plus whole grains and beans, we have a varied diet, which we need because no one food has all 50 nutrients.

Flavors Are Synthetic

What flavor do you want? The answer used to be chocolate, strawberry or vanilla. Now you can take your choice of many, and you'll have to, to tolerate the processed, refined food that has very little flavor left after the natural flavors were destroyed by heat or other processing. One fluid ounce of liquid coconut flavoring can replace natural coconut flavor in 100 pounds of candy (Hunter, 1978).

Most of the 1,500 flavors are synthetic or imitation. Would you like tomato flavor? You have several choices of tomato flavor, and you might not get one bite of real tomato in the whole recipe.

Natural garlic and onion flavors don't last long in foods, so flavors are made by putting artificial oils in capsules that dissolve quickly when blended with moist food. The artificial oils last on the shelf for a year, whereas fresh onion or garlic may sprout or mold.

Bread Additives

Bread can be fortified with non-instant powdered milk to furnish excellent protein, if *we* make the bread. If the factories make it, 50 percent of the powdered milk is often replaced by vegetable oils, whey and modified starch, which are cheaper but not so nutritious. The replacement is used in cakes, doughnuts, muffins, biscuits, pancake mixes, cookies, cream fillings and icings.

Synthetic Fish Sticks

Are you having frozen fish sticks for dinner? Here's what you may be eating. Blocks of frozen fish are sawed into diagonal pieces that make them look like natural fillets. They are put on a conveyer belt and battered, breaded and fried. Then they are refrozen, packaged, heat sealed, stored and shipped. Later you buy them and thaw and reheat them for your family. At every step of the processing, food value is lost; the result is nutritionally deficient fish.

Maybe you'd rather have shrimp. A factory worker pours tons of tiny thawed shrimp into one end of a machine. At the other end, out come 20 or so large "shrimp" for every 300 to 400 tiny shrimp that went in. They can also be shaped into cutlets or rounds. Clams are also treated this way.

The FDA requires the label to tell the shopper that the food is "restructured," but the same food has no labels in restaurants (Hunter, 1978).

Imitation Fruits and Vegetables

The cherry on your grapefruit or your cupcake may not be real. Synthetic fruit is made by dropping tiny amounts of colored and flavored sodium alginate into calcium chloride. A "skin" forms on the outside of each drop. When the drops cure, the substance inside of the skin gels. Such cherries are also used in fruit cakes and pie fillings. Many other fruits and vegetables are made the same way. They are popular because they may be cooked but still stay crisp. The only thing wrong is that they have almost no food value (Hunter, 1978).

Raisins can be cheaply and easily made of sugar, corn syrup, vegetable oils and fats, other ingredients and raisin flavor. It's impossible to know if the raisins are real or make-believe.

Are the Potato Chips Real?

A potato chip used to be a potato chip. Then along came chips made from dried potatoes. They're the ones that are all the same shape and are neatly packed in a small container. Are those newcomers potato chips?

The original chips break easily and don't keep well on the shelf; they become rancid in a month or two. The new chips, with their preservatives, last up to one year.

Manufacturers of the original chips ridiculed the newcomers, and said they weren't really chips, but the courts ruled that there was no major difference, so the newcomers are also called potato chips. However, since 1977, the label has to say, "made from dried potatoes" in letters half as large as the words "potato chips." Often the new chips cost more than the old, and according to a survey, some people can't really tell the difference. Other people, however, report that the natural potato flavor is not there, or that the new chip is a "lousy product" (Hunter, 1978).

"Anything" Food

"Anything" food is my name for a mass of something that can be flavored with chocolate and be called chocolate pudding; with cheese and be called cheese sauce; with fish and be called fish sticks. The list goes on and on—sausages, bacon bits, turkey rolls and ice cream.

It can be dried, extruded, baked, shaped, flavored and stretched. It is the "silly putty" of the food world (Hightower, 1976). "Anything" food can be mixed with Colby cheese or fig bars, so-called strawberry filling in pastries and even brownies.

ADDITIVES

Additives of all kinds are put into our foods in great amounts. Even the FDA doesn't know how many are being used or who is using them and why. It is estimated that from 3,000 to 10,000 additives are in use. It's impossible to get an accurate number because there are no complete records of the additives approved before 1958 (Verrett, 1976).

Possibly no more than 7 percent of the additives have any vitamin or mineral value. All the rest are used to change the appearance, taste or texture of the food.

Many flavors are used because processing destroys the natural flavors in foods. Preservatives keep meat from changing color, bread from molding and fats from becoming rancid. More than 90 percent of the colors used are synthetic. Those and other synthetic agents make foods firm, clear or crisp, and make them foam or not foam. Others are just to make the food look like what it is not.

Most of the additives have been tested very little, but there are three tests that all chemical additives are given:

1. To determine whether the chemicals are toxic or lethal for short periods.
2. To determine toxicity for longer lengths of time.
3. To determine if the chemical causes cancer or organ damage over a lifetime.

Other tests examine the reproductive organs for birth defects and genetic damage, but very few chemicals have been subjected to this test.

Sweeteners should undergo all the tests, since people eat a lot of sugar over a long period of time. However, one widely used sweetener, Nutra-Sweet, was evidently tested only by the company that sells it—G. D. Searle and Company.

Nutra-Sweet is also called aspartame, and it is made from two amino acids. Here's the bad news: For each molecule of Nutri-Sweet consumed, we release into the blood one molecule of wood alcohol, also called methanol. During Prohibition, when the alcoholics could not get their usual drink, they drank wood alcohol. Some of them died, and some of them went blind. In the body, wood alcohol is oxidized to formaldehyde, a known carcinogen, and it produces squamous-cell carcinomas in experimental animals when they inhale it. It can cause mutations, birth defects and brain damage in laboratory animals and, in humans, confusion, leg cramps, severe headache and loss of vision (*Journal of Applied Nutrition,* Vol. 36, No. 1, pp. 42–54).

Packaging material would not ordinarily be tested with long-term tests because it would be unlikely that people would be exposed for any length of time. However, vinyl chloride was approved for meat wrapping, but it was found to cause cancer when workers in the factory where the meat was packaged developed liver cancer.

Test animals are given doses of the chemicals that range from 100 to 1,000 times higher than humans could receive in ordinary circumstances. The companies whose products are being tested ridicule the massive amounts of the chemical given to test animals, saying no one would ever be exposed to such large doses, but the large doses are used to try to compensate for the small numbers and the short life spans of the animals. The large doses are needed to reveal all possible adverse effects that might happen in a lifetime. If a chemical caused cancer in 1 percent of the population of 50 rats, the cancer might be overlooked in the experiment. Yet, if that percentage of humans died of cancer, two million people would die. Researchers multiply the safe dosage by 10 to allow for sensitivity in animal species, and then multiply it by an additional 10 to allow for individual animal sensitivities. That gives a 100-fold safety margin, which may not be enough.

Besides that, animals in studies are exposed to only one additive at a time, but humans are exposed to hundreds at all times in air, food and water, as well as to industrial chemicals and to drugs given by doctors. It is well known that chemicals can cause worse damage when more than one is ingested or breathed in, but they have never been tested completely.

The company that markets the chemical must submit proof to the FDA that the additive is safe. However, the FDA can set tolerance levels for the additives. According to the Delaney Clause, the only chemical that cannot have tolerance levels set is a cancer-causing agent. That clause rules that no chemical can be used if it is shown to cause cancer at any potency in either man or animal.

Many tested chemicals and some not tested but Generally Recognized As Safe (GRAS) have been withdrawn from the market because new tests showed toxicity (Verrett, 1976).

Two examples are Red Dye #2, which was used for 50 years, and cyclamate, an artificial sweetener. Both were taken off the market when tests showed the additive caused cancer and other ailments in animals. After the ban on cyclamate, the company and independent laboratories kept testing, and finally asked again for acceptance. The request was turned down, so another additive that had been used for years was taken off the market. Hundreds of other additives are still on the market, no doubt without sufficient testing, and sufficient testing may never be done. Our best bet is to eat natural foods that don't have additives.

AUTOMATED FOOD DISPENSING

Some institutions such as schools have to serve so many people in such a short time that they run cafeteria trays on a conveyer belt, stop them under one nozzle that drops a serving of mashed potatoes, then under the next nozzle for a squirt of gravy, then on down the row for the rest of the meal (Hunter, 1978). Some items squirted on the tray are rather liquid, but they solidify when exposed to air.

Several years ago, I attended a meeting of a school food service organization and heard about this serving method. One of the speakers said, "Sometimes the gravy gets squirted on the salad instead of the potatoes, but we're improving our service all the time." Everybody laughed, but I wondered what the kids at school thought about salad with gravy.

SOIL DETERMINES THE HEALTH OF FOODS

If you'll imagine a cubic foot of soil, then replace two pounds, about four cups, of that soil with organic matter, that's what it takes to make good soil. The soil will then contain nutrients needed to make healthy plants. Water will penetrate to the roots of the plants, and there won't be much runoff or erosion. Organisms in the soil will change nutrients present into other compounds as needed by the plants (Ebeling, 1981).

If plants can't get nutrients from the soil, they will not live, and animals and humans in that area will not be healthy. Soil, plants, animals and humans must all be given food supplements (called fertilizers, when given to plants).

Crop yield is limited by whatever nutrient is present in the smallest amount. If only one nutrient is missing, completely or in part, it will not grow. This is called the "law of the minimum." We've long known that a nutrient missing in a human diet causes death or disease; now we realize it's the same for plants. And plants need vitamins and minerals, as humans do.

Some parts of Australia are called "trace element deserts" because one or more elements are missing, even in small amounts, and plants can't grow.

The Florida citrus industry could not exist in Florida's sandy soil unless trace elements were added to the soil or sprayed on the foliage. Such small amounts are needed that the missing elements can be absorbed through the leaves.

Vary Your Diet

Certain plants require a lot of some elements, moderate amounts of others and small amounts of still others, the same way that humans obtain different amounts in different foods we eat. That is why Rule 4 of the *Home Study Course* is "vary your diet." If you eat only a few foods, you might be eating foods that have the smallest amounts of certain nutrients, and deficiencies of those nutrients can lead to disease.

Too little magnesium in the diet is known to cause heart disease. It also causes potassium to be lost from the body, and potassium is important for a healthy heart. Finland has a very high rate of heart disease and a very low content of magnesium in the soil. Arteries go into spasm when magnesium is deficient, and also when a lot of fertilizers high in nitrogen, phosphorus and potassium are used.

Years ago (before I became interested in nutrition and changed my diet), I used to have muscular spasms and fast heartbeat, and when I took moderate amounts of all nutrients in supplement form along with my good diet of natural foods, the spasms quickly disappeared. Now, I see many people who have such spasms, often in their feet and legs. My diet plan, which includes all the nutrients, eliminates the problem.

Other nutrients that are deficient in soils have been noted. Sulfur and sulfur-containing amino acids are required for the manufacture of proteins. Plants that are deficient are spindly and stunted, and they have yellowish leaves. If your tomato plants look sickly, they might need more sulfur.

Selenium in Soil

Selenium is required for plants and animals, but in some areas certain plants accumulate so much selenium that when cattle graze on them, they get alkali disease. However, cattle won't eat those plants if any other plants are available.

A deficiency of selenium in humans affects the heart muscle; the heart enlarges, and it can fail and cause death. This is called Keshan disease, and it was very common in China where the selenium had leached out of the soil. Crops, especially corn, soybeans and sweet potatoes, are low in selenium. Selenium was given to thousands of children at the rate of one-half to one microgram a week. After about five years, not one new case of Keshan disease was reported.

In many areas, animals don't get enough selenium in their feed crops. The tiny differences in one study showed that states that had 0.06 ppm or more selenium in crops had a significantly lower death rate from cancer than the states that had 0.05 ppm or less.

An infant's death is always tragic, especially when it dies of SIDS (Sudden Infant Death Syndrome). Infants' blood is low in selenium and vitamin E, and this deficiency may be related to the disease. Infants who are breast-fed in the first month of life receive 10 times more vitamin E and more than twice as much selenium as infants fed cow's milk formulas (Ebeling, 1981).

Agriculture and Nutrition

In addition to the nutritional value of plant crops to the animals and humans who eat them, the business of agriculture has an influence on the food humans eat.

To make sure vegetables and fruits are available and the competition is squelched, big combines are taking over the farms and produce. They grow the produce and process it themselves or sell it if they don't need it. They produce 10 percent of what they process, but they have 78 percent more of the producers on contract, with is 88 percent of the total. Is anything wrong with that? Maybe nothing, but the contract is prepared by the corporation lawyer, printed and delivered on a take-it-or-leave-it basis.

Vegetable growers sign up with big food corporations that have 69 percent of their vegetables grown under contract with the growers. The corporation decides what part of the crop is acceptable, and it buys that part at, say, 23 cents a pound. In 1972, the farmer got paid only 0.0005 cents for 8 percent of his crop of asparagus. The corporation has sole power to decide whether the crop is worth 23 cents or 0.0005 cents. The farmer can offer his unacceptable asparagus only to the corporation. If the corporation doesn't want to buy it, the farmer can sell it for any price he can get. But there is nowhere else to sell it.

The farmer may have to give his crop away to the corporation, but the corporation sells it at a pretty penny to be used as asparagus soup, asparagus cuts and asparagus tips (Hightower, 1975).

THE FUTURE

The future holds great promise for people who

want to be well. We should eat natural foods and take moderate amounts of all food supplements to allow for any loss of food value in shipping or in poison sprays that we may not be able to avoid, and for the unusual stresses of the environment that we're all subjected to. In the 18 years that I've been interested in nutrition, I have seen great changes made. More and more people are realizing the importance of nutrition and are assuming the responsibility for their own health. Many physicians and other health professionals are suggesting changes in diet and supplements of vitamins and minerals to obtain and maintain health. Let's each one tell someone else about the delight of waking up every morning without pain, with no damaging stress to worry us, and with the unlimited energy to work and play that we deserve.

We can be healthy, energetic and slim, and we *deserve* to be.

QUESTIONS

TRUE/FALSE

1. Lead, mercury and cadmium in our drinking water can take the place of required minerals and damage our bodies.

2. Studies show that people who live in soft water areas have more poisonous lead in their bones than people who live in hard water areas.

3. Side effects of niacin include a flush that causes red, stinging skin for 30 to 40 minutes.

4. Some investigators think that caffeine will some day be recognized as one of our major health hazards.

5. The most important thing about protein is to eat a varied intake of plant and animal protein and to digest it well.

6. Fast-food hamburger chains and schools are often the first users of synthetic foods.

7. Microbes are becoming resistant to the antibiotics in animal feed, and the animals and humans have to be fed larger and larger amounts of the antibiotics.

8. Soy, which is added to beef to make patties, absorbs up to four times its weight in water.

9. We never fry anything. Instead, we "frizzle" (a little butter in a moderate skillet).

10. Hardened fat such as margarine raises the melting point of the fat above body temperature, and it becomes saturated in our blood.

11. More fatty deposits in the arteries are caused by margarine than by butter and eggs.

12. Worthless carbohydrates are made from cotton, paper waste, rayon and cellophane, and added to food, but no one can tell they are there.

13. High-cellulose bread, made with a large amount of fiber, may have a severe shortage of nutrients.

14. Diets containing sugar rather than starch can lead to 300 percent more triglycerides in the blood, which can lead to heart attack and stroke.

15. The average American thinks fruit juice is good for us, but fructose (the sugar in fruit) increases the levels of triglycerides that lead to heart attack and strokes.

MULTIPLE CHOICE

1. Water must be available for life itself because: (a) the blood is mostly water, (b) the urine contains wastes dissolved in water, (c) we die in a few days if we have no water, (d) most everything in our cells is dissolved in water.

2. The following conditions may be symptoms of early alcoholism: (a) sneaking drinks, (b) low self-esteem, (c) self-pity, (d) reduction of sex drive.

3. Alcohol leads to: (a) cirrhosis of the liver, (b) birth defects, (c) tendency to add weight.

4. Caffeine has adverse reactions that can lead to: (a) heart disease, (b) cataracts, (c) diabetes, (d) stress damage.

5. Cholesterol—good or bad? (a) eggs are good food, and we can eat one or two a day, (b) cholesterol will not harm us unless we get too much, (c) we manufacture cholesterol in every cell, (d) cholesterol is required for life itself.

6. Vegetable oils can be detrimental to our health because of: (a) high heat, (b) solvent (such as gasoline) left in the oil, (c) fatty acids removed from the oil, (d) a preservative that is added.

7. To be used as margarine, oil is hardened by: (a) adding hydrogen to the oil, (b) heating it to a high temperature, (c) pressing it, (d) making it into saturated fats.

8. Oils can cause cell damage: (a) by being exposed to oxygen and becoming rancid, (b) by having a preservative added, (c) by being reheated, (d) by being kept in a cooker for long periods of time.

9. Hardened vegetable oil is dangerous because it contributes to the incidence of: (a) nerve disease, (b) heart disease, (c) hardening of the arteries, and (d) cancer.

10. Imitation food includes: (a) sausage with more than a little cereal and water, (b) cheese if it doesn't have enough fat, (c) jelly if it doesn't have enough fruit.

ANSWERS

True/False

1. T 2. T 3. T 4. T 5. T 6. T 7. T 8. T
9. T 10. T 11. T 12. T 13. T 14. T 15. T

Multiple Choice

1. a,b,c,d 2. a,b,c,d 3. a,b,c 4. a,b,c,d 5. a,b,c,d
6. a,b,c,d 7. a,b,c,d 8. a,b,c,d 9. a,b,c,d 10. a,b,c,

REFERENCES

Abrams, H.L. Jr. *J. Appl. Nutr.*, 28(2–3):33–40, Summer 1976.

———. *J. Appl. Nutr.*, 32(2):53–87, Nov. 1980.

Brewster, L. and Jacobson, M.F. *The Changing American Diet*, Center for Science in the Public Interest, 1755 S. Street, N.W., Washington, DC 20009, 1978.

Cheraskin, E. and Ringsdorf, W.M. Jr., *New Hope for Incurable Diseases*. New York: Exposition Press, 1971.

Cheraskin, E., Ringsdorf, W.M., and Medford, F. H. *JIAPM.*, 2(2):9–17, Second Quarter, 1975.

Ebeling, W. *J. Appl. Nutr.*, 33(1): 19–34, Spring 1981.

Frazier, C.A., *J. Appl. Nutr.* 31(1–2):8–13, 1979.

Hall, R.H. *Food for Nought*. New York: Vintage, 1976.

Hightower, J. *Eat Your Heart Out*. New York: Vintage, 1976.

Horrobin, D.F. *Essential Biochemistry, Endocrinology, and Nutrition*. Aylesbury, Bucks.: M.T.P., 1971.

Hunter, B.T. *The Great Nutrition Robbery*. New York: Charles Scribner's Sons, 1978.

Pauling, L. *How to Live Longer and Feel Better*. New York: W. H. Freeman, 1986.

Pfeiffer, C.C. *J. Appl. Nutr.*, 27(4):43–49, Winter 1975.

Reiser, S. Physical Differences between Starches and Sugars. In: *Medical Applications of Clinical Nutrition* (ed. J. Bland). New Canaan, CT: Keats, 1983.

Verrett, M.J. *J. Appl. Nutr.*, 28(2–3), Summer 1976.

Williams, R.J. *The Prevention of Alcoholism Through Nutrition*. New York: Bantam, 1981.

Lesson 6

VITAMINS FOR HEALTH AND ENERGY

LESSON 6—VITAMINS FOR HEALTH AND ENERGY

MILLIONS OF words have been written about vitamins. This lesson will discuss vitamins A through E. Since my nutrition students are always most interested in knowing the deficiency symptoms of the vitamins, that is what we'll emphasize in this lesson.

IMPORTANCE OF VITAMINS

Of course, we must get vitamins into our food program. If we miss getting even one, we might die. People are more interested now than ever before in the vitamin content of food, and many of them are taking vitamin supplements.

The average American probably realizes that he doesn't feel well, but he thinks his ailments, especially fatigue and stress damage, are normal, so he just puts up with feeling bad all his life. After all, everyone he knows feels bad, and he thinks that's the normal way to feel. It isn't normal, but it surely is average.

The tragedy of being tired, depressed or having heart disease or cancer is that people who suffer from these ailments are probably not getting enough vitamins and minerals, which are so easy to obtain that it is tragic for anyone to miss getting what he needs.

Vitamins function in the body as coenzymes. Enzymes direct and carry out all reactions in the body, first breaking down the food we eat into its nutritional parts, then using those parts to build up our tissue—eyes, muscles, organs and the whole person.

Each vitamin serves a different enzyme system. When we speak of a vitamin deficiency, we mean that there is not enough of that vitamin to activate all its enzyme systems. This action is not chemical but physical. A spark plug in a car is a physical thing, but what a spark plug does is something else.

Thus if we miss getting a vitamin we need, the enzyme system will not work, and some of our cells will not be made correctly. We will have disease because we didn't eat the food that contains the vitamin that makes the enzyme system work.

We all have about 15,000 enzymes, all of which function with the help of coenzymes—vitamins. Sick people need much larger amounts of vitamins than other people to make sure their enzyme systems work well. This information is based on research done by Dr. Roger J. Williams, University of Texas at Austin, who originated the genetotrophic theory of disease. This means that a person may have in his genes a requirement for larger amounts of one or more nutrients than the average person needs. If he doesn't get the larger amount, he gets sick.

His ailment may be cardiovascular disease, cancer, maturity-onset diabetes or Alzheimer's disease (our four top killer diseases), arthritis or possibly any other disease you can name. Some infants are born with illness, probably caused by not getting the nutrients they need in the womb, but many people with these diseases cause their own illnesses by not getting enough of the nutrients required for their particular genes (Bland, 1981).

The amount of the enzyme cannot be increased because its pattern is in the genes, but the amount of the coenzyme can be increased so that the entire enzyme system is prodded to function better.

It is known that 17 diseases are caused by such deficiencies of vitamins, including homocysteinuria (an inborn error in the use of amino acids, causing mental retardation, enlarged liver and cardiovascular and skeletal disorders). For those with homocysteinuria, death usually occurs in the teens.

Homocysteinuria is caused by a deficiency of an enzyme. When vitamin B12, its coenzyme, is given in an amount 1,000 times the usual dose, there is no retardation; the child lives normally. Also, it is probable that other less serious and less recognizable diseases are caused by slight deficiencies of the same coenzyme, B12.

Only one in 10,000 live births in this country results in these 17 diseases, but a deficiency of another nutrient may also cause disease. Enzymes themselves are made of amino acids, but if one of the amino acids is damaged by prescribed drugs, by X-rays, by severe infections or by the lack of one or more nutrients, a mutant is made, and every amino acid made by the same pattern will be the mutated form. As more and more of the cells are made with mutated amino acids, the organ deteriorates, and cancer or some other disease can develop (Bland, 1981).

Other conditions demand larger than usual doses of vitamins: pregnancy, liver disease, diabetes mellitus, malabsorption syndrome, effects of medication (which causes vitamin deficiency) and any illness, plus stress. There is no way to be sure that what seems like an adequate diet is really adequate (Altschule, 1974).

Also, when anyone has eaten poorly and his resistance is low, megadoses of vitamins may be needed for a short while. Later, the intake can be cut down to a maintenance dose.

The important thing is to supply enough coenzymes (vitamins). They may correct the deficiency if the need is discovered early enough.

Next, let's say a few words about dosages and about vitamins in general.

Dosages for Children

Most dosages given on labels of food supplements are for adults. Vitamin dosage for children, in general, is as follows:

1. Children age 1 to 6, ¼ the adult dose.
2. Children age 6 to 12, ½ the adult dose.
3. Children age 13 and up, take the adult dose.

Infants less than one year old usually take baby vitamins in liquid form from the health food store in amounts suggested on the label. If the child is on the borderline, say age one, six or 12, go by his size and weight, or give one-third or one-sixth of the adult dose.

Ground Rules for Vitamins

A good diet is not enough unless we're 25 years old and in excellent health. And we wouldn't stay that way very long if we were on the Standard American Diet (SAD). So many protective nutrients are missing completely or in part that it is very rare if anyone can stay healthy on that diet.

Any problem, especially stress, brings a need for added vitamins and minerals. Supplements must be used consistently by most people. Although a good diet is of utmost importance for health, we cannot stay well by eating the food from the marketplace because it is too processed and refined. So we take moderate amounts of food supplements as insurance.

Here are some ground rules for taking supplements.

1. If you're not in good health, begin with small amounts of all vitamins and minerals ground up, gradually increase to large amounts temporarily, and when your health problems are solved, cut back to maintenance doses. If the digestive system is not in good condition, suddenly putting large amounts of tablets in your stomach might cause gas, abdominal cramps or other reactions. See Lesson 1 for detailed instructions for beginning your supplement program.

2. Since no one vitamin works alone, we need all vitamins and minerals. Dr. Roger J. Williams (1971) says that all nutrients work as a team.

3. If one vitamin is given, its complex should be given—the B complex, C complex (which includes bioflavanoids) and E complex (which

includes all the tocopherols—alpha, beta, delta and gamma). The label on the E complex will say "mixed tocopherols."

4. It's best to take vitamin and mineral supplements with meals because digestive enzymes help digest the supplements along with the food.

5. Minerals are essential, both the major and trace minerals. Minerals function as vitamin-enzyme activators, so the enzyme cannot work without a mineral to activate it.

When we're starved for vitamins, we get infectious diseases. Then the endocrine glands work overtime to fight the disease. That uses up all the vitamins in the glands, and the glands become exhausted. The exhausted glands are more subject to infections, so the vicious cycle continues.

If the cells are mature, they will not suffer greatly at first if the supply of vitamins is decreased. The old cells will break down if they don't get vitamins for a long time. But new cells being made need a lot of nutrients or they won't be made correctly.

Some tissues of the body manufacture new cells continually to replace old cells. Some of these are the skin, pancreas, the lining of the intestines and the red and many of the white blood cells. All these cells are always being worn out and replaced.

Because of this, most vitamin deficiencies show up first in damage to the skin, the lining of the intestines and the bone marrow where the red cells are made. Thus anemia and skin diseases are commonly seen in vitamin deficiencies, as are digestive problems, even those as simple as gas and bloating caused by lack of assimilation of nutrients in the small intestine (Horrobin, 1973).

Vitamin and mineral deficiencies are first shown as depletions, then as changes in the cells. But we can't see those changes. Finally, the changes are severe, and they are recognized as disease. For example, after vitamin B1 depletion, no changes were found in an experimental study for five to 10 days. After 10 days, cells changed, but classical signs of disease weren't seen for 200 days. Between 10 and 200 days, there was gradually increasing ill health, with loss of weight, loss of appetite, malaise (body weakness or discomfort often marking the onset of disease), insomnia and increased irritability (Marks, 1975).

If the diet had been improved and all vitamins and minerals given, chances are the classical signs would never have been seen because the disease would never have developed.

The RDA (Recommended Daily Allowance) for nutrients is set by the Food and Nutrition Board of the National Research Council, National Academy of Sciences. It is supposedly set for a 25-year-old male in excellent health and adjusted for all other ages. But it is very unusual for *anyone* to be healthy on such small amounts of vitamins and minerals, especially if he eats the Standard American Diet.

It is not known how much is required for sick people, those under stress or those suffering from fatigue.

If anyone has *any* ailment, nutritionists agree that he has a vitamin-mineral deficiency, especially if he has an ailment and his doctor says he has "nothing organically wrong." In that case, his doctor obviously doesn't know to test for a deficiency of a nutrient, because he hasn't studied nutrition in medical school, and he doesn't realize that nutritional deficiencies cause all diseases.

How Vitamins Work

There are only about 20 known vitamins, and they influence thousands of happenings. As coenzymes, they cause reactions at the rate of a thousand times a second. An example is what happens when peroxide is poured on the skin—it bubbles because an enzyme, peroxidase, is present on the skin and it speeds up the breakdown of peroxide. This doesn't happen when peroxide is poured on glass or wood. Trillions of similar reactions occur in the body every second.

Synthetic vs. Natural Vitamins

The controversy over whether we should take natural or synthetic vitamins goes on and on. The answer seems to be that natural is better, and we should especially get natural vitamins A, D and E. Most of us can't get enough natural B and C from supplements to give us the amount we need—the tablet would be as big as a golf ball.

Natural vitamin A is from beta-carotene, found in red, yellow and green fruits and vegetables or as retinol from meat, eggs and dairy products. Beta-carotene is really not a vitamin—it is a provitamin, and it will be changed into vitamin A by a healthy liver when the body needs it. Since it isn't stored, it can't become toxic.

Vitamin A (and D) can be assimilated more easily if our digestive systems work well enough to assimilate oils. Thus, researchers suggest that we take a little butter or cream when we take beta-carotene in order to activate enzymes to digest the fat-soluble vitamins along with the food we're eating. A small amount of butter on vegetables would be enough fat.

Synthetic D made from irradiated ergosterol is not recommended. The studies performed on humans, usually children, that showed adverse reactions from large doses of vitamin D used irradiated ergosterol, which is the kind of vitamin D added to milk. The natural vitamin D3 should be used in supplements.

Vitamin E: The suggested form is d-alpha tocopherol (or tocopheryl), acetate or succinate, not the synthetic dl-alpha.

Vitamins B and C, which are water soluble, are used up and replenished daily. It is difficult to get recommended amounts of natural B and C in tablet form, so we take synthetic B and C in tablets and depend on our food to give us natural B and C. Food is the most important part of this program, but we can't be well without food supplements.

A synthetic vitamin contains one or more pure substances. The natural product—desiccated liver, for example—that is a good source of all known and possibly some unknown B vitamins contains other vitamins, minerals, trace elements, enzymes and coenzymes, as well as other important nutritional elements. These substances may determine the degree to which the entire B complex, or whatever portion of it is in liver, is absorbed and used. Medical literature contains many reports that natural liver has more value than synthetic vitamins (Hunter, 1974).

However, it is well to remember what Dr. Roger J. Williams says about the differences in "natural," "artificial" and "synthetic" vitamins. Dr. Williams is the discoverer of the B vitamin pantothenic acid. He says: "First, we need to realize that each ingredient of our diets, including water, is a chemical. Natural chemicals include all those that enter into the makeup of living animals and plants. Artificial chemicals include those that are foreign to our bodies and to our food. Synthetic chemicals are those produced in the laboratory and may be either natural or artificial.

"When we produced natural pantothenic acid in the laboratory, we separated about 10 milligrams of slightly impure pantothenic acid from hundreds of pounds of liver at a cost of approximately $20,000. This was a natural vitamin.

"We then determined its chemical structure and duplicated its molecules exactly. The two products are identical and cannot be told apart by any means whatever. The advantage of the synthetic product made in the laboratory is obvious when we compare costs. The wholesale price of the amount that cost us $20,000 to produce from liver is now less than one-tenth of one cent" (Williams, Bronson).

"Let's consider something else. If you have a vitamin C product that states on the label, 'From rose hips,' you have either a product of very small potency or one that has synthetic vitamin C combined with a small amount of natural rose hips. If the product were of high potency, it would be too big to swallow. When vitamins are chewed, they have to be made to taste good. Thus, they have sugar and other flavorings in them. It is better to swallow a small tablet to get a big amount of vitamin C than to have to chew many tablets containing sugar to get the dosages of vitamin C recommended these days to ward off all the pollution, the excess cholesterol and hundreds of other problems that humans get when they don't get enough vitamin C."

Probably most important of all to remember is that these foods we take in tablet form to supplement our diet are just that—supplements. If we eat only junk food and take vitamin-mineral tablets, we can't be well. Food is still more important than tablets. When we eat nutritious food, we will get natural vitamins. To those nutrients, let's add supplements in tablet form and let's remember we can never maintain health with a diet of junk foods and vitamin tablets.

Once in a while, when I meet new people interested in nutrition, someone will say, "I'm taking all vitamins and minerals, but I don't feel any better." I ask them if they're taking digestive enzymes. Nutrients may pass unabsorbed through the entire digestive system. We must have bile to emulsify fats; plus hydrochloric acid, manufactured in the stomach and also available at all health food stores in tablet form. We also need digestive enzymes from the pancreas, which change the food we eat into substances that go into our blood, then into our cells to repair tissue and to furnish energy.

The body's ability to metabolize (use) foods decreases with age; thus, people might not be able to absorb the nutrients they're so carefully taking. That's because the digestive tract doesn't have the vitamins and minerals needed to make healthy cells.

Also, if anyone has liver disease, his tissues will be unable to use the vitamins he takes, because the liver will not be able to process them—or to make enzymes and hormones needed to use the vitamins. Other diseases such as tropical sprue can have the same effect. In this condition, the lining of the intestines becomes diseased and people are unable to absorb food. Also, doctors' drugs and alcohol interfere with the use of various nutrients (Herbert, 1975).

VITAMIN A

Vitamin A is needed for growth, health and life in humans. Without it, we would die. It is especially important for vision, reproduction and secretion of mucus to keep our mucous membranes healthy in order to avoid colds and other infections, and to keep cells that line blood vessels and tubes anywhere in the body from becoming sick.

The sick cells cause fat to build up in the arteries, which leads to heart disease. We also must have vitamin A to manufacture differentiated cells. When cells grow from one fertilized egg cell, the same kind of cell is made during several cell divisions. Later, cells begin to change to muscle, skin, hair, liver and all other tissue cells. These are differentiated cells. Cancer is said to be caused by the loss of our ability to make differentiated cells—tumors are cells that are similar to the egg cell we began life with. So if vitamin A is plentiful enough, it will make cells that are different from each other rather than all alike as are cancer cells.

Another special use of liquid emulsified vitamin A is to apply it on the skin in cases of eczema or skin lesions such as psoriasis or even hemorrhoids. When applying, first test the liquid on a small area of the skin.

The relatively new supplement form of vitamin A, beta-carotene, is now being used much more than vitamin A from fish liver oil or in the liquid emulsified form. Beta-carotene is a provitamin and is not changed to vitamin A until the body needs it; therefore, it is not stored and it is nontoxic. Vitamin A is often deficient in the American diet. It is found in liver, cream, eggs and butter. Carotene or provitamin A is found in dark green and yellow vegetables. Only one percent of the carotene in raw carrots can be absorbed when we eat carrots, because the teeth can't break down the cellular structure of the carrots. About 30 percent can be absorbed from steamed carrots because hot steam breaks open the cells of the plant and releases the nutrients. Carrot juice is a good source of carotene. Vitamin A is destroyed by blood-thinning medications such as Dicumarol or by mineral oil.

Deficiencies

Night blindness is often the first symptom of a vitamin A deficiency. Such a deficiency is also one of the main causes of blindness in the United States (Rosenberg, 1974). Vitamin A is especially important for the health of the retina and the pigment layer of the eye. The cornea gets calcified and opaque without A and blindness may occur. There is sensitivity to bright lights, itching, burning and inflammation of the eyelids. Some eye changes may be irreversible (Robinson, 1972).

Babies are born with low stores of vitamin A because A can't pass easily through the placenta. Beta-carotene might help during pregnancy. Many infants are born malformed because of deficiencies of A (Jennings, 1970). Vitamin A is essential for the normal growth and development of bone. Without it, the skull and the holes in the skull that the nerves go through don't enlarge normally. The brain and nerves therefore are damaged (Horrobin, 1973), and the baby can be born with a birth defect.

Skin damage is common. Along with deficiencies of B and D, vitamin A deficiencies can cause the skin surface to be in such poor condition that the cells can't fight the bacteria that are always on the skin inside and outside the body. Deficiencies also cause dry, rough, scaly skin; acne; and goose-pimple-like bumps that first appear along the upper forearms and thighs, then on the shoulders.

Vitamin A improves acne, but zinc is needed to get A out of storage in the liver and send it to the blood for circulation to all cells, so zinc may help acne more than A does (Ballentine, 1978).

The skin and mucous membranes in the respiratory passages and all over the body thicken and become dry in a deficiency, which leads to infections. The skin of the intestines is damaged without sufficient vitamin A. Therefore, if digestion is not good, there can be frequent infections of the stomach and intestines.

Moisture protects the inner skin so bacteria, viruses and allergens (substances that cause allergies) can't get in. Without vitamin A, the moisture is not secreted, and the inner skin dries out. The dried skin cells flatten out and look more like outside skin. When these unusual flat cells are found in the cervix or entrance to the uterus in a Pap smear, the patient is told she is in danger of developing cancer. Thus one of the most frequent cancers in women is partly caused by a deficiency of vitamin A, which stops the secretion of mucus in the cells of the cervix. The dried-out cells are abnormal and can turn into cancer cells (Ballentine, 1978).

The same thing happens in the lungs. Lung cancer starts in the cells that line the respiratory tract when vitamin A is deficient, and the mucus-secreting cells dry out, become abnormal and change to cancer cells (Ballentine, 1978).

Vitamin A deficiency causes thickening of the cells that line tubules that go from one organ to another; the tubules close up. If the tube from the pancreas to the small intestine closes, the digestive enzymes in the pancreas, which should go to the small intestine to digest food, can't get out of the pancreas and they become activated there. They then do what all enzymes are supposed to do—digest something. They digest the pancreas itself, causing holes to appear and disease of the pancreas. This ailment is called pancreatitis.

In general, vitamin A deficiency can cause damage to tissues all over the body: kidney stones are caused partly by a deficiency of A, probably because the deficiency causes lesions (sores) in the kidney (Guyton, 1976). Vitamin A protects us from infection at every point where bacteria, viruses or pollutants from air, water or food can enter the body. Dry, brittle hair; loss of appetite and weight; sterility; and damage to the enamel of the teeth are common deficiency symptoms (Rosenberg, 1970). Stomach ulcers are also common, as are infections of the tonsils, sinuses, bronchial passages, mouth and lungs (Jennings, 1970). Mucous membranes and all other lining surfaces of the body from mouth to anus need vitamin A.

Damage to the lungs can cause pneumonia and other respiratory infections (Horrobin, 1973). This has been known since 1930 (Ballentine, 1978). Other ailments are hemeralopia (day blindness—defective vision in bright light), keratomalacia (dry spots that cause the cornea to become soft) and hyperkeratosis (overgrowth of cells in the cornea).

Probably the most exciting information pertains to cancer and vitamin A. The first time I heard about this relationship was on March 11, 1977, when a lecturer from M.D. Anderson Hospital and Tumor Institute of Houston, Texas, said it would be almost impossible to get cancer of the skin or mouth if we ate enough vitamin A. The mouth is lined with epithelial cells—the same kind of cells that line all body cavities. The cancers of these cells are called carcinoma, and they make up about 85 percent of our cancers.

Two researchers in Germany, Wolf and Ransberger, have used vitamin A treatment for cancer for about 40 years with great success.

Toxicity

Vitamin A from fish liver oil is one of the two vitamins that are toxic in large amounts. (Vitamin D is the other one.) Symptoms of toxicity are dry, rough skin; enlarged liver (it will cause pain at the right side of the waist); and painful joint swellings.

Also, itchy rash, severe headache, loss of appetite and pain in the long bones are signs of too much of the vitamin, as well as nausea, irritability, headaches, hair loss and increased pressure in the cranium. The condition may be mistaken for a brain tumor. All these symptoms and signs disappear when vitamin A is reduced (Marks, 1975). In all the history of medicine, only about two dozen cases of overdose have been recorded (Rosenberg, 1970).

In recent years, beta-carotene has been used when large doses are needed, because beta-carotene is a provitamin, and it isn't changed to vitamin A until the body needs it. Thus it is not toxic.

Dosage

Investigators suggest dosages ranging from 10,000 IU to 50,000 IU as the ideal daily allowance. Cheraskin (1976) suggests about 33,000 IU a day. If you're in a good health, probably 25,000 IU would

be enough for a maintenance dose. If you have any symptoms or signs of vitamin A deficiency, you may want to take as much as 100,000 IU—half with breakfast, half with dinner for a while. Take beta-carotene if you take more than 25,000 IU. However, some nutritionists suggest dividing the amount between beta-carotene and fish liver oil. When your symptoms clear, reduce to 25,000 IU and stay on that amount indefinitely.

If vitamin A is needed for a severe condition, several methods will increase absorption without increasing the amount of A. Lecithin, an emulsifying agent, will help. Pancreatic enzymes, which contain an enzyme that breaks down oil, will help, and taking hydrochloric acid tablets will improve the digestion of protein, which will improve vitamin A absorption. It is best not to take vitamin A on an empty stomach (Bland, 1981).

VITAMIN B COMPLEX

One of the most important things to remember about the B vitamins is that they all must be taken together. If one is taken in large doses, it might cause a deficiency of others.

We need more B vitamins when we're under stress or when we have infections. Also, people who drink a lot of alcohol or coffee or eat a lot of refined carbohydrates need more. Children and pregnant women need more than usual for normal growth (Kirschmann, 1973).

Some of the recent research on suicides in adolescents points to deficiencies of B vitamins in the diet. Suicide is now ranked as the second leading cause of death in persons from 10 to 20 years of age, according to officials of the American Association of Suicidology. Signs that a teenager or even an adult might be thinking about suicide are mental depression, sleeplessness, loss of appetite, weight loss, headache and general aches and pains, as well as psychological symptoms like lethargy, crying, apathy and an inability to concentrate. These correspond to symptoms of B vitamin deficiencies. It may be difficult to get a person in this condition to change his diet, but the rewards are so great that it should be attempted (*Houston Chronicle*, 1978). Our brain and nervous system couldn't work without the B complex, so if you know someone who can't think clearly or a child who is hyperactive or sluggish, B complex should help.

Also, all the following tissues depend on B complex: hair, skin, eyes, mouth, liver and smooth muscles of the intestines.

In one double-blind study (Jooli and Eswaran, 1980) injections of vitamins B1, B6 and B12 were given to a group of 30 schizophrenics. Results showed such improvement that the investigators recommended giving injections of the three vitamins to all acute schizophrenics. They said the vitamins obviously provided nutrients needed by the brain because deficiencies had led to the inability of the brain to form neurotransmitters, substances which send messages along nerves so we can think.

Sources

Best sources of the B complex are brewer's yeast, wheat germ and liver. Others are whole grains, meat, fresh vegetables, legumes, eggs, nuts and seeds. There are smaller amounts in many other foods. Yeast and liver should be balanced with calcium and magnesium because of their high phosphorus content.

Yogurt is a good source of the Bs because it provides friendly bacteria that manufacture B vitamins in the intestines. Buy yogurt that says "live culture" on the label. Some yogurt is combined with the culture first, then pasteurized, which kills the bacteria. If the milk is pasteurized first and the culture added later, the friendly bacteria are still alive. This yogurt can be used as a starter to make your own.

Deficiencies

If we're a little deficient in B vitamins, we lack energy, and our brains are tired. We can't think well, and our nerves are joggled (Pfeiffer, 1975). These signs and symptoms appear before any physical symptoms show up (Jennings, 1970).

Soon, we can't digest food, we aren't hungry, our stomach tissues are not healthy and we become constipated. When people come to me for counseling, they tell me their ailments, and almost without fail, they are tired, depressed and constipated. Just think how many people are extremely deficient in B vitamins.

There are plenty of B vitamins in complex carbohydrates such as whole grains, vegetables, fruits, nuts, seeds and dairy products, but the B's have been processed out of white flour and white sugar. Enriched bread isn't really good because only B1, B2 and B3 plus iron are added. That makes a poor ratio, and it can cause a deficiency of those that aren't added.

On a poor food program, muscles waste away and become paralyzed. The heart may not be able to pump blood around the body. Then the kidneys can't excrete enough urine, and large amounts of water accumulate in the tissues. This is called edema. Heart irregularities are common. The heart muscle weakens and can cause cardiac failure. The right side of the heart becomes enlarged. Three times the normal amount of blood may return to the heart, and the muscles are so weak they can't pump it out.

Other signs of deficiency are redness of the mouth and tongue; the patient may vomit and have severe diarrhea. These conditions can cause death. Still other deficiencies are an enlarged, flabby colon and hemorrhoids. The blood vessels change. Small vessels disappear, and large ones become larger, thus some cells may be so far from a capillary they can't get food.

The heart, blood vessels and nerves use a tremendous amount of energy; thus they need a lot of B vitamins. There might be enough B's to allow the heart muscle to beat, but not enough to furnish energy for every brain cell. Thus someone might be forgetful or irritable, yet his heart beats on and on (Horrobin, 1973).

If the adrenal glands don't get enough B's to make the energy they need, cortisone might not be made in sufficient amounts to make the immune system work to keep us from having allergies (Jennings, 1970). Also, output of sex hormones is decreased without B, and then the sex organs can't function well (Horrobin, 1973).

Dosage

The B vitamins should be taken in a certain ratio to each other. B1, B2 and B6 are usually given in equal amounts. B3 (niacin or niacinamide) and pantothenic acid are usually given in doses five to seven times more than those of B1, B2 and B6. Check with Lesson 1 of this course.

Most important, if you take large doses of any vitamin for a short time, reduce to the dosage for maintenance by tapering down.

Even if we eat plenty of B vitamins, we may lose them if we take drugs. Vitamins B and C are partially destroyed by aspirin, antibiotics, diuretics and refined sugar. B-complex vitamins are needed to process alcohol and coffee, yet most alcoholics and coffee drinkers do not eat foods high in vitamin B.

VITAMIN B1 (THIAMINE)

Vitamin B1, thiamine, is a coenzyme. That is, it works with an enzyme to break down carbohydrates into glucose, particularly for brain food. It is called the morale vitamin because it gives us a good attitude and mental disposition. We must have it for growth as well as good muscle tone, especially in the stomach, intestines and heart.

Think what happens if our muscle tone in these three organs isn't good. The muscles in our stomach walls couldn't churn food to mix it with stomach acid, and we couldn't digest and assimilate proteins. Thus we couldn't turn the proteins we eat into amino acids to repair tissue and to replace cells that wear out every day. The heart is a muscle, and without tone, the heart couldn't beat. Without muscle tone, the intestines couldn't push the fecal matter along so that it can finally be excreted. People who are constipated understand that very well.

If we eat the average American intake of sugar—which is much too much—128 pounds per person per year—or if we drink too much alcohol, we will destroy our thiamine. Also, if we have to submit to surgery or if we suffer from stress, fever or diarrhea, we need more thiamine than usual.

Deficiencies

Let's begin our long list of thiamine deficiency symptoms with early symptoms: loss of appetite, vomiting, fatigue, lack of vigor, loss of weight. Deficiency is widespread in elderly people (Marks, 1975).

Mild deficiencies include sleeplessness, headache, numbness, burning and aching hands and feet, fatigue, insomnia, diarrhea, debility, plugged hair follicles, stomach and intestinal disturbances, weak and sore muscles, enlarged liver and swollen and weak heart with palpitations. These also can be severe. Our emotions will be unstable, and we'll be depressed. Alcoholics have so much alcohol in the blood that thiamine can't be absorbed. Deficiencies often show up after surgery or after diseases that cause fever (Pfeiffer, 1975).

The tissues that suffer most from thiamine deficiencies are those that depend the most on carbohydrates for energy: the cardiovascular system and the nerves (Jennings, 1970).

Early heart symptoms are fast heartbeat, shortness of breath, dizziness, irregularities in the heartbeat and being conscious of every beat. The heart rate may be slowed. Patients with advanced disease have edema (retention of fluid) in the abdomen or in the extremities. This is called ascites. The inside of the blood vessels swell and some capillaries are blocked; others have too much blood (Jennings, 1970). The patient stays in bed to avoid sudden circulatory failure and death (Sebrell, 1973).

The earliest symptoms of nerve damage are in the brain and spinal cord, causing neurasthenia (a nerve disease marked by chronic abnormal fatigue, feelings of inadequacy and insomnia), loss of attention, irritability, vague fears and inflammation of the nerves beginning as an abnormal sensation of the extremities, especially of the toes and feet (Sebrell, 1973).

The nerve cells swell, the myelin sheaths of the nerves (the coverings that protect the nerves) degenerate. Pain can radiate along the nerves in the extremities. In severe deficiency, nerves can degenerate and cause paralysis; if there is no paralysis, the muscles wither and cause severe weakness (Guyton, 1976). These conditions can return to normal within one to 14 days after B1 is given (Pfeiffer, 1975).

Gastrointestinal disturbances include loss of appetite, indigestion, constipation, occasional vomiting and a colon that is loose and floppy because the muscles are not healthy. Expectant mothers may be free of severe symptoms yet the baby's nerves can be affected (Sebrell, 1973).

Deficiencies can affect the mental processes, resulting in apathy, confusion, emotional instability, irritability, depression, fear of impending disaster, failure to concentrate and defective memory. Sometimes the mental symptoms are seen after only a few days of deficiency (Pfeiffer, 1975).

These symptoms must sound very familiar to many persons who have gone on crash diets to lose weight. If we don't get enough B1, the unpleasant symptoms can appear in a few days. That's why so many people give up their diets, saying, "Losing weight isn't worth feeling like that." They're right, it isn't. Weight loss can be pleasant. If we get all the nutrients we need, we won't be hungry. Also, if anyone in your family is an alcoholic, you probably recognize these symptoms: listlessness, apprehension, lack of appetite and fatigue. Manual dexterity is lost, the patient becomes irritable, confused and inattentive to detail (Marks, 1975). Early brain damage can occur that is irreversible, so early treatment is important. A sudden severe deficiency can cause profound mental changes (Marks, 1975).

Probably the saddest group of people with some of these symptoms are the schoolchildren, who are continually fussed at by teachers and parents. The poor child doesn't want to suffer from his poor coordination or his inability to concentrate, but often a child's diet is low enough in B1 to cause these problems.

Two diseases thought to be caused by alcohol poisoning are now known to be due to thiamine deficiency: Wernicke's syndrome, (characterized by lack of muscular coordination and mental changes) and Korsakoff's syndrome (loss of memory of the immediate past). These respond well to thiamine. Public health suggestions include fortifying alcoholic beverages with thiamine and serving thiamine-rich snacks on bar counters.

Dimness of vision similar to that found in prisoner-of-war camps can be attributed to thiamine deficiency. Without thiamine, the adrenal glands overproduce, then they get exhausted and don't produce enough hormones; therefore there is a deficiency of cortisone. The thymus—the source of immunity—withers away (Guyton, 1976). Headaches can be caused by a slight deficiency of thiamine.

Much of the thiamine is lost when a diuretic is taken. A woman I met briefly told me she was pleased that she had to take only two drugs prescribed by her doctor when most of her friends took six! Then she remembered, "Oh, I take three. I forgot about the water pills."

Water pills are taken almost universally by elderly people who lose thiamine and other nutrients just when they need them the most—when they begin to slow down due to the aging process. Waste water will be picked up and excreted if every nutrient is furnished in plentiful amounts, especially protein. If protein is digested to amino acids with the help of hydrochloric acid in the stomach, our livers will manufacture the protein, which will pick up the water, and we won't need water pills (diuretics).

VITAMIN B2 (RIBOFLAVIN)

Vitamin B2, riboflavin, helps turn proteins, carbohydrates and fats into our bodily tissues, especially eyes, hair and skin. We usually don't get enough if we don't take food supplements. But remember that we generally should take moderate amounts of all Bs rather than large amounts of only one.

There are several reasons why we don't get enough riboflavin—we drink too much alcohol, we don't have a good diet because we have ulcers or diabetes or we eat too much white sugar and white flour.

You can often notice these symptoms of deficiency:

1. Feeling of grit and sand under the eyelids
2. Sores and cracks in the corners of the mouth
3. Sore, red tongue
4. Burning of the eyes and tired eyes
5. Sensitivity to bright lights
6. Scaling around lips, nose, forehead and ears
7. Trembling, dropsy, inability to urinate
8. Dizziness, vaginal itching, oily skin.

Riboflavin deficiency is usually combined with a deficiency of B1 and B3. Many diseases such as beriberi, pellagra and sprue (inability to digest fats) are due to a deficiency of several B vitamins (Guyton, 1976).

Early B2 deficiency symptoms and signs often relate to the mouth and eyes. There is soreness and burning of the mouth and tongue that make it hard for the patient to swallow. Then the lips get shiny, red, and scaly like chapped lips and cracks appear in the corners of the mouth (Marks, 1975).

Vertical wrinkles radiate up from the upper lip, and the upper lip even "disappears" (Ballentine, 1978). The lips can also become dry, red and slick where they close. If the deficiency is severe, ulcers can form. There is sometimes discomfort when eating and swallowing (Marks, 1975). The tongue changes may be severe. The tongue becomes purple-red. The papillae (the little bumps on the tongue) stick together in clumps with slick places in between. This is called a geographic tongue because it looks like a river and its tributaries.

The eyes are sensitive to light, a condition called photophobia. They shed tears, burn, hurt and itch. They get tired and bloodshot and vision is blurred. The cornea can become hard and cause almost total blindness (Marks, 1975).

The skin becomes inflamed, scaly and oily, especially in the folds around the nose and in the creases between the nose and cheek. Little whiteheads form, and the skin resembles sharkskin (Sebrell, 1973). Deficiencies may cause a fungus such as athlete's foot, and the skin on the external sex organs can become scaly. Problems can arise in the bone marrow. Not enough red blood cells are made, so a person may have aplastic anemia (Marks, 1975).

Deep-seated deficiencies of B2 may begin with the adrenal glands and the thyroid. The adrenals direct the use of food in the body (metabolism). The thyroid sets the speed at which the body works. Without B2, much fat accumulates in the adrenals, the liver, the kidneys and the artery walls, and these tissues can't do their work. Not enough glucose can be stored in the liver and muscles, a condition that can lead to low blood sugar (Jennings, 1970).

If we eat a lot of sugar, a deficiency of B2 can lead to accumulation of sugar products that can cause cataracts. Lesser (1980) tells of a woman whose cataracts slowly receded on a dosage of 10,000 IU of vitamin A and 400 mg of riboflavin daily. The cornea can become opaque (Marks, 1975). A B2 deficiency can result in depression, forgetfulness and headaches (Guyton, 1976). Deficiency signs show up the most when patients have been burned or wounded and repair is needed. Protein is also needed in larger amounts at this time (Goodhart and Shils, 1973), but it may not be available because the stomach doesn't make enough hydrochloric acid when nutrients are deficient, and we can't turn protein into amino acids for repair of tissue without the acid. There will be a lot of gas and bloating, which can be helped by taking supplements of hydrochloric acid and by eating yogurt (Lesser, 1980) or by taking acidophilus from the health food store.

VITAMIN B3 (NIACIN)

Vitamin B3 helps improve blood circulation and helps lower excessive cholesterol in the blood. If we eat too much sugar, niacin will be eliminated from the cells.

For about 50 years, it has been known that a deficiency of niacin causes pellagra. Early signs of the disease are in the skin and the mouth. The tongue becomes red and ulcerated. Muscles are weak. The lining of the intestines is inflamed, and vomiting and diarrhea are common. There is brain damage and finally insanity and death (Horrobin, 1973).

There is very little out-and-out pellagra in this country now, but many common signs of the illness are seen in minor deficiencies of the vitamin, which show up as problems with the nerves, the skin and the digestive tract.

Early stages of deficiency are muscular weakness and poor glandular secretion. For example, the adrenal glands may not be able to secrete cortisone; the sex glands may not be able to secrete estrogen and other sex hormones. In severe deficiency, there is actual death of tissues. Diseased lesions appear in many parts of the central nervous system (CNS) and permanent mental disease or many different types of psychosis may result. Skin cracks and pigments appear in areas exposed to mechanical irritation, radiant heat, fires or sunlight. Deficiency causes irritation and inflammation of mucous membranes and other parts of the gastrointestinal tract, leading to digestive problems, partly because there is not enough breakdown of foods in the intestines so the breakdown products can repair and feed the tissues (Goodhart and Shils, 1973).

Damaged tissues cause burning of the mouth, glossitis (shiny red tongue) and stomatitis (cracks in the lips), and the skin wears off the tongue. Tartar may be deposited in the mouth (Marks, 1975).

There is loss of weight, weakness, mental depression, gas and indigestion followed by diarrhea, constipation, nausea and vomiting and achlorhydria (lack of hydrochloric acid in the stomach, without which we cannot digest protein).

Skin lesions are common. The elbows and knees are dry, scaly and have dark pigmented areas. The darkened area may spread to the legs or forearms. It seems that the skin can't repair the damage (Guyton, 1976), which begins like sunburn. The lesion may become fiery red and painful and it usually becomes infected. It is frequently found on the genitalia. The pigmentation gets worse during healing, and it may persist for a long time after lesions are healed.

Mental changes are depression, fear, confusion and impaired memory. About 2 percent have serious mental disturbances. Another type of mental change is grasping and sucking reflexes and disorientation. Laziness, then hysteria and maniacal outbursts occur (Marks, 1975).

VITAMIN B6 (PYRIDOXINE)

We know how important hydrochloric acid (HCl) is to help us digest and assimilate protein, but without B6, we can't produce the hydrochloric acid. Nor can we absorb vitamin B12. Linoleic acid, the one essential fatty acid the body can't manufacture and we have to get from food, can't function well without B6. B6 also helps digest proteins, carbohydrates and fats; it helps produce antibodies so we won't have infections or allergies, and it helps make red blood cells so we won't be anemic. With the help of B6, sugar that has been stored in the muscles and liver is released to the blood so we won't have low blood sugar.

When we're under stress, sugar is also released to our adrenal glands to furnish energy to manufacture hormones.

B6 also helps change tryptophan—an amino acid—into niacin, which then has a calming effect on the nervous system. B6 must be present for the manufacture and function of DNA and RNA, which makes new cells when our old ones wear out. B6 must be given with all other B's to avoid an imbalance or deficiency of the other B's. Larger than usual amounts should be taken during pregnancy, heart failure, aging, radiation and during the use of birth control pills.

Deficiencies

Deficiencies of B6 cause low blood sugar, water retention, numbness or cramps in arms and legs, crankiness, tremors in hands, forgetfulness, slow learning, crippling rheumatoid arthritis, neuritis, high cholesterol, kidney stones and eczema.

B6 combines with vitamin E to use polyunsaturated fats correctly. These fats must be changed by the body into prostaglandins, which are hormone-like substances that have many duties in our tissues, including preventing the fatty deposits in the arteries that lead to heart attacks.

It is thought that convulsions in infants are partly caused by B6 deficiency because nerves are damaged (Jennings, 1970). Deficiency of B6 in the brain and nervous system causes long-lasting mental problems. These problems can include degeneration of the myelin sheath of the nerves. Humans may have epileptic seizures (Ballentine, 1978). Other deficiency symptoms are mental depression, apathy, sleepiness and nausea and vomiting in children and in pregnant women (Goodhart and Shils, 1973).

Recent studies of mental problems show neuritis (inflammation of the nerves), abnormal encephalograms and loss of a sense of responsibility, plus personality changes marked by irritability and depression. Doesn't this make you wonder how many divorces and lost jobs are caused by a deficiency of B6?

The vitamin is essential for making red blood cells, and we can't absorb iron, one of the major components of the cells, without it. Blood vessel walls in the adrenal glands get thick, and nutrients can't pass easily from the blood to adrenal cells to make our natural cortisone and other hormones (Jennings, 1970).

Kidneys are affected by B6 deficiency. A kidney disease called uremia can be caused by lack of B6, which causes vomiting and loss of nutrients. B6 supplements plus a natural food diet should be given to uremic patients. Uremia damages nephrons in the kidneys and they can no longer excrete the poisonous waste products of proteins. Symptoms and signs are nausea, vomiting, headache, vertigo (a feeling that the world is spinning around), dimness of vision and coma or convulsions (Stone, 1975).

Many women suffer from lack of B6. A deficiency may cause the acne that appears before the menstrual period. Morning sickness may be due to a lack of B6, partly because more B6 is needed in pregnancy. Later, symptoms may lead to toxemia of pregnancy (high blood pressure, protein in the urine, edema, convulsions and coma), with the loss of nearly half of the pregnancies in which toxemia occurs. The mother's life is also endangered. Diabetes that occurs during pregnancy may be caused by a deficiency of B6 (Ballentine, 1978).

Other studies (Schler and Pfeiffer, 1982) showed that the vitamin most lacking in diets of the elderly is B6. Aging appears to be associated with low levels of B6, even when the diet is presumably adequate.

A young mother in one of my nutrition classes told the class that she had toxemia of pregnancy before her two-year-old child was born. She seemed happy to report that she had suffered from a serious disease. I asked her (rather tactlessly, I'm afraid) what in the world she ate at that time. Her eyebrows went up, and she said, incredulously, "Was my toxemia caused by what I ate?" Obviously, many of us have a long way to go before we understand that what we eat determines how healthy (or sick) we are!

Varied tissues all over the body are damaged by deficiencies of B6. Greasy sores show up around the eyes, nose and mouth, forehead, eyebrows and even behind the ears (Jennings, 1970), and there are cracks in the corners of the lips as with B2 (Marks, 1975). Intertrigo is a skin disease occurring on surfaces of the skin that rub together, such as in creases of the neck or folds of the groin and armpit and beneath the breasts. It is common where there is moisture, warmth and friction. It can burn, itch and cause fissures. Sometimes deficiencies cause dizziness, weakness, nervousness, insomnia and difficulty in breathing. Relief is possible in 24 hours with B6 (Goodhart and Shils, 1973). Without B6,

protein is lost from tissues, and the muscles waste away. There are many infections, plus a scaly skin condition, loss of motor functions and weight loss.

Prescribed drugs interfere with the work of B6, which is one reason people can have a deficiency—oral contraceptive pills are one outstanding example. Estrogens increase the requirements of B6. Studies show that 80 percent of a group of women taking the Pill had a relative B6 deficiency, and 20 percent had an absolute B6 deficiency. Mental depression that often goes with taking contraceptives can be relieved by B6. Such depression causes pessimism, anxiety, dissatisfaction, lethargy and loss of the life force.

B6 deficiency is particularly noted in alcoholics, and requirements are increased in patients with hyperthyroidism (Goodhart and Shils, 1973).

In some organs, deficiencies occur rapidly if we don't get enough B6. Especially affected are skin, mucous membranes and bone marrow. The immune response doesn't work well without B6 because a lack of protein causes atrophy of the thymus, an important part of the immune system (Stone et al., 1975). Also, B6 is needed to make DNA and RNA, and without those nucleic acids, which plan and carry out the orders of the body to manufacture needed substances, antibodies cannot be made. A reduction in lymphocyte count is fairly common in B6 deficiency (Marks, 1975). Lymphocytes (white blood cells) are part of the immune system.

Anyone who eats a lot of white sugar, white flour and fat builds up a B6 debt that is hard to pay off (Ballentine, 1978). When white flour is milled, more than 75 percent of the B6 is lost, and it is not returned. White sugar and fat have no B6. Thus these foods, common in the Standard American Diet, lead to deficiencies of B6 and many other nutrients. Also, anyone who regularly eats big steaks and other meats should take more B6 than the average person.

PANTOTHENIC ACID

If you're under stress but can roll with the punches, you probably have enough pantothenic acid, a B vitamin needed for healthy adrenal glands; thus the stress does not damage your cells.

Many people, however, don't get enough pantothenic acid (panto), and their adrenals begin to wither away and are finally destroyed. You can anticipate stress and feed your glands so they won't become exhausted. If you have frequent infections, you need panto. Even people who grind their teeth in their sleep may need panto (Lesser, 1980).

The adrenal cortex can't work without panto. The glands should produce cortisone and other adrenal hormones important for healthy nerves. If our nerves are not working well, we can't withstand stress. In a mild deficiency of panto, cell membranes can break down, and the fat cells can fuse and finally die (Jennings, 1970).

Panto is an important part of the Krebs cycle, the main energy-producing system in the body (Jennings, 1970). Also required are folic acid and biotin, two other B vitamins. If the cells lack these three vitamins, the cells switch to another energy system called glycolysis, which has much less power. The body can't live well on the amount of energy available from glycolysis. However, cancer cells, which require very little energy or vitamins or minerals, *can* live on this kind of energy.

If the Krebs cycle isn't working well, lecithin and other substances can't be made. We need lecithin to make the myelin sheaths that protect the nerves. Without lecithin, the sheaths may deteriorate and the nerves will not function.

A chemical called acetylcholine, which is manufactured in the body with the help of panto, transmits messages at nerve endings. Without the chemical, the nerves can't control the muscles. Some muscles must squeeze the fecal matter through the intestines; thus anyone who suffers from constipation may need more panto.

Acetylcholine also directs nerves that determine our mental attitudes. Without panto, we may become depressed. The brain can be damaged without panto because aminobutyric acid, which regulates the activity of neurons, can't be produced. Infants without enough panto may have convulsions.

Many cells show damage in panto deficiency. Membranes of lysosomes (tiny organelles in the cell) tear, and the enzymes spill out and eat the cells. The lysosomes' job is to "eat" dead cells so the cells won't clog our tissues, but the lysosomes are not supposed to eat the cells *until* they die.

In the gonads (sex organs) of mice that are deficient in panto, the cells in the testicles swell up, then they degenerate and disappear. In females, the cells of the ovary degenerate.

All of this damage usually results in severe stress, which causes the adrenal glands to swell. They fill up with blood and dead cells and cortisone can't be produced. Thus, when a person is under stress, he will not be able to throw off the stress because his adrenal glands can't produce the hormones needed. The pituitary, adrenal and sex hormones are all made from cholesterol, but these hormones are used up during stress, and the cholesterol to make new hormones can't be replaced without pantothenic acid. Sometimes it takes months to replace the hormones. Sometimes the glands will begin to function within 24 hours (Jennings, 1970).

Damaged tissues anywhere in the body are common when the adrenals are exhausted. The adrenals should call out antibodies to get rid of the damaged cells, but exhausted adrenals can't call out antibodies, and the tissues become more and more damaged.

Often the first deficiency symptom of panto is headache, then fatigue, impaired motor coordination, muscle cramp, gastrointestinal problems, fast heartbeat, lack of white cells and especially hypoglycemia (Marks, 1975).

Other disorders of panto deficiency are bed sores, varicose ulcers, burning feet, vomiting, abdominal distress, cramps, tenderness in the heels, fatigue and insomnia (Goodhart and Shils, 1973).

Other signs are herpes simplex (cold sores and fever blisters) and herpes zoster (shingles), which respond well to treatment with the vitamin plus a good diet.

There can be pain and soreness in the abdomen; nausea, burning and prickling in hands and feet (called paresthesia); and less function of antibodies. If panto and B6 are both deficient, antibodies against bacteria aren't produced.

Other symptoms are retarded growth, failure of reproduction, graying hair, skin inflammations, fatty liver and others. These deficiencies lead to loss of adrenal function, then to ulcers in the stomach and mucous membranes of the intestines (Jennings, 1970).

Persons who have gout may not realize the importance of panto. The vitamin helps convert uric acid to urea and ammonia, which are then excreted in the urine. If there's not enough panto, the uric acid crystals settle in the soft tissues around the joints and cause gout.

Many patients who have had abdominal operations lose the ability to move their bowels or urinate. This loss of movement can be corrected by panto (Williams, 1971).

Without panto, we can't make enough bile acids to digest fat, we can't make enough antibodies to ward off infections and we can't use proteins, carbohydrates and fats because our livers degenerate and don't perform their 500 or so jobs, some of which are to make intermediate products of proteins, carbohydrates and fats. The products are then used as building blocks of our tissues. If these products are in the blood, they'll get to every cell, and every cell and organ will be healthy.

The cells that line our intestines wither without panto, and we can't digest and assimilate foods well enough to repair tissue. We become physically weak and mentally depressed.

FOLIC ACID

Folic acid, a B vitamin, gets its name from foliage, because foliage plants are good sources of the vitamin. If all people ate one fresh fruit or one fresh vegetable every day, it is said that folic acid deficiency would be wiped off the face of the earth. As it is, one-third of all pregnant women are deficient in the vitamin (Goodhart and Shils, 1973). It is said to be the most common vitamin deficiency in the world (Howard, 1974).

Folic acid can be manufactured in the intestines, but if we have taken antibiotics, or if we can't absorb our food well, this source may be lost (Jennings, 1970). Folic acid must be changed in the liver to folacin before the cells can use it. This change can be made only if we have plenty of vitamin C.

Many green vegetables, especially spinach and peas, are good sources, as are liver and kidney. Cooking reduces the content in foods considerably (Marks, 1975). Folic acid is easily destroyed in the refining and canning of foods (Goodhart and Shils, 1973).

Deficiencies

Some early deficiency symptoms of folic acid are irritability, forgetfulness, hostility and paranoid behavior, all of which are strikingly improved 24 hours after folic acid is given.

Deficiencies of folic acid can cause macrocytic or megaloblastic anemia. This means that the red blood cells can't mature, and they become too large, but more important, they are fragile, so they don't live as long as healthy red blood cells. The same result is found in B12 deficiency.

A folic acid deficiency often accompanies alcoholism. Also, other nutrients may not be absorbed from the intestine.

If folic acid is in short supply early in the pregnancy of experimental animals, anemia may occur (Jennings, 1970), or the fetus may just stop developing and be reabsorbed. If deficiency begins later, the young are born, but 95 percent of them have abnormalities such as undeveloped organs and malformations of the bones, heart and blood vessels. Sometimes the brain is outside the body or the brain cavity is swollen with fluid. This seems to indicate that many of the birth abnormalities in humans may be due to a deficiency of folic acid and other nutrients (Ballentine, 1978).

Low levels of folic acid and of vitamin A, B2 and C in the blood of expectant mothers may result in birth defects such as spina bifida. This is called a neural tube defect, which means that the spinal cord is damaged, and the baby is crippled for life.

The World Health Organization reports that from one-third to one-half of all expectant mothers suffer from folic acid deficiency the last three months of pregnancy, which causes many instances of mental retardation.

Many patients in psychiatric institutions show low levels of folic acid. Their usual symptoms are indifference, withdrawal, lack of motivation and depression. People who are eating average, balanced diets get from 0.15 to 0.2 mg per day, which is less than half the recommended dosage of 0.5 mg. Many nutrition scientists say the recommended dosage may be far too low (Ballentine, 1978).

In infants, deficiencies may become severe before the normal bacteria that protect the colon are built up. Many babies have suffered mental retardation because their mothers did not get enough folic acid (Horrobin, 1973). A prolonged deficiency causes the end of the pregnancy.

VITAMIN B12

B12 is required for healthy skin cells inside and outside the body. It helps to make DNA and RNA, as do B6 and folic acid. It helps manufacture the fats that surround and protect the nerves, as well as those that maintain the bone marrow, the digestive tract and the central nervous system. B12 helps the growth and repair of tissue. To absorb B12, we must have calcium, hydrochloric acid and the intrinsic factor. B12 is called the "extrinsic factor" that the body gets in food. B12 cannot be absorbed by itself because it is actually too large a molecule to pass through any of the openings in the digestive tract, and it gets through only by linking with a carrier called the "intrinsic factor" found in the gastric juice. The B12 is carried to the ileum (last section of the small intestine), where it is absorbed into the blood. It is then stored in the liver. It is used with folic acid to form parts of the nucleic acids—DNA and RNA.

Deficiencies

Although some people may not get enough B12 in their diets, most B12 deficiencies are due to lack of absorption, which means that there's not enough intrinsic factor (Goodhart and Shils, 1973).

A B12 deficiency keeps sperm cells from maturing; women may be sterile and fetuses abnormal. The brain does not function normally without B12. Generally, improvement is rapid when B12 is given, but nerve damage improves slowly.

B12 deficiency can cause numbness and tingling in the hands and feet. Persons can lack position sense; they can be unsteady; have poor muscle coordination; be moody, mentally slow; have a poor memory; be confused, agitated, depressed; have delusions, hallucinations and rather severe psychoses (Goodhart and Shils, 1973).

In a severe deficiency of B12 there is damage to the large nerve fibers in the spinal cord. The patients lose feeling in their arms and legs and may become paralyzed. This damage takes a long time to develop unless there is damage to the stomach or ileum, then disease could occur in three to six years (Goodhart and Shils, 1973).

Of course, there's no way to know how long the deficiency of either B12 or the intrinsic factor has gone on.

BIOTIN

It was formerly thought that biotin was destroyed by avidin in raw egg whites. The study that was supposed to prove that case used massive amounts of raw egg whites (30 percent of the total diet) and no yolks, which are rich in biotin (Lesser, 1981). Now, Cordas (1981) suggests a raw egg a day for extra nourishment for anyone, especially for the elderly.

Deficiencies

In humans, deficiency of biotin is rare, except in infants (Marks, 1975). Infants deficient in biotin have seborrheic dermatitis (skin disease with yellow, greasy, itchy patches on the scalp, face and ears). Even breast-fed infants may have skin disease that resembles eczema (Marks, 1975).

Deficiencies at any age include grayish, dry, scaly skin with mild inflammation. The tongue papillae waste away. There are signs of nausea, loss of appetite, muscular pains, gastrointestinal problems and changes in the EKG. In a study, all signs and symptoms disappeared in five days after biotin was given by intravenous injection (Jennings, 1970).

In a deficiency of biotin, cholesterol in the liver is not metabolized, so blood cholesterol rises (Jennings, 1970). Also, amino acids may not be changed to proteins; the use of glucose and fatty acids is impaired, which leads to lack of energy and many other deficiencies.

Biotin-deficient rats suffered from a deficiency of male sex hormones, which caused degeneration of the testes with delayed manufacture of sperm cells and abnormal sperm cells.

Kirshmann (1975) reports that biotin has been beneficial in treating baldness.

CHOLINE

Choline, a vitamin B cousin, is a precursor of the neurotransmitter acetylcholine. That means it is required to send messages along the nerves, so it helps our brains work well. One of its most important actions is to prevent or eliminate depression. It also helps us think.

One study reported in the *American Journal of Psychiatry* told of a woman who had been severely depressed for many years. She was put into a hospi-

tal, and physicians first gave her all drugs ever used to relieve depression, one after the other. She got worse. Then they used choline chloride, a synthetic choline, but it did not help.

Next they used the natural form of choline—lecithin. She improved greatly; she said she had never felt so good before. Then, as a further test, the physicians took her off lecithin and she became depressed again.

Choline also helps regulate gall bladder function and prevent gallstones. It can be used in kidney damage and in eye conditions such as glaucoma.

The richest source of choline in food is egg yolk, and an even more concentrated source is lecithin, from the health food store. Ask for the highest percentage of phosphatidyl choline. Check the label for this potency.

Deficiencies

Studies have been done with animals that were given a high-carbohydrate diet deficient in choline. The animals developed fatty livers. If the young animals lived, they later developed cirrhosis of the liver. This disease is characterized by death of liver cells and buildup of nodules and fiber. Usually the disease signs take a long time to show up, but suddenly the patient has abdominal swelling and pain, edema and/or jaundice.

Dr. Burton Combes, a researcher at the University of Texas Health Science Center in Dallas, says that liver diseases will have gone up from fifth place to third place as a cause of death by the time you read this. Cirrhosis of the liver alone is now the seventh leading cause of death. Drinking alcohol is one of the main causes of cirrhosis. Others include prescription and street drugs, industrial pollutants and consumption of white sugar and white flour products that lead to excess fat in our tissues.

Carlton Fredericks conducted a study with college girls who had nervous symptoms before their menstrual periods. Most of the girls taking 1,000 mg of choline a day and 500 mg of inositol became calm before their periods, with no feelings of "climbing the wall." The first period after beginning therapy was sometimes worse, but later periods were much better (Fredericks, 1965).

INOSITOL

Inositol (also related to the B complex) keeps triglycerides from stacking up as fat on artery walls. It also works with choline to help people withdraw from tranquilizers.

Fredericks (1965) states that the inositol content of falling hair is about 50 percent below that in healthy hair. He comments, however, that he has never seen inositol cause hair growth on bald spots.

Deficiencies in humans cause a mild dermatitis, lassitude, muscle pains, digestive problems and sensitivity of skin or sensory organs (Guyton, 1976).

Three nutrients (inositol, choline and methionine) work together to keep cholesterol and fat from stacking up in the arteries and in liver cells. They also change harmful, cancer-causing estrogens to estrones, which are nontoxic. Women on the Pill, plus anyone with uterine or fibroid tumors, would do well to make sure their food program includes these three important nutrients.

PARA-AMINOBENZOIC ACID

PABA (para-aminobenzoic acid) ointment helps lighten the pain of burns and sunburn immediately. It is used as a sunscreen. It may delay old-age skin signs such as wrinkles, dry skin and dark spots. Studies show that PABA helps improve lupus erythematosus and scleroderma. It is also a B cousin.

PABA is important as a growth factor (Fredericks, 1975), and it works in the intestines to stimulate the bacteria to make folic acid (Kirshmann, 1973).

PABA also helps make red blood cells. It protects the skin from ultraviolet light. Fredericks (1965) says he has used PABA to stimulate fertility in both sexes. It inhibits destruction of estrogen by the liver, which would be of help in women who need to make more. It is helpful in arthritic diseases and in slowing down the aging process.

VITAMIN C

Vitamin C (ascorbic acid) helps our bodies produce interferon, which helps us fight infection, and which recently has been used to fight cancer.

The poisonous aluminum deposits that often collect in our brains can be lessened with C. If we get enough C, our blood vessels are more elastic, and that protects us from ruptured vessels as in heart attacks or strokes.

Cholesterol doesn't stack up in arteries, and toxic drugs aren't so dangerous if we have plenty of C. C is a natural antibiotic, but it doesn't damage the liver as do man-made chemical antibiotics. The liver works better with C, and our wounds heal faster.

Klenner (1974) suggested large amounts of vitamin C for strep and staph infections, measles, viral hepatitis, certain types of cancer (cervical, lung and bladder) and radiation burns, cystic mastitis, dental cavities, mononucleosis, schizophrenia, arthritis, poison oak and ivy, prickly heat and heat stroke, surgical wounds, rheumatic hearts, tuberculosis, pneumonia, pancreatitis and virus pancarditis (inflammation of the heart).

The late Irwin Stone, another of the vitamin C "greats," said that large doses of C helped polio, hepatitis, herpes, rabies, whooping cough, leprosy, typhoid fever and dysentery.

Dr. Linus Pauling's research shows that vitamin C helps us make more white blood cells to fight infections and it also helps us manufacture collagen (connective tissue that strengthens the tissues and holds our organs in place).

Phagocytes, the white blood cells that "eat" foreign invaders such as bacteria and viruses, depend on ascorbic acid. They are the garbage men of the cells. If ascorbic acid is at too low a level, the phagocytes won't attack or digest invading microorganisms.

Leukemia patients have large amounts of ascorbic acid locked in their leukocytes (white cells). Thus, the patients develop scurvy because they do not have enough freely moving ascorbic acid. The suggested amount is 25,000 mg a day (Stone, 1972).

Ascorbic acid is needed for breakdown of cholesterol to bile salts, thus atherosclerosis is a long-term deficiency of ascorbic acid that permits the cholesterol levels to build up in the arteries. Dramatic effects have been obtained with small 500-mg injections of C for 60 days. Plaques may disappear entirely.

Arthritis and rheumatism cost their 39 million victims more than $1.3 billion a year. With one to 10 grams a day of C, there has been complete recovery within three to four weeks with no heart complications.

To avoid infections such as colds, flu, pneumonia and cystitis (bladder infection), Irwin Stone (1972) suggested the following.

At the first hint that you are getting a cold, begin taking vitamin C. The hint may be a runny nose, a tickle in the throat or a chill. If it's cystitis, you'll know immediately if you're going to develop the infection if you've ever had cystitis before, because there is a burning sensation on urination.

Take the C at this rate: 1,500 to 2,000 milligrams (mg) immediately. (The bigger doses are for bigger people.) After 20 minutes, take the same amount; after another 20 minutes, take the same amount. You have taken 4,500 to 6,000 mg of vitamin C within 40 minutes. That amount will kill all the weak bugs, and you'll think you're well. But the strong, powerful bugs will begin to multiply, and the next morning you'll wake up with a full-blown cold that will probably last three days regardless of how much vitamin C you take. That's because the powerful bugs are much harder to kill.

To avoid a return of the cold, take 1,000 to 2,000 mg of vitamin C every hour or two for two or three more days. Recent research shows that the cold could return after a week and be a very severe infection if you stop the vitamin C too soon.

Large doses of vitamin C may result in intestinal gas or diarrhea. When we take vitamin C in larger and larger amounts, the cells get saturated. After that, if you take more, the cells can't accept it, so the C spills over into the intestines and causes gas or diarrhea. If you begin to get gas, cut back 1,000 to 2,000 mg a day and take that amount every day. This is bowel tolerance, and everyone should be taking bowel tolerance of vitamin C. If you ever cut down on your C, do it gradually.

You should never develop another infection if you take vitamin C the way Irwin Stone has suggested. But remember, start the C at the first sign, no matter how small the sign. If you sit around to see if you develop a cold tomorrow, you will not be able to avoid the cold. It may be a much more severe infection and last days longer.

When you're on this vitamin C program, be sure not to miss taking the C for even one day. The powerful bugs will multiply and it may take hundreds more milligrams to kill them off.

Linus Pauling (1986) says if you're on his suggested dose of 6,000 to 18,000 mg a day and you develop a cold, you weren't taking enough vitamin C.

VITAMIN D

Vitamin D is essential for the absorption of the calcium we eat to make our bones and teeth. Without it, not enough calcium can be absorbed to replace the small amounts that are lost daily into the urine and feces (Horrobin, 1973).

Vitamin D is one of the vitamins of which we can get too much. Symptoms of too much D are general depression and diarrhea and abnormal calcium deposits in soft tissues (blood vessel walls, liver, lung, kidney and stomach) (Rosenberg, 1974). There are very few cases of vitamin D overdose compared to the cases of vitamin D deficiency (Jennings, 1970).

Deficiencies

The earliest symptoms of deficiencies are restlessness, irritability and swelling of the head. Months later, X-rays of bones show lesions. In advanced cases, there are such conditions as square heads, deformed chests, potbellies and constipation (Sebrell, 1971).

Many older women and men have osteoporosis (porous bones), which is now treated with vitamin D (Fredericks, 1965) and hydrochloric acid—the digestive acid in the stomach that helps us assimilate calcium.

It is important for patients with poor bones to take vitamin D supplements, especially if they are taking cortisone. Poor bones and teeth are a sign of deficiency; calcium and phosphorus can't be used by the body unless vitamin D is present.

Osteomalacia is much the same as rickets. There is a lack of minerals that shows up especially in the pelvis, the chest and the extremities. Spontaneous fractures occur. Many elderly people have some degree of osteomalacia. All should receive adequate amounts of D (Marks, 1975), plus all minerals and vitamins as part of a natural food diet.

Deficiency symptoms in infants that are born with low stores of D because of the mother not getting enough in her diet when pregnant show up as birth injuries. Later these infants develop poor bones structure and crooked teeth.

It has never been determined officially how much D adults need a day. Suggestions range from 400 IU for children to 800 IU for women during the last half of pregnancy, and 1,000 IU for severe deficiency.

If you expose 20 percent of your skin surface to sunlight for 30 minutes, you'll get about 400 IU of vitamin D (Bland, 1981).

VITAMIN E

Do you take vitamin E and feel that it isn't working for you? It may not be, but not because of the E. If we don't make enough pancreatic enzymes or bile, the E can't be assimilated. It must be emulsified and taken up through the lymphatic system and distributed throughout the body.

Even in the best of conditions, a person absorbs only 20 to 30 percent of the E. The Harvard Medical School has found a high risk of heart disease and cancer in animals on average levels of E. Anyone who eats a lot of vegetable oil should be sure to take extra E, otherwise the extra oil may cause the fat in the cells to become rancid. The rule of thumb is to take about 50 IU of vitamin E for every three extra tablespoons of oil (Bland, 1981).

Deficiencies

In a study in *Lancet*, investigators withheld both selenium and vitamin E from the diets of laboratory animals, and they developed cystic fibrosis. They also had the same degeneration of the pancreas that children with cystic fibrosis have. Nutritional treatment should be tried as soon as the condition is discovered in children. Dosage should be 400 to 800 IU a day of vitamin E and 100 to 300 micrograms of selenium. Lecithin is an emulsifying agent, and it helps with the uptake of E into the lymphatic system. See your nutrition-minded physician for information about dosage.

Vitamin E is essential for reproduction in both men and women and also for growth and vigor. We can't resist infections without E, we lose weight, we don't grow normally, we're weak, our muscles waste away and our nerves cannot make our muscles move correctly.

We can't make cortisone unless there's plenty of E in the adrenal glands. Without E we can't resist stress, we age rapidly and our skin becomes wrinkled because the deeper skin layers lose their elasticity.

Vitamin E helps keep the heart muscle from degenerating and the arteries from being stacked up with fat. It strengthens the heartbeat by supplying extra oxygen to the cells in the heart muscle. Probably most important of all is that it keeps the polyunsaturated fat in the cells from becoming rancid. Rancidity causes holes to form in cell membranes, and the cells cannot work normally. Thus many different diseases can be caused, based on the location of the cells that were damaged.

Vitamin E in Man and Animals

In animals, a deficiency of vitamin E shows greater disease states than with a deficiency of any other vitamin. It affects reproduction, muscles, skeleton, circulation and breathing, and produces disturbances of the liver, kidney and blood, and a shortened life span. Specialists on aging believe that taking supplements of vitamin E can lengthen the life span in man by five to 10 years. Animal cells kept in a solution of E in test tubes lived for 120 cell divisions (the usual is 50) (Di Cyan, 1972).

Vitamin E deficiency causes a special type of anemia in premature infants. If iron is given, the anemia is worse. In chicks, the most brain damage is caused when 5 percent corn oil is fed and no vitamin E is given. Infants have low stores of E at birth. If they don't get enough soon, they show the same symptoms as chicks—brain damage and damage to the nervous system.

Jaundice in newborn infants can be caused by deficiencies of E. As red blood cells are destroyed, their coloring matter forms a pigment called bilirubin, which is usually excreted in bile. When vitamin E is deficient, many blood cells are destroyed so fast that the pigment can't be excreted fast enough. The pigment accumulates, settles in the tissues and the baby becomes jaundiced (Jennings, 1970).

In E deficiency, male rats can't produce sperm that move; females resorb their embryos. Damage to males is often irreversible, to females reversible. But vitamin C may help the males.

Vitamin E can't be absorbed or transported without bile, present only when fat is eaten. Thus skim milk and low-fat milk may allow vitamin E deficiency to develop. If inorganic iron is eaten, E is destroyed so take one supplement in the morning and the other at night. Cereals fortified with iron may be dangerous. Healthful mineral tablets that contain iron as an amino acid chelate are available at health food stores.

E is a powerful anticoagulant; in a deficiency, clots form easily in blood vessels. Infantile softening of the brain seems to be caused by clots in blood vessels (Jennings, 1970).

SUMMARY

This lesson should be used with Lesson 1, which is the basic diet and food supplement plan. Suggested amounts of vitamins and other supplements are given in that lesson.

Most of the counselees I see are very ill. They have been to four or five physicians before coming to me to improve their nutrition. They need large doses of supplements for a few weeks. However, their digestive systems are often not in good enough condition to metabolize the supplements. In such cases, they should start with small amounts and build up to the amounts that allow the body to heal itself. Later, they can reduce the amounts to maintenance doses. Details of how much to take are given in the chart at the end of Lesson 1, "*A Basic Diet Plan and Use of Food Supplements.*"

Listen to your body, and let it tell you how much to take. You may want to increase at any time you're under stress, either physical, mental or emotional.

QUESTIONS

TRUE/FALSE

1. Fatigue, depression, heart disease and cancer are all related to deficiency of vitamins.

2. Deficiency of nutrients means that more enzymes are needed but can't be supplied, but more coenzymes (vitamins) can be consumed, which relieves the deficiency.

3. Without vitamins, our glands get infected, infections cause exhaustion, exhaustion causes more infections, so we have a vicious cycle.

4. Nutritionists recommend natural vitamins A, D and E, but synthetic B and C are often suggested.

5. Food is the most important part of our program, but we can't be well without food supplements.

6. Nutrients may pass unabsorbed through the entire digestive system.

7. As people age, they don't use food well; thus, they may not be able to absorb nutrients.

8. Vitamin A is especially important for the health of the eyes and skin.

9. Zinc is needed to get vitamin A out of storage in the liver, so zinc may help acne more than vitamin A does.

10. Vitamin A can be toxic in enormous doses, especially in the form of fish liver oil, but the toxicity is reversed when the vitamin is withheld.

11. B vitamins must usually be taken together, because if one is taken in large doses, it might cause a deficiency of others.

12. If B vitamins are in short supply, there might be enough B's for the heart muscle to beat, but not enough to furnish energy for every brain cell. Thus, someone may be forgetful, but his heart beats on and on.

13. The tissues that suffer most from B1 deficiency are the cardiovascular system and the nerves.

14. Deficiencies of B2 may show up first in the adrenal glands, as cataracts or as wrinkles in the upper lip.

15. Vitamin B3 deficiencies show up as central nervous system problems.

16. B6 helps us produce hydrochloric acid, which is required for digestion of protein and repair of all tissue.

MULTIPLE CHOICE

1. Vitamins are needed to: (a) help an enzyme system work, (b) make healthy cells.

2. Larger doses of vitamins are needed by persons with these conditions: (a) pregnancy, (b) liver disease, (c) diabetes, (d) stress, (e) malabsorption.

3. New cells are always being made in these tissues: (a) muscles, (b) pancreas, (c) lining of the intestines, (d) red and white blood cells.

4. Vitamin A: (a) helps make mucus, required for healthy cells, (b) prevents the drying of cells that makes cells precancerous.

5. The following conditions require extra B complex: (a) stress, (b) infections, (c) alcoholism, (d) eating excess sugar.

6. All the following tissues depend on B complex: (a) hair, (b) skin, (c) eyes, (d) mouth, (e) liver.

7. These mental problems appear first in deficiencies of B complex: (a) tired brains, (b) inability to think, (c) jangled nerves.

8. The following drugs partially destroy vitamins B and C: (a) aspirin, (b) antibiotics, (c) diuretics, (d) refined sugar.

ANSWERS

True/False

1. T.   2. T   3. T   4. T   5. T   6. T   7. T   8. T
9. T   10. T   11. T   12. T   13. T   14. T   15. T
16. T

Multiple Choice

1. a,b   2. a,b,c,d,e   3. b,c,d   4. a,b   5. a,b,c,d
6. a,b,c,d,e   7. a,b,c,   8. a,b,c,d

REFERENCES

Altschule, M.D. *Preventive Medicine* 3:180–183, 1974.

Baker and Frank. *J. of Appl. Nutr.* 33(1):3–18, 1981.

Ballentine, R. *Diet and Nutrition, A Holistic Approach.* Honesdale, PA: The Himalayan International Institute, 1978.

Bland, J. Tapes of Seminar at International College of Applied Nutrition. Dec. 1981.

Brin, M. *N. E. J. Med.* 289:979, 1973.

Cheraskin, E., Ringsdorf, W.M. and Brecher, A. *Psychodietetics.* New York: Bantam, 1974.

Cheraskin, E. et al. The "Ideal" Daily Vitamin A Intake. *Inter. J. Vit. Nutr. Res.* 46(1):11–13, 1976.

Cohen and Duncan. *British Med. J.* 4:516–518, 1967.

Cordas, S. Tape from Fifth Annual Nutrition Education Conference, Houston, Texas, 1981.

Davis, A. *Let's Have Healthy Children.* New York: Signet, 1972.

DiCyan, E. *Vitamin E and Aging.* New York: Pyramid, 1972.

Fredericks, C. *Eating Right for You.* New York: Today Press, 1975.

——— and Bailey, H. *Food Facts and Fallacies.* New York: ARC, 1965.

Goodhart, R.S. and Shils, M.E. *Modern Nutrition in Health and Disease.* Philadelphia: Lea and Febiger, 1973.

Guyton, A.C. *Textbook of Physiology.* Philadelphia: Saunders, 1976.

Herbert, V. *The Rationale of Massive-Dose Vitamin Therapy.* Proceedings, Western Hemisphere Nutrition Congress IV; Acton, MA: Publishing Sciences Group, Inc., 84–91, 1975.

Horrobin, D.F. *An Introduction to Human Physiology.* Davis, 1973.

Horwitt, M.K. Vitamin E: A Reexamination. *Am. J. Clin. Nutr.*, 29:569–578, May 1976.

Houston Chronicle, section 1, p. 24; Jan. 22, 1978.

Howard. *J. of Nutr.* 104:1024, Aug. 1974.

Hunter, B.T. *Consumer's Research*. March 1974.

International Symposium on Vitamin E. Tokyo: Kyoritsu, Shuppan Co. 1972.

Jennings, I. *Vitamins and the Endocrine Metabolism*. London: Heinemann, 1970.

Jooli and Eswaran. *J. Ortho. Psych.* 9(1):35–40, 1980.

Jukes, T.E. Fact and Fancy in Nutrition and Food Sciences (in) *The Nutrition Crisis*, A Reader: Ed. T.P. Labuza, St. Paul: West, 1975.

Kirshmann, J.D. *Nutrition Almanac*. New York: McGraw-Hill, 1973.

Klenner, F. *JIAPM*. 1:45–69, 1974.

Krebs, E.T. Jr. John Beard Memorial Foundation. San Francisco, CA 94101.

Lesser, M. *Nutrition and Vitamin Therapy*. New York: Grove Press, Inc., 1980.

Marks, J. *A Guide to the Vitamins*. Baltimore Univ.: Park Press, 1975.

Passwater, R. *Supernutrition*. New York: Pocket, 1976.

Pauling, L. *How to Live Longer and Feel Better*. New York: W. H. Freeman, 1986.

Pfeiffer, C.C. *Mental and Elemental Nutrients*. New Canaan, CT: Keats, 1975.

Philpott and Khaleeluddin. *JIAPM* 6(2):29–35.

Pike and Brown. *Nutrition: An Integrated Approach*. New York: Wiley and Sons, 1975.

Robinson, C. H. *Normal and Therapeutic Nutrition*. New York: Macmillan, 1972.

Rosenberg, H. and Beldzman, A. N. *The Doctor's Book of Vitamin Therapy*. New York: Putnam, 1974.

Sebrell, W. H. *Malnutrition, Preventive Medicine and pH*. New York: Appleton-Century-Crofts, 1973.

———, and Harris, R.S. *The Vitamins*, Vol. 1. New York: Academic Press, 1967.

Schler, A. and Pfeiffer, C.C. *J. Ortho. Psych.*, 11(2):81–86, 1982.

Stone, Irwin. *The Healing Factor: Vitamin C Against Disease*. New York: Grosset and Dunlap, 1972.

Williams, R. J. *Nutrition Against Disease*. New York: Pitman, 1971.

———. Pamphlet. La Canada, Cal.: Bronson Pharmaceuticals.

Lesson 7

MINERALS AND THEIR IMPORTANCE IN NUTRITION

LESSON 7—MINERALS AND THEIR IMPORTANCE IN NUTRITION

MINERALS ARE IMPORTANT

CHELATED MINERALS

MAJOR MINERALS

Calcium
Calcium and Bones
  Hydrochloric Acid Needed
  Bones Lose Calcium
  Chelation Therapy
  Chelation Removes Lead
  Choosing Chelation Therapy
  Selection of Patients
  Good Foods Can Chelate
Magnesium
  Studies on Magnesium
  Magnesium Deficiency Symptoms
Phosphorus
Potassium
  Babies Are Vulnerable
  Potassium Deficiency
  Sources of Potassium
Sodium

TRACE MINERALS

Chromium
  Chromium in Childhood
  Chromium in Foods

Cobalt
Copper
Germanium
Iodine
Iron
Manganese
  Manganese and the Brain
Molybdenum
Selenium
Silicon
Zinc
  Zinc and Wound Healing

DANGEROUS MINERALS

Aluminum
  No More Aluminum
Arsenic
  Arsenic Kills Cells
Cadmium
  Cadmium, A Mistake
Lead
Mercury
  Mercury Changes Cells

HAIR ANALYSIS

FOOD AND FOOD SUPPLEMENT PROGRAM

QUESTIONS AND ANSWERS

MINERALS ARE IMPORTANT

MINERALS ARE of great importance in the diet because they activate chemical reactions in the body and enzyme systems that help to digest food. Many people do not get enough minerals to do all this work, so they get sick.

There are two groups of needed minerals—major and trace. The designation refers to how much of each group is required in the diet. The major minerals we'll discuss are calcium, magnesium, phosphorus, potassium and sodium. The trace minerals we'll talk about are chromium, copper, cobalt, iron, iodine, manganese, selenium, zinc, germanium, silicon and molybdenum. Other trace minerals required by the body are fluorine, silicon, sulfur, tin and vanadium, all of which have recently been added to the list of important nutrients. Our food must contain all the essential minerals. They are required

for life itself. If one is missing, even in trace amounts, our diet will not be complete, and we'll get sick. We may die young because we've been missing tiny amounts of minerals and didn't even know it.

Many Americans have severe deficiencies of minerals. Minerals help form proteins, and they help the body to balance its fluids. We need a constant supply of minerals to replace what is lost every day in urine, feces and sweat.

If anyone has anything wrong with him, it is wise to consider deficiencies of minerals or vitamins and to add to the diet natural foods or food supplements containing these nutrients. Most people think only of vitamins as food supplements, not realizing that minerals are just as important.

Minerals must be transported around the body to the specific locations inside the cells where each mineral is needed. Calcium, phosphorus, magnesium and vitamin D must be transported into the bones and cartilage to help prevent osteoporosis (porous bones). Minerals help people with slipped discs, rheumatoid and other forms of arthritis and osteochondrosis (disease of the growth centers in children) to recover from many of their ailments.

All minerals must be obtained from the food we eat, and each cell must get the amount it needs. Although trace minerals are used in tiny amounts, they are nonetheless essential.

I once heard a hospital dietician speak. She was urging her audience to eat white enriched bread! After the talk, I asked her if she didn't think whole-grain bread would be better because so many nutrients were removed in the processing. She replied, "Oh, they're just trace elements."

Trace or major, the nutrients are essential to life, so if you've been hearing that trace elements aren't important, we'll review some of the latest research on what trace elements do in the body.

First, let's discuss chelated minerals, a term that is being used more and more in nutrition. Then we'll talk about major minerals, trace minerals, the toxic minerals (and how to avoid them) and finally, hair analysis—is it necessary?

CHELATED MINERALS

Minerals must be chelated (pronounced key-lated) to amino acids so they can be transported through the blood to the cells. "Chelate" is from a Greek word meaning crab's claw. The amino acids surround the minerals and join to them as if they were being held in a claw, because they can't get across membranes by themselves.

The combined minerals and amino acids go to the duodenum (first eight to 11 inches of the small intestine), where they are taken across the intestinal wall to the capillaries. Then they enter the bloodstream (Fouad, 1976). Fouad notes that the first requirement in the digestion and assimilation of minerals is a normal, healthy gastrointestinal tract, especially the upper portions (the duodenum/jejunum), where proteins are broken down to amino acids and where absorption of minerals takes place.

But often the minerals don't get chelated to amino acids because the digestive tract isn't healthy or because we have eaten too much junk food and too little protein, and some of the amino acids are missing. Maybe we took diuretics and washed out the minerals. In any case, the minerals don't reach our cells.

But minerals can be chelated in the laboratory—the amino acids are "clawed" to the minerals and put in tablet form. Then when we take the tablet, the chelation process is already formed, and the minerals joined to amino acids go right through the

membranes of the capillaries and the cells to the exact spot where they're needed.

Iron in chelated iron tablets, for example, is joined with three different amino acids, each of which helps move the iron along to the parts of the body where it is needed. Much of the iron goes to the liver, which is the main storage depot for iron used to make hemoglobin (the part of the red blood cell that carries oxygen). Chelated iron is no longer an inorganic iron; it is a natural organic iron called transferrin (Fouad, 1976).

Some antibiotics are chelates. They enclose or bind the minerals that bacteria live on, so the bacteria die from a deficiency. Antibiotics can likewise keep our bodies from using minerals. Have you ever heard anyone say, "I got over the flu in 10 days, but it took me six weeks to get over the antibiotics"?

Other inorganic compounds that minerals combine with, such as fumerates, citrates and gluconates, go through one of the following pathways (Fouad, 1976):

1. About four-fifths of the compound is insoluble and passes through the intestinal tract unused and is excreted. If nutrients don't get into our blood and tissues, they're not really being used.

2. Part of the remaining one-fifth should go through the lining of the small intestine into the bloodstream, but the lining is negatively charged, and the inorganic mineral adheres to the lining and can't be absorbed. Poisonous inorganic minerals (lead, cadmium, etc.) may adhere to the membranes of the small intestine and cause severe irritation and bleeding if too much of those poisons get into our system (Fouad, 1976).

3. The remaining small amount of the free minerals may combine with amino acids (which have been broken down from protein digestion) and form a mineral chelate that is absorbed immediately. This amount is between 1 and 6 percent of the total inorganic mineral intake (Fouad, 1976). Thus very small amounts are actually absorbed into the blood.

The label on the mineral supplement should state that it is an amino acid chelate. Miller (1974) tested many vitamin-mineral supplements and found that more than half the sugar-coated tablets were not absorbable. He suggests uncoated tablets.

MAJOR MINERALS

Calcium

Calcium is necessary for reproduction and growth. It helps maintain the cell membranes so nutrients can pass through if they need to, or be kept out if they should be kept out.

Calcium has a significant effect on the nervous system, the heart and on bone formation (Guyton, 1976). It also helps to conduct nerve impulses. When there is too little calcium, the nervous system becomes more and more excitable because the brain cell membranes become very permeable. The nerve fibers "fire" spontaneously, and nerve impulses go to the muscles and cause tetany (muscle twitching, cramps and convulsions). Sometimes the nerves become so excitable that the muscles in the lower arm and hand go into spasm. Tetany is a severe disease that can kill.

When there is too much calcium in the fluids, the nervous system is depressed, and the reflex actions of the central nervous system are sluggish. The muscles get weak and we become constipated. We often lose our appetites, probably because the muscles in the walls of the intestine can't contract well enough to send the fecal matter out of the body (Guyton, 1976).

Calcium helps to maintain the proper rhythm of the heart and it helps muscles to contract. The heart is a muscle, and it can't beat without calcium. Investigators have deprived laboratory animals of calcium and found that the heart enlarges, enzymes don't work and blood doesn't clot. We might bleed to death without calcium. If calcium reserves become dangerously low, the heart flutters.

Calcium and Bones

The 99 percent of the calcium that is in our bones and teeth is like money in the bank. If we don't eat enough calcium, it is drawn out of the bones so the heart will keep on beating, but the bones may then become porous because they contain less and less calcium. Then the soft bones break easily. We can live with broken bones, but we can't live if our hearts don't beat.

This fragile bone condition is called osteoporosis, with symptoms of low back or rib pain and with frequent fractures, especially of the ribs, wrists and hips. The number of hip fractures doubles in women over age 50 with each five-year addition of age. Porous bones may break spontaneously when we turn over in bed or when we cough, sneeze, stand up or walk downstairs. Fourteen million women and one-fourth as many men have osteoporosis. Some investigators say it is as common as having gray hair when we get old (Arnow).

Jennifer Jowsey of the Mayo Clinic recommended that everyone 25 years old or older take 1,000 mg of calcium as a supplement in order to avoid osteoporosis in later years. By the time the bone condition shows up in an X-ray examination, 30 percent

of the normal amount of calcium may have been withdrawn from the bone (McBean, 1974).

This bone loss can sometimes be reversed, but it may take a long time. We need more calcium with a corresponding increase in magnesium. For every 1,000 mg of calcium in supplement form, 400 to 500 mg of magnesium is suggested.

Hydrochloric Acid Needed. To make sure the minerals are assimilated, we need hydrochloric acid (HCl), the acid normally secreted by cells in the stomach to help break down proteins and dissolve minerals. The older we get, the less HCl we make. Therefore, many people take supplements of HCl. Much of the new therapy for arthritis is based on increasing the HCl so that calcium can be assimilated and put into the bones and teeth where it belongs rather than stacking up in the blood vessel walls (hardening of the arteries) or in the joints (arthritis) where it doesn't belong.

We don't assimilate calcium well if we eat a lot of oxalic acid. This acid is found in raw vegetables, especially spinach, beet tops and Swiss chard. As a rule, we should cook these vegetables. Cocoa also contains oxalic acid (McBean, 1974).

Some investigators say that phytic acid binds calcium and excretes it in the feces. Phytic acid is found in whole grains, especially in the bran and husks. In leavened bread (raised with yeast), an enzyme in the grain destroys phytic acid, but the enzyme doesn't work, they say, in baking-powder bread (McBean, 1974). However, Ballentine (1978) says that when we're on a good diet and get enough calcium, we have no problem eating whole grains. In fact, the intestinal tract may contain an enzyme that splits phytic acid (McBean, 1974). Also, if we get the vitamin D we need, there will be no problem with phytates.

A group of drug and alcohol addicts was treated with high doses of multiminerals, especially calcium and magnesium, plus vitamin C. Another group was given only vitamin C and a third group only the usual medication. Results were best in the group that took minerals plus vitamin C. They had more energy, they no longer craved drugs and they had stayed off drugs for up to six months when this report went to press.

Calcium can pass through our intestines without being absorbed if we have diarrhea, take laxatives or eat too much high-fiber food. Also, coffee can wash calcium out of the alimentary tract in urine and feces. If our kidneys don't work well, they allow calcium to pour out in the urine.

Bones Lose Calcium. An excess of phosphorus in the tissues can make us lose calcium from our bones. Soft drinks with or without sugar contain phosphorus, and when we drink them, we lose so much calcium that we may have osteoporosis or arthritis. I met a young man one day who asked me if the 12 bottles of soft drinks a day he was drinking were doing him any harm. I mentioned numbness in fingers and lips, and nerves that can't be calm when calcium is being washed out of the digestive tract by soft drinks. He said, "I don't have those symptoms, but I do have severe arthritis." Thus, at age 24 or so, this young man had an old man's disease—arthritis—partly because he drank so many soft drinks.

When calcium is in short supply in body fluids, tetany results (Guyton, 1976). Vitamin D increases the depositing of calcium in the bones. In fact, without vitamin D, the bones don't have enough calcium; they get soft and they bend, as in rickets or osteomalacia (bad bones—adult rickets).

Some people can't absorb vitamin D because they don't have enough bile or pancreatic enzymes to digest fat. Vitamin D is a fat-soluble vitamin that helps deposit calcium in bones (Horrobin, 1973).

Calcium and other minerals must be dissolved in the strong digestive juice in the stomach so they can be taken into the blood and reach the bones. Many people have kidney stones because undissolved calcium and phosphorus clump up and form stones. Also, the urine is too alkaline, and alkaline urine will not dissolve the stones. An acid-producing diet should be eaten (Guyton, 1976), and supplements of HCl should be taken. Elderly people may want to take HCl indefinitely.

Chelation Therapy. There's a lot of information in medical journals and health magazines about chelation therapy to get rid of calcium and other minerals that are stacking up in blood vessels and causing hardening of the arteries, which leads to heart attack and stroke. This therapy is not the same as the chelated minerals we talked about earlier; it is another chelation process.

I don't believe that it is the treatment of choice. I believe that good nutrition will keep us from needing such drastic treatments as chelation, but it is definitely better than heart bypass operations to get relief from arteriosclerosis. Thus, I'll briefly describe the chelation therapy and when it is used. Please remember, if you eat the natural food way, you won't need chelation therapy because you won't have arteriosclerosis.

Chelation therapy is used to get deposits of calcium out of the arteries and other parts of the body. Of course, the only time we need to get rid of calcium is when it's in the wrong place. It is removed by injecting an amino acid, ethylenediaminotetracetic acid (EDTA), into the bloodstream by a slow drip. Each treatment takes several hours, and the patient has to be watched carefully to make sure that not too many other minerals in addition to the excess calcium are being excreted. Since the minerals that belong in the blood are also excreted with the calcium, mineral supplements are given (Halstead, 1979). This process is called chelation, which means a "clawing." The EDTA grabs the calcium, holds it like a claw and excretes it from the body.

Chelation Removes Lead. Chelation has been used for years to remove lead, a poisonous metal, from the body. One patient who was given this treatment for lead also had arteriosclerosis, which was greatly improved. After that, chelation therapy was used in thousands of patients without one death due directly to the treatment. Excellent results have been claimed in treating hardened heart valves, intermittent claudication (pain in the calves of the legs caused by blood clots), gangrene, angina, heart attacks, stroke, senility and many other conditions. These ailments are usually caused by poor circulation due to hardening of the arteries. Nutritional deficiencies can lead to deposits of unwanted calcium in the soft tissues.

We must realize that this treatment is not without danger, and it is expensive. So we don't want to eat junk food and get our blood vessels filled with calcium, then have to submit to this treatment. One thing in its favor, as we've said, is that it's much better than the heart bypass operation. A good diet would have prevented the calcium deposits in the first place.

Are you wondering whether or not your bones and teeth will be chelated out of your body? They won't. Calcium in the bones and teeth is so tightly bound to proteins and other substances that it can't be pulled out by chelation therapy. But the calcium that has been abnormally laid down in the arteries can be reduced over a period of weeks with chelation treatment. As we've said, not only calcium but other minerals are removed. When the mineral deposits in the artery walls begin to break up, the rest of the materials, which are mostly fats, are released into the bloodsteam and are excreted. Getting rid of the deposits makes the opening of the arteries larger, and more blood flows through, bringing nutrients to the cells.

Choosing Chelation Therapy. You should know what to expect if you choose chelation therapy. Following this procedure, a patient should completely change his way of eating to avoid recurrence of fatty plaques in the arteries that start the calcium deposits. A success rate of about 75 percent has been experienced in the last 20 years or so with this therapy. Another 15 percent show mild improvement, but 10 percent show no improvement (Halstead, 1979). You may recover from arteriosclerosis with this treatment, but you have solved only one problem. If you change your way of eating, you may not only recover from arteriosclerosis but also prevent intestinal ailments, allergies, osteoporosis, Parkinson's disease, cancer, AIDS and other chronic degenerative diseases. A natural food diet will relieve and prevent most of our ailments.

Selection of Patients. Everyone can't take chelation therapy. If the liver and kidneys aren't working well, the waste products can't be eliminated. There are other risks. As the EDTA is dripped into the blood vessels, the patient may have muscle cramps, fever, joint aches, headaches and nausea; some reactions are quite toxic.

Patients undergo one treatment, then are observed for three days before being given another treatment. If there are no adverse reactions, a series of 20 three- to four-hour treatments is given, usually once or twice a week. Some people need 50 treatments. With chelation therapy, calcium deposits anywhere in the body can be dissolved. With surgery, one vessel at a time must be repaired at great expense and with severe trauma to the patient.

Good Foods Can Chelate. May I emphasize the importance of good nutrition! A good diet often will completely eliminate angina pains and all symptoms and signs of heart disease and other circulation problems.

I remember a physician who called me for a counseling appointment. He had talked to me before about coming, but he had never made a definite appointment. This time he said, "I'm desperate." He had had many heart scares and had been rushed to the hospital for treatment. But he obviously wasn't getting better. The attacks were more frequent and more severe. He went on my food and food supplement program and became so much better that, after about two months, I got a postcard from him. He had gone to Canada and was enjoying a lovely vacation.

Another friend was so ill with heart disease that he couldn't walk across his living room. After changing to a new diet and a food supplement program, he felt so well that he dug up his backyard and planted a garden.

See Lesson 3, "Heart Disease and Nutrition," for specifics of the diet and food supplements for the heart.

Our bodies contain only small amounts of minerals, but those small amounts are absolutely essential for skin, hair, muscles, blood, bone and brain cells; in fact, for every body tissue.

Let's look at the cells under a microscope. Inside are "organelles," little organs called mitochondria,

which are the powerhouses of the cells, where we get our energy. Heart cells, which work so hard to pump blood, need a lot of power, so each cell may have as many as 1,000 mitochondria. Each mitochondrion contains 500 or more enzymes that release energy from the food we eat. That's one-half million enzymes in each cell, and we have about 70 trillion cells. The total number of enzymes boggles the mind!

Each enzyme must have a mineral to activate it. It's like a car. We put in gas, water and oil, but the car doesn't move until we turn the key in the ignition. The "key" in an enzyme system is the mineral that makes the system work.

Magnesium

If you get plenty of magnesium, you should get the following benefits: strong bones, teeth, muscles and heartbeat. Your personality should improve, and you'll have a healthy nervous system. Your enzyme systems will work better (Hall and Jaffe, 1973).

We mentioned strong bones and teeth, which everyone knows have a lot of calcium in them. Calcium is the basic ingredient in chalk, and you remember the chalk you used to use in school—it crumbled to dust. When magnesium, phosphorus and vitamin D are added to calcium, teeth become dense and tough (Ashmead).

Magnesium also keeps calcium from being deposited where it shouldn't be, such as in the arteries, where it causes arteriosclerosis, and in the kidneys where it causes painful kidney stones (Ashmead).

The average American diet is 200 mg short every day of the required amount of magnesium set by experts such as Dr. Mildred Seelig (1964). Besides that, if we're under stress or eat the average American intake of sugar (about 128 pounds per person per year), we use more magnesium and are more deficient. The average American diet often supplies no more than 120 mg of magnesium a day. The suggested amount (Cheraskin and Ringsdorf, 1977) is 400 to 500 mg for adults. People who drink coffee or alcohol, or who take diuretics, may flush magnesium out of their systems with the extra liquids.

Studies on Magnesium. Magnesium catalyzes more enzymes by far than any other mineral—more than 100 (Miller, 1974). Magnesium (with calcium, potassium and manganese) largely controls the activities of the nerves of the brain as well as the rest of the body.

Magnesium activates most of the enzymes that use vitamins B1, B2 and B6. Therefore, what is thought to be a deficiency of any of those vitamins might really be a deficiency of magnesium (Lee,

1983). Menstrual cramps, for example, may be caused by lack of magnesium.

Magnesium also relaxes our muscles, whereas calcium helps them contract. If there isn't enough magnesium, the muscle can't relax, and it twitches and trembles. If there is a severe shortage, the muscle cramps and goes into spasms.

Think how important magnesium and calcium are for the heart. First, the heart muscles must contract, then relax, and this goes on about 72 times a minute for 24 hours a day, hopefully for 80 or 90 years. If the minerals are not available, the heart can slowly stop beating. Studies show that at least 20 percent of the people who die of heart attacks have blood flowing through all their arteries, so the attacks weren't caused by fatty deposits; they were caused by lack of calcium and/or magnesium.

Magnesium stops the abnormal heartbeats caused by digitalis. If magnesium is depleted, there are changes in the heart muscle (Classen, 1979). Magnesium is used to treat seizures associated with kidney inflammation and eclampsia of pregnancy (convulsions and coma). Anyone with healthy kidneys would not be likely to be deficient in magnesium, but magnesium deficiency is common in man. Some of the reasons magnesium is so lacking is that it is lost in the urine when people take medication or ingest chemicals from the environment. It may also be low because we don't have enough hydrochloric acid in the stomach to dissolve it so it can go into the blood.

Sometimes magnesium deficiencies have no symptoms, but common symptoms are muscular twitching and mild or moderate delirium. Heart symptoms include abnormal rhythms, fast heartbeat and increased toxicity from digitalis. In a study of seven people, four had abnormal ECGs, which were completely reversed when magnesium was given. Magnesium deficiencies show up as changes in heart function, but they are usually not severe unless the person is under a great deal of stress. Also, if the person increases his resistance by exercise and good nutrition, including magnesium, he should not have a major heart problem.

When there is an overload of calcium and a loss of magnesium, the stage is set for heart cell death. Loss of the magnesium keeps enzyme systems from working, especially the systems that furnish energy for the heart to beat. Thus, heart cells will break down.

In raising livestock, the animals sometimes die suddenly from heart disease when they're being fattened or transported to the slaughterhouse. Experiments show that fewer animals died if magnesium and chloride were increased. The death rate was reduced significantly, and the animals were much less excitable. The treatment reduced the amount of calcium and sodium in the heart, and increased the amount of magnesium and possibly potassium (Classen, 1979).

That information has probably been broadcast widely to farmers. I've never read much about the importance of magnesium for human hearts except in medical journals, and very few people read those. Hopefully, we can spread the word about good nutrition and reduce the death rate in humans, as was done in livestock.

Magnesium and calcium share the same transport system when they travel around the body. If we take large doses of calcium without magnesium, calcium takes up all the space on the "bus," and magnesium doesn't get to ride! We need about twice as much calcium as magnesium, and the recommended multimineral supplement given in Lesson 1 is in that ratio.

It is difficult to get enough magnesium in our food. For example, magnesium is plentiful in whole wheat; almost all of it is removed from white flour. Some magnesium is lost when food is cooked, and water softeners remove both calcium and magnesium. Alcohol binds magnesium so the body can't use it.

Magnesium is needed to maintain the correct potassium level. Potassium is essential for proper working of muscles, especially in the heart. Also, a deficiency of magnesium may cause blood clotting.

The most consistent adverse reaction caused by a magnesium deficiency is that calcium is deposited in soft tissues. It concentrates particularly in the kidneys and causes kidney stones.

A deficiency of magnesium causes the nerves in the arms and legs to be irritated. In infants, a deficiency causes convulsions. It causes anyone to be hyperirritable; there are abnormal reactions of nerves on muscles and abnormal heart rhythms (Goodhart and Shils, 1973).

A 55-year-old man with magnesium deficiency was irritable, uncooperative; had cramps in his muscles, tremor, weakness, hallucinations and lapse of memory. Then he was given magnesium sulfate. Thirty-six hours later he was much better, but it was several more days before his mind returned to normal (Hall and Jaffe, 1973).

Magnesium Deficiency Symptoms. Magnesium deficiency symptoms range from mental fatigue and feelings of being unable to cope (Do you know any young mothers, housewives or businessmen or women who have these symptoms?) to excitability, irritability, agitation, depression and anxiety (Hall and Jaffe, 1973).

Eating large amounts of calcium, sugar or protein can cause deficiencies because these foods don't add magnesium to our diets. There will be a loss of muscle tone in the intestines, which can't contract well enough to expel gas as fast as it is formed. Severe deficiency is found in cirrhosis of the liver, malabsorption, digestive disturbances and chronic alcoholism. Prescribing a little more magnesium should go a long way to prevent muscular disease, including muscular dystrophy. The human heart depends especially on magnesium, and heart failure is still the number one cause of death (Miller, 1974). Coffee, tea and colas are strong diuretics, which cause the loss of magnesium and potassium, leading to a deficiency and upsetting the entire nervous system.

Magnesium is found in many foods, but the richest sources are green vegetables, molasses, nuts and whole grains, which many people don't eat. Butter is a good source, as are bananas, oranges, grapes, chicken and seeds. You can harvest your own fresh magnesium by growing carrot tops in a dish and mixing them with your salad greens. Hard water contains magnesium, which is much better for us than soft water, which contains sodium. Diets high in calcium are likely to be low in magnesium because there's so much calcium that magnesium may not be absorbed.

Phosphorus

Phosphorus is a mineral in such large supply in the average American diet that deficiencies are seldom found.

It is common to get too much phosphorus, however, and the ratio of calcium to phosphorus and other minerals is what's important. Osteoporosis develops when a person takes in more phosphorus than calcium (Jowsey, 1975).

When people take antacids for a long time, phosphorus can't be absorbed in the intestinal tract. This causes weakness, bone pain and a definite deficiency of calcium, which is lost in the urine (Lotz, 1964). This may cause osteomalacia. People should usually substitute hydrochloric acid for the antacid. Symptoms of too little acid are gas, bloating and a too-full feeling after meals. Hydrochloric acid and pancreatic enzymes usually relieve the symptoms quickly.

Food sources of phosphorus are the most common foods—meat, milk, eggs, cheese, grains, legumes and nuts.

Potassium

If experimental animals don't get potassium, heart muscle cells die, and kidney tubules fill up with fiber and can't filter wastes. It is thought that this damage is reversible, but studies have never been done on humans because the deficiency causes damage so fast.

Rheumatoid arthritis is also related to potassium deficiency. Raw vegetable diets, high in potassium, have helped many patients. Potassium is lost in perspiration, not usually enough to do any harm, but when people take steam baths, they might lose enough to cause pain. The Finns take steam baths and have one of the highest rates of arthritis in the world.

Heart disease has been treated with potassium by several investigators since 1957. When the therapy first started, it was thought that the improvement in symptoms was because of low sodium, but now it is thought that if enough potassium is given, the cells take it up, and sodium leaves the cells, as it should, since it belongs outside the cells. Also, anyone who takes a lot of sodium loses potassium in the urine. Just by cutting down on sodium (salt), more potassium is left in the cells (Weber, 1974).

Potassium deficiency is found in congestive heart failure, cirrhosis and steatorrhea (inability to absorb fats). The brain cells of epileptics are deficient in potassium. If we eat too much sodium chloride (salt), our blood shows too little potassium, and our blood sugar will be low. With supplements of potassium we can absorb glucose from storage in the liver and keep our blood sugar normal.

Potassium can be toxic in large amounts. Some investigators say any amount over 100 mg in tablet form is toxic.

When anyone has diarrhea or vomiting, the potassium reserves can be seriously depleted, and supplements in liquid form should be given because it might not be possible to get enough from food.

Babies Are Vulnerable. Babies are especially vulnerable to potassium deficiency because they are growing so fast. When we go without water, we need more potassium, and babies can't drink when they want to, so they may need more than they get. Babies who die from diarrhea lose up to 40 percent of muscle potassium. When babies with diarrhea were given supplements of potassium, the death rate went down from 34 percent to 6 percent.

Any shock can cause a loss of potassium, especially surgical shock. Potassium supplements are being used now in surgery. A burn or injury can cause excess loss of potassium. It is known that negative ions in the air cause twice as much potassium as usual to be lost in the urine of rats. If this is true for humans, they would excrete more potassium during thunderstorms. Also, people who use certain types of electric ionizing heaters may need supplements.

Diuretics are used to wash excess calcium out of

the blood vessels so it won't block the arteries and cause fatty plaques that lead to heart attack and stroke. However, when diuretics are used, potassium is washed out too, and potassium supplements should be taken. Formerly, tablets of potassium chloride were used, but now it is known that they cause strictures and ulcers of the bowel. It is better to eat high-potassium foods to get extra potassium.

Patients given cortisone lose potassium and retain sodium. They should eat less sodium and eat high-potassium foods. Patients who have chronic kidney failure should not take potassium supplements (Glazener, 1974). Anyone using laxatives or enemas for a long period of time loses potassium, especially if the enemas are retained for a long time.

Potassium Deficiency. In a potassium deficiency, people lose weight, the acid in the stomach is weakened so it is difficult to digest proteins and kidney function is impaired. Sometimes people have edema (retention of fluid) during a potassium deficiency, and glucose tolerance is impaired in diabetics, possibly because insulin can't be excreted. The kidneys are more subject to infection if they're deficient in potassium, which helps defend against bacteria.

The potassium in blood plasma should be in medium amounts. If the potassium is too low or too high, death is almost certain. Too high an amount is worse than too low. Symptoms of too much potassium in cells are listlessness, mental confusion, numbness, a cold gray pallor, low blood pressure and a slow heartbeat.

There are several diseases in which the patient has a toxic level of potassium. They are kidney failure, extreme dehydration, shock and Addison's disease. These diseases can cause nerve problems—mental confusion, tingling in the arms and legs, numbness and so slow a heartbeat that the heart often stops beating. The episode seems the same as a heart attack, but blood is still flowing through the blood vessels. Even if this is not a typical heart attack caused by fatty plaques in the arteries, the person is just as dead.

Sugar and salt drive potassium out of the cells (Kirshmann, 1984). When we eat sugar, our urine becomes alkaline, and minerals aren't held in solution; they may combine with fat to cause atherosclerosis. We perspire potassium out of our tissues. Rather than taking salt tablets, we should take potassium.

Symptoms of deficiency are fatigue, constipation, muscle cramps, lack of appetite and mental apathy. More serious effects are depression, weakness, disorientation, irritability and abnormal heart rhythms (Lesser, 1977).

To absorb potassium, we need vitamin B6, sodium and magnesium, which will help the nerves work. This is especially important for the elderly, who are often weak and unable to concentrate. In one study, 86 percent improved.

Sources of Potassium. Fruits and vegetables are excellent sources of potassium. Bananas are famous for the mineral, but they don't contain as much potassium as other foods, especially butternut squash, lima beans and green leafy vegetables.

There is no potassium in white sugar, and only one-fourth mg per calorie in white flour. A food must have one milligram per calorie to carry its weight, and if any food is less than one, we must obtain potassium from other foods. Best sources are celery at 20 mg per calories; spinach, 29 mg and blackstrap molasses at 13.5 mg per calorie.

Meat eaters have a lower intake of potassium than vegetarians. Fat eaters have an even lower intake because fat cells are very low in potassium and very high in calories. Beef animals are raised to furnish three parts of fat to one of protein, whereas in the old days, the ratio was three parts of protein to one of fat. Fat in bacon has only 0.2 mg of potassium to a calorie, and there is no potassium in vegetable oil. Fat as corn oil causes great deterioration of heart tissue if potassium is marginal. (We already know that we shouldn't eat corn oil margarine!)

Unrefined seeds and nuts have a high rate of potassium to low sodium. Humans who eat natural foods get plenty of potassium, but refined foods do not furnish the amounts needed. For example, 99 percent of the potassium is removed when sugar is refined. Seventy-five percent of the potassium in whole-wheat flour is removed when it's made into white flour. Canned and frozen vegetables lose up to 50 percent of their potassium when processed. When vegetables are blanched for freezing, the heat destroys the cell membrane, and the potassium spills into the water.

When we know such details about the food we're putting into our bodies, isn't it amazing that people think they can stay well by eating junk food? Where are they going to get the B vitamins they need to get the energy to keep sodium out of the cells so the potassium balance will be correct?

We should not try to suddenly change our diets without a little study of the food and food supplements outlined in Lesson 1 of this course. Our wonderful bloodstream will take the nutrients through the blood vessels to all the cells so they will function the way nature planned for them to.

Sodium

It seems that everybody knows the most important thing about sodium—don't eat too much of it!

But that's really brushing sodium off too lightly. Sodium and its partner, potassium, transmit messages along our nerves (Ballentine, 1978).

We need very little sodium. Many people live better when they reduce their salt intake to as little as one-eighth teaspoon a day. The average American eats from one to two teaspoons a day— 5,000 to 10,000 mg of salt. People who eat a lot of processed snack foods may eat as much as four teaspoons a day. This may be so hard on the body, if it is continued for a long time, that high blood pressure may *force* those people to reduce their salt intake.

It would help to get optimum amounts of potassium because a high intake of potassium seems to result in lowered sodium. We should stay away from canned foods. There are 2 mg of sodium and 316 mg of potassium in fresh peas; but in canned peas, there are 236 mg of sodium and only 96 mg of potassium (Ballentine, 1978).

TRACE MINERALS

Trace minerals are used in the body in tiny amounts, but without them we would die. All of them work together, and we need more when we're under physical or emotional stress.

Trace minerals known for years to be needed by man are manganese, iron, cobalt, copper, zinc and iodine. Added to that list in the last 30 years are molybdenum, selenium and chromium, and in the last 10 years, silicon, vanadium and nickel.

All of these elements are judged essential because we get sick if we don't get enough of them, and our ailment is prevented or cured when we get them. Every one of these elements can be toxic if we get too much. That applies, of course, to water and air as well, but we are careful about the amounts we take of all of them (Mertz, 1981).

Trace elements help enzymes work with vitamins and vice versa. They depend on each other, but they are required in different amounts; for example, 400 mg of magnesium is suggested each day for the average adult, but only about 15 mg of zinc. The body cannot manufacture any trace mineral; we must get them all from food or food supplements.

Trace minerals help activate thousands of enzyme systems in the body, so each mineral helps out in more than one enzyme system. All of these elements are specific; that means a deficiency of one element can be prevented or cured only by the element that is deficient; no other element can re-

pair the damage. Special carriers recognize the mineral as it enters the body, and deliver it to the specific cells and parts of the cells where the mineral is needed. The carriers usually carry about one-third of their maximum load. This is probably nature's way of getting rid of an overload. If we eat too much of a mineral, the excess will be excreted in urine and feces.

Of greatest importance is absorbing the minerals we eat. Proteins (mineral carriers) are partly digested in an acid medium (pH 2) in the stomach. Their digestion is finished, and the digestion of carbohydrates and fats, which supply nutrients that help absorb the minerals, takes place in an alkaline medium (pH 8 to 9) in the small intestine. From there, the minerals go to the blood and then to every cell in the body (Mertz, 1981).

If we don't eat the nutrients needed to maintain the correct acidity and alkalinity, we can't assimilate minerals. But these nutrients are found in the natural food diet we advocate.

Chromium

A chromium deficiency can lead to low or high blood sugar. Chromium is a cofactor for insulin and is a part of the glucose tolerance factor, which is what regulates our blood sugar level so we won't have hypoglycemia or diabetes. Diabetics, who obviously have low stores of chromium or they wouldn't have the disease, absorb an abnormal amount of chromium if it becomes available. A deficiency is also related to atherosclerosis. Sugar and chromium are related in that too much sugar helps cause fatty plaques in the arteries. A deficiency of chromium keeps us from using sugar correctly.

"Well-balanced" diets of Americans were found to be remarkably low in chromium. To determine if there was any relationship between low chromium stores and blood sugar levels, researchers studied glucose tolerance because so many people had either diabetes or hypoglycemia, and the cause of their illnesses couldn't be explained. As many as 50 percent of the patients with abnormal blood sugar levels regained normal glucose tolerance with chromium supplements. Later a supplement called Glucose Tolerance Factor was developed that contains chromium, three amino acids and vitamin B3, which has been successfully used to help control diabetes.

Chromium in Childhood. Children who have juvenile diabetes mellitus have smaller amounts of chromium in their hair than normal children have. Hair is often tested to determine its mineral content, as excess minerals in the hair usually mean that excess minerals in the body are being released to avoid a toxic buildup in the cells. Also, women who have several children have less chromium in their hair than women who have no children. The longer a woman has been pregnant, the less chromium she has in her hair. Thus if pregnant women don't take chromium supplements, they will have less chromium the more times they get pregnant, and their offspring may be deficient in chromium.

Infants whose mothers were given chromium can use carbohydrates better than those whose mothers were not given chromium. Thus the children may avoid low and high blood sugar.

Chromium in Foods. When cereals are refined, they lose 84 percent of their chromium. When sugars are refined, they lose 100 percent. Thus diets high in refined foods may lead to a deficiency of chromium. Brown sugars containing molasses are a fair source. Yeast is a rich source of the mineral. Vegetables are estimated to supply 30 to 50 parts per billion; grains, 40 ppb; and fruit, 20 ppb. The best food sources are brewer's yeast (not torula), black pepper, liver, cheese, bread, mushrooms and beef. The lowest amounts are in skim milk, chicken breast, white flour and haddock.

Most people should take supplements to be sure they have enough, but they should allow for a lag period before they feel the effects.

Cobalt

The main purpose of cobalt in the body, so far as is known, is to make B12 a good working vitamin. B12 activates enzymes and helps make red blood cells. It doesn't take much cobalt—just 0.1 mcg a day—that's the amount of graphite that would be in a period at the end of this sentence if I were writing with a pencil. The normal diet of meat eaters supplies five to eight mcg a day.

A deficiency of cobalt causes impaired growth and listlessness; people become emaciated and anemic. Three hundred micrograms a week of B12 will eliminate the symptoms.

Too much cobalt causes polycythemia (too many red blood cells). At one time, beer glasses were dipped in cobalt chloride to help stabilize the foam on the beer. This poisoned the beer drinkers, who got polycythemia, abnormal nerve function and degenerated muscles. They had 10 times the normal amount of cobalt in their tissues.

Copper

One of the most important things copper does is to help make red blood cells. Iron can't function without copper, which helps release iron and transport it around the body (Hambidge, 1974). There also may be deficiencies of copper if there is too much zinc or cadmium. Enzyme systems that need copper may not get it. In farm animals, the deficiencies cause slow growth and poor reproduction.

Nerves don't function well without copper, but if large doses of copper are given, seizures can occur. Fourteen times as much zinc should be eaten as copper (Pfeiffer, 1975), so if you're taking food supplements, note the amounts of each on the label.

Deficiencies cause lesions in bones, osteoporosis, enlargement of the cartilage of the ribs, cupping and flaring of the ends of the long bones, spur formation, spontaneous fractures of the ribs, decreased pigmentation of the hair and skin, dilated veins near the surface, seborrheic dermatitis (a skin disease with patches of dry, moist or greasy scales on the face, genitals and especially on the scalp, sometimes spreading over the entire scalp and causing dandruff and itching). Also, diarrhea, nerve problems (especially in premature infants), and abnormal growth.

Copper deficiency may be the reason why some people, mostly young women, become anorexic (go without food until they lose so much weight that their lives are threatened). Copper is needed to make a neurotransmitter that sends messages needed for a normal intake of food. Thus the cause of anorexia is partly a deficiency of copper (Hoes, 1980).

A copper deficiency in children can be caused by an all-milk diet and can lead to anemia. They will need both copper and iron to correct it. Too little copper has caused disease in animals similar to stroke and heart attack in humans.

Pfeiffer (1975) has studied schizophrenia for many years, and he believes that schizophrenics have too much copper for the amount of zinc. He emphasizes strongly that we should get 14 times as much zinc as copper. Also, excess copper is often found in cancer patients' blood. Copper is an antagonist of vitamin C and zinc (Braverman and Pfeiffer, 1982).

Germanium

Germanium is a mineral that may be very important in the treatment of cancer and other diseases. It greatly enriches the oxygen content in the body. All diseases are partly caused by a deficiency of oxygen—each disease strikes when oxygen is lacking. Germanium helps the brain and heart, which need more oxygen than any other parts of the body. The mineral should be taken with an excellent diet of natural foods. Asai (1976) says he has used germanium-rich garlic to treat cancers of the lung, bladder and breast, as well as asthma, diabetes, high blood pressure, neuralgia, leukemia, softening of the brain and cirrhosis of the liver. American journals state that 40 percent of high blood pressure cases can be improved with garlic.

Iodine

Iodine is essential for man because, without iodine, the thyroid gland can't produce its hormone, thyroxin, which regulates the rate of metabolism (how fast we use foods). If we don't eat enough iodine, the gland enlarges to try to produce more thyroxin, and the enlarged gland is called goiter. Too little thyroxin makes a person overweight and sluggish. Essential processes of the body slow down: the rate of the heartbeat, conduction of nerve impulses and thinking.

Iodine deficiency in pregnancy causes stillbirths, malformed infants and, if severe, idiots called cretins. A slight deficiency causes mental retardation. Raw legumes (beans, peas and peanuts) can cause goiters, but cooking destroys the substance that causes the goiter. Deficiencies of iodine may be caused by doctors' drugs. Some are very potent inhibitors: sulfonamide tolbutamide, propelthiouracil, and methimazole.

Lack of iodine at puberty may cause heavy hips and thick legs. In women, it may cause ovarian damage and inability to become pregnant. A lack also causes headaches, listlessness and sluggishness.

"Myxedema" is hypothyroidism (low thyroid hormone output). Early symptoms are so vague that the disease may not be recognized. They are lethargy, frequent tiredness, sensitivity to cold and general ill feeling. Later the patient has a bloated appearance, with puffiness in the face, thick dry skin, sparse coarse hair, muscle weakness, slow thinking and hoarseness. Edema (collection of fluids) is common. The heart is often dilated and flabby, and the patient may rapidly develop atherosclerosis (fatty plaques in the arteries).

Excess iodine may contribute to a disease called Hashimoto's thyroiditis. Cells are damaged and as the disease continues, they are replaced by fibrous tissue (*Medical World News*, 1974). An excess may also make a person underweight and very active. He may not sleep well.

The Recommended Daily Allowance (RDA) of iodine is set by the Food and Nutrition Board of the National Academy of Sciences at 100 mcg a day for adults. One research team, after several years of research with 1,010 doctors and their wives, determined that the optimal intake of iodine would be about 10 times more than the RDA. When the subjects consumed 1,000 mcg a day, they had many fewer symptoms and signs of deficiency. This group of investigators has found that many other nutrients are required in amounts two to 10 times the amount suggested by the RDA.

The mineral is found in fish and other seafood and in sea vegetables (kelp, for example).

Iron

Iron is carried in the red blood cells combined with protein as hemoglobin. Hemoglobin delivers oxygen to the cells and picks up waste matter (carbon dioxide) and returns it to the lungs to be breathed out. Iron is one of the most important elements in nutrition. It is in many enzyme systems. It is absolutely essential for maintenance of energy systems within the tissue cells, without which life would cease within a few seconds (Guyton, 1976).

Iron is thought to be the nutrient that is the most scarce in human populations. Women are most affected by deficiencies (Hall, 1978). Although men need only about six to nine millograms a day, women need more—from 14 to 28 mg because of the loss of iron during menstrual periods. A conservative estimate is that 60 percent of all women in the United States suffer from iron deficiency anemia. Anemia is frequent during infancy, and especially common in prematures and twins. Sometimes anemic babies need folic acid rather than iron, and iron supplements make the baby worse. When people don't eat enough animal protein, the deficiency of iron is greater, and it is greatest among the poor and among children who are growing fast (Goodhart and Shils, 1973). Many adolescent girls who diet to lose weight or choose a diet of junk foods become anemic. Iron deficiency anemia contributes to weakness, ill health and substandard performance, but there are few deaths.

Studies show that iron-deficient rats that developed anemia could not perform "intellectual processes" as well as rats which were well nourished (*ICAN Update*, 1980). The investigators say that a deficiency of iron in humans may cause a decline in intelligence. This is true of many other minerals and vitamins as well. If any one of the nutrients needed to make a healthy cell is missing, the cell cannot function properly.

Deficiency symptoms include fatigue, weakness, lassitude, "dead-tiredness," vague gastrointestinal complaints, flatulence, constipation, diarrhea, nausea, craving for unnatural foods (common in pregnancy), eating clay or earth or ice, glossitis (inflammation of the tongue), stomatitis (inflammation of the mouth), dysphagia (difficulty in swallowing) and lack of hydrochloric acid in the stomach. Fingernails and sometimes toenails become ridged, easily broken, thin, lusterless, brittle and flattened, then spoonshaped. In severe cases, the heart may become dilated, and heart murmurs may be heard.

Sometimes there are light spots on the skin (vitiligo) and edema (Goodhart and Shils, 1973). The eyes show irritation of the delicate membrane lining the eyelids and the tongue is sore. The skin is pale. The external genital organs of the female are inflamed, and there is a chronic fungus infection of the mucous membranes (Bland, 1983).

We build back our stores of iron very slowly because, as we increase our iron intake, we absorb less of it. Small amounts of iron as found in multimineral supplements are recommended. However, even small amounts of iron cannot be absorbed without plenty of hydrochloric acid in the stomach. Iron isn't usually thought of as toxic, but it can build up in the body to poisonous levels. Siderosis and hemochromatosis are both diseases caused by too much iron. When cells are damaged by a deficiency of any vitamin or mineral, altered body chemistry can result in an overload of iron.

Manganese

Manganese is not as well researched as other minerals, but it is found throughout the entire body, especially in the liver, pancreas, pituitary, mammary glands and bones. Thus, deficiencies may show up as fragile bones or as abnormal growth of bones. Deficiencies slow down bone healing and the ability to reproduce. Backaches due to disc problems are common in deficiencies, but, of course, other deficiencies relate to backaches, especially deficiencies of vitamin C (Lee, 1983).

Probably the most important use of manganese is that it combines with superoxide dismutase, an enzyme that protects the cell membrane from attack by free radicals. Free radicals are parts of molecules that have been separated from their partners. They bounce around in the cell trying to join up with another partner. At every bounce, they damage the cell, and damaged cells cause aging and almost any other ailment you can name. Fast-growing cancer cells have little or no manganese or superoxide dismutase (Lee, 1983).

Man cannot live without manganese because important enzymes require the mineral. One of the most important is the enzyme that forms urea. If urea isn't made, ammonia collects in the body fluids and causes toxicity (Guyton, 1976).

Laboratory animals deficient in manganese do not grow correctly, they have bone abnormalities, they don't reproduce normally and the central nervous system doesn't work well.

Manganese is in many foods we eat, but as with animals, if we don't get the right amount, our bones, tendons and nerves will suffer. Many schizophrenics have excess copper in their blood, which can be corrected with zinc and manganese. It also may mean that anyone with an excess of copper is subject to schizophrenia (Aston, 1980).

Manganese and zinc help excrete excess copper in the blood, which is common in such diseases as depression, epilepsy, alcoholism, infectious diseases, heart problems and some cancers.

Deficiencies of manganese show up in children as poor development of bones, joints and cartilage. Physicians may interpret it as "growing pains." In older people, deficiencies may lead to diabetes, low blood sugar, arthritis, epilepsy, schizophrenia, weight loss, dermatitis, nausea, slow growth of hair, changes in hair color and very low amounts of cholesterol in the blood.

Athletes often have manganese and zinc deficiencies that cause cartilage problems, especially in the knees. Wherever in the bones the disease strikes, it responds well to a natural food diet with emphasis on zinc, B6 and manganese (Aston, 1980).

Inner ear problems may be caused by a manganese deficiency. The tiny crystals in the inner ear are the balance mechanisms of the body. A baby with manganese deficiency might not be able to balance himself and stand until he is three or four years old. Later he would not be good at sports.

If animals vary greatly in requirements of minerals, it seems obvious that humans do too. It cannot be tested, because it would be impossible to feed deficient diets on purpose to humans.

Manganese and the Brain. Manganese helps the brain to work well by helping hormones send messages. Manganese may prevent and cure cases of tardive dyskinesia (a rhythmic movement of muscles anywhere in the body, often in the face and mouth), if given in doses of 15 to 60 mg a day. Niacin (vitamin B3) sometimes helps in this disease if given at doses of 100 to 500 mg a day.

Manganese deficiency may cause lupus erythematosus and other collagen diseases. Epileptic patients are deficient in blood manganese. Animals have more seizures from manganese deficiencies, probably because the cell membranes are not stable. The investigators say that dietary supplements of manganese should be used to control seizures.

Manganese is absorbed slowly, and months may go by before manganese supplements help the patient. Occasionally, manganese taken by mouth may cause blood pressure to go up, but, otherwise, oral manganese is harmless, and food supplements may be helpful in diseases that have not been conquered.

Good sources of manganese are nuts, tropical fruit, whole grains, spices and legumes. Poor sources are refined sugar, vegetables, fruits, meats and other animal proteins. The germ of cereal grains is the richest source, and if people don't eat whole grains, they should consider taking supplements of manganese (Aston, 1980). Wheat germ, a good source, may be eaten as a cereal with milk.

The amount of manganese recommended for a 118-pound woman ranges from 1.1 to 16.5 mg a day; for a 154-pound man, 1.4 to 21 mg. However, the maximum might be much more. If we eat too much calcium and phosphorus, we can aggravate a manganese deficiency, so we should take more manganese. Lactose (milk sugar) may help us absorb manganese. It is rare that oral supplements of manganese are toxic, but manganese is better absorbed if taken in chelated form (Aston, 1980). Many multimineral supplements contain five to 10 mg, the amount suggested for one day.

Molybdenum

Molybdenum helps to furnish us energy. That statement alone should assure your interest in molybdenum, because almost everyone I talk to is tired and needs more energy. Most of the body's molybdenum is concentrated in the liver, kidneys, adrenals, skin and bones. People who eat refined foods may suffer from ailments of those tissues. If you've switched from red meat to plant proteins, you've found a good source of molybdenum—beans. Others are whole grains and organ meats. The suggested amount of molybdenum to take as a supplement is from 150 to 500 mcg a day (Lee, 1983).

Selenium

Selenium was thought to be toxic until 1957. Of course that was in large amounts. But it is now known to protect against cancer and many other diseases (Schwarz, 1975). Selenium, sulfur-containing amino acids and vitamin E work together very closely. Vitamin E and selenium break down and detoxify peroxides and keep free radicals from doing their dirty work. Free radicals damage: (1) connective tissue, (2) the elastin in artery walls and other tissue, (3) the lubricant that should protect your joints so that you won't have arthritis and (4) tissue cells, which accumulate age pigments (brown spots on skin and also in brain cells, which you can't see but which cause clots to form in blood vessels).

One of the most exciting studies I've found is on selenium and its effect on cancer in laboratory animals. Schrauzer and Ishmael (1974) used mice that are bred to get breast cancer spontaneously (the way humans get it—not by injections of chemicals). On a normal diet of laboratory chow, 82 percent of the mice developed breast cancer. But on the same diet, with two ppm of selenium in their drinking water, only 10 percent of the mice developed cancer. Let's shout that from the housetops.

Deficiencies of selenium cause growth impairment. But possibly the most tragic diseases related to selenium deficiency are muscular dystrophy, heart muscle degeneration, death of liver cells and kidney damage. The more blood vessels there are in one location, the more selenium is needed. Blood vessels congregate in the lungs and heart. Studies show that these areas of the body degenerate without selenium (Hunter and Lusk, 1973). If anyone has these problems and is not taking selenium, he is missing the protection he deserves.

High blood pressure, which often leads to heart attack and stroke, responds to selenium. Eyes that have cataracts have only about one-sixth as much selenium as normal eyes. Selenium also may help people who are extra-sensitive to light (Hunter and Lusk). Selenium neutralizes heavy metals such as mercury, cadmium, silver and probably lead, by binding them so they can't react dangerously in the body. But since selenium is bound to the metals, it can't do the work that it usually does, and we should probably take more during bad pollution times or if we live or work in a heavily polluted area.

Oxygen reacting on fat makes the fat rancid, whether the fat is butter sitting on your table at home or inside the membranes of your cells. That's why selenium and other antioxidants are so valuable to the body—they keep the body fats from becoming rancid. Rancidity in membranes leads to free radicals and all the damage they do. Selenium helps to destroy rancid fats before they attack the cell membranes. It works with vitamin E, which acts inside the membranes to prevent rancidity at that point. Rancid fats greatly damage cells, causing premature aging, cancer and heart disease (Fouad, 1979).

We can get too much selenium, just as we can get too much of anything. Large amounts inhibit certain enzymes and adversely affect the fetus. Bone and cartilage can be abnormal.

Silicon

Silicon is a trace mineral recently found to be essential. During a short period of bone formation, it is concentrated in bone in even higher amounts than calcium. Animals deficient in silicon developed severe bone deformities, especially in the skull. It is also needed in collagen, the tissue that holds our cells together.

It isn't yet known how much silicon man needs or how it is used, but it may be important for the health of the heart. It is known that silicon is missing to a great extent in the aortas of animals that have atherosclerosis. Supplements of silicon improved the health of these animals (Mertz, 1981).

Zinc

Zinc is needed in three ways: (1) for healing of burns and wounds, (2) for normal growth and (3) for sexual maturity. The prostate gland and sperm cells have more zinc than any other organs or tissues. This is reflected in the many men who have prostate problems and low zinc stores. Symptoms of prostate ailments are frequent urination, especially at night, the feeling of never quite emptying the bladder so there is dribbling of urine or a weak stream of urine (Wright, 1977). Dr. Wright's treatment includes:

(1) chelated zinc, 50 mg, 1 tablet three times a day,

(2) essential fatty acids, 400 mg, 1 capsule three times a day,

(3) tablets from whole-animal prostate gland, 2 tablets, three times a day,

(4) pollen tablets, 3 a day.

A physician I met on a tour told me, "Every man gets prostate trouble if he lives long enough." Surely, our nutritious diet that includes zinc supplements can prove that statement false.

If we don't get enough zinc, our senses of smell and taste are not good. People salt their food too much because they can't taste a little bit of salt. Then they drink a lot of water to quench their thirst and get the salt out of their bodies. Some people who react this way have been given 100 mg of zinc sulfate a day, and their taste returns (Cott, 1973). When I counsel people in nutrition, I am startled by the large number of people who have lost their sense of smell. On a diet of natural foods and food supplements, they usually regain it.

Zinc and Wound Healing. It has long been known that zinc is needed to heal wounds. The number of days women had to stay in the hospital after gynecological surgery was cut in half when they were given zinc supplements. In the women who were not given zinc, 75 percent of surgical wounds broke apart after healing had started. Only 20 percent of zinc-treated women had this happen (Pories et al., 1974).

Zinc is needed for DNA and protein to be manufactured. It helps keep transplants of tissue from being rejected. Zinc levels are lower in women who use the Pill. Without zinc, our skin will not be healthy, and we won't have an appetite. We can't grow without zinc. Many schizophrenics are deficient in zinc and manganese, and have too much copper and iron (DiCyan, 1983).

It is obvious what when anyone is sick enough to go to a hospital, he's deficient in nutrients, probably many nutrients. Zinc supplements combined with a good diet and moderate amounts of all other nutrients would undoubtedly shorten or maybe prevent hospital stays. New cells can't be produced without zinc (or without other nutrients). So it is especially important to get plenty of zinc when in surgery. Zinc quickly heals leg ulcers in an average of 32 days, compared to 77 days without zinc treatment. Stress destroys zinc in the body during the stress of surgery, of driving the freeways or of an accident or burn. We require more zinc when we breathe in air polluted with cadmium. The answer is to get all nutrients with optimal amounts of zinc.

Zinc helps to keep hair in good condition; it prevents dull, dry, brittle, stiff hair. Without zinc, hair can be painlessly pulled out (Bland, 1983).

A woman in one of my early nutrition classes had two sons, ages four and two years. The four-year-old had been allowed to drink up to 10 glasses of apple juice a day, which was the main source of his calories. He became deficient in many nutrients, and his little two-year-old brother took great pleasure in pulling his hair out in chunks. The boy didn't even cry; it didn't hurt. Obviously, he was deficient in zinc as well as in many other nutrients.

Zinc is refined out of many of our foods, but fish, meat and eggs are good sources, as are pumpkin seeds.

DANGEROUS MINERALS

What are heavy metals? What harm do they cause?

The dangerous metals are aluminum, arsenic, cadmium, lead and mercury. They're dangerous because they are toxic, and they shouldn't be taken into the body. But with the pollution of air, food and water we take in a lot of them. Here are some of the bad things they do:

(1) Destroy brain and nerve cells.

(2) Increase the permeability of the cells, allowing nutrients to leak out and poisons to get in.

(3) Inhibit the work of enzymes. This leads to fewer enzymes and hormones. We can't break down proteins to make enough amino acids or make enough energy for all our cells (Alseben and Shute, 1973).

Living things have evolved in a world with very few toxic elements; therefore, the body hasn't been required to detoxify these poisons until the present time. Now, there's a great deal of lead, cadmium and arsenic in our polluted air, food and water because those metals are used in industry. A renowned authority on the subject says we are killing ourselves with toxic minerals. Pollution and food processing, says Dr. Henry A. Schroeder (1975) of Dartmouth Medical School, are the major killers of man. The pollution from pesticides, weed killers, carbon monoxide and many other things people worry about is degradable because they are from organic substances. But no metal is degradable. Once metals are dug from the earth, they stay with us, and they'll be around as long as we are.

Aluminum

Aluminum could be the one substance in the universe that will ultimately end all human life. Aluminum makes up 8.4 percent of the earth's crust, so it is in almost everything we eat (Bjorksten, 1981).

The aluminum accumulates in the tissues at a steady rate, increasing continuously, which could cause death (if it continues long enough) in 100 percent of the people within 120 years. Aluminum congeals the brain, causing severe nerve symptoms, and immobilizing the proteins the body needs. It is found in large amounts in cases of senile dementia (Pfeiffer, 1975). Chelation, which is the joining of toxic metals to an agent that draws them out of the body, doesn't work with aluminum. Now, most people die of heart and blood vessel diseases and cancer, but in the future, it may be that most of us may die of aluminum poisoning (Bjorksten, 1981).

No More Aluminum. We may not realize how we take it into our bodies. Schroeder says the aluminum in baking powder and cooking utensils does not damage our tissues—it is usually excreted. However, Pfeiffer (1975) warns us against cooking acid foods in aluminum pans. Mineral deposits on the pans may go into the food and then into the "unsuspecting consumer."

The most common sources of the poisonous metal are processed cheese, table salt (aluminum is added to keep salt from caking) and white flour (aluminum is part of the bleaching material).

Two major sources of aluminum are antacids, which contain aluminum hydroxide gel and are available as many trade names and deodorants, which get into the body through the pores.

The first person who had poisoning attributed to aluminum was a metal worker who had loss of memory, tremor, jerking movements and incoordination. Later studies showed that various medicines contained aluminum and could cause a health hazard.

Aluminum is known to accumulate in the brain, and a tragic disease that relates presenility to aluminum toxicity is Alzheimer's disease. The usual program of natural foods and moderate amounts of food supplements may well prevent this ailment, now becoming more and more common. As of now, most researchers say that once the brain cells are filled with aluminum fiber, the disease cannot be reversed. The time to start your nutritional therapy is now.

Arsenic

Arsenic is used to feed chickens and swine to make them fat, to deworm animals, to control weeds and insects and to make cigarettes. Most of the arsenic entering the body is changed to arsine oxide, which keeps the cells from using oxygen. Symptoms of the gas are headache, loss of appetite, vomiting, blood in urine, numbness, abdominal pain

and yellowing skin. It is said that all of us have all these symptoms from time to time—the difference is in degree (Alsleben and Shute, 1973).

Arsenic's major effect is to kill capillaries, especially in the blood supply to the pancreas and adrenals. When capillaries are damaged, plasma and proteins leak out and cause sclerosis (hardening) and fibrosis (formation of fibrous tissue), which can lead to scleroderma (hardening of the skin), multiple sclerosis, arthritis, even heart damage. The linings of the stomach, intestines and kidney tubules can be so damaged that they bleed and destroy cells.

Arsenic Kills Cells. Arsenic is used to treat cancer because it kills cells. Of course, it kills good cells as well as bad ones. It is hard to find arsenic in the body when it is used as a poison, thus it's hard to find it when it is eaten in contaminated food. The compounds have little or no taste, and the symptoms are similar to those of other illnesses. Arsenic pesticides kill more children than any other such substance. Fish often contain more arsenic than other foods, especially saltwater fish. Arsenic is a potential cancer-causing agent, especially cancer of the skin, lungs and liver. Arsenic accumulates in the hair, so hair analysis can help diagnose arsenic poisoning.

Cadmium

The most dangerous of the heavy minerals is cadmium because it replaces zinc in the body. The zinc is needed to break down fat in the tissues, but when cadmium takes up space needed by zinc, the fat can't be broken down and it piles up in the blood vessels. Then we have high blood pressure and heart disease. Cadmium is leached out of water pipes by soft water, which is usually acid. When we drink the water, we are drinking cadmium.

Symptoms of cadmium poisoning are lung damage similar to emphysema, kidney damage (stones) and anemias. Cadmium has probably more lethal possibilities than any other element. An estimated two million pounds of cadmium are released into the atmosphere a year when scrap steel is melted down. Phosphate fertilizer contains cadmium. The sprays used on apples leave a considerable amount of cadmium on the fruit. Tobacco smoke is especially dangerous, and it is estimated that each cigarette has enough cadmium to cause emphysema. The smoke that curls around the cigarette and is inhaled by others rather than by the smoker can cause cadmium poisoning.

Cadmium, a Mistake. When an enzyme system needs zinc, it can accept cadmium by mistake. When it realizes its mistake, it can't release cadmium so the enzyme reaction does not take place, and more cadmium collects in the cells. When this happens over and over, many cells are put out of commission, and tissues and organs eventually don't work (Pfeiffer and Iliev, 1977). Whole grains have six times more zinc than cadmium. But white flour has six times more cadmium than zinc. So when we eat white bread, we have only about a 16 percent chance of getting zinc, which we need, and we have an 84 percent chance of getting cadmium, which we don't need (Ballentine, 1978).

If the diet is good enough, we will have enough resistance to throw off the effects of small amounts of toxic metals. Ballentine (1978) suggests a diet rich in iron and zinc, whole-grain flour, plenty of vitamin C and milk protein. Selenium will help defend our bodies against cadmium toxicity. Cadmium collects in the kidneys and causes kidney damage. Another good defense is to take predigested amino acid supplements (Alsleben and Shute, 1973).

Lead

Lead is the second worst mineral. As it is now taken into the body, lead reduces life spans by 20 percent, increases infant mortality rates and increases the incidence of abnormal offspring (Schroeder, 1975).

Most of the lead poisoning in the general public is unrecognized. One of the most common sources of poisoning used to be from canned food because the seams of the cans were soldered with lead, and the lead leached into the food. The FDA realized this, and they ruled that all cans should be made without soldered seams. Symptoms of lead poisoning are achy feeling, heartburn or upset stomach, mental sluggishness and fatigue. This is the result of years of lead buildup. We take in lead from food, water and air, but the most dangerous is from air. Lead damages living organs, especially membranes of red blood cells and smooth muscles, such as those in the walls of the blood vessels and bronchial tubes.

Lead can cause anemia; the whites of the eyes can get slightly yellow. Other symptoms: irritability, insomnia, headaches, dizziness; finally twitching of the face and eyelid muscles, trembling of hands and fingers, tingling, numbness, neck and shoulder muscle pains and arm pains. Stomach problems are common, with nausea and vomiting. Leukemic children always have high blood levels of lead. The best treatment is to take vitamins and amino acid-chelated minerals and to eat a lot of beans and whole grains, which will combine with the lead and excrete it. Sulfur-containing amino acids help counteract the lead as do vitamin C and calcium. So we should eat eggs and add vitamin C and calcium tablets. We should also avoid breathing lead and try to stay out of traffic! (Alsleben and Shute).

Mercury

Most Americans have filled teeth. They probably think the fillings are silver but they are 50 percent mercury and only 33 to 37 percent silver, with moderate amounts of tin, copper and zinc. Many studies show that the mercury from the fillings leaches into the blood and poisons the body. People have mental illnesses, the "shakes," emotional problems and a disease that resembles multiple sclerosis (Huggins, 1982).

A 17-year old-girl with a high IQ, who was formerly a cheerleader and had a lot of friends, suddenly changed. She would never leave her mother, she dropped out of school, was highly introverted and mildly discouraged with life. She had severe chest pains and was worried about dying. She had been to 50 psychiatrists without any help. Her dentist replaced mercury amalgam fillings with "composite." For the next four days, as the stored mercury was dumped into her urine, she had attacks, but after that, the attacks stopped and her health problems disappeared. If you're already on a natural food program and you still have these problems, you might want to see your dentist about replacing mercury fillings with some other substance.

Mercury Changes Cells. Mercury changes every cell with which it comes in contact. It affects mucous membranes of the mouth, esophagus, stomach and intestinal walls. The damage is especially ominous if it occurs in the brain, liver and kidneys. Early mercury poisoning symptoms are the same as those of the flu: dry throat, hacking cough, headache, chills, fever. To detoxify, take all nutrients plus nucleic acids (Alsleben and Shute). This sounds like our diet and food supplement program as given in Lesson 1.

Many diuretics are made with mercury; the kidneys eliminate not only the mercury but also excess water and water-soluble nutrients. Mercury is attracted to sulfur; therefore it destroys many of the sulfur-containing amino acids. Selenium is helpful in detoxifying mercury. If you've ever wondered why fish that have so much mercury in their tissues aren't poisoned, it's because they also have much more selenium, which keeps the mercury from being toxic (Pfeiffer, 1975).

HAIR ANALYSIS

Let's consider hair analysis, since it is becoming so widely advertised that many people request it. First, people think they will be told what vitamins and minerals to take. No, vitamins are not included, just minerals.

I have had counselees tell me, "Don't start me on hair analysis. I've been that route. If calcium is low, they put you on calcium; three months later, another analysis shows that calcium is too high and phosphorus too low; so they take you off calcium and put you on phosphorus. Three months later, I have to have another analysis, and three months later, another, and I'm on a merry-go-round." I agree. In most cases it is not necessary.

Here's what a typical booklet furnished by a hair analysis laboratory says: "High calcium and magnesium with relatively low sodium and potassium is a classic pattern for low blood sugar. A six-hour glucose tolerance test should be run to confirm it."

Any good nutritionist or physician should be able to tell by talking with a counselee that symptoms of low blood sugar are present. In my food and food supplement plan, everybody eats a diet of natural foods and takes moderate amounts of all food supplements. The body will take the nutrients it needs and excrete the rest. Thus, the body will heal itself. Following the six basic rules listed in Lesson 1 will make sure that our cells get the nutrients they need.

How do we get rid of the heavy metals that might be present? By taking vitamins A, C, E, selenium and especially legumes—beans, peas and peanuts. These are the best foods known to rid the body of toxic metals, and besides that, they furnish nutrients to build up our cells.

When people are sick, they obviously haven't been getting the nutrients they need. Their body chemistry is upset or they wouldn't be sick. On my program, they will be taking all nutrients; their body chemistry will become normal, and they will improve. Therefore, it seems unnecessary to have a hair analysis.

I spoke with a representative of a hair analysis company recently, and he said, "Hair analysis hasn't been as helpful as we thought it would be."

FOOD AND FOOD SUPPLEMENT PROGRAM

One of my counselees complained of headaches, allergies and other ailments. She improved on the diet, but her headaches recurred often enough so that she had to continue painkilling drugs. Finally, she told me she worked at a drive-in bank window that had a roof over it and very poor circulation of air. The combination of a previously poor diet and the constant exhaust fumes in the enclosed area had started her on a vicious cycle of headaches and drug poisoning along with the lead poisoning from the exhaust. The girl changed her job, stayed on her diet and supplements and recovered.

The diet and food supplement program I'm talking about is in Lesson 1 of this course. Another helpful book is my cookbook, *Switchover! The Anti-Cancer Cooking Plan for Today's Parents and Their Children*. If you need drastic changes in your diet, it's obviously because you have drastic health problems. I counseled a lovely woman recently. She said she had only a few minor ailments, but her daughter had been in one of my nutrition classes, and she had given her mother a counseling session with me as a birthday present. That's really the time to start doing something about our health, before anything serious happens. And isn't it nice to know that a loving daughter wants her mother to be around a long time in excellent health.

When we become interested enough in our health, we will be glad to make the easy changes we've noted throughout this course. The food tastes so good and the results of this food program are so exciting, we'll know we're giving our bodies the best possible care.

QUESTIONS

TRUE/FALSE

1. Minerals are divided into two groups—major and trace, depending on the amounts needed by the body.

2. Chelated minerals are minerals that have been joined to amino acids so they will pass across membranes as needed.

3. Without magnesium, the intestines can't squeeze the feces along well enough to expel gas as fast as it is formed.

4. Osteoporosis develops when our diets contain more phosphorus than calcium.

5. The average American eats one to 2 teaspoons of sodium a day; people who eat a lot of snack foods may eat four teaspoons a day.

6. Trace elements help activate thousands of enzyme systems.

7. Iodine is required for a healthy thyroid gland, which regulates how fast we use food.

8. Without iron, life would cease within a few seconds.

9. Symptoms of manganese deficiency may be called "growing pains."

10. Zinc is especially important for the health of the sex glands.

11. Arsenic is fed to chickens and swine to make them fat, but it keeps the cells from using oxygen.

12. Cadmium is the most dangerous of the heavy metals because it replaces zinc in the body.

13. Sulfur-containing amino acids help counteract lead poisoning, so we should eat eggs and take vitamin C and calcium.

MULTIPLE CHOICE

1. Calcium: (a) helps conduct nerve impulses, (b) needs to be dissolved by hydrochloric acid, (c) helps the heart beat, (d) must be used in the correct ratio with magnesium.

2. Loss of calcium can result from: (a) coffee washing calcium out of the intestines, (b) drinking too many high-phosphorus soft drinks, (c) deficiency of vitamin D.

3. Sufficient magnesium helps: (a) provide strong bones, (b) improve your personality, (c) provide healthy nerves, (d) improve your enzyme system.

4. Magnesium deficiencies include: (a) muscle twitching, (b) delirium, (c) abnormal heart rhythms, (d) change in the heart muscle.

5. Signs and symptoms of potassium deficiency include: (a) heart disease, (b) rheumatoid arthritis, (c) cirrhosis.

6. Chromium relates to: (a) high or low blood sugar, (b) insulin, (c) atherosclerosis.

7. Too much or too little cobalt relates to: (a) poor growth, (b) anemia, (c) poor nerve function, (d) listlessness.

8. Deficiencies of copper cause: (a) osteoporosis, (b) spurs, (c) diarrhea, (d) nerve problems.

9. Germanium helps prevent: (a) cirrhosis of the liver, (b) asthma, (c) diabetes.

10. Manganese deficiencies may show up as: (a) fragile bones, (b) slow bone healing, (c) inability to reproduce.

11. Heavy metals are toxic and they: (a) destroy brain and nerve cells, (b) stop enzymes from working, (c) possibly cause Alzheimer's disease.

ANSWERS

True/False

1. T 2. T 3. T 4. T 5. T 6. T 7. T 8. T
9. T 10. T 11. T 12. T 13. T

Multiple Choice

1. a,b,c,d 2. a,b,c 3. a,b,c,d 4. a,b,c,d 5. a,b,c
6. a,b,c 7. a,b,c,d 8. a,b,c,d 9. a,b,c 10. a,b,c
11. a,b,c

REFERENCES

Alsleben and Shute. *How to Survive the New Health Catastrophes.* Anaheim, CA: Survival Publications, 1973.

Aston, B. Manganese and Man, *J. Ortho. Psych.* 9(4):237–249, 1980.

Asai, K. *On the Medical Properties of Germanium.* Tokyo: Asai Germanium Research, 1976.

Ashmead, DeWayne. *Chelated Magnesium.* Albion Laboratories.

Ballentine, R. *Diet and Nutrition.* Honesdale, PA: The Himalayan Institute, 1978.

Bestways. Oct. 1973, p. 27.

Bjorksten, J. *Rejuvenation* 9(4):76–77, Dec. 1981.

Bland, J. Editor, *Medical Applications of Clinical Nutrition.* New Canaan, CT: Keats, 1983.

Braverman, E.R. and Pfeiffer, C.C. *J. Ortho. Psych.* 11(1):28–41, 1982.

Cheraskin, E., Ringsdorf, W.M. and Medford, F.H. *Soc. and Occup. Med.* 5:558, 1977.

Classen, H.-G. Magnesium and Cardiac Necroses. *J. Int. Acad. Prev. Med.,* 6(1):118–138, 1979.

Cott, Allan. *J. App. Nutr.* 25(1,2):15–24, 1973.

Davis, A. *Let's Have Healthy Children.* New York: Signet, 1972.

DiCyan, E. *Your Good Health* 1(2):23, July 1983.

Dines Letter. P.O. Box 22, Belvedere, CA 94920, p. 14, May 1979.

Ellis, F.R. et al. *Am. J. Clin. Nutr.,* 25:555, 1972.

Flynn, A. *Am. J. Clin. Nutr.* 29(4–5):51–57, 1977.

Fouad, M.T. *J.Ap.Nutr.,* 28(1):6013, 1976.

———. *J. Ap. Nutr.* 31(1–2):14–23, 1979.

Galton, L. *Houston Post, Parade,* Feb. 8, 1976.

Glazener, E.J.H. *J. Appl. Nutr.* 26(1–2):28–33, 1974.

Goodhart and Shils. *Modern Nutrition in Health and Disease.* Philadelphia: Lea and Febiger, 1973.

Guyton, A.C. *Textbook of Medical Physiology.* Philadelphia: Saunders, 1976.

Hall and Jaffe. *JAMA,* June 25, 1973.

Halstead, B.W. *Public Scrutiny,* July 1979.

Hambidge, K.M. *Proc. Nutr. Soc.* 33:249, 1974.

———. *Am. J. Clin. Nutr.* 27:505–14, 1974.

Hoes, M.J. *J. Ortho. Psych.* 9(1):41–47, 1980.

Horrobin, D.F. *An Introduction to Human Physiology.* Davis, 1973.

Huggins, H.A. *J. Ortho. Psych.* 11(1):3–16, 1982.

Hunter, H. and Lusk, G.J. *Bestways,* Oct. 1973, p. 22.

International College of Applied Nutrition Update, p. 2; August 1980.

Jowsey, J.O. *Proc. Western Hemi. Nutr. Congress* IF 155–61, 1975.

Kirshmann, J. D. *Nutrition Almanac.* New York: McGraw-Hil, 1984.

Lee, W.H. *Your Good Health* 1(1):15–17, May 1983.

Lesser, M. *Select Committee Report.* Washington, DC: U.S. Govt. Printing Ofc., 1977.

Levander, O.A. *JADA* 66 (4):338–345, 1975.

Lichtman, et al. *N. Eng. J. Med.* 280:40, 1969.

Lotz, Ney, and Bartter. *Trans. Amer. Physicians* 77:281, 1964.

McBean, L.D. *Am. J. Clin. Nutr.* 27:603; June 1974.

Medical World News. Vol. 15:8k; Nov. 8, 1974.

Mertz, W. *Science*, 213:1332–1338, Sept. 18, 1981.

Miller, J. J. *JIAPM*, pp. 80–97, 1974.

Nieper, H. *JIAPM* 2(2):18–22, 1975.

———. *Mineral Transporters*. The Silbersee Hospital, Hannover, German Federal Republic, n. d.

Passwater, R. A. and Cranton, E. M. *Trace Elements, Hair Analysis and Nutrition*. New Canaan, Conn.: Keats, 1983.

Pfeiffer, C. C. *Mental and Elemental Nutrients*. New Canaan, Conn.: Keats, 1975.

——— et al. A. *J. Ortho. Psych.*, (9(2):79–89, 1980.

——— and Iliev, P. A Study of Zinc Deficiency and Copper Excess in Schizophrenias. (in) *Diet Related to Killer Diseases V: Nutrition and Mental Health*. Washington: U.S. Government Printing Office, 1977, pp. 143–150.

Schrauzer, G.H. and Ishmael, D. *Ann. Clin. Lab. Sci.*, 4:441–47. 1974.

Schroeder, H.A. (in) Labuza, T.P. *The Nutrition Crisis*. St. Paul, Minn.: West, 1975.

Seelig, M. The Requirements of Magnesium by the Normal Adult. *Am. J. Clin. Nutr.*, 14(6):342–390, 1964.

Shamburger and Willis. *CRC Reviews*, 6–71.

Schler, A. and Pfeiffer, C.C. *J. Ortho. Psych.*, 9(1):6–10, 1980.

Vesen, P. et al. *Lancet* II, 74, p. 110, July 13, 1974.

Wills, M.R. and Savory, J. *Lancet*, p. 29, July 2, 1983.

Wright, J. V. A Case of Prostate Enlargement. *Prevention*, July 1977, pp. 69–73.

Lesson 8

ARTHRITIS AND NUTRITION

LESSON 8—ARTHRITIS AND NUTRITION

THE WHAT AND WHY OF ARTHRITIS

ONE SUNDAY a few years ago, a big-city newspaper ran a full-page story about children who were suffering from rheumatoid arthritis. They were undergoing painful physical therapy. Among others pictured was a cute little two-year-old girl I'll call Mary.

As therapy, Mary was placed on a table and her knees and elbows were forcefully bent and moved to try to keep the joints flexible. She was described thusly: "Mary howls. Her bones crack. Her knees are crimson and swollen. Her face is puffy from drugs."

This medical treatment does absolutely nothing to get at the cause of the disease.

Others Are Helped

But thousands of children and adults who suffer from arthritis have been helped to normal or near-normal health with good nutrition. Their agony has been relieved, they go back to school or work free from pain.

However, very few physicians know that good nutrition can heal swollen and aching joints. Pain can be lightened; people can live out their lives without the misery of arthritis and other rheumatic diseases such as gout and bursitis.

The doctor who treated Mary didn't know about nutrition. I asked him what kind of diet his patients were on. He answered, "I don't know. I hope they get three squares a day."

Most physicians use this terse comment when speaking about arthritis: "We don't know what causes it. We don't know how to cure it. You'll have to learn to live with it. Take 12 aspirins a day and come back to see me in three months."

Obviously, this treatment does absolutely nothing to determine the cause of the disease.

Arthritis Attacks Joints

Arthritis, a disease of the joints, is one of the fastest increasing degenerative diseases. You probably don't think about your joints unless you have arthritis; then you think of them all the time because they hurt.

When they don't hurt, joints work beautifully as hinges of our bones. Each hinge consists of two ends of bones, shaped perfectly to allow smooth motion. Connective tissue (which holds our cells together), ligaments and tendons connect the bones. The ends of the bones inside the joint are covered by a thin layer of cartilage that the bones glide on very smoothly every time you move your elbow, knee and all other joints.

Also, another membrane, called the synovial membrane, surrounds the ends of the bones and secretes a fluid that "oils" the hinge and provides even smoother motion. Since these joints are used so much in movement, and since some of them are major weight-bearing joints, they are often injured. Many people think the injury is caused by day-to-day wear and tear, but it is now known that good food oils the hinges and makes the membranes and bones work well for a lifetime. Thus the injury is usually caused by poor nutrition.

Symptoms to Watch for

The following warning signs may help you recognize the danger of developing arthritis and you'll be able to stop eating junk food and change to a natural food diet before the disease progresses.

1. Stiff, painful joints when you wake up in the morning.
2. Pain and tenderness in any joint at any time.
3. Swelling.
4. Pain and stiffness in the lower back, knees and other joints.
5. Tingling sensations in the fingertips, hands and feet.
6. Fever, weakness, tired feeling, loss of weight.

Nutrition and Arthritis

It is easy, then, to figure out why our joints are injured. It's because the tiny damaged cells in any of the tissues surrounding the hinge could not be repaired because one or more vitamins, minerals or amino acids needed for repair were missing. Arthritis, is, therefore, a nutritional deficiency disease. If we eat all the nutrients we need, we can prevent or control arthritis.

Arthritis and many other diseases may run in families. This doesn't mean you inherit it and can't do anything about it. You may inherit a vitamin dependency, which means that some of your family members need an unusually high intake of one or more specific nutrients. But if you get these nutrients in your diet in sufficient amounts, you won't have the ailment. If you don't get these nutrients, any ailment your parents had may show up in you.

The arthritis patient has a known negative nitrogen and calcium balance. This means that his system can't use food well. Thus his body deteriorates a little every day. His muscles wither, his bones lose calcium and he lacks energy because he can't use sugar well.

The patient with rheumatoid arthritis has a systemic disease and is a sick individual. Most arthritics begin to improve quickly if they take hydrochloric acid (HCl). That strong acid will assure the conversion of proteins to amino acids needed to strengthen muscles and to make mucus to lubricate the joints. The acid will also dissolve the calcium and send it to the bloodstream, then to the bones and teeth where it belongs. If the calcium is not dissolved, it will be deposited in the joints. That's arthritis. The HCl is available at health food stores in tablet form.

Dr. Robert Bingham of the Arthritis Center in Desert Hot Springs, California, says (1972), "No person who is in good nutritional health develops rheumatoid or osteoarthritis."

KINDS OF ARTHRITIS

There are many forms of arthritis—rheumatoid and osteo, gout, bursitis, ankylosing spondylitis (arthritis of the spine, a variety of rheumatoid arthritis) and pyorrhea, also called arthritis of the teeth. We will discuss, primarily, rheumatoid and osteoarthritis. About 35,000,000 people suffer from those two common forms, but all forms respond to nutritional therapy.

Rheumatoid Arthritis

Rheumatoid arthritis (RA) usually strikes people in their thirties and forties. It causes crippling and destroys the cartilage and tissues inside the joints. Sometimes the bone is destroyed. Scar tissue forms between the joints that can fuse together. Soft tissues swell and are very painful.

Dr. Roger Williams (1971) explains what RA is. "Our joints and all other movable structures in our bodies must be lubricated, and the lubricant used is called synovial fluid. This fluid is mostly a solution of various mineral salts, but it contains mucus which gives it lubricating properties. The water in the fluid comes from the water we drink, and the minerals are supplied in our food. The mucus must be produced in our bodies by living cells from raw materials furnished by food. If we don't have enough of any mineral, amino acid or vitamin, or if the cells are poisoned by bacterial toxins or allergens, the cells can't make mucus, so the joints won't be well enough lubricated. Then every movement is accompanied by friction and pain."

Pain like that of the little girl in the newspaper story.

When the membranes aren't lubricated sufficiently and the smooth surface of the cartilage gets rough, the cartilage softens and eventually wears away until the bone is exposed.

Half a million children in this country are handicapped by RA and other ailments that often go with it: heart disease, strep infections in the throat, scarlet fever and infections in the upper respiratory tract. About 17,000,000 suffer from rheumatoid arthritis, mild or severe.

Osteoarthritis

Osteoarthritis (OA), a disease of the cartilage, strikes people in their fifties and sixties, and causes bony spurs and nodes in the hands, knees and spine.

When we have OA, here's what happens in the joints. The cartilage is destroyed, and the bone underneath is exposed. Small pieces of the cartilage remain in the joint. They become calcified and stick out above the surface of the joint. When these bony spurs get big, they may rub against each other and cause pain and keep us from moving the joint. Sometimes the joint is fused with scar tissue and it won't move at all.

Rheumatism

Rheumatism, also called fibrositis, is a condition of the muscles that usually attacks adults. It is caused by deficiencies of nutrients needed to make healthy muscles, but the pain of rheumatism can be caused by exposure to cold weather or by a direct draft of cold air. It causes pain and stiff and sore tissues, but it doesn't attack joints. In muscles it is called myositis; in bursae, bursitis; and in the back, lumbago. It can appear in the neck muscles. Sometimes old people have night cramps.

Gout

Gout is an arthritislike disease in which deposits of uric acid stack up in and near the joints. This keeps the joints from being well lubricated. Many more men than women have gout. Certain foods form acid crystals, which accumulate in large masses around joints. Some of these foods are fish and shellfish, sausage, goose liver and almost any meat product such as gravy, meat soups and meat sauces. It isn't just meat and fat foods that do the damage; it is "junk foods"—sweets of all kinds—pie, cake, ice cream and even strong spices.

Gout also occurs with constipation, indigestion, headache, neuralgia, depression, irritability, eczema, hives and heart symptoms; so gout is not just a pain in the big toe (where symptoms often originate), it is part of a general illness of the whole body. Uric acid crystals form in such large amounts that the patient is finally severely crippled. Sometimes the skin breaks and discharges the chalky crystals. Sometimes gout patients develop nodules about the size of a pea on their ears. Those are deposits of uric acid crystals.

Gout is related to kidney stones and gallstones in that the accumulation of this gravel is similar in all ailments (Warmbrand, 1974). It seems that hardening of the arteries is a similar deposit of calcium that has not been kept in solution because of a deficiency of hydrochloric acid in the stomach. Thus the damage may be caused by drinking water with meals and diluting the acid digestive juices.

Polymyalgia Rheumatica

Polymyalgia rheumatica (PMR) is marked by rheumatic pain in several muscles. It usually is found in elderly people, especially in the neck, shoulders and sometimes in the hips. The patients suffer from fatigue, they lose weight and they have low-grade fever.

Ankylosing Spondylitis

Ankylosing spondylitis (AS) is arthritis of the spine, although knees and shoulders may be painful. Even the eyes become inflamed in about one-third of the patients. Ten times more young adult men than women suffer from this disease. How many times have I heard people complain of low back pain! This is the way AS starts. It can proceed to a curvature of the spine that makes the patient hunch over. If you have low back pain, start the new nutrition now.

All these conditions are relieved by diet. Basically, the diet for all forms of rheumatism and arthritis is the same, but cherries in any form—juice, canned and especially fresh—are recommended specifically for gout, apparently because of their vitamin C content.

Medical students are taught, "There is no satisfactory treatment for these conditions and no known way to stop them from getting worse, which they do, gradually, during the rest of the patient's life" (Robbins, 1974).

It would be interesting to have the authors of medical textbooks meet some of the many people I know who have conquered their arthritis with good food and food supplements.

STRESS PROBLEMS

Stress and Arthritis

Maybe you've heard that arthritis usually develops after a person has suffered an unusual stress, which might be physical, such as an illness; mental, such as depression; or emotional (one of my counselees said she had been jilted by her boyfriend just before her arthritis developed).

Since I first heard this, I've been asking arthritics if they were under extreme stress before the illness developed. Many of them recall that something traumatic happened in their lives. Even if a trauma does happen, we don't have to suffer the pain of arthritis—we just need to eat better so that the stress we're going through won't damage our tissues.

When people are under stress they often don't feel like eating at the very time they need protective foods the most—and more of the food, not less. Since their livers, joints and all other organs don't get the nutrients they need, disease is caused somewhere in the body. Stress also causes poor digestion of foods. We can digest and assimilate foods better if our minds and emotions are working well.

We can compare the stress of arthritis to starting a car. When the motor is cold, it needs a lot of gas and not much air. The carburetor adjusts the mixture so it is "rich" in gas. If we kept up this amount too long, the car wouldn't run well. There would be "side effects" such as excess carbon or a foul-up of the electrical system.

The adrenal glands use a rich mixture containing all of the 32 hormones they make when there is stress. This is cortisone. But if we get too much of this mixture, it causes side effects just as taking too much cortisone—as a drug—causes side effects. It causes the adrenal glands to wither and it can even cause death.

When the automobile warms up and runs smoothly, the carburetor adjusts the fuel so more air and less gas go to the motor. When the body runs smoothly without much stress, the adrenal glands adjust the production of hormones to a combination that does not damage the body. If we eat well, we get the nutrients that the adrenal glands need. Hans Selye, a stress expert, says, "Poor foods certainly induce stress that can delay recovery."

Once I found a picture of a man in a medical textbook. His greatest claim to fame and the reason his picture was in the book was that he was the first man to be treated with cortisone for rheumatoid arthritis. That was soon after cortisone had first been manufactured in the laboratory. At that time, physicians thought they had the final answer to arthritis. The pain was relieved, patients were joyful—surely this was the hoped-for cure. But their joy was short-lived. Patients built up a tolerance to the drug, so that the dosage of cortisone had to be increased drastically to kill the pain. Such large doses caused poisoning, and the man pictured in the textbook was the first man to die of cortisone treatment for arthritis.

It is still important for the arthritic to have plenty of cortisone, but it must be manufactured in his own adrenal glands so that the right amount will be released at the right time. The only way we can make our own is to get the needed nutrients from our food. One of the most important of these nutrients is pantothenic acid, one of the B vitamins that we'll talk more about later.

Aspirin and Other Dangerous Therapies

Although aspirin is known to have severe side effects, a recent newspaper report from a medical conference tells physicians that the best treatment for arthritis is aspirin. The article says that aspirin has been used to treat arthritis for 100 years without a clear understanding of how it works. That probably means without a clear understanding of what it does to people. The newspaper report also said, "Aspirin can have toxic side effects. It may cause or aggravate ulcers and harm the liver, especially in children." All aspirin causes bleeding of the delicate membranes that line the stomach. A little aspirin causes a little bleeding; a lot of aspirin causes a lot of bleeding.

One of my friends, who was taking from 12 to 30 aspirin tablets a day because of his rheumatoid arthritis, was rushed to the hospital bleeding from both ends. The bleeding finally stopped and my friend lived, but the "treatment" he had undergone had made him worse for the 10 years or so he had been on it.

When anyone takes a lot of aspirin, vitamin C is

destroyed more quickly than without the aspirin. Thus anyone on a high-aspirin intake may get relief from pain, but he's making his condition worse.

It is generally accepted that the use of aspirin over long periods of time depresses the immune system. The patient may then suffer from chronic arthritis the rest of his life. The drug (acetylsalicylic acid), even in very small amounts, has caused numerous cases of poisoning in humans. One patient was reported to suffer from a heart weakness with a pulse rate of 136 and swelling of the face and mucous membranes. Other patients experienced profuse sweating, cold hands and feet and rapid pulse.

Other popular drugs aren't any better, especially cortisone. Many people have developed ulcers in the colon because of cortisone and other steroids such as ergosterol, progesterone, testosterone and aldosterone. Those drugs cause powerful side effects such as mental problems, diabetes, high blood pressure, peptic ulcers, lack of resistance to infection, fluid retention, cataracts, fragile bones and fat deposits, especially in the face. Another painful disease, osteoporosis (porous bones), is often a side effect of doctors' drugs. Cortisone does suppress the symptoms of RA, but when the drug is stopped, all the symptoms return.

Anti-inflammatory drugs cause some of the worst side effects, such as hearing problems, brain disorders, bleeding, skin rash, sore throat, shortness of breath and severe headache. The drugs also destroy red blood cells, and blood counts must be analyzed from time to time.

One more drug that suppresses the immune system is a gold compound. It has serious side effects. Nobody knows exactly how the body reacts to the gold shots. Some people think the gold acts as a stimulant, rather like shock therapy (Warmbrand, 1974). Everybody agrees that gold therapy is highly toxic. After using it, patients complain of skin diseases, stomach and digestive problems, kidney and liver ailments, headache, dizziness, severe anemia, ulcers in the mouth and general weakness. One percent of the people die from inflammation of the brain.

ENVIRONMENTAL POLLUTANTS AS A CAUSE OF ARTHRITIS

Environmental pollutants can destroy so many of the vitamins and minerals in our bodies that they can help cause arthritis.

Cigarettes. Smoking is known to use up vitamin C with every cigarette smoked. It upsets the vitamin balance and causes nutritional deficiencies that can lead to joint pain.

Alcohol. Anyone who drinks alcohol may destroy so much B1, B6 and folic acid (another B vitamin) that arthritis might develop. Magnesium is easily destroyed by alcohol, and magnesium is needed in dozens of enzyme systems. Everything in our bodies works through enzymes, and the manufacture of synovial fluid and healthy cartilage is no exception.

Stress. We talk a lot about stress in this course, because stress can cause damage to every cell in our bodies. As we said before, adrenal glands wither without needed nutrients, and they can't help us withstand damage from stress. Extra vitamin B and C plus minerals are needed, and if they're not taken in food and supplements, our joints can suffer. We need half as much magnesium as calcium. If we don't eat enough magnesium, calcium may be increased in the blood, which might cause bone spurs to form.

Medication. More than 90 percent of all the 100 top-selling drugs in this country can cause deficiencies of vitamins and minerals. All doctors' drugs have adverse side effects. One reason is that certain drugs compete for vitamins and minerals in the body. Thus, arthritics cannot absorb and use the nutrients needed for healthy joints and cartilage.

Mineral Oil. A laxative, mineral oil keeps calcium, phosphorus and vitamin D, all essential for the manufacture of healthy bones and teeth, from being absorbed. Mineral oil should never be used as a laxative.

Antacids. Antacids keep minerals from being dissolved, therefore the minerals can't go into the blood and cells. When calcium, for example, is dissolved in the stomach, it builds up bones so they won't be porous. Undissolved calcium can stack up in our bones as spurs. Antacids bind phosphorus in the digestive tract and it is not available to help make bones.

If your doctor tells you he doesn't know the cause or cure of arthritis, it's because he may not have studied nutrition, and he doesn't realize the importance of minerals and vitamins for healthy bones and joints. If and when he runs tests, he might not test for magnesium, zinc or phosphorus, because he probably has never read anything about the real cause of arthritis. This information is in medical journals and books in every medical library in the world, but is almost ignored in medical textbooks.

If we realize the importance of these vitamins and minerals, we will know to change to a natural food diet plus all known supplements so our bodies can heal themselves. Then we will no longer suffer from the pain and swelling of arthritis.

THE LIVER AND ITS INFLUENCE ON ARTHRITIS

Much of the stress of arthritis is actually caused

by a damaged liver—one that is not functioning well enough to process nutrients needed for the adrenal glands and for joints and tissues all over the body.

We have discussed the liver in Lesson 4, "Allergies and Nutrition." Let's review it here.

Three organs that are important in any discussion of arthritis are the liver, the pancreas and the adrenal glands. Arthritis is not just a disease of the joints—it affects all tissues, especially those three glands. They and the rest of the body will be well and we will not have arthritis if we get plenty of good, natural food and enough vitamins and minerals to make healthy cells.

Digestion and the Liver

When we eat, some of the starch is digested in the mouth and becomes sugar. You'll notice the sweetness if you eat a piece of bread or other starch. If you chew it long enough, it will taste sweet.

The partially digested starch goes to the stomach with the rest of the food. Starch digestion stops for the time being, and protein digestion begins. Protein is first broken down into small pieces called peptides when we chew it, and later the peptides are broken apart into amino acids.

Enzymes in the stomach, which work in a very strong acid medium, break the peptides apart, so if the acid in the stomach is strong enough, the big proteins are partially digested there.

The calcium we eat in milk, cheese, green leafy vegetables and other foods must also be dissolved in the strong acid of the stomach or it will not go into the bones and teeth. Instead, it will go to the soft tissues such as the cartilage and joints, where it can cause arthritis.

The foods next go into the small intestine where they must be digested in an alkaline medium with the help of the pancreatic enzymes. Here the digestion of all proteins, carbohydrates and fats is completed. The proteins are broken apart with different enzymes, and the amino acids inside the proteins are released. The amino acids are combined with vitamins, minerals, hormones and enzymes to make healthy tissue, including joints. The carbohydrates are changed to simple sugars, and the fats to fatty acids. Some of the fats are used as structural material to build cells, but most of them and all of the carbohydrates are used as energy, which we need in tremendous amounts to help our 70 trillion cells do their work.

The proteins, carbohydrates and fats then go through the walls of the small intestines into capillaries in the villi (fingerlike projections that stick out into the open part of the intestine). All the capillaries of the entire 20 feet of small intestine converge into larger and larger blood vessels until they all flow into one large vein that leads into the liver. This is called the portal vein.

The portal vein then spreads out into thousands of capillaries as the blood goes through the liver. On the top side of the liver, the blood converges into one vein again—the hepatic vein, which then goes into larger veins until it gets to the heart. There, the blood enters the systemic circulation and takes the food we've just eaten to cells all over the body.

Work of the Liver

As the blood goes through the liver, the food is changed into many substances that the body needs: the amino acids that comprise our hair, eyes, muscles bones and blood (if the liver is healthy). But several things can happen here to make us sick. For one thing, we may not have been able to break down the proteins into amino acids because the acid in our stomach wasn't strong enough for the enzymes to work. For another, the walls of the intestines may have been full of holes. Such unhealthy tissue may have released big molecules of undigested protein into the bloodstream. Those big molecules are not supposed to get in. When they do, they are foreign to the body and are poisonous.

Arthritis and allergies are both diseases that cause an inflammatory reaction. This reaction starts when a foreign invader gets in the body. In allergies it's dust, pollen or something we've eaten. In arthritis, it's a large molecule of food that didn't get digested and broken down to a simple substance that the body can use.

As early as 1913, some researchers reported that rheumatoid arthritis is a specific reaction to the presence of a foreign protein in the tissue (Blond, 1950).

The foreign proteins get into the tissues because we don't have enough enzymes in the stomach and small intestine to digest the big molecules down to amino acids to repair the muscles and bones, and to make new red and white blood cells. We really can't use the half-digested proteins—they're not good for anything. In fact, they're poisons, and our immune system has to destroy them. Also cells in the liver may be so weak that they can't detoxify the poisonous proteins in the bloodstream. Both conditions are caused when we eat junk food, which doesn't have the nutrients needed to make enzymes, and which can't make healthy liver cells.

In addition, weak liver cells can't send nutrients to the joints to make healthy synovial membranes, and they can't change the food we've eaten into mucus for lubrication.

How will we know if our livers are working well enough to handle all these jobs they must do to keep from having arthritis?

We won't know. The liver can be damaged without any symptoms or signs showing up, because one cell takes over for another cell and does its work. Thus our livers will function fairly well on fewer and fewer cells, until even a moderate stress can cause severe liver damage. We may have a swollen abdomen, the whites of our eyes may turn yellow, our legs may itch, we may have fever or be irritable, or we may have swollen eyelids in the morning because of retention of fluids in the tissues (dema). Our liver is supposed to make a special protein whose job is to pick up waste water from the tissues all over the body. If the liver doesn't have enough raw materials to make the protein, fluid collects. But long before these signs show up, we can have enough liver damage to allow arthritis to develop.

The pancreas must be healthy too, because a healthy pancreas makes enzymes to digest proteins, carbohydrates and fats in the small intestine. If we have eaten enough of the 50 or so nutrients needed for healthy joints, we will have enough nutrients to make the enzymes.

ARTHRITIS OF THE TEETH

If you have pyorrhea (periodontal disease) you may not realize it, but you have arthritis of the teeth. This is a disease of the gums and of the bones that support the teeth.

The bone deteriorates, the teeth get loose and fall out. Sometimes people have this condition, and it gradually gets worse for 10 to 20 years. It works so slowly that many people think it's part of the natural aging process. That is false. Neither man nor animals should lose their teeth when they get old.

Pyorrhea starts when tartar accumulates on the teeth. This pushes back the gum line, and the blood can't supply the tissues sufficiently. Thus, resistance is low, and the bacteria that are always in the mouth cause an infection. This infection gradually causes destruction of the bone. The condition is usually found with a general arthritis condition, often at about age 30 to 40. But here's the happy part—if nutrition is corrected, the disease can be completely reversed. It also helps to have regular dental checkups.

DIET IS OF FIRST IMPORTANCE

Eggs

Roger J. Williams (1971) reports that when guinea pigs are fed diets supplemented with egg yolk, they are protected from arthritis. Dr. Stevan Cordas, a physician in Bedford, Texas, spoke at the annual Nutrition Education Conference of the Nutrition Education Association, and he told of giving elderly people a raw egg and milk drink every day, and

of how helpful it was for general health. Many other researchers and nutrition-minded physicians advocate raw egg drinks, saying there seems to be special value in consuming raw eggs, especially for elderly people. Many of those people have arthritis. A recipe for a good drink is in the chart in Lesson 1.

If you're still afraid of eggs because of the cholesterol scare, see the detailed discussion of eggs in Lesson 3, *Heart Disease and Nutrition*. The cholesterol myth has been exploded. We can eat eggs in moderation (one or two a day) if we eat other nutritious foods.

Five Special Foods

Ruth Stout, a gardener who has written several books, says that when she was about 80 years old, she got arthritis. She had read somewhere about five foods people should eat every day to avoid or control arthritis. They are avocados, bananas, pecans, wheat germ and brewer's yeast—some of each every day, plus a good diet. She ate those foods, and, before long, her arthritis was gone. She has told many other people about the foods, and she gets letters from people everywhere who say the foods have greatly relieved the pain and swelling of arthritis.

Other Good Foods

Arthritics have to change from the average American diet of processed convenience foods to the diet given in Lesson 1 of this course:

First, proteins: fish, eggs, cheese, milk, grains and legumes (no red muscle meat—steaks, roasts, chops or hamburger). Fish is probably the best choice for an arthritic, plus frequent meals of grains and legumes. Eat about twice as much grain as legume (beans, peas and peanuts), which is the correct ratio to make complete proteins.

Second, carbohydrates: whole grains, vegetables both cooked and raw and whole fruits (except citrus—no oranges or grapefruit).

Third, fats: butter (no margarine, no hard white shortening, or bottled oil) plus seeds and nuts.

Alfalfa tea has helped many an arthritic, and it's easy to make. Heat for 30 minutes (but do not boil), one ounce of untreated alfalfa seed and two and a half cups of water. Strain well. Make one day's supply only, and store in fridge. Mix with an equal amount of water and drink four glasses a day, 30 minutes before meals and snacks so you won't dilute the hydrochloric acid in your stomach.

Although many Americans eat too much salt, arthritics profit by eating a special high-sodium food. It is celery. The sodium in celery helps keep inorganic calcium in solution so that it can be eliminated. The celery can be eaten raw or made into tea. Simmer two heaping tablespoons of celery seed in two quarts of water in a covered pan for three hours. Strain and drink as hot tea several times a day, 30 minutes before meals and snacks. Vary the celery drink with the alfalfa tea.

Poor Foods

Patients with arthritis have usually eaten too many foods made from refined flour and too many sweets and fats. The typical patient is middle-aged or elderly and overweight but poorly nourished. He is on a diet high in refined carbohydrates that are deficient in vitamins and minerals, and this deficiency has gone on for months to years before the onset of his arthritis.

Nervousness and mental and emotional stress interfere with appetite, digestion, absorption of food and the choices of food. Anything that goes wrong with a person's nerves and emotions can cause bodily changes that affect the bones and joints.

We can test ourselves for bodily changes in the hair, skin, eyes, teeth, finger- and toenails, in fat distribution and in muscular development. If any changes occur, arthritis may not be far behind. The best time to get rid of arthritis is before it starts. But it's possible to get rid of pain and swelling even if you've had arthritis a long time. New patients should eliminate red meat, maybe forever. Your body will tell you in a few weeks or months if you can eat meat again. One of my friends says she never has pain if she stays on her diet carefully, so once you get over the pain and swelling, let your body be your guide to foods that might cause a reaction.

FOOD SUPPLEMENTS

Everybody should be on a good vitamin-mineral supplement program. Researchers have tested individual vitamins, but no single vitamin deficiency has been found to cause arthritis. So there is no magic bullet. It takes all vitamins and minerals, some in large doses for a short time. B-complex vitamins and C are especially needed. Patients have increased requirements because of stress of the disease itself (Goodhart and Shils, 1973). The chart in Lesson 1 of this course will give you the amounts needed for the average diet. Specific nutrients are usually needed in larger amounts in case of disease such as arthritis. You'll find those in the chart in Lesson 1 and at the end of this lesson.

Let's look at recommendations from researchers who have done studies on individual food supplements.

Hydrochloric Acid

Dr. Alan Nittler, author of the book A New Breed of Doctor, says the first thing to take for arthritis is hydrochloric acid, which is available in tablet form at health foods stores. Sometimes the label reads, "Betaine Hydrochloride" (either with pepsin or without). The preferred form is with pepsin, a stomach enzyme that breaks down the proteins to smaller forms, if there is enough hydrochloric acid present in the stomach. The strong acid will allow calcium to go into solution so it can be assimilated and deposited in the bones where it belongs instead of in spurs where it doesn't belong. Next, Nittler suggests calcium and magnesium, plus a good diet. The multimineral suggested in the supplement program in Lesson 1 provides 1,000 mg of calcium and 500 mg of magnesium. Severely ill patients may need to increase those amounts. If you do, go up gradually; a total of more than 1,500 mg of calcium and 750 mg of magnesium is *seldom* needed. The more calcium you take, the more hydrochloric acid you need to assimilate it.

Nittler also says about bursitis, "Deposits of calcium in tendons, bursa and joints won't happen if enough hydrochloric acid is present. If it is, some of the deposits can be dissolved. It may take a long time to dissolve calcium deposits, but it can be done."

When we eat a lot of white sugar, white flour and fats, which make up about 70 percent of the average American diet, we can't make enough hydrochloric acid in our stomachs. A strange thing is that symptoms of too little and too much acid are the same, but it's easy to find out if we need more acid or less. If we take tablets of betaine hydrochloride with pepsin and we are relieved of our gas, bloating and heartburn, then we needed the acid. If we're not relieved, but the pain becomes worse, we have too much acid. All we need to do is drink two or three glasses of water to dilute the acid. It is very rare to find an arthritic patient who has enough HCl.

Adelle Davis in *Let's Get Well* (1965) says that she heard a doctor lecturing on nutrition state that "the hydrochloric acid of the stomach is so valuable that the sale of every antacid preparation should be prohibited by law."

With too little hydrochloric acid, we can't absorb vitamin C or the B complex; and minerals can't reach the blood or the synovial fluid.

Vitamin B Complex

Pantothenic Acid. Dr. Roger J. Williams (1971) says if there are weak links in our nutrition chains, there will be disease, including arthritis. He refers to a survey in London in which arthritics were tested for blood levels of pantothenic acid. In all subjects where there wasn't much pantothenic acid in the blood, arthritis was present. Some severely deficient patients were bedridden. Pantothenic acid is required to withstand stress; the pain of arthritis is a severe stress on the body. The lower the blood levels of pantothenic acid, the more severe are the symptoms of RA. Panto is helpful in preventing arthritis, and if the disease is present, daily injections of panto may lead to more of the nutrient in the blood that will then be available for cells in the joints.

It is known that a deficiency of pantothenic acid causes calcification of the joints and cartilage. The average daily intake is about five mg, but the minimum need is about 50 mg. Arthritics need large doses for a while. See the chart in Lesson 1 and the suggestions at the end of this lesson. You may eat your panto as brewer's yeast, liver, wheat germ, kidney, heart, salmon, eggs, brown rice, bran, soybeans and peanuts. How many average Americans eat anything on that list? Not many, but I believe they would if they knew they could get rid of their terrible pain.

It is probably impossible to get enough panto from those foods, although we should eat all of them. We need to fortify our cells with panto and all other vitamins and minerals in tablet form.

Vitamin B6. Dr. John Ellis in Mt. Pleasant, Texas, has worked with pyridoxine (vitamin B6) to relieve arthritic pain in hands, shoulders, hips and knees and especially carpal tunnel syndrome in the wrist. He has found great benefits and no side effects. Thus, says Dr. Ellis, B6 deficiency is another weak link in an arthritic's nutrition chain.

B6 is also especially recommended by Richard Passwater (1975). He says it is so important because it is removed in the refining of flour and it is not returned when flour is enriched. The amounts mentioned in the Diet Plan—Lesson 1—correspond to the amounts suggested by Passwater.

Lecithin. Lecithin is an excellent source of two very important relatives of the B vitamins, choline and inositol. Lecithin is used in industry to emulsify fats; therefore, it keeps fat in the blood flowing freely so that it doesn't combine with calcium and pile up in nodes or knots in the joints. Both arthritis and gout show unnatural mineral deposits in joints, and the nodes or knots sometimes contain cholesterol. Magnesium and lecithin help dissolve these deposits. Magnesium is found in raw green leafy vegetables, and it is deficient in the general population, says Dr. Williams.

Lecithin is found in egg yolk and soybeans and the preferred supplement is granular. Gelatine capsules are available, but they are not recommended because gelatin is a poor source of protein, and it ties up many enzymes for its digestion. The enzymes are better used to digest complete protein.

Folic Acid. Folic acid deficiency may well contribute to lack of well-being in arthritic patients. New, healthy cells can't be made without folic acid. The deficiency may lead to glossitis (inflammation of the tongue). The patient may be severely affected by the administration of drugs such as barbiturates, which interfere with the use of folic acid.

Dietary intake of ascorbic acid (vitamin C) is lower in RA patients than in controls. Folic acid deficiency can result from increased demand for vitamin C, because folic acid can't be changed to its active form, folacin, without vitamin C.

PABA. Carlton Fredericks tells us that the B vitamin cousin PABA (para-aminobenzoic acid) is a help against arthritis. Ads in the *Journal of the American Medical Association* recommend this vitamin in the form of a potassium salt. This form is available only on prescription. But the Arthritis Foundation still insists that no vitamin helps arthrits!

Niacinamide (Vitamin B3). Several reports of the importance of B3 are in the literature. Dr. William Kaufman studied joints and found that stiffening is relieved by the use of niacinamide (Williams, 1962).

Abram Hoffer, one of the originators of megavitamin therapy for schizophrenia, gave large doses of niacin to his mother when she had a severe case of arthritis. Later, he got a letter from her that said, "The pain and swelling are gone, the little bumps on my fingers are going away, and I feel marvelous." And that was just six weeks after she started taking the vitamin (Hoffer, 1977).

Vitamin B12. Several investigators say that a vitamin B12 deficiency may be found frequently in arthritic patients if specifically looked for. Patients should be given sufficient B12, plus hydrochloric acid, to assimilate it. Our need for HC1 was confirmed by D. J. Deller in the *British Medical Journal*, 1966.

Vitamin C

Vitamin C is required in larger than usual amounts (Passwater, 1975) when we're fighting a crippling disease such as arthritis. As the late Irwin Stone said (1973), collagen protein is essential for health of the joints; collagen requires plenty of vitamin C for its manufacture. Stone reports on studies from the 1950s in which six grams (6,000 mg) a day of ascorbic acid were given with "astonishing results" to people who had rheumatism. Other reports show that one to 10 grams of ascorbic acid daily brought about a rapid and complete recovery in three to four weeks from rheumatic fever.

Another big help from vitamin C is to keep the synovial fluid thin, so the joints will move more easily. Synovial fluid is also produced with the help of B2, B3, vitamin A, magnesium, phosphorus, calcium and B6.

B6 helps prevent numbness and tingling of the hands and feet and the pains so common at night in arthritics.

Importance of Vitamin C. Berkley (1982)) says, "Of all the vitamins, vitamin C is probably the one needed most by people with arthritis." He points out that C plays a part in practically all the reactions that take place in the human body, especially in the reactions that protect the body from disease. Linus Pauling says he has taken 18,000 mg a day for several years. Dr. James Greenwood reported in 1964 that he had used vitamin C to help prevent and overcome spinal disc problems and in treating osteoarthritis. He also said that the disease was not completely cured, but "vitamin C can do much to help."

A group of researchers in Boston induced osteoarthritis in guinea pigs. They then gave 2.4 mg of vitamin C a day—the recommended dose for an animal that size—to some of the pigs. They gave 150 mg a day to the rest. That is the equivalent of giving a 150-pound mn 15,000 mg of C, about 400 times more than the RDA. When the animals were examined later, those on 150 mg had far less damage to the cartilage in the joints than the ones on 2.4 mg.

How to Take Vitamin C. If you want to try vitamin C, keep in mind that it goes through the system and is used up quickly. It's best to take the C several times a day, possibly work up to 1,000 mg every hour. If you're awake for 15 hours a day, this amount would correspond to the amount given the guinea pigs that improved so much.

Some nutritionists recommend that time-release capsules be taken, but that might not be a good idea. It is essential that the capsules dissolve in the right place in the digestive tract so the C will get to the cells. Sometimes my counselees tell me they take a lot of vitamin C, but it doesn't do them any good. It may be that the timed-release capsules do not dissolve at the right time and place, whereas straight C does.

How Much to Take? "Bowel tolerance" is the suggested amount to take. This means, to begin with, take 500 mg three or four times a day and work up. Eventually, as you increase, you will get gas or diarrhea, because the cells become saturated, and when you take more, the cells cannot absorb it, so it spills over into the intestines and causes gas or diarrhea (usually gas first). Your bowels can't toler-

ate that much, so you cut back 500 or 1,000 mg and take that much every day. That amount is *your* bowel tolerance.

Vitamin C is the only vitamin that tells us how much we need. Sometimes people forget that they need to increase the amount of C, and they stay on 500 mg four times a day. It is important to increase to bowel tolerance. Reread this lesson and Lesson 1 so you will help yourself elminate the pain and swelling of arthritis.

Pauling (1986) says that you should take vitamin C every day, because there is a rebound effect if you stop and the risk of disease is increased.

Vitamin C should always be taken with its complex—the bioflavonoids. Get them from your health food store, and take about 100 mg for every 500 mg of vitamin C you take. They may be bought as citrus bioflavonoids. If you get rutin and hesperidin as your bioflavonoids, you may take less. Check the label and take what it recommends. Maybe in six months or so, you'll be able to eat whole oranges or grapefruit occasionally again. Always eat some of the white rind or the membrane surrounding the sections of fruit. These are good sources of the bioflavonoids.

The form of vitamin C you take can vary from tablets to powder, but the usual recommendation is to take powder, buffered with calcium, sodium or several minerals, all available at health food stores. Sometimes, tablets don't dissolve where they should, and if C is taken in powder form dissolved in water, it can no doubt be better assimilated.

Early Work with Vitamin C. Humans and guinea pigs have a lot in common. Neither animal can manufacture vitamin C in his cells as can most of the rest of the living creatures. In the 1920s, a great deal of research was done on vitamin C using guinea pigs to try to find out how vitamin C was used in human bodies.

It was found that C is required to manufacture collagen—the most plentiful protein in our bodies. Collagen sticks the cells together. Read any physiology book and collagen is always spoken of as "glue." Without collagen our teeth fall out because the glue is missing. In scurvy, caused by a deficiency of vitamin C, tissues do not hold together to make healthy organs. Imagine a heart that doesn't hold together. In the past, sailors on long voyages were unable to get fresh fruits and vegetables, good sources of vitamin C. Many reports tell of deaths among the sailors similar to modern heart attacks.

When guinea pigs were deprived of vitamin C for only 14 days, their tissue contained only 2 to 3 percent collagen. The pigs given the vitamin C contained 14 to 16 percent collagen. Think of the teenagers you know. Do you suppose they get enough vitamin C to make healthy collagen? Think of the adults you know. Many of them have aches and pains that are the beginning of arthritis, caused partly by a deficiency of vitamin C.

Vitamin C was discovered by Albert Szent-Györgyi in 1928, and soon after that, many studies were done using small amounts of vitamin C, from 100 to 250 mg, with little or no success. Finally, in the 1950s, several successful studies were reported. Private investigators used larger amounts of C than had ever been used before. Six grams (6,000 mg) gave "astonishing" results in some cases of acute and chronic rheumatism and in patients with lumbago, sciatica and bronchial asthma.

Another physician successfully used eight to 12 grams of C plus antibiotics against rheumatic fever. Others used one to 10 grams of C daily against beginning arthritis. After the 1950s, there was silence. What happened? If more research had been done, the collagen diseases that cripple so many sick people might have been eliminated from the population (Stone, 1973).

Vitamin D

Vitamin D is noted for stimulating the absorption of calcium. In fact, the process of absorption depends on the amount of vitamin D in the tissues (*Present Knowledge in Nutrition*, 1967).

Adelle Davis (1965) recommended 2,500 units of vitamin D in the diet for arthritics during critical stages of the disease. The amount can be reduced to one-half when the patient improves.

Minerals

Calcium. Although it seems strange that anyone who has calcium spurs on his hands would need more calcium, that is exactly the case. The problem is that the stress of arthritis pulls calcium out of the bones, so the person may suffer from osteoporosis (porous bones). Obviously, there is not enough calcium, but more important, it is not being assimilated and put where it should be—in the bones and teeth; thus it stacks up in the joints.

Osteoporosis expert Dr. Jennifer Jowsey says that anyone 25 years old or up should take 1,000 mg of calcium as a supplement every day in order to avoid osteoporosis later. This would also help an arthritic avoid further development of his disease.

Amounts suggested as supplements of calcium range from 1,000 mg to 2,000 mg a day, depending on the length of time the disease has been evident and how severe it is. Twice as much calcium as magnesium is the suggested ratio. Hydrochloric acid should be taken with the minerals so that they will be assimilated.

Potassium. Potassium deficiency is related to arthritis.

The Masai tribesmen in Africa have a diet fairly high in blood, which may cause potassium deficiency; they have higher incidence of RA than surrounding tribes. Eskimos who have moved to towns have a fairly high rate of rheumatoid arthritis. Thirty percent of their food is bought from a store; it is probably high in fat. Much of the other 70 percent is fat from fish. Fat is low in potassium, as are processed foods, especially sugar and white flour.

The sodium pump, which keeps sodium outside the cell and potassium inside, slows down in cold weather; therefore potassium leaves the cell. This may cause the feet and fingers to hurt when the weather is cold.

Foods high in potassium are seaweed, celery, bamboo shoots, spinach, blackstrap molasses, pumpkin, broccoli, tomatoes, cucumber, carrots and many other vegetables. Oranges contain fair amounts of potassium, but oranges and other citrus fruits are not recommended for arthritics.

Zinc. One researcher ran studies on humans with arthritis, giving them supplements of zinc. Compared to the controls, the patients on zinc showed:

1. Less joint swelling
2. Less tenderness of involved joints
3. Less morning stiffness
4. Better walking time over 50 feet

This was a small study of 24 patients, but all of them had had long-standing diseases. They were an older group, they had many joints involved and they had not improved by using drug therapy previously.

In a report at a convention on zinc, it was mentioned that juvenile RA patients usually tested low in zinc (*Zinc Metabolism*, 1977).

It is obvious that zinc is not the complete answer to arthritis, but only one of the nutrients needed in the diet. We don't want "less" joint swelling, tenderness and stiffness; we want "no" symptoms and signs of arthritis. How can we accomplish this? By getting all the nutrients in our diets.

Good sources of zinc in foods are sunflower seeds, seafoods, organ meats and brewer's yeast.

Why Larger Amounts of Supplements Are Needed

As we've seen, much research shows that nutritional deficiencies cause arthritis; on the other hand, arthritis causes the deficiencies to be worse. To balance this cycle, arthritics should accept the fact that, because of their ailment, they need large doses of all nutrients for an indefinite period of time (Baker and Frank, 1982).

People who eat the average American diet of processed, refined, canned and frozen food, and probably too much red meat, white sugar, white flour and any citrus fruit or juice are subject to arthritis. Nonfoods cause poor absorption of food and inability to change vitamins into their active forms, inability to store sufficient vitamins, increased use of vitamins in tissues and excessive loss in the urine. Some vitamin antagonists take the place of the vitamin in an enzyme system; the enzyme is then faulty, and the system jams.

Any trauma (injury) as disastrous as severe arthritis will increase vitamin requirements. Studies show that 45 percent of the patients in hospitals need more folic acid, and that it is the most common vitamin deficiency. It is needed more than ever during illness, because new cells need to be made, and it is impossible to make a new cell without folic acid. Thirty-nine percent of the patients are low in several vitamins, especially A, C and B6. Often, people who take drugs or drink alcohol, socially or otherwise, develop deficiencies of folic acid. The livers of these people are damaged, and they need folic acid for repair and manufacture of new cells.

A person on the average American diet probably has never heard of such deficiencies, yet they lead to years of pain due to arthritis. B2 and B3 are needed for energy; B1, B6 and biotin are especially important for people who drink alcohol. Vitamin E is needed for fatty liver; vitamin C, folic acid, B12 and B6 for the manufacture and use of proteins. It's impossible to repair damaged joints without protein.

Dr. Williams sums up the nutrients to emphasize in treatment, along with all the rest of the 50 or more: niacin, pantothenic acid, riboflavin (vitamin B2), vitamins A, B6, C and the minerals magnesium, calcium, phosphorus and trace minerals. These nutrients will feed all cells that produce synovial fluid and will keep bones, joints and muscles healthy.

Baker and Frank emphasize that a shotgun approach to adding supplements to the diet is undesirable because natural food and food supplement therapy succeeds only in persons receiving a balanced diet. If enough proteins, minerals and vitamins are taken, the enzymes and hormones can be properly made. If the liver is not working well enough to store the nutrients, a severe deficiency can develop, and the nutrients should be replaced continuously.

If the supplements cannot be absorbed because of sick cells in the digestive tract, recovery will take longer, but the patient will gradually improve as he digests more nutrients. Vitamins must always be combined with excellent, natural food, plus proteins, fatty acids and minerals. Vitamins by themselves cannot prevent or correct a deficiency, and a deficiency of one vitamin may lead to malabsorption of another.

The excitement about this program is that the pain and swelling of arthritis can be relieved. First food, then food supplements will help improve all arthritic conditions.

I had arthritis 18 years ago when I first went on my natural food diet. My doctor had told me there was nothing to be done about it. I would have good days and bad days, but I would never be free of the disease. I have been free of arthritis for about 17 years and 9 months—no pain, no swelling. It was easy and pleasant. And, of course, I stay on my food program.

SUGGESTIONS FOR NUTRITIONAL THERAPY

Two nutrition-minded therapists have been successful in treating arthritis.

Dr. Collin H. Dong's 30-Year Success Story.

Dr. Dong is a practicing physician who has had outstanding success in treating arthritis. He says he was afflicted with the baffling disease at the age of 35 after he had practiced medicine for seven years. For the next three years, the only relief he got was from taking large doses of aspirin and related painkillers ordered by his doctors. His arthritis became progressively worse, with wracking pain in various joints and with severe skin disease. His last doctor had nothing to suggest to further treat these two ailments.

Until then, Dr. Dong had not thought much about nutrition, except that he had to eat to live. In his youth, he had been on a more or less simple Chinese diet of *small* amounts of beef, pork, chicken and fish with *large* amounts of vegetables and rice. When he started the practice of medicine in 1931, he gradually changed to a diet like that of most affluent Americans.

To treat his arthritis, Dr. Dong went on a simple diet of fish, vegetables and rice. He still took medication, but he didn't improve rapidly. However, when he eliminated drugs, especially aspirin, and certain combinations of foods, he began to feel better. The best diet for him was a seafood, vegetable and rice combination.

He says, "To my utter amazement, in a few short weeks, there was a complete change." He could sleep again, he was agile, could shave, he played golf, and he had almost a complete remission from the crippling disease. This remission has lasted 31 years (Dong, 1973).

Since his rejuvenation, he has treated hundreds of cases of rheumatic diseases with remarkable results. He reminds us that medication alone will not cure disease. We must not forget that an affluent society consumes many foods, food components and preservatives, any one of which may cause allergies. He thinks that arthritics lack the ability to produce antibodies to protect themselves against allergens that cause arthritis.

Jane Banks, Dr. Dong's collaborator, had a family history of arthritis. She had the disease, and her brother died from the effects of medications for RA. She began Dr. Dong's diet with only fish and vegetables. Two weeks later she was almost completely free from pain. Now she can hardly remember what the pain was like.

I know many people who have changed their food programs to the natural food diet. Besides feeling better, they enjoy the taste of the food. One woman commented: "The taste and nutrition of natural food meals are superior. Processed food doesn't even taste good after you've had the real thing."

Suggestions from Adelle Davis

Adelle Davis was one of the researchers who knew years ago that nutritional treatment relieved the pain and swelling of arthritis. This information is from her book, *Let's Get Well* (pages 106 to 117 of the paperback edition, 1965).

She suggests a diet high in protein because stress destroys protein in the body. Most researchers suggest no red meat; the protein should be obtained from other animal sources as well as from plant proteins.

To build up the adrenal glands, the essential fatty acid, linoleic acid, can be obtained from nuts and seeds—mostly raw. Be sure to roast peanuts. Raw peanuts contain a harmful substance that destroys one of the pancreatic enzymes that digests protein. The substance is destroyed when peanuts are roasted. This also applies to other legumes—beans and peas. They must be cooked.

Pantothenic acid has long been known to help make our own cortisone, an important hormone made by the adrenal glands.

Stress causes pantothenic acid and vitamin B2 and C to be depleted. It may take several weeks to build up the glands before we notice improvement. Large doses of vitamin C may be needed; Davis suggests about 60 times the normal amount recommended. That would be about 3,600 mg, which nowadays is not considered a large amount after all.

Calcium is needed in large doses of up to two grams (2,000 mg) with about half that much magnesium and one-third that much phosphorus. Usually people who take extra wheat germ, lecithin, yeast and desiccated liver, however, get enough phosphorous and do not need phosphorus supplements.

Vitamins E and B6 help withstand the stress of the disease.

These nutrients are the ones we've already mentioned as relieving arthritis or any form of rheumatic disease. Obviously, a diet containing all nutrients and no junk foods will bring relief. My counselees tell me that their gout seems to be manageable by proper eating plus vitamins and minerals.

ARTHRITIS AS ALLERGY

Mandell and Conte (1982) say that the majority of the health professionals do not realize that arthritis results from allergies. However, other health professionals do not realize that arthritis, allergies and all other ailments are caused by nutritional deficiencies.

Some investigators believe that up to 50 percent of the 39,000,000 people who have arthritis are allergic to the nightshade vegetables: (potatoes, tomatoes, eggplant and peppers). They also say that arthritics who react to one or more nightshade plants may do so because such plants make up such a large percentage of their diet. One of our major basic rules in this course is to vary your diet. The nightshades will not be a problem if we go by that rule.

Mandell and Conte suggest that all their patients fast for four days to begin their treatment. After this fast, many patients had no symptoms of arthritic pain even if they had the disease for years. This corresponds to my suggestions in this course that everyone—for relief of any ailment—stop eating the average American diet and, instead, eat natural food and take food supplements.

Obviously, anyone who has arthritis has been eating foods that do not contain the nutrients needed for health of the joints, thus they are better off if they don't eat anything for a while. However, instead of fasting, if they eat small amounts of natural, unprocessed, unrefined foods and take moderate amounts of all vitamins and minerals in supplement form, they recover faster, because they replace nutrients and build health rather than going through the intermediate stage of fasting and waiting to get started on good food.

The body must throw off poisons that may have accumulated for months and years, which it can do faster if it has plentiful amounts of carbohydrates and small amounts of fats for energy and moderate amounts of proteins for making enzymes and hormones and for repair of tissues.

I have dozens of letters from arthritics who have been to me for counseling and from others who have bought my books who say they have no more pain and swelling. Occasionally, I even hear from some people who have straightened slightly bent fingers with this food and food supplement program.

After the fast, some investigators allow their patients to again eat foods that might have caused the allergic-arthritic reaction. Sometimes, one food, they say, can cause a reaction like they had before the fast. That reaction is probably the result of poor digestion, especially a deficiency of hydrochloric acid that is essential to digest proteins.

The reaction could also be caused by a deficiency of pancreatic enzymes that digest proteins, carbohydrates and fats in the small intestine. Also, since these enzymes require an alkaline medium, it may be that the pancreas was unable to manufacture the needed sodium bicarbonate to change the strong acid in the stomach (pH 2) to a strong alkaline (pH 8.8) in the small intestine.

We've already mentioned that when we're under stress, we don't manufacture enough sodium bicarbonate, and it is well known that arthritis is a very stressful disease. It is a vicious cycle—the stress of arthritis keeps us from making sodium bicarbonate to digest foods so we won't suffer from stress and develop arthritis.

Imagine that you've burned your arm. Your flesh is red and raw and sensitive to anything that touches it—soft cotton, gauze or even to a light touch of your own finger. When cells inside the body are red and raw—damaged because they didn't get the nutrients needed to make healthy cells, they are sensitive to anything that touches them. That includes almost any food, especially undigested food, and what the cells need is amino acid (proteins) that will repair tissues, plus fats and carbohydrates for energy. Our 70 trillion cells use a lot of energy daily to breathe, to maintain a heartbeat and to do all the work they must do to keep our bodies functioning.

Mandell and Conte found that many of their arthritis patients had other ailments such as fatigue, weakness and lack of appetite. They were cold and weak, and their hands and feet burned and prickled. Others suffered from hay fever, asthma, hives, eczema, migraine headaches and colitis.

Most of my arthritic counselees tell me they're allergic to certain foods. I ask them how the foods affect them, and most of them say, "I can't tell any difference when I eat them, but the tests showed I'm allergic."

I believe that if people will eat only food that repairs cells or furnishes energy, they will never be allergic to anything. Most nutrition-minded physicians know how important it is not to overeat. Too much of anything can cause an allergic reaction that could result in arthritis pain and swelling. When we eat three small meals and three smaller snacks a day of only natural food—nothing processed by man such as soft drinks, potato chips, dough-nuts, coffee and all other nonfoods—we digest our food well, and we don't suffer from allergies or arthritis.

Coffee, milk and white sugar are said to be major causes of arthritis, and of these three, coffee and sugar are not allowed on my food program for anyone. The other, milk, is allowed in only small amounts, one to two glasses a day of pasteurized, homogenized milk or yogurt, a little more if the milk is raw. Thus, we do not eliminate some foods because people are allergic to them, we eliminate foods that have no food value. As we improve our diet, we gradually eat more and more foods that we have formerly been allergic to, and before long, we can eat all healthful, natural foods and we won't be allergic to anything.

Other nonfoods tested by these investigators included chlorinated water, artificial food color, mothballs and disinfectant sprays. Whether these are ingested or inhaled, they are not allowed in a program for health.

Our plan allows only natural foods. If any allergy tests are performed or considered when the patient is allowed to smoke, inhale poisons *or eat junk food*, the principles of good health are being compromised.

PERSONAL EXPERIENCES

A Child with Rheumatoid Arthritis

One day a woman called me about her child with RA. Under drug treatment, he had become worse. Finally, he was given gold shots. He had a bad reaction to these shots, and his kidneys were damaged. Next he was put on cortisone with all of its possible severe side effects, including death. The mother was looking for another way.

It should be obvious to everyone, especially to physicians who specialize in arthritis, that the disease is caused by lack of nutrients in the entire body. However, drugs and chemicals were given to this poor child, and his liver, pancreas and adrenals (which were already partially damaged by a poor diet), were overwhelmed by the toxins in these foreign chemicals, and the child's body could not fight off the disease. This child was changed to a natural food diet, and he no longer suffers from arthritis.

A Woman with Osteoarthritis

A woman in one of my nutrition classes showed us her twisted fingers. After about six weeks on her good diet, the pain and swelling in her joints was gone. But what was most surprising was that the first joint on her forefinger had been bent and now it was almost completely straight!

And they say that nothing can be done about arthritis!

A Better Than Average Diet?

One comment that so many of my counselees make when they come to me wanting relief from arthritis, heart disease, cancer and all the rest is, "My diet is much better than the average. I don't eat much sugar." One woman with cancer spoke those very words. Then she admitted, "But I smoke, have a cocktail or two every evening and eat convenience foods. . . ." She realized that even if her diet were better than the average, it wasn't good enough for her.

Robert, Age Eight

The most rewarding letter that I have received from a counselee with arthritis is from a woman who brought her eight-year-old son to see me several years ago. She wrote this letter when he was 10.

When I first brought Robert to you, his rheumatoid arthritis had spread to every joint including the spine. He had been under Dr. X's care for five years (the same doctor who treated the children in the newspaper story). Dr. X and his five associates at the clinic treated Robert with physical therapy every four weeks at Z Hospital. Robert was in the hospital four months out of every year. Due to the experimental medication he was on for three years, he developed stomach ulcers, internal bleeding and allergies. This is when I withdrew him from the experimental study and brought him to you. You did a workup and suggested a number of healthful foods that I gave him in the form of milkshakes—four daily—adding fresh organic fruit and yogurt—no meat, no sugar.

He has thrived. No more ulcers, no more allergies, no more visible arthritis. His weight had never passed 30 pounds. Now he weighs 54 pounds. [Robert's mother said he had not gained a pound in three years on his old medical therapy, from the time he was five until he was eight.] His cheeks are rosy; he is healthy. No more rheumatoid fever that always lasted for months. He took P.E. for the first time last year. He went from bed to running and playing, and is as active as any 10-year-old.

The change was so remarkable that his teachers didn't recognize him after that first summer on your nutrition program. The doctor even had him on Darvon for pain in his head because of spine involvement, but that pain stopped. Not even an allergy! He takes no medication whatsoever since our consultation.

The drink that Robert's mother made for him contained about one cup of whole milk, one raw egg (from the health food store), one teaspoon to one tablespoon of lecithin and from one-fourth teaspoon (for beginners) to one tablespoon of brewer's yeast. She added any whole, fresh fruit Robert liked and also added ground vitamin and mineral tablets plus wheat germ and bran if he needed it. This recipe is also in Lesson 1 of this course. Let's remember that all the rest of the natural foods must be eaten: whole grains, vegetables, legumes (beans, peas and peanuts), and fish and eggs for protein.

Letters from Counselees

"I am happy to report that my general health was greatly improved by way of more energy (almost immediately) and almost an immediate improvement in my elimination and hemorrhoid condition. My nails hardened and lengthened considerably. *My stiff back is loosening.*"

"I no longer take medication for gout, nor follow the diet for gout. I've been eating an egg a day. I've lost about 10 pounds I needed to lose. As a salesperson, I can work on my feet for four hours a day. Gout appears to be manageable by proper eating and some 12 vitamin and mineral tablets a day."

"I've made only a limited transition to natural foods, but even that has helped. My arthritis is much better. I expected to have an operation for my gum problem, but I now think it will be avoided."

"The food supplements you outlined for my husband really made him feel so much better. He doesn't complain of arthritis any more, and he is able to engage in physical activity now. He has also lost 25 pounds this past year, and I think the food supplements were a great aid in this endeavor."

SPECIFICS OF ARTHRITIS/NUTRITION PROGRAM

Now just exactly what shall we eat to get rid of arthritis? The overall diet and food supplement program is found in Lesson 1 of this course. Begin the new food program immediately. Start with small amounts of the food supplements, and go up gradually.

1. No red meat (muscle meat—steaks, roasts, chops and hamburger). Proteins can be mostly eggs, and whole grain and legume combinations, both from the health food store, plus fish.
2. Vegetables, both cooked and raw. Many steamed vegetables are of great value. Steamed green leafy vegetables contain the greatest concentration of vitamins and min-

erals. If you have a juicer, juice organically grown carrots from the health food store and drink immediately. Drink carrot and apple juice combined. Don't drink juice made from green leaves unless you can get organically grown vegetables. Drink all juices freshly squeezed. Eat small amounts of potatoes often—put them in the steamer with other vegetables.

3. Eat fruits fresh, raw, and ripe. Don't eat citrus fruits. Don't drink any kind of fruit juice—it's too sweet.

4. A specific food supplement for arthritis is calcium combined with magnesium. The recommended amount for severe arthritis is about 2,000 mg of calcium a day, with half that amount of magnesium. After pain and swelling are gone, gradually decrease the amounts to about half. Go up later if your body tells you to.

5. Hydrochloric acid is needed to digest and assimilate the protein as well as the vitamins and minerals, especially calcium and magnesium. If you buy an all-purpose digestive enzyme, it will contain hydrochloric acid and pancreatic enzymes. Start with one early in each meal. Increase to four or five, depending on the reaction. If you have a burning sensation in the stomach, drink water and dilute the acid to stop the burning. But chances that this will happen in an arthritic are rare.

6. Pantothenic acid is usually not found in large enough amounts in the average B-complex vitamin tablet. I suggest about 750 mg a day in divided doses for people with any ailment. Arthritics should go up to about 1,000 mg a day in divided doses—1,500 mg total, if needed.

7. The intake of vitamin C should be at bowel tolerance. This means to start with about 500 mg four times a day. Increase the amount until you get gas. Cut back until you don't have gas, and take that much every day. The recommended form of vitamin C is ascorbic acid buffered with calcium or with several minerals. These forms are called calcium or mineral ascorbates. I think it's a good idea to take powdered ascorbate 30 minutes before meals with water, and carry tablets in your purse or pocket for meals and snacks when you're away from home.

8. Much research shows the value of taking amino acids to build up the cells damaged by deficiencies of protein because of the stress of arthritis. These can be obtained as powder, tablets, capsules or liquids. Take the amount recommended on the label. This will usually be about 1,500 mg three times a day with water before meals. Since these amino acids don't need to be digested, the water can wash them through the stomach into the small intestine where they will go through the intestinal wall into the bloodstream and then into every cell to build health.

You might need twice that much, later, if you've been deficient for a long time and your digestive system isn't working well. Eventually, you can go back to a smaller dose for maintenance. You may continue to take amino acids according to directions in the chart in Lesson 1. I use a (+) mark in that chart to mean "Take the supplement about one month out of three to avoid trouble in the future." These amino acids are already digested and eager to go to work on your depleted cells. They don't have to be changed by digestive enzymes (Philpott, 1977).

It's Your Body

There is no human being in the world who can tell you how much of every nutrient to take every hour all day long. Our middle names should be "Moderation" and "Listen-to-Your Body." You will begin to improve, but you may have setbacks from time to time. Carefully analyze what happened to cause the setback, and let your body tell you what to do.

You may be able to reduce the pantothenic acid to about half the amount suggested. We should maintain the vitamin C intake at bowel tolerance. If you're young, you probably will not need to stay on large amounts of digestive enzymes. When you get your body built up, your own cells will make the digestive enzymes you need. Older people may want to take the enzymes from now on—let your body tell you.

Start Slowly

As we say with all nutrition programs—start slowly. Your digestive system may not tolerate large amounts of these supplements. So take it easy. Although we say start slowly, go up as fast as you can. This program is mildly detoxifying. It will pull poisons out of your cells and tissues all over your body, and when the poisons get into the blood on the way to the urine and feces to be excreted, they can cause slightly uncomfortable reactions. That's why we say work in this program gradually. However, don't go too slowly.

Remember to listen to your body and let it tell

you how much of the nutrients you need. Especially—don't overeat!

Do it Yourself

I have talked to many people who say nothing in the world would make them go back to the old way of eating junk foods. You will probably feel that way too.

When you get where you want to be, you'll probably eat "off the diet" sometimes. Your body will let you know what you can tolerate of other foods such as red meat or citrus fruit. We have such a wide variety of delicious, healthful foods, we never need to long for the old way of eating junk. We will eat better, the food will taste better, we will feel better.

Don't be like the woman I talked to on the phone. She was bedridden with arthritis when she called me. I said "No junk food." She said, "If I have to give up cola drinks and potato chips, I'd rather be dead." Most people would rather not be dead; they're so eager to live a pain-free life that they are happy to prepare these tasty, nutritious meals and stay away from junk food forever.

The exciting thing about this whole therapy is that you can do it yourself. Recently a young man I'll call John came to my lecture in Phoenix. He stayed late after the meeting to talk. He said he had had a severe case of rheumatoid arthritis. He had finally heard about nutrition, and he found my books and went on the nutrition program. He said, "Within two weeks, I felt much better, and now I'm completely well. If people only knew how easy it is to get well, they would never put up with arthritis."

Remember, John, Robert and hundreds of others who have overcome their arthritis. You have the power. Use it.

QUESTIONS

TRUE/FALSE

1. Synovial fluid works as the oil on a hinge to provide smooth motion in the joints.

2. Arthritis is not a nutritional deficiency disease.

3. Most arthritics will improve if they take hydrochloric acid.

4. An arthritis expert says, "No person who is in good nutritional health develops rheumatoid or osteoarthritis (RA or OA)."

5. Pain is caused when the membranes aren't lubricated well enough, the cartilage wears away and bone rubs on bone.

6. Rheumatism, a disease of the muscles, usually attacks adults.

7. Gout is a disease caused by eating too many sweets.

8. Stress damage may cause arthritis to develop.

9. We must manufacture 32 hormones in the adrenal glands to help handle stress.

10. Hans Selye, a stress expert, says, "Poor foods certainly induce stress that can delay recovery."

11. Smoking uses up vitamin C, which can lead to joint pain.

12. Mineral oil is a healthful laxative for arthritics.

13. Foreign proteins get into our cells because we don't make enough enzymes in the stomach to destroy them there.

14. The liver can be severely damaged before any signs of damage show up.

15. Many nutritionists suggest that people with arthritis should supplement their diets with raw egg yolk.

16. The cholesterol myth has been exploded, and we can now eat one or two eggs a day if we eat all other good foods.

17. Although we eat as well as we can, we also need to take moderate amounts of all food supplements.

MULTIPLE CHOICE

1. Signs of arthritis include: (a) stiff, painful joints, (b) swelling, (c) tingling sensations in fingertips, hands and feet.

2. An arthritic patient can't: (a) digest and (b) assimilate calcium normally, so he (c) loses calcium from his bones.

3. RA affects people in the following ways: (a) crippling, (b) synovial membranes deteriorate, (c) soft tissues swell.

4. Aspirin: (a) causes ulcers, (b) harms the liver, (c) makes the stomach lining bleed.

5. Aspirin used over a long period of time can cause: (a) chronic arthritis for life, (b) heart weakness, (c) swelling of the face and mucous membranes.

6. Cortisone may cause: (a) colon ulcers, (b) mental problems, (c) diabetes, (d) high blood pressure.

7. Gold therapy can cause: (a) skin disease, (b) stomach problems, (c) headaches, (d) severe anemia.

8. Alcohol makes arthritis worse because it destroys: (a) magnesium, (b) synovial fluid, (c) cartilage.

9. Antacids cause the following: (a) inability to dissolve calcium so it will make healthy joints, (b) formation of spurs, (c) binding of phosphorus in the digestive tract.

10. Liver cells help prevent arthritis: (a) by detoxifying poisonous proteins in the bloodstream, (b) by making healthy synovial membranes, (c) by

changing some of the food we've eaten to mucus for lubrication.

11. Unhealthy liver signs: (a) swollen abdomen, (b) whites of eyes get yellow, (c) legs may itch, (d) possible swollen eyelids in the morning.

12. Junk food can lead to disastrous changes in: (a) nerves, (b) emotions, (c) bones, (d) joints.

ANSWERS

True/False

1. T 2. F 3. T 4. T 5. T 6. T 7. T 8. T
9. T 10. T 11. T 12. F 13. T 14. T 15. T
16. T 17. T

Multiple Choice

1. a,b,c 2. a,b,c 3. a,b,c 4. a,b,c 5. a,b,c 6. a,b,c,d
7. a,b,c,d 8. a,b,c 9. a,b,c 10, a,b,c 11. a,b,c,d
12. a,b,c,d

REFERENCES

Baker, J. H. and Frank, O. *JIAPM* 7(2):19–24, July 1982.

Berkley, G. *Arthritis Without Aspirin.* Englewood Cliffs, NJ: Prentice-Hall, 1982.

Bingham, R. *J. Appl. Nutr.,* Winter 1972.

Blond, K. *The Liver*: Porta Malorum—*"The Gateway to Disease."* Baltimore: Williams & Wilkins, 1950.

Davis, A. *Let's Get Well.* New York: Signet, 1965.

Deller, D.J. *British Med. J.* 1966.

Dong, C.H. *Woman's Day,* Aug. 1973.

Goodhart and Shils. *Modern Nutrition in Health and Disease.* Philadelphia: Lea & Febiger, 1973.

Hoffer, A. *Bestways.* April 1977, pp. 36–42.

Mandell, M. and Conte, A.A. *JIAPM* 7(2):5–18, July 1982.

Passwater, R.A. *Supernutrition.* New York: Pocket, 1975.

Pauling, L. *How to Live Longer and Feel Better.* New York: W. H. Freeman, 1986.

Philpott, W.H. *Supplement to A Physicians' Handbook on Orthomolecular Medicine,* 1977.

Present Knowledge in Nutrition, 1967.

Robbins, *Pathologic Basis of Disease,* 1974.

Selye, H. *Nutr.* Today, 5:2–10, 1970.

Seroy, W.H. *World Health and Ecology News,* 2(4).

Stone, I. *The Healing Factor, Vitamin C Against Disease.* New York: Grossett & Dunlap, 1974.

Warmbrand, M. *Encyclopedia of Health and Nutrition.* New York: Pyramid, 1974.

Williams, R.J. *Nutrition in a Nutshell.* New York: Dolphin, 1962.

———. *Nutrition Against Disease.* New York: Pitman, 1971.

Zinc Metabolism. Current Aspects in Health and Disease, 1977.

Lesson 9

STAYING YOUNG WITH GOOD NUTRITION

LESSON 9—STAYING YOUNG WITH GOOD NUTRITION

HOW TO STAY YOUNG

"AGING IS a process that occurs over a lifetime . . ." Nothing new and unusual there, eh? But the quotation (Winick, 1976) continues: ". . . how we eat will in part determine how fast we age and what diseases of the elderly we contract."

Are you staying young? Whatever your age now, you can live longer and be healthier if you eat natural food and take moderate amounts of all vitamins and minerals. The detailed food and food supplement program is in Lesson 1 of this *Home Study Course.*

Our whole approach to the subject of aging is to live longer and to age more slowly, but most important of all, to prolong the healthy middle years, *not* to spend more years at the end in a wheelchair. As many people say, "We add life to years and years to life."

According to Linus Pauling (1974), if we take vitamins E and C we should feel better and live eight years longer; if we eat half as much sugar as the average and improve our diets in other ways, we should live another eight years longer; if we don't smoke, we can add another four years. This is a total of 20 additional years of life—not at the end as senile old folks, but in the middle years, when we are up and moving.

The average length of life expected at birth has increased considerably—by about 20 years in this century, but this is because fewer babies and young children die. The life expectancy of 20-year-olds is almost no longer now than in 1950. Middle- and upper-class men do not live longer. In fact, in 1980, 40-year-olds didn't live as long as they did in 1900 (Bjorksten, 1980). Life expectancy for a 50-year-old man has increased only two years in the last two centuries. The maximum life span has not increased since Biblical times (Schloss, 1981). This is in spite of the amount of money spent on medical care. The cost went up from $12 billion a year in 1950 to $94 billion in 1973. By 1993, the bill for health care is expected to be one trillion dollars (*U.S. News and World Report*, August 22, 1983).

So the medical profession with its powerful drugs cannot claim credit for longer life expectancy except for the antibiotics that help against infectious diseases. However, we now know that all antibiotics damage the liver, and that we will contract another infectious disease sooner if we let our resistance get so low that we have to take antibiotics. As we grow older, we succumb to chronic degenerative diseases, for which medical science claims no answers as yet. But nutritionists justly claim that natural foods plus vitamins and minerals, all of which are virtually nontoxic, build the body, and that we can and must be responsible for our own health.

The three top killer diseases are heart and blood vessel problems, cancer and diabetes—all known to be nutritional deficiency diseases (Mayer, 1974). The fourth killer disease, according to health professionals, will jump from fourth place to first in about 15 years. What is that fast-moving disease? Alzheimer's.

Mayer (1974) says, "We have made very little or no progress in slowing down or preventing a great deal of suffering known to be avoidable. We haven't educated our people about nutrition. Older people do not need as many calories as they used to, but they need even more nutrients, especially protein, vitamin B6, magnesium, zinc, calcium, iron and all other vitamins and minerals. Sometimes they almost live on tea and toast without enough protein. They take mineral oil as a laxative, which drains away fat-soluble vitamins."

Life expectancy is much longer in some other countries. In Ecuador, records show that some people live to be 150 years old. Some people in the village of Vilcabamba in the Andes still work at the age of 100. Their diet consists of fresh fruit and vegetables, lean meat, very little fat and unstrained honey.

That's similar to my diet, except we use very little honey, no fruit juice and we eat moderate amounts of grains and legumes (beans, peas and peanuts). To get the nutrients from these foods distributed to every cell, we must have a good blood supply with plenty of oxygen. This can be assured if we eat all 50 nutrients in natural foods plus food supplements that will give us all eight essential amino acids (proteins), carbohydrates, fats, about 20 vitamins, 20 minerals and water. Not recommended are prepared package mixes or processed foods in bags, boxes, cans or frozen packages.

One of the most important diet principles is that we should never overeat. Rats fed less than their usual amount of food were, over a lifetime, smaller as adults, but they lived twice as long. Of course, we're not rats, but we can learn from them and apply this research to our own lives. I'm sure every reader has overeaten at one time or another, and felt gassy and bloated as a result. That's because if we eat too much at one time, we overload our digestive systems and we can't digest the food. Undigested food is poison in our bodies.

Recent studies showed that rats fed small amounts at a time (they were nibblers instead of gorgers) also lived twice as long. The rats that ate larger portions three times a day became sick with degenerative diseases just as humans so often do. My nutrition philosophy emphasizes six small meals a day because, if we nibble, we will have enough enzymes to digest and assimilate our food better.

Since our food is so processed and has so much food value destroyed, people interested in staying healthy and living longer usually take food supplements. Are they really worthwhile?

Hans Kugler (1973), an expert on aging, reports on an interesting experiment with white mice, whose metabolism is very much like that of humans. To one group of mice, he fed 5 percent wheat germ and 10 percent brewer's yeast. They exercised on a rotating drum for about 30 minutes twice a week. These mice lived 30 to 40 percent longer than the controls, which were on a diet containing all nutrients thought to be needed by mice. The experimental mice also looked younger, were more active and their hair was shinier. Another group of mice was given the same diet plus vitamin C, B complex, extra pantothenic acid (a B vitamin), calcium and magnesium. They lived 45 to 65 percent longer.

Kugler next studied mice that were not allowed to exercise and were exposed to smoking. They drank alcohol and ate a lot of sugar. This lifestyle is very similar to that of the average American. Their life spans were only about half as long as those of the mice on the regular laboratory diet.

THEORIES OF AGING

There are several major theories of aging, and all of them relate to nutritional deficiencies. If we begin now and eat the way this book suggests, we will eat all nutrients needed, and our cells and tissues will work well. We can extend our good years.

Cross-Linkage Theory

Cross-linkage is the major cause of aging, according to many researchers. It is primarily the binding together of proteins, nucleic acid molecules and many other substances such as carbohydrates, undigested food and abnormal cells that, during the course of a lifetime, are not made perfectly because some of the nutrients were not available. With an agent such as aluminum, all of those substances can become cross-linked (bound together), as can cells that are damaged by X-rays, by prescribed drugs and street drugs, by severe infections, and by malfunction of the immune system. There are tremendous amounts of damaged cells and other substances that get tangled in our tissues like garbage. The cells can't use the garbage, but they can't get rid of it either, and it accumulates for many years.

Many other ailments are caused by the cross-linking of other substances, one of which is lipofuscin, a brownish pigment similar to the spots on some people's hands. It also accumulates in the brain and damages brain cells.

We can't prevent the cross-linkages, but with a natural food diet and moderate amounts of all food supplements, we can slow the rate at which the cross-linkages occur, and we can break down the tangles before they become so knotted that nothing will help.

Cell Multiplication Theory

Some investigators think that a cell multiplies a certain number of times, and then dies because its DNA doesn't work right. DNA is the nucleic acid that controls our genes and sets the pattern for new cells. DNA also makes the pattern for all the enzymes, so if DNA doesn't work correctly, the enzymes don't work correctly. (Krehl, 1974).

Waste Products Theory

Another theory of aging is that we may not get rid of wastes from the cells. The wastes should be picked up by albumin, which is made by the liver for that purpose. If any of these processes aren't working well, our cells get full of garbage that they can't get rid of. Nutrition experts say that if we don't die of a killer disease, we die because our cells are so full of wastes that they can't function. These waste products are similar to the tangles already mentioned. I met a charming little lady recently who had such serious pitting edema (if the flesh is pressed, the print of the finger remains) that her legs from the hips down were swollen to about twice their normal size. She was not only miserable but also very ill. It is obvious that her liver couldn't manufacture enough albumin to pick up the waste water.

Damage to the Immune System Theory

Still another theory is that something goes wrong with the immune system. Antibodies made by the immune system protect the body from foreign substances. But sometimes antibodies attack the tissues of the body. This causes what's called autoimmune diseases (Krehl, 1974).

Free Radicals Theory

Another theory is that free radicals cause aging. This is a fascinating subject that we'll be hearing about more and more, so let's learn the details. Atoms in cells have electrons in pairs whirling around the nucleus of the atom. When our cells get hit by radiation, by viruses and bacteria, by doctors' or street drugs, by oxygen reacting on polyunsaturated fats in the cells (this causes the fats to become rancid) and by other injuries, one of the electrons can be knocked out of orbit. That leaves the other electron by itself, and it should be paired. So it whirls around looking for another electron to join up with.

It attacks practically anything and attaches itself to it. Sometimes the attack is so violent that it creates other free radicals and sets up a chain reaction. Free radicals can split molecules in half, knock pieces out of them, contribute to the buildup of lipofuscin pigment and garble the working orders to the cells such as correcting a shortage of insulin in the pancreas or releasing more blood-albumin to pick up waste water so that fingers and ankles won't swell. When there are many free radicals, the business of the cell is out of order.

Free radicals can also damage the genes. When a cell with a damaged gene divides to make two cells, the abnormal gene can obviously make the new cell abnormal. These cells can become cancer cells. Free radicals damage other tissues, especially elastin. Elastin is like elastic—it stretches and shrinks. There's a lot of elastin in blood vessels, because if the vessels weren't elastic, the extra surge of blood that goes through the vessels when we exercise might break the blood vessel and cause a hemorrhage. Elastin also helps our skin stay wrinkle-free if we're on a staying-young diet.

The word "antioxidant" appears over and over in medical literature on aging. An antioxidant is a substance that prevents free radicals from forming by protecting the cells from the oxygen that makes the fat in the cells rancid. Antioxidants are the vitamins C and E, the mineral selenium and the amino acids cysteine, methionine and cystine. (A good source of those amino acids is eggs.) It seems strange that although we can't live without oxygen, it can sometimes damage our tissues.

The joining of free radicals in a cell causes trouble. Proteins and nucleic acids link together and form huge molecules that can't be broken down by our enzymes. The cells can't get rid of the big molecules, and the molecules can't be changed to amino acids. But sometimes the mitochondria (little organs in the cells that make energy) accept the cross-linked proteins and later find out they can't use them (Rosenfeld, 1976). They're joined like two assembly-line workers lassoed together. They take up too much room, and they can't work well. What if billions of your cells were filled with these cross-links and/or free radicals. You'd not only have wrinkles, you'd probably have arthritis, digestive disorders and maybe even cancer. You would probably *not* live a long, happy life.

The answer to all this damage is to eat plenty of the antioxidants—vitamins E and C, selenium and sulfur-containing amino acids (found in good proteins) (Tappel, 1968). Animals in experimental studies had increased life spans when they were given antioxidants. Compared to a human life span, the animals lived to be 124 rather than 75 (Passwater, 1975).

AILMENTS OF THE AGING

The following ailments are often related to aging, although many of them are also found in young people.

Mental Diseases

"Lack of proper vitamins and minerals will insure brain malfunctions" (Corwin's emphasis, 1980). That is such a definite, striking statement from an expert on nutrition and the brain that no one could take it lightly. Corwin continues: "The root cause of degenerative diseases which are responsible for most of our deaths is malnutrition. Malnutrition is responsible for malfunction of the hormones and enzymes that control our brains. Because of this, many of the vital organs can become diseased, because many of them are controlled by the nervous system or by hormones under direct or indirect control of the brain. These malfunctions cause the degenerative diseases which kill 80 percent of our people. They can and must be prevented and cured."

Malnutrition of brain cells is common in people who do not eat to stay young. Brain cells use about 20 percent of the total energy from the food we eat, even though the brain weighs only about 2 percent of the total body weight. In the average adult, brain cells die off at the rate of about 100 an hour. Thus, a 40-year-old person has about 90 million fewer brain cells than he had 10 years before. But since we start with about 12 billion brain cells, we have enough to last till we're 125 if we live that long.

Cells usually die either because they don't get everything they need or because they get poisoned by something they don't need. Since brain cells may die of malnutrition, a person on a natural food diet will possibly lose fewer than the average, and those on a diet of junk food may lose many more.

When people get old, they often eat very poorly (the tea and toast group) and their blood vessels may be partly stopped up with fatty deposits. Thus less food and oxygen go to the brain, which causes confusion and loss of memory. If an abundance of minerals and vitamins is available, the cells can supply sufficient oxygen and food for the brain. Senile patients will be able to remember better and think more clearly and quickly.

The Brain Needs Nutrients. If you've ever read a list of deficiencies of B-complex vitamins, you'd think it was a list of symptoms of aging. Many of the symptoms are mental changes such as depression, fear, confusion and poor memory, with about 2 percent having serious mental problems (Sebrell, 1973). There is loss of attention, irritability, vague fears, emotional disturbances, nerve damage in the arms and legs and brain damage. There can be sores in the hypothalamus region in the brain that cause capillaries to thicken and become blocked, and blood can't get to all the brain cells—that's why we are depressed, afraid, confused and can't remember. The damage can be severe, with permanent dementia and many different types of psychoses if no treatment is given. The treatment needed is nutritious food.

Many old people are sent to psychiatrists because of these mental symptoms, but all they need is a good diet and food supplements. There may not be enough oxygen in the brain or enough glucose. A good way to get more oxygen in all cells is by taking supplements of pangamic acid (also called dimethyl-glycine). We should also do deep breathing exercises daily.

Depression in the second half of life is so frequent it is thought of as normal. Depression may be caused by lack of enzymes that we have to have to manufacture enough energy for our brain cells to think and to remember, but as we age, our enzyme systems deteriorate faster and faster; finally we lose our memory, become disoriented, can't think well and we become severely depressed. To keep the enzyme systems working, we need vitamins E, C, B3, B12 and pangamic acid. We also need oxygen. Linus Pauling says that if people can get enough oxygen to the brain, depression can be avoided altogether.

Two thousand years ago, Virgil wrote, "Age carries all things, even the mind, away." It is the same now. After all these years, there is very little improvement in the pitiful people who suffer from senility, whether mild or severe.

Most elderly people have for years been eating the average American diet that is so deprived of nutrients most of us cannot be mentally alert without taking food supplements. The complete diet and food supplement program are given in Lesson 1 of this book. Often the first sign of senility is loss of short-term memory. If you have this problem, nutrition experts advise moderate amounts of all food supplements with large amounts of vitamins C, E and A, plus selenium. Niacinamide (B3) should also be taken in large amounts, because it thins the blood, which will be able to flow through the brain to all the cells, bringing oxygen, which is vitally needed by forgetful people.

If you're responsible for the care of an elderly person, try those suggestions from some of the best nutritionists in the country. If you do not have this problem, begin now to open up the capillaries in your own brain so later on you will not become senile. This seems to be the most dreaded age change—to lose the power to think. It doesn't have to happen; we can eat well so our brains will stay young.

Alzheimer's Disease. Alzheimer's disease is presenile dementia; it is our fourth killer disease, and experts say it might be our first killer in the twenty-first century. Alzheimer's usually starts as early as age 30 with loss of short-term memory, and continues until the victims can't remember their children's names or how many children they have. I have heard many young people whose parents suffer from this disease say, "She [or he] was a brilliant lawyer [teacher, engineer, writer . . .]. It seems so tragic that this had to happen." Alzheimer's is no respecter of good brains. All brains deteriorate if they are not fed what they need.

Undigested food and cells that were made incorrectly combine as fibers with aluminum or another mineral and make a tight knot, something like a knot in your shoestring that is hard to untie. The loose ends and the loops of the fiber combine with more aluminum and get knotted again, and pretty soon there is such a tight tangle that it is impossible to get the knot untied. Aluminum is attracted to the brain, where the aluminum tangles accumulate and cause Alzheimer's disease.

Many middle-aged people are severely ill with Alzheimer's, and most of them die about 10 years after discovery of the disease. The victims had been accumulating aluminum and cross-linkages for 40 to 50 years.

The major part of the aluminum in the tissues can be removed, but so far, no one knows how to get the aluminum out of the nucleus of living cells. Researchers say that when hardening of the arteries, other blood vessel diseases and cancer are all cured or prevented, aluminum could become the next major life-ending scourge.

Aluminum makes up 8.4 percent of the earth's crust and is present in almost everything we eat. It accumulates in the human body at a steady rate, and it causes death if enough of it gets to the brain. There are two reasons why this happens.

1. Aluminum is a flocculant; it makes anything look and feel like wool. This is the woollike fiber that collects in the brain.
2. Aluminum is a powerful cross-linking agent, and it attaches itself to proteins and turns them into tangles so they are worthless to the body.

We can immediately remove several sources of aluminum from our cells. We can stop taking antacids. Some people dose themselves with from 800 to 5,000 mg of aluminum from antacids in one day. We rub aluminum from antiperspirants into our pores, then it goes to the blood, then to the brain. Aluminum from cooking utensils is not readily taken into our cells. Some package mixes for biscuits, cake and other foods contain 15 mg of aluminum in every serving; processed cheese may contain 50 mg in one slice.

Digestive Problems

Old people often have elimination problems. They need plenty of water plus fiber from whole grains, vegetables and fruits. Fiber helps keep our bowels regular. We can take unrefined bran from health food stores, and eat whole-grain breads we've made ourselves. I like to add bran to any bread, biscuit, cracker, muffin or cookie I make because it gives them a more "open" texture—not so dense. I add wheat germ too, for extra protein, B-vitamins and flavor. Try some of the good recipes in my cookbook, *Switchover!*

You may never have heard of one of the most important uses of fiber in the diet. It is to furnish food for the friendly bacteria that live in our colons (Cummings, 1983). These bacteria live on the products of fermentation (breakdown of carbohydrates into substances that can go into the blood and then into our cells).

About three pounds of the bacteria live in our intestines. That's more bacteria than there are cells in our bodies, and we have 70 trillion cells. The main carbohydrate going into the colon is fiber, and our colons need 20 to 40 grams of fiber to be digested every day and used for energy by friendly bacteria. If we eat more fiber, the bacteria produce more energy.

Stomach and intestinal gas (methane, hydrogen

and oxygen) is often a problem with oldsters, especially if they are constipated because they don't eat enough fiber or drink enough water. The gas can be expelled from the rectum or absorbed into the blood stream. When the blood with the gas in it goes through the lungs, the gas is exhaled and eliminated from the body. These gases are all odorless. If there is any gas expelled through the rectum or the mouth that has a bad odor (burping or bad breath), it probably comes from undigested protein that collects in the colon. If there is not enough fiber and water to push the feces through to be excreted, the feces stay packed in our intestines for weeks, months and sometimes years. They are literally poison in our bodies, and poisonous bacteria live happily in the intestines because that's the exact climate they like. They're happy, but we're not. We must get this encrusted, rotten mass out of our colons.

Here's how you can tell if you are digesting your protein well. If you are not, your stools will be dark colored, small around and hard (sometimes too soft), they will sink to the bottom of the bowl and they will smell bad. Our stools should be light colored, big around, soft yet well formed, they should float and should have almost no odor. If the stools are not soft, we might have to strain to pass bowel movements. Straining at stool is the cause of hemorrhoids and varicose veins. We can attain the desired stools by taking bran, cellulose from fruits and vegetables and soured milks such as yogurt and buttermilk.

The best and fastest way to attain the stools we want is to take *Lactobacillus acidophilus* from the health food store. It comes in liquid, powder or tablet form. It's a good idea to vary the form you take. Also, get the kind that contains no *bulgaricus* bacteria, because they are destroyed by the acid in the stomach. The acidophilus should get through the stomach and set up colonies of friendly bacteria in our intestines that will manufacture B vitamins for us. See dosage directions on the label. When your stools are as we described, you can stop taking the acidophilus, but if you notice an odor when you defecate, take more.

Studies in rats show that friendly bacteria in the intestines help the immune system work, and help us resist infection. The bacteria also detoxify certain cancer-causing agents by keeping them in circulation in the liver, where they are detoxified.

The bacteria are not controlled by nerves or hormones but by the amount of fiber in the diet. This is certainly a good reason for everyone to eat a lot of fiber. We can't have healthy intestines without fiber for bulk, without water to move the fiber along and without plenty of bacteria to furnish some of the vitamins we need.

Malabsorption

Our "stay-young" food program includes absorbing our food well. If food can't be absorbed, it's because the intestinal walls are diseased, and the nutrients can't get through into the blood stream. Protein, especially, must be digested to amino acids, which must be absorbed into the blood and assimilated into the diseased intestinal walls to repair those cells. Many of my counselees tell me in a confidential tone, "My doctor says my diet isn't so bad; I just don't assimilate my food." They don't realize that that complaint is almost universal, yet extremely easy to correct.

Hydrochloric Acid. Why don't we absorb and assimilate our food well? Researchers say that by age 30 (some say 20) we don't make enough strong digestive juice (another name for it is hydrochloric acid—HCl). HCl has to be strong to break down the big molecules of protein to tiny little amino acids that we use to build cells and tissues. By age 60, 30 percent of Americans make *no* hydrochloric acid. How do they live? In hospitals and nursing homes (Balecki and Dobbins, 1974).

After we've eaten the average American diet for many years, the cells in the stomach walls that make the acid are so sick from the junk food in our diet that they can't produce as much acid as we need.

Many other factors contribute to a deficiency of HCl. If there's not enough acid, the undigested proteins go on into the large intestine and stack up in the sigmoid colon, near the rectum. By that time, they're putrefied (a polite way of saying rotten), and they cause gas. The sigmoid colon is very muscular because it is supposed to store waste matter until it goes to the rectum to be excreted. Strong muscles are required to hold the wastes. But when a blood vessel goes into the colon to feed the colon itself, it makes a little weak spot in the muscle. The gas pushes up at the weak spot with tremendous pressure and forms a wedge shape sticking out from the colon into the abdominal cavity. The wedge stretches out as more undigested fecal matter collects and more gas is produced. The wedge gets as big as a grape, with a narrow neck. The "grape" is surrounded by only a thin membrane that was formerly the lining of the intestine. It has no muscles in it, so the "grape" is there for life because there aren't any muscles to push the rotten fecal matter back into the colon to be excreted. The only way to get rid of the "grapes" is by surgery. I know some of you realize that I'm describing a disease called diverticulosis; the "grapes" are diverticula, and if they get inflamed, the disease is called diverticulitis.

The diverticula stick out into the abdominal cavity from the sigmoid, from anywhere else in the colon, from the small intestine, from the stomach and even from the esophagus. Forty-five percent of adults have this disease; 60 percent of 60-year-olds. If we stay on a good diet, the diverticula will not become inflamed.

How can we avoid these dangerous diverticula that often lead to cancer? We should not drink water with meals, because that dilutes the hydrochloric acid in the stomach and we won't be able to digest and assimilate our proteins to repair tissues.

Probably the worst thing anyone does for his health is to take antacids, which do relieve the gas, bloating and too-full feeling after meals, but that keep us from digesting the protein we so sorely need to repair the cells so that we won't get diverticulosis. What we need is hydrochloric acid. It relieves the gas and bloating and helps us digest and assimilate our protein for repair of all tissues.

What other problems do we have if we can't digest food? We can't make the intrinsic factor needed with B12 without hydrochloric acid. Also strong acid in our stomach kills bad bacteria. They say that bugs can't live in an acid medium. Calcium that we eat has to be dissolved in the strong acid in the stomach so it will go to our bones and teeth rather than to our joints and cause arthritis or to our blood vessels and cause hardening of the arteries.

Reasons for Malabsorption. One more way to prevent malabsorption is to make sure that our food goes through our bodies from mouth to anus in about 36 hours. If we have enough water and plenty of fiber, especially bran from whole-grain cereal and cellulose from vegetables and whole fruit, our bowel movements will be regular, and wastes won't stack up in the colon to cause diverticulosis and maybe cancer of the colon.

Other reasons for malabsorption are surgeries. If anyone has had his stomach or intestines or any part of them removed, absorption will be poor. Also, if we don't make enough bile, we can't digest fats in the small intestine. We make bile out of cholesterol that we eat or out of the cholesterol that our cells make. We would die without bile, and nature knows that, so nature gave us a way to make cholesterol in every cell. We need good food to make it; we can't make cholesterol out of soft drinks and candy bars. Nutritionists recommend fat-dissolving pancreatic enzymes until we can begin to make our own bile. See the food supplement chart in Lesson 1.

Drugs such as alcohol, cathartics and diuretics keep people from absorbing nutrients. Alcohol interferes with the absorption of fat and of vitamins A, B1, B12 and folic acid. Malabsorption may last six weeks after giving up alcohol. Mineral oil absorbs the fat and the fat-soluble vitamins A, D, E and K and excretes them from the body. We can't

live without the fat-soluble vitamins, so we don't take mineral oil. Diuretics force water out of our tissues, and we lose minerals with the water, which can lead to many diseases caused by mineral deficiencies, among them osteoarthritis and osteoporosis. It seems that older people take diuretics—water pills—just as a matter of course. They don't realize they're making their health worse. The liver manufactures a protein that will pick up waste water if we eat all nutrients needed to make the protein, and if our livers are healthy enough to make it.

Anybody with congestive heart failure and pericarditis (inflammation of the sac that surrounds the heart) also has congested intestines, pancreas and liver. If the congestive heart failure lasts longer than three or four weeks, the body loses protein and fat. But needed nutrients will reverse the condition. If there is pain in the intestine, a major blood vessel in that area may be stopped up, which is always a result of malnutrition and malabsorption (Balecki and Dobbins, 1974).

If X-rays of the abdomen or pelvic area are taken, the bowel may be injured, regardless of how little radiation is given. Effects of radiation may occur within two years, but they may occur 15 to 30 years later. Whenever they occur, they cause malabsorption of fat, carbohydrate and protein, and they interfere with the circulation of bile that is needed to help absorb fats. The bowels don't have enough movement to pass feces along, so people become constipated. This same disorder is found in elderly diabetics.

Paget's disease of the bones is often found in the elderly. It is thought to be partly caused by a deficiency of folic acid. Without folic acid, nutrients can't be absorbed in the small intestine. Skin disorders such as psoriasis and eczema can be caused by malabsorption of folic acid and of vitamin B12.

The treatment for all these diseases of malabsorption is an excellent diet plus vitamin and mineral supplements (Balecki and Dobbins, 1974). The fact that disease is evident means there have been deficiencies of nutrients, but these problems can be reversed with a good diet.

Heart Disease

"In 90 percent of cases, death caused by hardening of the arteries is now avoidable. That statement has enormous significance (Carpenter, 1980).

Phase 1. The first symptoms and signs of arteriosclerosis are damage to some part of the blood vessel lining caused by:

1. Nutritional deficiencies.
2. Chemicals and pollutants in the environment inside and outside the body.

3. Radiation.

4. Allergens (foreign invaders in the body such as dust, pollen, asbestos and undigested food, plus fast food and junk food such as white bread, white rice and pasta), none of which furnish enough nutrients to take up space in our stomachs.

5. Refined sugar, the worst of the junk foods.

6. Physical stress—the adrenal glands protect us from stress damage if they are healthy enough to make the hormones we need to prevent stress.

The overall cause is poor nutrition, which actually causes all the rest.

Phase 2. Any substance floating in the blood sticks to the damaged lining of the blood vessels, especially where the vessels branch. These substances are a cholesterol called low density lipoprotein (the bad cholesterol), other fats, proteins (especially undigested proteins that the body can't use—they damage any tissue they adhere to), big molecules of sugar and minerals. Especially damaging is calcium that couldn't be dissolved and sent to the blood, then to bones and teeth, because the acid in the stomach was too weak to dissolve it (Carpenter, 1980). If there is enough vitamin E, C, B6, selenium and methionine (an amino acid), the body can defend itself against the damage; the substances will not stick to blood vessel walls (Carpenter, 1980).

Phase 3. The third phase is cross-linking of the substances already stuck to the walls. This means that the long molecules of undigested protein, bad cells and other substances are cross-linked with a metal; this time calcium is the cross-linking agent. The calcium and proteins are bound into tangles that stick to the fats on the artery walls, which makes the blood vessels brittle. They break easily and cause hemorrhages. The tangles must be dissolved and sent to the digestive tract to be excreted.

Enzymes will help get rid of the tangles, but anyone who has eaten so poorly that the tangling has occurred has probably been eating so poorly that he isn't making enough enzymes to dissolve the tangles. The more substances that stick to the walls, the more calcium is deposited, until finally there is a severe blockage.

Minerals. Our hearts need calcium to continue beating, because a muscle can't contract without calcium, and the heart is a muscle.

Also, if we don't get enough potassium the soft tissues may calcify. This is what happens when we have arteriosclerosis (hardening of the arteries). It isn't that we have too much calcium, it is just de-posited where it doesn't belong because of a lack of potassium and usually an excess of sodium. Everybody knows we can get too much sodium. The more sodium we eat in relation to potassium, the more heart cells are killed. Too much fat in the diet can cause fast heartbeat, irregular heartbeat or "heart consciousness," which means that we feel every beat of the heart, especially when we first lie down and get quiet.

The incidence of heart disease has actually gone down in this country and in England. Acheson and Williams (1983) think that it is because people are eating more fresh green vegetables and whole fresh fruits that contain many more vitamins and minerals than processed foods. Vitamin C, for example, protects against high blood pressure and strokes whether caused by hemorrhages or clots. The fragile capillaries in the brain are strengthened by the C in the fruit. Vitamin C also helps break down clots of fibrin—the protein deposits that form tangles and trap fat, which increases the size of the fatty plaques. Potassium, found in high amounts in vegetables and fruits, cuts down the incidence of strokes caused by hemorrhages because potassium helps keep the smooth muscles of the blood vessels strong and flexible. During exercise, when the blood pulses forcefully through the blood vessels, the muscles will stretch; they won't tear and cause strokes.

Lecithin. Lecithin deficiency is the real cause of heart disease, although excess cholesterol has been taking the blame (Rinse, 1981). Lecithin is a fat that dissolves cholesterol and takes it to the liver to be made into bile. Cholesterol does not stack up in our blood vessels if we eat enough lecithin to keep it melted and flowing in the blood.

If the lecithin content of the blood is higher than 36 percent, no atherosclerosis occurs, even if there are high amounts of cholesterol in the blood. Below 34 percent, atherosclerosis is found.

Other ailments caused by a shortage of lecithin pertain to the brain and nervous system. Fat stacks up in the capillaries in the brain and we can't think well. Our short-term memory suffers. We become depressed. Other specific nutrients needed to handle all those ailments are vitamins B6, C and E, and minerals calcium, magnesium, chromium, vanadium, copper and others.

We should eat lecithin in food and many of us should take it in supplement form every day of our lives. There is a lot of lecithin in the good kind of cholesterol called HDL (high density lipoprotein). Lecithin emulsifies cholesterol and sends it to the liver where it is changed to bile with the help of vitamin C. Bile helps us digest and assimilate fats. The bad lipoproteins are very low in lecithin and high in cholesterol and triglycerides, which they carry to fat storage cells in tissues and organs, where they build up and form plaques (Rinse, 1981). These are the LDLs (low density lipoproteins), which cause heart attacks and strokes.

We want to get rid of the LDL and build up the HDL. That's easy. We do it with eggs and other sources of lecithin, in order to melt away the hard fat that clings to the blood vessel walls. So instead of eggs being no-no's, they are excellent foods, and we should eat one or two a day. Eggs have five to seven times more lecithin than cholesterol. Lecithin makes our blood just the right consistency, not too thick and not too thin. When there is a deficiency of lecithin in the blood, heart disease can be severe. The main reason that people have heart attacks is that they don't eat enough lecithin. The National Heart, Lung and Blood Institute in Washington conducted an investigation that showed that a high HDL content of the blood is a sign that no atherosclerosis occurs, while high LDL usually means that the disease is present. Thus the answer to heart disease is in food—especially lecithin from egg yolk, wheat germ, yeast, nuts and seeds, plus vitamins and minerals to make the enzymes and hormones. The foods and food supplements needed are in Lesson 1 of this *Home Study Course*.

Cholesterol. It is known that cholesterol is needed in every cell in the body—it is 5 to 10 percent of our brain tissue and part of our sex glands and adrenal glands, so we can't live without it. Yet for 25 years or so, we were told not to eat eggs because they contain cholesterol. During those years, not one person's life was saved from heart disease, and more people died of cancer. If we eat cholesterol, our livers make less; if we don't eat it, our livers have to make more. Sometimes we don't make enough because we eat junk food and we don't have the ingredients needed to make it. We should eat moderate amounts of eggs, butter, whole milk (not required) and even liver.

If the cholesterol we eat doesn't stack up in our blood vessels, then where does the cholesterol in the arteries come from? Researchers found that a mutated cell from the inside wall of the artery divides and forms the plaques. Why does a cell become mutated? Because of any of the reasons mentioned in the section on "Theories of Aging." They include medical X-rays, doctors' drugs and garbled messages put out by hormones that are incomplete because all the nutrients needed to make them complete weren't eaten by the individual. Those mutated cells die and form cholesterol, which melts only at high temperatures; therefore it forms hard plaques at our body temperature of 98.6 degrees F. Cholesterol doesn't break down easily without leci-

thin, so it isn't excreted easily and it crystallizes in the plaques.

As long as 30 years ago, it was shown that as lecithin decreased in human arteries, calcium increased, thus causing arteriosclerosis (hardening of the arteries). Several studies long ago showed that people sick with heart disease got well when given lecithin orally or by injection. Then a study was done that showed why that was so. Lecithin keeps the cholesterol fluid at a body temperature of 98.6 degrees F, so cholesterol doesn't harden to fatty plaques.

Although cholesterol has been blamed for heart disease, many studies show that when people are on low-cholesterol diets or take cholesterol-lowering drugs, they have atherosclerosis as severely as before treatment. Lecithin works, and it is a food factor, not a drug.

Other Fats. Hydrogenated fats (margarine and hard white shortening) are the most deadly fats. They melt only at 114 degrees F, and they don't flow through the blood vessels; they congeal and stack up in the arteries, causing atherosclerosis. The depositing of calcium in these fatty plaques is called arteriosclerosis.

Studies with pigs fed a stock diet and four different foods showed that hydrogenated fats caused the worst arteriosclerosis, sugar the next worst, butter only a little and eggs almost none. This information should be widely publicized.

Polyunsaturated fatty acids (PUFA) cause early aging because the fats become rancid in the cells. A small amount of the PUFA is necessary, but we should get it from nuts and seeds rather than from bottled oil. And we should take the antioxidants to cut down on rancidity.

Stress

Stress exhausts our adrenal glands. The glands become covered with brown pigment and the energy cells don't make energy—all because we don't eat well enough to replace the nutrients destroyed by stress. Here are some of the changes: don't-carishness, depression, irritability, childish reasoning, loss of memory and confusion (Bourne, 1967). Does this sound like anyone you know?

Although most of the people I counsel blame stress for their ailments, they should blame themselves because they eat junk food and their adrenal glands become exhausted. Healthy adrenals protect us from stress damage, but exhausted adrenals *cause* stress damage. See Lesson 2 for more details.

Parkinson's Disease

Parkinson's disease is one of the most miserable diseases that afflicts older people. It is possible to prevent Parkinson's completely with diet, and the time to begin to treat the disease is before you have it. As early as 1965, Adelle Davis reported on some cases that improved with large amounts of B complex; a complete, natural food program; and all other nutrients in supplement form.

I talked with a man one day who had been told by his physicians that he had Parkinson's disease. He didn't have any tremor when I met him, and I asked him how the doctors had diagnosed the disease. He said they drew a line on a sheet of paper and told him to write on the line. His writing was cramped and illegible, and he wrote at a 45-degree angle. The doctors told him that was a sure test for Parkinson's, that he would develop the tremor in about two years and he would be dead in about 10 years. They also told him to go home; they could do nothing for him.

He went on a natural food diet and when I called him about two months later, he said, "Guess what! I can already write on a straight line." He wrote me a letter about two years later, and he said he had never had any more trouble writing on a line, and he had never had one tremor in all that time. I heard from him after another two years, and he was still in excellent health. His doctors told him they must have misdiagnosed!

The *AD Newsletter* (Spring 1986) reported that drugs with the bad side effects given for Parkinson's disease do not halt the progression of the disease. So what's our answer? Eat to prevent disease.

Diabetes

Chromium deficiency often leads to high amounts of sugar in the blood, which, of course, is diabetes. In the United States, the older we get, the less chromium we have in our blood, and the less sugar we can tolerate. Studies have shown poor glucose tolerance in a majority of persons older than 70 years of age, and in many people under 70.

Chromium is in yeast, butter and cream; the best source is brewer's yeast. The latest research reports that a high complex carbohydrate diet (as outlined in Lesson 1) plus chromium will relieve symptoms of diabetes and often allow diabetics to quit taking insulin (*MD*, March 1976).

The outdated treatment for diabetes was insulin injections. Patients were put on a high-protein, low-carbohydrate diet. That treatment allowed the patient to live, but it didn't cure the disease (Corwin, 1980). It led to increased incidence of diabetes until it has become our third killer disease. The new preferred treatment for diabetes is good nutrition—a moderate protein, low-fat and high *complex* carbohydrate diet, with plenty of fiber, and not one grain of white sugar or white flour. Juvenile diabetes is caused by destruction of the islets of Langerhans partly because of a severe shortage of vitamin B6.

Nutrients especially needed to prevent the onset of diabetes are B6, zinc, magnesium and vitamin C. It has been found many times that blood sugar in diabetics can become normal by providing the nutrients needed by the brain, which prods the pancreas to resume its normal activity.

Muscles

Often people get sagging, flabby muscles as an early sign of aging (Gutman, 1972). This is a deficiency of protein. If we don't eat enough protein, then protein in the skeletal muscles is broken down to make protein for the heart muscles. We can live with weak muscles in our arms and legs, but we can't live with weak heart muscles. We sometimes have to break down muscle protein to make energy, if we don't eat enough carbohydrates and fats. The best carbohydrates are whole grains, vegetables and whole fruits. The best fats are butter, nuts and seeds. The best proteins are chicken from health food stores, fish, dairy products and especially whole grain and legume combinations, as given in Lesson 1. We should eat very little red (muscle) meat— steaks, roasts, chops and hamburger. These meats still contain 20 to 50 percent fat even if we trim off all visible fat.

So any time our muscles waste away, it's because we didn't eat enough protein or we didn't eat enough complex carbohydrates and fats, and the body had to break down the protein in our muscles to furnish energy.

Osteoporosis

Bone diseases are common in old people. The main reason is that we don't eat enough minerals, especially calcium, phosphorus, magnesium and the sunshine vitamin—vitamin D. Older women often don't get out in the sun. Sometimes they wear long sleeves and hats, and their skin is not exposed to sunshine. We also need calcium all our lives, and many people don't get as much as they used to when they get old.

If we don't get the nutrients needed to make bones, we get osteoporosis—porous bones. Ninety-nine percent of the calcium in our bodies is in our bones and teeth, but the 1 percent that's left circulates in our blood to feed our soft tissues. Muscles can't contract without calcium. Nature made us so our hearts would get enough calcium even if our bones become weak and will break easily. So many older people get osteoporosis (four times as many women as men) that it is said to be as common as gray hair when we age. Brittle nails, nervousness, abnormal heartbeats, formation of tartar and inflammation of the gums are seen in early stages of osteoporosis—all caused by calcium deficiencies. When calcium is laid down in soft tissues, as in blood vessels, where it does not belong, it is usually because there is not enough phosphorus, magnesium and vitamin D to combine with the calcium to make bone (Molnar, 1972/3).

Osteoporosis doesn't show up when bones are X-rayed until 30 percent of the mineral in bone is gone. Many surveys show that by the time women are 55 and men 60, 30 percent of individuals have had at least one bone fracture.

Someone can be standing up and suddenly fall down. Everybody rushes to pick her up, and they discover a broken hip and think she broke it when she fell. The truth is, the weakened hip broke from the weight of her body and caused the fall. People with osteoporosis can break a hip by just turning over in bed.

When we take calcium supplements, we can rebuild bones. But we have to have all nutrients including hydrochloric acid, because we can't dissolve and absorb calcium without plenty of acid in the stomach. A researcher at Mayo Clinic, Jennifer Jowsey, says that people 25 years and older should take 1,000 mg of calcium as a supplement in order to avoid osteoporosis when they get old.

If we're past 25, we should start as soon as possible, always remembering to get magnesium, phosphorus and vitamin D with the calcium, and hydrochloric acid to assimilate all the nutrients.

One of my oldest friends came to me for counseling not long ago. I was shocked to hear her say that she had osteoporosis, and she had known it for several years. She obviously hadn't realized how serious it is, because she didn't change her diet until the pain got so bad she couldn't stand it any more. It pays to start at age 25, as Jennifer Jowsey says, and take all nutrients needed for good health. It takes a long time to build back bone, but it can be done.

When I first changed my own diet (I was a sugar-coffeeholic until about 18 years ago), I had so much new energy that I exercised without getting tired for the first time in my life. Evidently I hadn't been on the diet long enough to build my bones up, because the more I exercised, the more my bones ached. I had the energy to dig up the backyard and plant a garden but my bones hurt worse, and it took almost a year on my good food program before they stopped hurting. Some pathology books say it is impossible to replace the bone and to relieve the pain of osteoporosis, but I know it is possible; I've done it. Now, I would know to take larger doses of the minerals with hydrochloric acid, and my bones would get strong faster.

Laboratory studies also show that bones can be built back. Dogs were given diets low in calcium and high in phosphorus. The first bone to deteriorate was the jawbone. The teeth became loose and the gums bled. The poor dogs had periodontal disease, just as so many humans have because they eat the average American diet of junk foods. Other bones deteriorated more slowly. When dogs were given 10 times as much calcium, and other nutrients needed in the correct ratio, all the bones became normal. The first bone to recover was the jawbone, and the teeth and gums became strong (Lutwak, 1974).

The best combination of the nutrients is a large intake of calcium, up to 2,000 mg a day for a while, about one-half that amount or a little less of magnesium and about one-third as much phosphorus, with 1,000 to 2,500 units of vitamin D. Don't forget the hydrochloric acid to assimilate all of it.

If we eat or drink too much phosphorus, calcium is withdrawn from the bones. Many popular foods are very high in phosphorus, and they make our bones porous, especially bottled drinks with or without sugar. It's tragic to see people drink sugar-free drinks thinking they are not harming their bodies because they're not eating sugar. But they're ruining their bones and helping themselves develop arthritis. Other foods high in phosphorus are processed cheese, ice cream, snack foods such as crackers, potato chips and soft drinks, which have helped increase our phosphorus intake at least 200 percent in the last 20 years (Winick, 1976). Also, meat and potatoes are high in phosphorus and low in calcium. High-calcium foods are green leafy vegetables, sesame seeds, molasses and seaweed—foods not found in large amounts in the average diet. Jennifer Jowsey says that "only by dietary calcium supplements can a correct calcium-to-phosphorus ratio be maintained."

By age 60, 45 percent of the people in the United States have lost all their teeth, mostly because of periodontal disease (Krehl, 1974). Anyone who has periodontal disease should realize that osteoporosis is probably developing, and he should improve his diet and avoid the severe pain of porous bones. Other investigators (Molnar, 1972/3) have mentioned the importance of potassium, which reminds us that we need the entire team of nutrients. We can't leave any out.

We don't absorb more than 50 percent of the calcium we eat, and sometimes not more than 5 percent, depending on how much phosphorus, protein and magnesium we eat with it. If we absorb more than we lose, it goes to our bones. And if we lose more than we absorb, it is pulled out of our bones, which makes them weak and porous (Lutwak, 1974).

The bones most likely to lose calcium are the vertebrae, the heel bone and the jaw. At least 12 million women in this country have such porous bones that they've had fractured vertebrae. Even a small deficiency over many years causes osteoporosis. When we eat enough calcium and enough other nutrients to assimilate it, our bones become healthy. It takes a long time, but we *can* build back bones.

Osteomalacia

Osteomalacia (another bone disease) is called "adult rickets." Thus, even though we're no longer children, we can still suffer from "bad bones," which is what "osteomalacia" means. Childhood rickets is partly caused by a deficiency of vitamin D, and adult rickets is too. We should get vitamin D from the sun or from supplements of fish liver oils, plus all other nutrients.

Experimental Drugs

Elderly people have other problems besides lack of good food. They are often given experimental drugs so the doctor can observe the results. Doctors think that the elderly are a good group to try out new drugs on because they have high incidence of disease. But since there are so many ways that the elderly can suffer from lowered thinking ability, they should be protected from being exploited by physicians' experimenting with new drugs (Bernstein, 1975).

The elderly may not be able to think as well because of:

(1) Loss of neurons and decreased weight of the brain, especially from age 60 on. (Neurons are thinking cells.)
(2) Degeneration of the blood vessels and of circulation, especially in the brain.
(3) Vitamin deficiency states.
(4) Degenerative disease of the central nervous system.

Reports show (Hurwitz and Wade, 1969) that adverse drug reactions are two and one-half times higher in old people than in the young. The median age of patients hospitalized with drug reactions is 60.

Radiation

Radiation can make us get older faster. Radiation is always in the atmosphere and it can damage our cells. A study showed that irradiated insects age faster than controls. Sexual organs wither and brain tissues become spongy. There is degeneration of the cells in the brain that make energy for us to think (Miquel, 1972).

Radiation from X-rays causes the same trouble. There is "general acceleration of the normal aging process." Both animals and humans that have undergone a lot of X-rays get old-age diseases at younger ages. The experimental animals given high-fat diets, then X-rayed, had more destruction of tissue than those on low-fat diets. And the old animals had more tissue damage than young ones (Svojtkova, 1972).

The answer to radiation is never to have X-rays as a screening tool. Agree to radiation only in a matter of life and death, as in an accident. When X-rays are necessary, our best protection is a good diet with emphasis on antioxidants. These are vitamins E and C, the mineral selenium and the sulfur-containing amino acids methionine, cystine and cysteine.

Cataracts

Cataracts are so often found in oldsters that it may seem a normal part of aging. But it is not normal. It is average, but not normal. Here's one way to avoid cataracts: Take supplements of the minerals potassium and magnesium. If we don't assimilate calcium well, it stacks up in soft tissues such as blood vessel walls (arteriosclerosis), joints (arthritis) and the lens of the eye (cataracts). Other minerals help assimilate calcium. So if you want to avoid all the above conditions, add moderate amounts of all minerals (and vitamins) to your diet in supplement form. And whatever age you are, start now! We shouldn't eat much fat; the best fats and the amounts needed are given in Lesson 1 of this course. Remember, we must have all the nutrients because they all work together.

Cataract is the loss of transparency of the lens of the eye. A cataract does not hurt. It can be caused by aging, injury to the lens, eye infections, electric shock, exposure to X-rays, endocrine gland disturbances, prenatal infections and drug poisoning or therapy.

The only sensible way to treat cataracts is to eat all nutrients needed to make healthy lenses, but the usual treatment is surgery, which is often unsatisfactory. Blindness may follow surgery, especially if the patient is old and weak because of glaucoma, retinal detachment or cystoid macular edema. An intraocular lens can cause iritis or infection. Sometimes infection occurs, and the new lens has to be removed. Sometimes three new eyeglass prescriptions have to be bought within the first year after surgery. These eyeglasses may be uncomfortable, and it is hard to get used to changes in vision.

Thus it is best to prevent cataracts if at all possible. First, don't go out in the bright sunlight; it will cause the lenses to accumulate protein, which shows up as the yellow-brown color of some cataracts. Protective sunglasses will help by absorbing ultraviolet light if you're outdoors between 10 A.M. and 4 P.M. Plastic glasses tinted gray or gray-green are suggested (Duarte, 1982).

If you're a new patient and are developing cataracts, you have no doubt been deficient in glutathione and vitamin C, in enzymes requiring sodium and potassium and in other nutrients. Also, an increase of sodium and a decrease of potassium in the lens allows swelling caused by water accumulation. To correct the sodium-potassium balance, there must be plenty of energy to make the pump work to pump sodium out and to pump potassium into the lens. The most important nutrient that keeps the pump working is glutathione, a combination of three amino acids.

As your cataract grows, your vision will be blurred. Depending on the kind of cataract, the blurring will be in the center of your vision or around the edges. Often, people don't notice the blurring when it is around the edges, and they don't realize they are really developing cataracts.

Now is the time to improve your food and food supplement program so the condition will not develop or will be reversed. If nothing else, degeneration may stop and not get worse. Often when the cataract is stabilized, the patient's vision will improve but it is not guaranteed.

Glutathione is "the most powerful shield against aging that we know of" (Duarte, 1982). All membranes of the eye require glutathione, which consists of three amino acids: glycine, glutamic acid and cysteine. Glutathione keeps the free radicals from reacting against the eye tissue. When we get old, we don't have as much glutathione as when we were young. But if we eat the three ingredients, and if all other nutrients are in our bloodstream, we may be able to stop the progression of the disease. However, the best time to begin this anticataract program is before a cataract develops.

Vitamin C helps avoid or control cataracts in these ways (Duarte, 1982):

1. Vitamin C protects the delicate lens so it will remain transparent.
2. It helps form collagen, the connective tissue that sticks our cells together.
3. It helps stimulate the immune system.
4. It protects the lens from near ultraviolet light.
5. It protects against free radicals, which we've talked a lot about.

Vitamin C is 50 times more prevalent in the lens than in the blood.

Bioflavonoids are needed, especially for diabetics. The suggested amount is 100 mg of bioflavonoids to each 500 mg of vitamin C. If bioflavonoids are plentiful enough, they help keep water from collecting in the lens and causing swelling.

Vitamin B2, riboflavin, helps glutathione function. Suggested dosage is 100 to 300 mg a day.

Vitamin B6 helps RNA and DNA, which make the patterns for our proteins.

Inositol and other B vitamins, 100 to 150 mg. (Other nutritionists suggest five times more of niacinamide and pantothenic acid, as found in this *Home Study Course,* Lesson 1.)

Selenium. At least 200 mcg a day, as a supplement, plus the amount consumed in food. It is important for glutathione activity. You may need to increase to 300 to 400 mcg a day. Don't take sodium selenite (Duarte, 1982).

Vitamin E works with selenium. See Lesson 1 for potency.

Zinc. See Lesson 1 for potency.

Anemia

We don't want to develop anemia when we get old. Anemia is sometimes caused by lack of iron, but it is usually caused by a lack of other nutrients such as folic acid or vitamin B12 or both. Pernicious anemia, caused by a B12 deficiency, is found almost exclusively in older people. A deficiency of folic acid is one of the most common deficiencies, often found when vitamin C is in short supply, since both these vitamins come from fresh fruit and vegetables. Vitamin C is needed to change folic acid to folacin, which is the working substance in the cells. Folic acid deficiency combined with a diseased liver is also found in chronic alcoholism, which is common especially in older men.

Macrocytic anemia is a folic acid deficiency. The red blood cells are larger than normal. All these conditions can be reversed with a good diet and food supplements. That's the beauty of good nutrition—it's never too late to start.

In examining the patient who might not be getting a good diet, physicians should notice the number of times he eats foods with empty calories such as most alcoholic beverages, soft drinks, sugar, syrups, jellies, jams, etc. Does he eat or omit breakfast? What kind of snacks does he eat? This advice is from the journal *Geriatrics* (Krehl, 1974). It seems like good advice to me, but all my counselees tell me that their physicians never ask what they've been eating.

Hemorrhoids

Many of us are bothered, some mildly, some severely, by the aggravating disease of hemorrhoids. They are caused primarily by straining at stool because of constipation. The veins of the anus and lower rectum swell, sometimes they enlarge suddenly and are filled with clots of blood. They may bleed and be very painful for a few days. Although most rectal bleeding is caused by hemorrhoids, the bleeding can be a warning sign of cancer and colitis (Pauling, 1980), so the diet should be changed, since all three of these conditions are nutritional deficiency diseases.

To prevent or control hemorrhoids, the first thing needed is to soften the stools, which is easy with a stool softener containing psyllium seed. This is available at any health food store. Also, vitamin C in large doses can be used as a stool softener. It also keeps walls of the blood vessels strong because it is needed for the manufacture of collagen, the protein that makes all of our connective tissue healthy. The dosage recommended for most people is from six to 18 grams of vitamin C a day in divided doses (Pauling, 1986). People who are ill may need more. Begin with about 500 mg four times a day, then work up till you get to as much as you can take without getting severe gas or diarrhea.

At the same time that you increase your vitamin C, apply topically a solution of sodium ascorbate (vitamin C powder buffered with sodium) mixed with vitamin E (Pauling, 1980). Straight ascorbic acid is too strong to use on tender skin.

I have letters from people who have completely eliminated their hemorrhoids with total nutritional therapy. A lovely woman came for counseling not long ago. She later said that one blessing she had realized from the new food and food supplement program was healing of her hemorrhoids.

The entire food and food supplement program is required for total therapy; there are no magic bullets. If all nutrients are not supplied, our ailments will not improve satisfactorily.

NUTRIENTS NEEDED

Let's go over some of the nutrients that are especially important to people who want to live a long time without looking old. That ought to be everybody!

Proteins

Protein deficiencies often show up as edema, pellagra, liver disease and macrocytic anemia. Some people have only one of these, but others have all. And all the ailments are caused by deficiencies of vitamins and minerals as well as protein.

We cause our edema (retention of fluids) by not eating enough protein and other nutrients needed by the liver to make albumin to pick up the waste water.

Albumin picks up waste fluids all over the body and excretes them. If there isn't enough albumin, the wastes don't get picked up and fluid collects in the tissues. The fluid usually appears first in the scrotum and labia, and then as a swelling in the legs. This is "pittable," which means that if you press your finger on the leg, it leaves an indentation. Also the tissues inside the body may be swollen.

This means that fluid is accumulating in feet, legs, fingers and eye bags. When I speak at club meetings, I hear people talk about taking "water pills." These are dangerous because they take away the good minerals and water-soluble vitamins, and the person gets worse instead of better. Anybody on water pills should be eating more protein and taking hydrochloric acid to assimilate it. Then they can probably phase out the dangerous water pills.

Symptoms of pellagra are skin disease, inflammation of the mucous membranes, diarrhea and psychic disturbances. Pellagra is usually a deficiency of niacin (B3). But if the person gets enough protein, he can make niacin from the amino acid tryptophan. People with this deficiency often get plenty of calories but lack vitamins and protein. The simplest form of the disease shows an enlarged fatty liver, and it can be reversed by supplying the missing nutrients. If the nutrients aren't supplied, however, the damage to the liver may be severe and irreversible (Dreizen, 1974).

Vitamins A, D and E

The following information about the dosage of nutrients is from medical and nutrition books and journals. Please check with your nutrition-minded physician to determine the amount needed in individual cases.

We often have deficiencies of fat-soluble vitamins A, D and E because we don't eat enough fat. Anyone who is in the "tea and toast" group should drink herb tea instead of the usual tea with or without caffeine, and should eat homemade wholegrain bread with butter (not margarine) on it. A few spoonfuls of ground-up pecans or walnuts, or any other nuts and seeds increase the food value. Sometimes older people take mineral oil as a laxative. The oil binds to the fats and drains them away, taking the fat-soluble vitamins with the oil (Mayer, 1974) and causing a vitamin deficiency.

Fat-soluble vitamins won't be absorbed if there aren't enough pancreatic enzymes, if the liver doesn't work well or if there are too many bad bacteria in the intestines. Yogurt will help keep away the bad bacteria, but there is something more powerful now—*Lactobacillus acidophilus*, available at health food stores in tablet, liquid and powder form. Don't buy the kind that has *bulgaricus* in it. See the section called "Digestive Problems" in this lesson.

Vitamin A. Nutritionists are now suggesting beta-carotene as the preferred form of vitamin A supplements. It is a provitamin, and it is not changed to vitamin A until the body needs it. Then the change is made in the liver, if the liver is healthy. It is almost impossible to get a toxic level of beta-carotene. Vitamin A from extremely large amounts of fish liver oil can be toxic, but the toxicity is reversed when the vitamin is withdrawn.

We don't realize we're deficient in vitamin A until we've been deficient for a fairly long time. The main signs of deficiency are in the skin and eyes, such as night blindness and dryness of the eyes. The skin gets dry and rough like the skin of a toad, especially on the hands, feet, shoulders and to a lesser extent on the chest, back and buttocks. The lesions are dry, horny, round to oval and all sizes (Dreizen, 1974).

Most researchers suggest 25,000 IU of beta-carotene for the average adult. People who have symptoms of deficiency may need more for a time, until their symptoms are gone, then they may decrease to 25,000 IU for a maintenance dose.

Vitamin D. Vitamin D deficiency is apparent in bone diseases. Vitamin D capsules can be given—possibly 1,000 to 2,500 IU for a short while, then decrease to 400 IU for maintenance.

Vitamin E. Probably the most pitiful older people are those whose brains are deteriorating. It is extremely difficult to do anything about someone whose mind is affected and who is belligerent and non-cooperative about a new diet. But for others, tremendous improvements can be made with good nutrition. Vitamin E is one of the most important nutrients to help avoid strokes and senility (Harai and Yoshikawa, 1972).

It is well known that a discoloration (lipofuscin pigment) takes place in the nervous systems of animals when they get old. The pigment is believed to be caused by the reaction of polyunsaturated fats on cells that are deficient in vitamin E, which we've talked about before.

Studies have been done with animals that show that any time vitamin E is in short supply in the diet, there is a greater possibility of having more pigment in the nervous system with fewer nerve impulses traveling to and from the brain. When animals were given injections of vitamin E, there was improvement in both conditions, which meant that the animals stayed young longer. The investigators said that older animals may require more than the usual supply of vitamin E to perform normal functions and to slow down the aging pro-

cess and prolong life (Harai and Yoshikawa, 1972).

Vitamin E can help make cells that are able to divide more than the average number of times. In a study, the cells from a human embryo that normally live for about 50 divisions lived for about 120 divisions and had "youthful characteristics." Thus if our cells have an environment that is as perfect as possible, including the maximum amount of vitamin E that we need, our cells will live longer and be more youthful! Wouldn't it be especially nice to keep our brain cells alive and working as long as we're here?

Vitamin E is one of the most important vitamins against premature aging because it is an antioxidant. It keeps oxygen from reacting on fats in the body and damaging cells. Selenium works with vitamin E, and vitamin C is the water-soluble vitamin that works as an antioxidant to protect our cells (*Science*, 1974).

Vitamin C

Vitamin C deficiencies often start with exhaustion, weakness, irritability and loss of weight. There is often a hemorrhage where there is a small injury. Bleeding into the muscles may make the muscles hard and more liable to injury. Petechiae (pinpoint, flat, round, purplish red spots) and ecchymoses (spots larger than petechiae and blue or purplish in color) respond to vitamin C. They are most common in the legs, lower body, face, neck and forearms.

Vitamin C deficiencies usually include gingivitis, which is inflammation of the gums, causing them to swell and change to a dark red or purple color. The gums glisten, bleed easily and become soft. The bones that hold the teeth decay, and the teeth may get loose and fall out.

In one study (Schorah, 1979), a group of elderly patients were given 1,000 mg of vitamin C a day for 28 days. The patients showed a slight but significant gain in weight and health compared to controls. Older people don't have as much vitamin C in their white blood cells as younger people do. Since white blood cells are part of the body's immune system, the older folks may not resist infection without supplements of vitamin C. As everyone knows, vitamin C keeps us from getting scurvy. These elderly people don't actually have scurvy, but they have subtle or severe ill effects from the deficiency of vitamin C (*Lancet*, 1979).

Vitamin B1

A B1 (thiamine) deficiency symptom is inflammation of the nerves that begins in the feet and goes up. There is weakness, cramping, burning or prickling of the skin, tenderness of the calf, impaired reflexes, toe and foot drop and withering of muscles. The leg complaints usually become severe before the rest of the body is involved; then the nerves of the trunk and diaphragm suffer.

Thiamine deficiency includes edema (retention of fluids), which also begins in the feet and legs and gradually moves up the body into the abdomen. Swelling of the abdomen is called ascites, and the swelling moves up into the chest. Heart failure can be caused by, among others, a deficiency of B1. Signs include pain in the chest, fast heartbeat, difficulty in breathing and what Dreizen calls "a bounding pulse with pistol-shot sounds over the large arteries." The heart gets very large, especially on the right side, and the pressure is high in the veins. The lungs are congested.

Encephalopathy means degenerative disease of the brain. This can be due to B1 deficiency. It usually shows up in people who drink too much and who eat junk foods. Symptoms are signs of vertigo (feeling that the world is spinning around you), headaches, nystagmus (rapid movement of the eyeball—horizontal, vertical or around and around), inability to tolerate light, disease of the optic nerve, clouding of consciousness, lack of muscular coordination and paralysis of the lips, tongue, mouth, pharynx (the space between the mouth and nose on the inside) and the upper part of the windpipe (Dreizen, 1974).

Vitamin B2

Deficiencies of B2 (riboflavin) often show up in elderly people. The most common sites are the tongue, lips, eyes and skin. The lips become pearly gray at the angles of the mouth. Later the gray pallor changes to a softening of the tissue with piling up of white matter on a pink background with cracks that radiate and may extend into the natural wrinkles at the corners of the lips. When these sores become chronic, they form a yellowish crust. The lips are often too red, slick and cracked.

The papillae (little bumps on the tongue) are swollen at first, then flattened and mushroom-shaped. The tongue looks pebbly. Later, the papillae wither. Sometimes the tongue becomes purplish red or magenta-colored, similar to the look the tongue gets when there isn't enough oxygen in the blood.

Eyes develop extra blood vessels in the cornea that move toward the center. Later the cornea may become opaque. Other eye signs are conjunctivitis (inflammation of the delicate membrane that lines the eyelids and covers the eyeball), inflammation of the eyelids, inability to tolerate light, the shedding of tears, burning and itching and inability to see well. Skin disease caused by deficiency of B2 usually begins in the folds around the nose and lips and spreads upward. The skin rash is scaly and greasy with a red base, and it spreads to the eyelids, chin and forehead. It can also cause rash on the scrotum and vulva.

Vitamin B3

Vitamin B3 (niacin) is important for elderly people. It helps the circulation in the capillaries so nutrients can get to the cells. This helps prevent clots in the brain (strokes), clogging and hemorrhages. Blood flows more forcefully through the brain and prevents senility. Niacin helps eliminate the fatty deposits on the skin. Hoffer says that people who come to him for treatment in a presenile state usually improve quickly on large doses of niacin and vitamin C along with moderate doses of all other nutrients. To test yourself to see if you need niacin, Hoffer says if you have to grope for words, if you ask the same question every few minutes and if you forget what subject you were discussing, you need niacin.

When we get older, the red blood cells stick together. They should go through the capillaries in single file; big clumps of cells can't squeeze through. The big clumps cause "sludging." The capillaries disappear and oxygen can't reach all the brain cells. Niacin keeps the blood cells from sludging so they get more oxygen and better circulation in the brain. This keeps us from becoming senile.

The person who wants to take niacin just for insurance should begin with doses as low as 15 mg a day. Some people take timed-release tablets that release 30 mg at first. Others take as much as 250 to 500 mg a day by working up gradually. The supplements must also contain all vitamins and minerals as found in the chart in Lesson 1. It's probably best to take the tablets in the morning and at noon. They might cause wakefulness if taken at night.

Vitamin B6

B6 is used in so many reactions that it can reasonably be called the "master vitamin" (Corwin, 1980). We can't manufacture human protein from the animal and plant proteins we eat without vitamin B6. *All* of the enzymes and many hormones depend on B6 (Corwin's emphasis). Without B6, calcium and phosphorus cannot be used properly. Calcium is required in more than three dozen reactions, some essential for proper nerve and brain functions. Are you sure your elderly relatives are getting the B6 they need to help them remember the question they just asked, and not ask it again every five minutes? Do you suppose your children are making poor grades on their tests in school because they lack the B6 they need to think with?

Are you taking supplements of B6 so when you get old you won't become forgetful or suffer from any of the other ailments that B6 can prevent?

The four best sources of B6 in food are desiccated liver, brewer's yeast, lecithin and wheat germ. How many of the general public ever heard of those foods? Maybe you think we can get the B6 we need from the small amount in green beans or other canned or frozen foods. Not so. Sixty to 80 percent of the B6 is lost in the canning process, 40 to 60 percent in freezing.

In the last few days, I have talked with two mothers of fine young men who did well all the way through school and college; one was a Phi Beta Kappa at Yale. He began to eat junk food when he went away to school. By age 25, he was manic-depressive and had been given tranquilizers and lithium. For 10 years he took those drastic drugs into his body. At 35, when his mother came to see me, he was completely unable to work. The tranquilizers had caused tardive dyskinesia. He couldn't control his muscles; they "fired" constantly, and his hands and arms jerked continuously. The lithium had damaged his brain over the 10-year period. One day he walked into the den where his parents were sitting and announced, "I've just taken a lethal dose of lithium, but now I've decided I want to live." He was rushed to the hospital, where the doctors managed to save his life, but he has permanent brain damage and will probably never hold a job or be able to care for himself again.

Other B vitamins (especially B1, B2 and B3) cannot work well without B6, and all four are essential for the brain and nerves to act normally.

Can we get enough B6 in the average American diet? No—there is no natural food that contains large amounts of B6 except those "health foods" I mentioned. Twenty to 70 percent of the small amount present in other foods is destroyed by cooking. As we said, white flour, white sugar and fat make up 70 percent of our calories; those nonfoods contain no B6. The only possible conclusion to draw from this information is that probably all Americans, even those who eat as correctly as possible, should be taking moderate amounts of all food supplements.

Dr. John Ellis of Texas gave 50 mg of B6 a day plus magnesium to pregnant women suffering from toxemia of pregnancy. Their toxemia was relieved. Forty percent of all pregnant women in the United States suffer from toxemia of pregnancy, which could undoubtedly be relieved by B6 and magnesium supplements. The requirement for such a large amount of a nutrient is called a "dependency," which means that an individual can't function on the amount most people need. Their health is dependent on their getting a larger amount. Thus 40 percent of American women may be B6 dependent.

A region in our brain called the hypothalamus, right in the middle of our heads and very well protected by the skull, determines whether or not insulin will be manufactured and released, in order that our blood sugar will be level, and we'll be able to think. Whether or not the hypothalamus functions depends partly on the amount of B6 flowing through the capillaries in our brains. If you want to make an impression on the intellectual fellow or girl you met last week, you might want to be fortified with good food containing B6 so your hypothalamus will make you intelligent.

The adrenal glands are also stimulated by the hypothalamus. If the adrenals do not function well, the liver can't make glucose from stored glycogen, and fatal hypoglycemia may result (Corwin, 1980). Stress control depends on the release of hormones by the adrenal glands, which are now known to depend directly on nerves in the hypothalamus, which depend on B6.

When our hypothalamus is working poorly, we can no longer control our brains. Hormones don't send messages; and diseases show up as bone disorders, dermatitis, poor growth, weight problems, poor reproduction, poor teeth, nerve disorders, progressive paralysis, lethargy and finally convulsions. The lack of a few milligrams of vitamin B6 and other nutrients can cause all these problems.

Heart disease was produced in animals by a deficiency of B6 alone and was prevented in a control group on the same diet with B6. Another of the most widespread nutritional deficiencies in the United States is that of magnesium. B6 and magnesium are both required for the manufacture of lecithin. If one or both are not available, blood vessel disease sets in. To make lecithin, we also need choline, which requires an amino acid, methionine. A good source of methionine is eggs, but so many people are afraid to eat eggs because of the cholesterol scare that it's difficult to get enough methionine.

Folic Acid

People with folic acid deficiency have anemia and signs of disease similar to those of a deficiency of other B vitamins: inflammation of the tongue, lips, palate and floor of the mouth; lesions in the stomach and intestines; diarrhea; malabsorption of foods from the intestines; and fat in the feces with stools that smell foul and are greasy and somewhat liquid. The tongue eventually becomes slick and pale to fiery red (Dreizen, 1974).

PABA

Para-aminobenzoic acid is a B vitamin cousin

that helps us to stay young. It tends to slow down or even reverse loss of muscle tone, wrinkling and graying of hair. It's in the B complex and must not be taken alone, but always with complete B complex vitamins or with liver, yeast or wheat germ. Enriched flour doesn't retain any significant amount (Fredericks, 1975).

Pantothenic Acid

Pantothenic acid is known to prolong life if we get it in optimal amounts. Roger J. Williams (1971) gave experimental mice extra amounts of pantothenic acid, and they lived longer than the controls. Their length of life, compared to the lifetime of humans, increased from 75 years to 89 years.

Vitamin B12

Pernicious anemia is a deficiency of vitamin B12, often caused by a deficiency of hydrochloric acid. Numbness and tingling of the extremities are common, with pallor, digestive problems and even heart and blood vessel ailments. Severe symptoms can include burning and prickling of the arms and legs. The person has poor muscle coordination when he walks. He may suffer from dribbling urine. In this vitamin deficiency, as in other B deficiencies, the patient may have shallow white ulcers on the tongue, the papillae may disappear and the tongue may be glazed. The lining of the stomach may have the same signs (Dreizen, 1974).

Calcium

Mid-back and low back pain is so common in older people, especially women, that all of them should take extra calcium. Older people lose height, they have deformed bones and often have spontaneous fractures and spasms in the muscles beside the backbone if their diets are deficient in calcium *and in hydrochloric acid to help assimilate it* (my emphasis) (Dreizen, 1974).

Magnesium

Drugs given to elderly patients can cause loss of magnesium in the urine. Also, if we don't get enough magnesium in the diet, we may have muscle tremors, nervous reaction to sights and sounds, delirium, convulsions, spasms in the wrists and feet and jerky or writhing movements of the hands (Dreizen, 1974).

Iron

Iron deficiency in the elderly shows up as a large reduction in red blood cells, which causes anemia. Weakness, easy tiredness, irritability, sore mouth and sore tongue are common symptoms. The fingernails get ridges down the length of the nail, and some patients develop flat or spoon-shaped nails. If

people are very pale and listless, their anemia is severe. Mouth signs are similar to deficiencies of B vitamins—the papillae get smooth and people have difficulty swallowing.

Iodine

Many symptoms of aging and of atherosclerosis can be eliminated with B vitamins and iodine. Try kelp or iodine supplements to help your thyroid make its hormone (thyroxin), and set the proper rate to use food so your energy level will be high. You may need thyroxin, but researchers suggest that many doctors are too eager to put their patients on thyroxin when many need only a good source of iodine in the diet. You may be able to make your own hormone. So try iodine, as kelp. Be sure you continue a good diet and all other food supplements. Since reading this reference, I've asked many people who take thyroxin if their doctors give them B vitamins so the hormone will be safe and effective. I have yet to find someone who answers, "Yes."

WHAT WE DON'T EAT

Let's summarize what we should not eat or drink: alcohol, white sugar, white flour and all processed foods that are canned, frozen or packaged, such as chips and commercial crackers. We eliminate cigarette smoke (this means that we don't smoke and we don't stay near people who do). We stay out of polluted areas as much as possible. We don't drink bottled drinks with sugar or without. The average American diet is about 70 percent white flour and white sugar products and fat with very little food value. The other 30 percent is canned and frozen vegetables and other foods that have also had much of the food value processed out.

This means we'll have to prepare food from scratch. Often a woman from my audience will tell me, "I'm a widow, and I don't like to prepare food just for myself." Thus she excuses her diet of processed convenience foods. But I have no sympathy for this kind of reasoning. This woman should have enough pride in her own body and enough interest in her own health to prepare her own food.

WHAT WE DO EAT

To extend our young years, we need all the nutrients in the diet as outlined in Lesson 1. As we always say, diet is of first importance. We can't stay well and live long on a junk-food diet and vitamin and mineral tablets. Supplements are required even when food is as good as we can get.

Along with the new diet, we exercise according to our age and condition, and we eat only natural foods; we take food supplements (vitamins, minerals and special foods such as liver, brewer's yeast and yogurt). A food supplement program is imperative because commercial food is so processed and refined. The best way to start a food supplement program is to take all supplements as listed in the chart in Lesson 1. Sometimes people have stomach pains if they start on too large amounts of vitamin and mineral tablets. So if you're new to supplements, start with the lower amount on the chart and grind them up as the directions say. After three or four weeks, you may find that you can tolerate the supplements in tablet form. However, you may prefer to grind up your supplements indefinitely. They are easier to digest and assimilate if you do. You'll notice that the supplements given in the chart have a higher and a lower amount suggested. You may need to go up for your particular condition. Listen to your body; it will tell you what to do. When you feel really great, stay at that level. Keep all supplements in balance as in the chart. If you have specific reasons for taking more, do so. You're different from everyone else; you may need more or less.

The amounts of nutrients should stay rather high from now on, because, as we age, our bodies slow down and don't work as efficiently, so they need all the help they can get.

We've mentioned the special importance of vitamins C and E and of hydrochloric acid to assimilate foods and supplements.

Our food intake will concentrate on eggs and dairy products, fish, chicken from the health food store, whole grain and legume combinations, and nuts and seeds, plus raw and steamed vegetables and whole fruits, but no fruit juice—it's a highly concentrated form of fructose.

The excitement of this diet is that it allows us to be responsible for our own health. We'll be able to withstand disease, both degenerative and infectious, and we'll be able to REVERSE THE AGING PROCESS.

QUESTIONS

TRUE/FALSE

1. The three top killer diseases are heart and blood vessel diseases, cancer and diabetes, all of which are nutritional deficiency diseases.

2. One of the most important diet principles is that we should never overeat.

3. When a group of experimental mice were exposed to smoking, they drank alcohol, ate sugar and lived only half as long as the controls.

4. Cross-linking is the binding together of such substances as proteins, carbohydrates, undigested foods and abnormal cells with an agent such as aluminum.

5. Straining at stool is one of the major causes of hemorrhoids and varicose veins.

6. After many years of treatment of diabetes with insulin, many nutrition-minded physicians are now treating the disease with a complex carbohydrate diet.

7. Ninety percent of the calcium in our bodies is in our bones and teeth, but the other 10 percent is used in the soft tissues such as the muscles to help the heart beat.

8. Osteoporosis shows up in X-rays as soon as calcium is lost from the bones, so everyone, especially women, should have X-rays every year to discover the disease when it first starts.

9. The high levels of phosphorus found in sugar-free drinks and in many other foods build healthy bones.

10. Many people develop cataracts but don't realize it because they don't notice that their vision is blurred around the edges, one of the signs of cataract.

11. When people get old, they will never be able to heal their hemorrhoids because the old tissue cannot be renewed.

12. Pitting edema is a sign of protein deficiency brought about by inability of the liver to make enough albumin to pick up and eliminate waste water.

13. All the following are symptoms of vitamin A deficiency: night blindness; dry, rough skin; dry eyes; loose bowels.

14. As we get older, deficiencies of iron show up as ridges in nails, pale complexions and difficulty in swallowing.

MULTIPLE CHOICE

1. We can live longer and be healthier if we: (a) eat natural foods and take moderate amounts of all food supplements, (b) eat steak every night for supper.

2. The average length of life has increased by about 20 years in this country because: (a) 20-year-olds live longer, (b) upper-class men live longer, (c) more money is spent for medications, (d) fewer babies and young children die.

3. To distribute nutrients from the food we eat to every cell, we should: (a) eat prepared mixes, (b) eat half our nutrients from natural foods and half from processed foods, (c) eat food supplements to get the four amino acids we need, (d) have a good blood supply with plenty of oxygen.

4. The reason we should not overeat is that: (a) we can't digest food well if we eat too much at one time, (b) we may not have enough enzymes to break the food to fragments that go into our cells, (c)

undigested food is poison to our bodies, (d) all of the above.

5. Our two major sources of aluminum are: (a) red meat and cheese, (b) black-eyed peas and cornbread, (c) antacids and antiperspirants, (d) aluminum cooking utensils and perfume.

6. Which of the following nutrients serve as antioxidants? (a) vitamin C, (b) vitamin E, (c) selenium, (d) amino acids that contain sulphur, such as cysteine.

7. Fiber is important in several ways: (a) to keep our bowels regular, (b) to furnish a carbohydrate that is used for energy by friendly bacteria, (c) to slow down passage of wastes, (d) to make us fat if we need to gain.

8. Cholesterol is required in our bodies to furnish: (a) 5 to 10 percent of our brain tissue, (b) part of our sex glands, (c) transportation to move dust and pollen out of the body, (d) part of our adrenal gland tissue.

9. To improve the tissues so hemorrhoids will be controlled: (a) soften the stools, (b) take vitamin C, (c) fast on fruit juice for one week, (d) apply on the inflamed skin a mixture of vitamins E and C.

10. Protein deficiencies often show up as: (a) retention of fluids (edema), (b) pellagra, (c) liver disease, (d) anemia.

11. Fat-soluble vitamins cannot be absorbed: (a) if the pancreas isn't healthy enough to make its digestive enzymes, (b) if the muscles aren't working well, (c) if the liver doesn't have enough healthy cells to make bile, (d) if there are too many unfriendly bacteria in the intestine.

12. People who stay young need calcium so they won't: (a) lose height, (b) have deformed bones, (c) have spontaneous fractures, (d) have spasms in their muscles.

ANSWERS

True/False

1. T 2. T 3. T 4. T 5. T 6. T 7. F 8. F
9. F 10. T 11. F 12. T 13. F 14. T

Multiple Choice

1. a 2. d 3. d 4. d 5. c 6. a,b,c,d 7. a,b
8. a, b, d 9. a,b,d 10. a,b,c,d 11. a,c,d 12. a,b,c,d

REFERENCES

Acheson, R. M. and Williams, D.R.R. Does Consumption of Fruit and Vegetables Protect Against Stroke? *Lancet* 1(8335), May 28, 1983.

AD Newsletter, Vol. 6 # 1, Spring 1986, p. 9.

Balecki, J.A. and Dobbins, W.O. Maldigestion and Malabsorption, *Geriatrics* 29(5):157–66, 1974.

Bernstein, J.E. and Nelson, F.K. Medical Experimentation in the Elderly. *J.Am.Ger.*Soc. 23:327–29, 1975.

Bjorksten, J. Longevity "A Quest." *Rejuvenation* 9(3):47–52, Sept. 1981.

Bourne, G.H. Aging Changes in the Endocrines. In: Leo Gitman, ed., *Endocrines and Aging.* Springfield, IL: Thomas, 1967.

Carpenter, D.G. Correction of Biological Aging. *Rejuvenation* 8(2):31–49, June 1980.

Corwin,. A.H. Civilization and Health. *Rejuvenation* 8(4):89–99, Dec. 1980.

Cummings, J.H. Fermentation in the Human Large Intestine. *Lancet* 1(8335), May 28, 1983.

Cysteine. Kal Self Education Series # 6.

Davis, A. *Let's Get Well.* New York: Signet, 1965.

Dreizen, S. Clinical Manifestations of Malnutrition. *Geriatrics* 29(5):97–103, 1974.

Duarte, A. *Cataract Breakthrough.* International Institute of Natural Health Sciences, Huntington Beach, CA, 1982.

Fredericks, C. *Eating Right for You.* New York: Today Press, 1975.

Gutman, E. and Hanzlikova, V. *Age Changes in the Neuromuscular System.* Bristol: Scientechnica, 1972.

Harai, S. and Yoshikawa, M. Vitamin E and Aging of the Nervous System. International Symposium on Vitamin E, Tokyo, Kyoritou Shuppan Co. Ltd. Tokyo: 1972.

Hurwitz, N. and Wade, O.L. *British Med. J.,* 1:531, 1969.

Krehl, W.A. The Influence of the Nutritional Environment on Aging. *Geriatrics* 29(5):65–76, 1974.

Kugler, H. *The Disease of Aging.* New Canaan, Conn.: Keats, 1984.

Lancet. p. 403, Feb. 24, 1979.

Lutwak, L. Continuing Need for Dietary Calcium Throughout Life. *Geriatrics,* 29(5):171–78, 1974.

MD. March 1976.

Mayer, J. Aging and Nutrition. *Geriatrics,* 29(5):57–59, 1974.

Miquel, J., et al. Natural Aging and Radiation-Induced Life Shortening in Drosophila Melanogaster. *Mech. Age. Dev.,* 1:71-97, 1972.

Molnar, K. Subbiological Aspects of Aging and the Concept of Biological Cathode Protection. *Mech. Age Dev.,* 1:319–26, 1972/3.

Passwater, R.A. *Supernutrition*. New York: Pocket, 1975.

Pauling, L. *New Dynamics of Preventive Medicine*. New York: Int'l Medical Book Corp. 1974.

———Hemorrhoids. *Linus Pauling Institute Newsletter* 1(10):6, Winter 1980.

Rinse, J. Food Deficiencies and Atherosclerosis. *Rejuvenation*, 9(2):33–34, June 1981.

Rosenfield, A. *Prolongevity*. New York: Knopf, 1976.

Schloss, B. Possibilities for Prolonging Life in the Near Future. *Rejuvenation*, 9(2):30–32, July 1981.

Schorah. *Lancet*, p. 403, Feb. 24, 1979.

Science. Aging Research (1): Cellular Theories of Senescence 186(4169):1105–07, 1974.

Sebrell, W.H. Malnutrition. *Preventive Medicine and pH*, New York: Appleton-Century-Crofts, 1973.

Svojtkova, E.J. et al. Aging of Connective Tissue. The Effect of Diet and X-Irradiation. *Exp. Gerontol.* 7:157–67, 1972.

Tappel, A.L. Will Antioxidant Nutrients Slow the Aging Process? *Geriatrics*, 23(97), 1968.

Williams, R.J. *Nutrition Against Disease*. New York: Pitman, 1971.

Winick, M. (Ed.) *Nutrition and Aging*. New York: John Wiley and Sons, 1976.

Lesson 10

BLOOD SUGAR LEVELS
AND NUTRITION

LESSON 10—BLOOD SUGAR LEVELS AND NUTRITION

NEW DIETS FOR BLOOD SUGAR DISEASES

ARE YOU one of the estimated 50 to 150 million Americans who have hypoglycemia or diabetes? Some of these people have mild diseases, but some suffer tremendously from accidents, family break-ups, blindness, gangrenous limbs, suicides and death.

Diabetes is the third ranking killer disease in this country, right after heart disease and cancer. The major cause of both low and high blood sugar is eating refined sugar.

Here's what Cheraskin (1968) says about sugar:

The sugar-laden American diet has led to a national epidemic of hypoglycemia, an ailment characterized by irrational behavior, emotional instability, distorted judgment, and nasty personality defects.

Airola says:

White sugar and white flour are more devastating to a person's health on an individual level and to the physical, mental and social health of the whole human society than any other single factor.

Low and high blood sugar should be discussed one after the other, because that's the way they often happen—one after the other. They are not opposite diseases. Low blood sugar (hypoglycemia) is usually a forerunner of high blood sugar (diabetes), and low blood sugar will often turn into high blood sugar if it isn't treated. The only treatment is diet.

The diet should include complex carbohydrates instead of refined sugars. Almost everyone thinks all sugars are the same but they're not. Glucose is the main sugar in our blood, brain and other tissues, but we never eat pure glucose; our bodies split almost anything we eat into simple sugars (Hoffer and Walker, 1978). Sucrose is white table sugar; it has no vitamins, minerals or fats to slow down digestion and to furnish nutrients to assimilate the sugar. It has been described as poison in the amounts that Americans eat, about 128 pounds per person per year. The only safe way to eat sugar is when it is combined with nutrients in food as glucose is, and eaten as complex carbohydrates.

Eating refined sugar (sucrose) causes addiction as severe as heroin addiction. The only difference between heroin and sugar addiction is that sugar is taken orally and heroin is injected. Sugar is easy to get and it is socially acceptable. People who withdraw from sugar have withdrawal symptoms just as severe as withdrawal from drugs. They shouldn't stop eating sugar quickly; they may have severe depression or anxiety.

Eating too much sugar causes many other diseases in addition to low blood sugar and diabetes. It increases dental caries and periodontal disease, it partly causes inability to digest food and it causes seborrheic dermatitis, a skin disease.

THE PHYSIOLOGY OF BLOOD SUGAR

Let's review what goes on in the body to cause swings of blood sugar, either too high or too low or both.

When we eat, we start digesting starch in the mouth in an alkaline medium. If we chew bread or other starchy foods a long time, they will taste sweet because they are being turned into sugar to furnish energy for our brains and other cells.

We swallow that food, and digestion of starch continues in the stomach for a short time. As soon as we have eaten enough food that contains protein, hydrochloric acid (HCl) is secreted by the stomach walls to help digest the protein. Starch digestion stops because the stomach contents are too acid to digest the starch.

The total contents of the stomach, with its partially digested carbohydrate and protein, goes on into the small intestine. There, the digestion of protein, carbohydrate and fat is completed, and the amino acids from protein and the simple sugars from carbohydrate go through the walls of the intestine into the bloodstream. All the blood vessels of the small intestine carry the protein, carbohydrate and 10 percent of the fat into the liver. The other 90 percent of the fat goes into lymph vessels, and it bypasses the liver on the first circuit of the body. Later, the fat joins the blood circulation and goes through the liver.

If the liver is healthy, it makes enzymes, hormones and many other substances from the amino acids, sugars and fatty acids in our food. But most of the carbohydrate, which is now glucose (a simple sugar), is either stored in the liver as glycogen (starch) or released to the blood if the person needs sugar immediately for energy.

The Liver

If the liver is healthy, it can store the glucose and release it little by little into the blood as our blood sugar gets low after a meal. This storage and slow release is the ideal way for the liver to keep the blood sugar at the right level—not too high and not too low.

Thus, if the liver works well, the nervous system (the brain, spinal cord and other nerves) will get the food they need a little at a time, so they will not easily become exhausted. We will not suffer from "nerves" (Ballentine, 1978).

Although a high-protein diet was formerly suggested for blood sugar problems, it is no longer used. Large amounts of protein put a strain on the liver and the ailment becomes worse. If we eat white sugar, it is rapidly absorbed from the intestine and sent to the liver in amounts too large for the liver to store. But if we eat starch, a complex carbohydrate, it is broken down slowly and does not overload the liver. Thus, with the combination of starchy foods such as whole grains, legumes and potatoes, plus a little fat such as butter, nuts and seeds, the sugar gets to the blood slowly, and wide fluctuations of blood sugar don't occur (Ballentine, 1978).

But if the liver is not healthy, the situation is far from ideal, and the liver can't turn the load of sugar into glycogen and store it. It has to release it into the blood. The sugar goes directly into the heart, which sends it in the blood all over the body. As it goes through the pancreas, insulin pours out. Insulin's job is to take sugar out of the blood so we won't have diabetes, but there is so much sugar in the blood that too much insulin pours out and takes too much sugar out of the blood. This keeps us from having diabetes, but it makes us have hypoglycemia.

If the blood sugar level drops too low, we may become unconscious or even die. Insulin does not think, and it does not know when to stop working. So nature gave us other hormones to come in and block the insulin. These hormones release sugar from the liver to build up the sugar level again. Hopefully, the level is balanced, and everything settles down nicely until the next meal and the whole thing starts over.

The Adrenal Glands

The adrenal glands play a key role in the control of blood sugar. The inside section of the gland, called the medulla, prepares us to handle stress. At a signal from the pituitary gland, it pours out adrenaline, which routes blood away from the organs whose work can wait (such as the digestive tract and kidneys) in order to supply more blood to the heart and lungs, because those organs can't wait for the nutrients they need. If our hearts don't beat and our lungs don't breathe, we may die suddenly. If we are severely stressed physically, mentally or emotionally, we need energy for our adrenal glands so we can fight or run away from the stressful situation.

The outside section of the gland, called the cortex, affects almost every system of the body. The major hormone is cortisol (similar to cortisone), which influences the blood sugar level and many other systems. If our adrenals don't secrete enough cortisol, our blood sugar and blood pressure are low, and we're mentally tired—we can't concentrate. We don't produce enough red blood cells, and we may be anemic. Allergies get worse. We can't respond to stress. Our adrenals can't make the cortisol if we didn't eat the nutrients needed to make it.

Healthy adrenals, then, make cortisol, which raises blood sugar so we can be mentally alert, respond to stress and solve other health problems.

The first symptoms of low blood sugar usually pertain to the brain—depression, headache, irritability, and inability to concentrate. Our brains need glucose. People usually react by eating a doughnut or drinking a soft drink. Both bring up the blood sugar quickly, but the sugar calls out insulin, which lowers the blood sugar again. Eventually the adrenals wither and can't make cortisol; we're on the miserable merry-go-round called hypoglycemia.

What causes the problem is a fast rise in blood sugar, because that always means a fast drop, maybe to a new low. A fast rise is most often caused by eating refined carbohydrates—white sugar and/or white flour, fruit juice and bottled or canned drinks.

The recommended diet is a high complex carbohydrate diet—whole grains, legumes (beans, peas and peanuts), vegetables and whole fruits, plus one or two eggs a day, fish, natural cheese, nuts, seeds and a small amount of red meat and butter (Goldwag, 1981).

Blood Sugar Regulation

Another gland that helps regulate blood sugar is the pituitary. It must be well nourished to make enough energy to activate its enzymes and hormones. One of the pituitary hormones raises blood sugar; another hormone in the adrenal glands breaks down stored sugar so it can be sent to the blood when needed. Other hormones help to make use of all carbohydrates, and the pancreas makes insulin so all those other hormones won't lead to an overload of blood sugar and cause diabetes (Williams and Kalita, 1977).

HYPOGLYCEMIA

The question is often asked, "Why has hypoglycemia been such a problem in recent years?" Here are some of the answers.

1. People have substituted "convenience foods" (which are deficient in vitamins, minerals, amino acids and essential fatty acids) for natural foods.

2. Farm soils have been depleted of their essential minerals, so even fresh fruits and vegetables don't have the quality they should.

3. Public water supplies are treated with alum, iron compounds, chlorine, ammonia, phosphates and fluorine. With all those additives, the body can't absorb added minerals, and it even excretes too much of the ones it gets.

4. The public consumes diuretic beverages—coffee, tea, cola—that cause loss of precious minerals.

5. Good-quality protein has declined—cheaper substitutes have been used, such as luncheon meats and hot dogs.

6. Dairy products have been changed so they'll be cheaper; for example, yogurt has increased levels of galactose, a kind of sugar that can start or aggravate hypoglycemia, as can excessive fructose (Miller, *JAN*, 1974).

7. Fructose is being used more and more in manufactured products.

Linus Pauling (1986) tells us why we should not eat fructose. Humans have been used to eating about 300 grams of glucose a day from starch for millions of years. They used to eat only about 8 grams of fructose from fruit and honey. When ordinary sugar (sucrose—table sugar, from sugarcane and sugar beets) became easy to get, humans started eating about 75 grams per day of fructose, which makes up half the content of sucrose. The human body can't take on a tenfold increase without having problems.

There's a great deal of misinformation about fructose that should be publicized. People would be glad to change to other sweeteners, especially fresh fruits, if they knew the disadvantages of fructose.

Early Treatments

Some physicians still have not accepted hypoglycemia as an illness. They call it a fad disease or they say there is no such thing or "I don't believe in it" (Vance, 1975).

You will probably tell your physician about your symptoms, and he may say you have emotional problems or a psychosomatic illness or nerves! But you are physically ill, with a disease that reacts on both body and mind.

"The medical mismanagement of the hypoglycemia syndrome is shocking to contemplate," said Vance (1975). There are many treatments used (incorrectly), such as sedatives, tranquilizers, stimulants, antidepressants, antacids, hours on the analytical couch, electroconvulsive treatments and others, ad nauseam. The cost of all this in money is staggering, but the tragedy is in the human misery and agony it causes.

One of the early treatments was especially drastic. When hypoglycemia was first discovered, it was thought to be caused only by tumors in the pancreas (which caused excess insulin to be secreted), because this condition was found in a few early cases. Later, when researchers realized that the finding was rare, they decided that low blood sugar must be caused by the pancreas being larger than usual, so the favorite method of treatment was to cut away part of the organ. In fact, early reports tell of one patient who had 65 percent of his pancreas cut away (Lyle, 1981).

Hypoglycemia plays a role in juvenile delinquency, anxiety neurosis, divorce, migraine, premenstrual syndrome, school dropouts, brain dysfunction, hyperactivity, suicide, stomach ulcers, narcolepsy (an uncontrollable desire to sleep), chronic insomnia, menopause, alcoholism, epilepsy, chronic fatigue, drug addiction, antisocial behavior, acute heart attacks and strokes (Vance, 1975).

If you have low blood sugar and don't know it, you may feel like getting a divorce, you may lose your job or you may fail a course in school.

If you know you have low blood sugar, you'll eat better and these problems won't bother you. Many people with hypoglycemia go from doctor to doctor and some are told to see a psychiatrist. Hypoglycemics need good food and food supplements.

Nutritional Causes of Hypoglycemia

The basic cause of hypoglycemia is poor diet. When every cell in the body does not get the nutrition it needs, we have problems.

1. We use up our carbohydrates (glucose) too fast by exercising strenuously. (Lack of nutrients needed for exercise.)
2. Nursing a baby causes the mother to use glucose fast. (Lack of nutrients needed for the stress of milk production.)
3. The pancreas may not make enough digestive enzymes to digest the food. (Lack of nutrients to make enzymes out of.)
4. The liver may not be healthy enough to store the glycogen. (Lack of nutrients to make healthy liver cells.)
5. The adrenal glands may not work well enough to raise the blood sugar when it gets too low. (Lack of nutrients needed to make healthy adrenal glands.)
6. There may be a tumor in the pancreas which keeps it from functioning. This is rare (Ibarra, 1972). (Lack of nutrients to make a healthy immune system to prevent cancer.)

White Sugar and White Flour

We've mentioned often not to eat refined white sugar and flour. Here are some good reasons:

1. They cause nutritional deficiencies.
2. We can handle best only whole, natural foods. If foods don't contain vitamins and minerals, the body uses stored nutrients to digest food that doesn't even provide nutrients for replacement of those used—a net loss.
3. Without enough nutrients, the glands don't work well. They become damaged, and damaged glands malfunction. Hypoglycemia is a sure sign that some glands are malfunctioning, especially the pancreas, the liver and the adrenals.
4. Refined sugars and starches are absorbed into the bloodstream quickly and call out too much insulin, which brings the blood sugar down. The level drops too fast and it goes too low.

Here's what happens next (Airola, 1977):

1. Heart and muscle action are weakened.
2. Brain and nerve cells don't work well.
3. Energy and endurance are lowered.
4. Emotional control and stability are lost.

All those reactions make the hypoglycemic crave a quick pickup—sugar, coffee, cola, alcohol or a cigarette. All these raise blood sugar levels quickly, but they call out insulin, which lowers the levels quickly.

What the body needs is whole complex carbohydrates (whole grains, vegetables and whole fruits), which are digested slowly and are slowly changed to sugar a little at a time.

The body handles these small amounts of sugar well. But when a load of refined carbohydrates (white sugar and white flour) is dumped into the system, symptoms of low blood sugar appear.

Symptoms of Hypoglycemia

It is estimated that there are about 100 symptoms of hypoglycemia. Some of them are (Vance, 1975):

Personality changes
Inward and outward trembling

Excessive perspiration
Hunger
Apprehension
Depression or sadness
Twitching muscles
Dribbling bladder
Convulsions
Unconsciousness
Extra heartbeats
Skipped heartbeats
Increased blood pressure
Excessive activity
Difficulty in concentration
Difficulty in speaking
Fainting
Emotional disturbances
Chilliness
Mental cloudiness
Prickly feeling on the skin
Headache
Visual disturbances
Awkward movements
Dizziness
Double vision
Blank expressions
Fast heartbeat
Throbbing pulse
Dilated pupils
Staring
Occasional muscle spasms
Loss of voice
Restlessness

A low blood sugar attack is often accompanied by sweating and a rapid heartbeat. Fainting and many other symptoms are caused by a lack of energy in the nerve cells (Horrobin, 1973). Most hypoglycemics don't have all of these symptoms, but if you have even one of them, you may have hypoglycemia. Many people have one or more of these symptoms. They can change their diets immediately without tests to verify the diagnosis, because the natural food diet will provide all nutrients needed for a healthy body, and the body heals itself. There will be no side effects or adverse reactions if you work into the program gradually (see Lesson 1). This program furnishes all nutrients in food, plus all known nutrients in supplement form.

If anyone wishes to take a test to find out his blood sugar curve, here's the way it is now being given by many physicians.

Hypoglycemia Tests

Although the old-fashioned, six-hour glucose tolerance test (GTT) has been used for years, it is becoming less and less popular with physicians be-cause of the side effects many people have. After fasting overnight, the usual test meal is a 75-gram load of liquid sugar. The problems patients have with this amount of sugar are potentially dangerous: headache, dizziness, fainting, weakness, nausea and vomiting. Some people even go into a coma. Often the test has to be stopped before it is finished.

Other investigators say that this GTT is not physiological, because free glucose is not found in the usual diet, and eating 50 to 100 grams of carbohydrates without protein or fat is rare in normal life.

Dr. Michael Walczak (1979) suggests a normal intake of food before the test, such as a meal of ham and eggs, whole-grain pancakes and syrup or bread and butter. He takes a history of how the patient feels at each hour after eating the suggested meal. The glucose values by themselves do not diagnose hypoglycemia.

Walczak reported that at a clinical refresher course he attended, the consensus was that "the oral GTT as it is now used is obsolete. But it will probably take 15 years to bury it!"

Reactions to the Glucose Test. Two of my friends who were given the liquid glucose say, "I will never take that test again." One had a two-hour test after the glucose. Her physician said that it is important to know if a person has diabetes, and a two-hour test shows that. This friend vomited up the glucose, but submitted to the test again on the advice of her physician.

The other friend said she took the glucose load followed by a blood sugar reading every hour for six hours. Her blood sugar went so low that she couldn't walk to the bathroom alone. She had a nurse on each side, practically carrying her. She could hardly sit up on the commode to urinate because of severe muscle spasms. She asked the nurse if anyone ever passed out, because she felt as if she would. The nurse said, "Yes, every once in a while. That's why we have this oxygen tent right here." My friend says, "The GTT is bad, very bad."

Incidentally, this same friend is now on the low animal-protein, high-carbohydrate diet, and says, "You really did me a favor when you told me about that diet. It has really helped me. You can't go wrong if you follow it, but you have to stick to it and do what it says. However, it is so easy to follow that now I don't even have to think about it. I have plenty of energy. I wake up in the morning ready to go, and I go to sleep at night very easily and sleep soundly."

Review of the Old Six-Hour Glucose Tolerance Test. The International Science Foundation furnished a reprint on hypoglycemia in which a physician (unnamed) described the GTT using 50 to 100 grams of liquid sugar. Although many physicians have quit using it, some still do. Here it is, for the record.

The patient comes to the laboratory for the test in the morning after having fasted for 12 hours. A sample of blood is taken, usually from a vein in the arm. This blood is checked to see what the "fasting blood sugar level" is. The body tries to maintain a good level, even if a person hasn't eaten recently. No two people are alike, so there's no level that's "normal" for everyone. We'll talk about an "average" level, around 90.

Next, the physician gives a specific amount of sugar. A half hour or an hour later, another blood sample is taken. The blood sugar will be about 140. These numbers mean the milligrams of sugar in every 100 milliliters of blood (about ⅜ cup). That is called 140 mg percent.

At the second hour, the level should be 120. At the third hour, the level of sugar should be down to its lowest point, about 85. (The body is now sending hormones to change glycogen to glucose to bring it up again.)

At the fourth hour, the level is around 95, and at the fifth and sixth hours, about 90, which is the fasting level we started with. If all these figures are plotted on a graph, a curve is shown. To "see" this curve, let's list the figures this way:

Fasting	90
First hour	140
Second hour	120
Third hour	85
Fourth hour	95
Fifth hour	90
Sixth hour	90

Hypoglycemics and diabetics have abnormal curves. Some are very erratic, as in "relative hypoglycemia," and the figures look like this:

Fasting	110 to 120
First hour	300
Second hour	330
Third hour	270
Fourth hour	250
Fifth hour	60 to 65
Sixth hour	100

At first, this curve looks like diabetes, because it goes so high, but it goes dangerously low in the fifth hour. The early curve is found in more than half of the confirmed diabetics, but the fifth-hour figure confirms hypoglycemia. This shows the importance of using a six-hour GTT rather than a three-hour test.

A flat curve, often found, is one in which the blood sugar level is rather constant; it doesn't vary more than 5 to 10 mg percent. The "curve" looks more like a straight line. The curves change in any patient.

You can test yourself well enough to decide if you have hypoglycemia. The following little list of symptoms will most likely be all the test you need.

1. My mind sometimes goes blank.
2. I lose my temper easily.
3. I am very impatient.
4. Certain things irritate me very much.
5. I am depressed and blue.
6. I feel very restless.
7. I need the stimulation of alcohol, coffee, cigarettes or drugs.
8. Occasionally I am ravenously hungry.
9. I drink cola and other soft drinks daily.
10. My mouth is very dry.

Many symptoms of hypoglycemia are the same as nervous symptoms: anxiety, tension, depression, fatigue and "jitters." All of these are usually felt after eating junk food, drinking too much coffee or missing a meal (Reed, 1977).

Hypoglycemia and Alcoholism

It is claimed that more than 95 percent of alcoholics have low blood sugar. It is safe to say that all alcoholics are malnourished; they lack proteins and carbohydrates for energy, and other nutrients such as vitamins and minerals. They need much more of these protective foods than nonalcoholics. They also lack healthy cells in their digestive tracts to digest and absorb the small amount of good food they get. The digestive system is damaged by alcohol; therefore, many nutrients cannot be absorbed, especially folic acid (a B vitamin) and thiamine (B1), B6 and B12. Certain psychotic states develop when those nutrients are missing, along with deficiencies of ascorbic acid, magnesium, zinc and protein. Delirium tremens is probably caused by deficiencies of magnesium during withdrawal from alcohol.

Colby-Morley (1982) lists the symptoms of alcoholism that were found with a battery of tests on 300 consecutive private patients in one clinic. The symptoms are the same as the symptoms of low blood sugar; apathy, irritability, restlessness, fatigue, anxiety, being negative about everything, confusion, depression, stupor, sluggish thinking, uncontrolled emotional outburst and coma.

Fredericks says that, since the brain and nervous system are very sensitive to changes in blood sugar, alcoholism may be a problem even if no physical symptoms are evident. Also, Roger J. Williams (1981) says that malnutrition is possibly a forerunner of alcoholism and that true alcoholism doesn't appear until the brain cells are severely deprived of food. He also says, "No one who follows good nutritional practices will ever become an alcoholic."

The major reason alcoholics become addicted is that they substitute beer, wine and/or whiskey for food. Most of them can be "cured" of alcoholism by eating the hypoglycemia diet. Rather than substituting candy and other sweets to phase out alcohol, which is common practice, the preferred snacks would be nuts, seeds, cheese and other natural foods. Many alcoholics become "dry," but on the sweet snacks, they are unhappy, depressed and even neurotic. These feelings lead again to drink.

The Wernicke-Korsakoff syndrome is a common nerve disorder associated with nutritional deficiencies in alcoholics. The acute stage of the syndrome responds to intravenous thiamine (B1). If the disease isn't recognized in early stages, the patient may develop an irreversible, chronic brain problem. He may lose his memory and not be able to function independently.

Dr. Williams has shown that alcoholics on the hypoglycemic diet may stop drinking or may take one drink and then stop. Dr. Williams says, "The elimination of alcoholic craving can be assured, provided the recommendations which we have made are followed" (Williams, 1981).

One nutrient especially needed by alcoholics is L-glutamine. It is a brain food and an amino acid. It goes through the blood-brain barrier, and when it gets into the brain, it is changed into glutamic acid.

Colby-Morley (1982) treated a group of physicians who had been referred by their colleagues because they drank too much. Her program corresponds to the complete diet in Lesson 1, plus the specific nutrients needed for hypoglycemics at the end of this lesson. After a year, the physicians were sober and reported unusual ability to concentrate, remember names, relax and quit smoking. They had feelings of well-being they had not known for years.

Hypoglycemia and Crime

Alexander G. Schauss, when director of the County Probation Department in Pierce County, Washington, used nutritional education and counseling in working with probationers. He set up a study (Schauss, 1978) using two experimental groups and two control groups. Each probationer had a sentence of from six to 12 months. Participants filled out a questionnaire to check on their physical health and behavior. The questionnaire also revealed the possibility of hypoglycemia, and some persons

were given GTTs. They also attended six classes in nutrition and then had nutrition counseling sessions with their probation officers.

There was a highly significant decrease in arrest rates in the nutrition education group. There was no significant change in the control group using the usual casework. Those probationers were on their regular diet and did not attend the nutrition classes.

The entire program was set up to educate probationers to balance their blood sugar levels. In one study of prison inmates, the estimated intake of sugar was several hundred pounds a year. Schauss said, "One of the easiest measures for preventing crime would be to eliminate all non-essential sources of sugar in the diet."

Hypoglycemia as a cause of crime has been studied in Cuyahoga Falls, Ohio. Barbara Reed (now Barbara Stitt), former chief probation officer in the municipal court, has proved that low blood sugar is the cause of much crime in this country today.

The reason she thought that criminals might be hypoglycemic, and that the disease is the cause of their criminal behavior, is that she herself had hypoglycemia. She found that when she ate a nutritious diet, eliminating junk foods, her health improved, and she no longer had symptoms of the disease. Later, after she got well, she realized that many of the probationers under her jurisdiction had the same symptoms she had when she was ill.

With the cooperation of an interested judge, she gave 106 persons a two-page written test that lists a total of 89 symptoms of low blood sugar. Of the 106 persons, 82 percent checked 15 or more symptoms, and 33 percent checked more than 25 symptoms. Some had as many as 50 to 70 symptoms. Mrs. Reed worked with each probationer to determine a better diet, free from alcohol, drugs, sweets, coffee, tobacco and soft drinks. Seven persons were referred to a clinic for testing for glucose tolerance-blood sugar levels.

All seven had previously been committed to mental hospitals several times, spanning periods of four to 10 years. Six of these people became healthy, productive citizens. (One improved dramatically, but returned to alcohol after his son committed suicide.)

Dozens of others, by simply following Mrs. Reed's suggestions, have become healthy and in control of their lives. None of the persons who cooperated with the program had further problems with the court. Entire families have been helped. Their children's schoolwork improved; husbands, parents, wives and other relatives have called the office to say how much happier they are.

Mrs. Reed observed, "Never before has the court had such a tool for working with the many ill people who find themselves in court. We wonder what the results would be if this method of treatment could also be applied to those sentenced to jail" (Reed, 1977).

Mrs. Reed reported on the diet for probationers to the Senate Select Committee on Nutrition and Human Needs on June 22, 1977. Her work was written up on Page 1 of the *Wall Street Journal* that month. Since then, she has traveled over the United States speaking before police and law enforcement agencies about the phenomenal success of this diet with probationers. It would undoubtedly be just as successful with people who have problems that may lead to criminal acts and with those who have had to go to jail.

Barbara Reed Stitt's work was also written up in *Prevention*. Here is a letter to the editor published a few months later. (Reprinted by permission of *Prevention*, September 1978):

I enjoyed your May article on probation officer Barbara Reed, "The Court Where Junk Food Goes on Trial." I happen to be one of the junk food addicts she helped.

Barbara Reed not only saved my life, but she had faith in my worth as a human being while others were skeptical. She came to my aid more than once, going above and beyond the call of duty. She used her own money to buy me and my children the vitamins we so badly needed, gave us her own food blender, and loaned us other materials needed for our no-sugar diet.

I asked her once what possible reward she could receive from helping the poor and public offenders. She told me that she expected no reward. My child suffered from hypoglycemia. Symptoms included lack of attention, forgetfulness, sleeplessness, and at times very bad behavior problems along with speech problems. He had seen many different doctors and had been refused entry into first grade. Mrs. Reed suggested a no-sugar, no-preservative, no-artificial-anything diet. My son's speech improved, and his other symptoms vanished. He also takes vitamin B complex daily. Soon he will be entering the second grade. I don't like to think of the terrible future he would have been facing if it were not for Barbara Reed.

When something as simple as diet can be so helpful to these people, why can't it be part of the program in every law enforcement agency in the land?

When deprived of blood sugar, the brain has no alternate food supply, and when brain metabolism slows down, the brain doesn't work well. Ninety percent of convicted murderers are diagnosed as paranoid schizophrenics suffering from low blood sugar or some vitamin deficiency.

Prisoners are restless when given coffee, white sugar and alcohol. A good diet reduces the number of discipline cases, and prisoners improve in academic and vocational classes.

Hypoglycemia and Mental Problems

Our brains feed on glucose, so our brains and nerves usually feel the effects of low blood sugar first. We can't reason well, we get sleepy, our hands and feet may tingle and get numb, we may tremble or feel butterflies in the stomach.

All these reactions are caused by nerve and brain deficiencies. When we don't have enough sugar in the blood, our nerves can't send messages to our brains because it takes energy for an impulse to move along the nerves. Without glucose, we don't have energy.

All parts of the brain need glucose to make the brain cells work. The thinking cells, the emotional center and the social center all work well with the right amount of glucose, but if there isn't enough, we can be stupid, emotionally drained and antisocial. We don't need tranquilizers or other medication, we need excellent nutrients to help make hormones to activate cells that control the levels of sugar in the blood.

Women may not realize that low blood sugar may cause many of their premenstrual tensions, including nervousness and hysteria. Children also have psychiatric symptoms, learning problems and sometimes psychotic and neurotic reactions when their blood sugar is low.

A mental problem common in hypoglycemia is depression, which is sadness combined with hopelessness. The answer is to treat patients for hypoglycemia, then give massive doses of vitamins, especially B complex and C. Probably hypoglycemia is one of the most overlooked causes of depression (Ross, 1975).

With a hypoglycemic, the physician may get a negative test and then diagnose psychiatric problems, which is certainly no help to the patient (Vance, 1975). If you think your mental symptoms are unusual, you may not know that patients have been diagnosed as schizophrenics, manic depressives and psychopaths, yet when their blood sugar was corrected, they got over their symptoms (Salzer, 1966). Psychiatrists usually don't recognize low blood sugar as causing psychiatric problems (Paterson, 1982), and, sad to say, some other branches of the medical profession have come to accept their judgment.

Paterson tested two groups of patients who came to him for help with mental or emotional problems.

The first group had symptoms of alcoholism, depression and schizophrenia. They were tested for low blood sugar because their symptoms seemed to be caused by changes in their eating habits. The second group were students and some staff members of a school. For breakfast, these people usually had coffee and a cigarette, and they chose other poor foods during the day. Eighty-one percent of both groups showed hypoglycemia on tests.

In both groups, symptoms were severe when insulin was excessively high. We've said that when blood sugar is low, it is because a load of sugar has been dumped into the blood, and it has caused the pancreas to overreact and secret excess insulin, which then takes sugar out of the blood.

Paterson's conclusion is that large-scale studies should be done in psychiatric institutions to determine blood sugar levels so proper treatment can be used. That treatment is good nutritious food. If it is not given, the patient may degenerate to either more psychiatric problems or diabetes or both.

If psychiatric patients are put in hospitals or other institutions and someone finds that they have low blood sugar, the usual advice given by physicians is to add sugar to the diet to bring up the blood sugar, which is the opposite of what is needed: a diet containing moderate protein, low fat and high complex carbohydrate. Patients should eliminate caffeine. They would spend less time in hospitals, where their diseases are made worse by the usual hospital diet that often allows lots of coffee, cigarettes and sweets between meals.

DIABETES

As we've said, hypoglycemia often turns into diabetes if it isn't treated. The first symptom of diabetes may be low blood sugar right after meals because so much insulin is released that it takes too much sugar out of the blood.

In juvenile diabetes, as more and more episodes of hypoglycemia occur, the cells that produce insulin are so exhausted that they can't make any more, and the low blood sugar becomes high blood sugar because there's no insulin to take the sugar out of the blood. This was formerly thought to be inherited, but it is now realized that nutritional deficiencies are the cause of juvenile diabetes.

In maturity-onset diabetes, the most common kind, there is usually plenty of insulin, but it just can't transport sugar to the cells. To get it there, we need vitamins and minerals in maximum amounts for all cells to function (Bland, 1981). The cells are surrounded by sugar, but they are literally starving for it because the nutrients needed to put it in the cells are not available. This condition causes the cells to break down the protein and fat they're made of to use for energy. It also causes water to be removed from the cells, taking minerals with it. The cells dry out, the kidneys and their tissues are overworked because they have to excrete all the wastes, and diabetes patients develop kidney or nerve damage (Bland, 1981).

Prevalence of Diabetes

The prevalence of diabetes in Western countries is increasing rapidly. In the United States, it is going up faster than the total population. The United States is one of the leaders in deaths from diabetes among the developed countries. During the last few years, it has become the third killer disease (right after heart disease with 3,000 deaths a day, and cancer with 1,100). There are about 1,000 deaths every day from diabetes and its complications (Cohen, 1975). If it continues to increase the way it is now, one in five people will eventually have the disease (Bland, 1981).

The complications of diabetes cut our life expectancy by as much as one-third. For every 10 years we live, we double our chances of having diabetes. Thus, if we are 40 years old this year, we'll be twice as likely to have diabetes 10 years from now just by living until we're 50 (Bland, 1981).

Complications of Diabetes

The most common complications of the disease are the following:

1. Fat is deposited in the arteries, causing poor circulation, which leads to heart attacks. Clots in the major arteries, especially in the legs, lead to gangrene in the feet and many patients must have their feet amputated.
2. Damage to the kidney ends in kidney failure. There is a seven times greater chance of kidney disease in diabetics than in nondiabetics.
3. Damage to the retina leads to blindness. This is the major cause of blindness in the developed countries. It amounts to 20 percent of all cases. It is really the result of deposits of fat in capillaries of the retina. This disease is 25 times more common in diabetics than in nondiabetics (Bland, 1981).
4. Infections are common, especially in the skin and urinary tract.
5. Ketosis and diabetic coma are common. Ketosis is a condition in which fats rather than carbohydrates are used for energy. When cells use fats, ketone bodies are formed. These make the blood acid and poison the brain; the patient may become comatose.
6. Physical and mental breakdown may occur.

Diabetics develop certain conditions.

1. High levels of ketone bodies make the blood too acid.
2. High levels of blood sugar make sugar appear in the urine.
3. Massive fluid loss causes severe dehydration of the patient.
4. The patient complains of passing large amounts of urine because there must be a lot of water to carry the excess sugar away. Thus the patient is always thirsty.
5. The patient eats excessively to furnish more calories and glucose (Horrobin, 1973).

In early diabetes, the patient will probably not have all these symptoms, but the diet should be changed immediately to the natural food diet.

The Role of Insulin in Diabetes

It is well known that insulin plays a major role in diabetes. When insulin was discovered, it was thought that the pancreas could not make enough insulin to take sugar out of the blood and put it into the cells. Now it is thought that the defect is not in the ability of the pancreas to manufacture insulin, but in the mechanism of getting insulin into the cells. Also, we need to know why so much sugar is put into the blood. Recent research shows that the amount of sugar in the blood depends on the *kind* of carbohydrate that we eat (Reiser, 1983). We should eat starch (complex carbohydrate such as whole grains, potatoes and sweet potatoes) rather than refined sugars such as sucrose (white table sugar) or fructose (fruit sugar and honey).

A special hormone (GIP—gastric inhibitory peptide) causes the pancreas to secrete more insulin when we eat a lot of carbohydrates at a meal (Reiser, 1983). The amount of insulin was found to be much greater if the carbohydrate was sucrose or fructose than if it was wheat starch. Both those simple sugars are absorbed faster and higher up in the intestines than starch is, which might explain why so much insulin is secreted so fast. More than twice as much of the insulin was secreted when sucrose rather than glucose was eaten.

The investigator notes: (1) sucrose is absorbed much faster than sugar made from starch; and (2) the more sucrose we eat, the faster it is digested and absorbed through the small intestine, probably because of the hormone GIP. People who constantly eat sucrose might eventually not be able to manufacture enough insulin to take sugar out of the blood. Thus they might become diabetic.

The blood sugar of laboratory rats given high sucrose or fructose meals rose about twice as fast as the levels in rats given starch meals. Although we need plentiful amounts of glucose to feed our brains, humans do not eat pure glucose. They eat starch that the body breaks down to glucose.

Other studies show that when human volunteers were fed drinks or meals containing 50 grams of carbohydrate, insulin responses were 35 to 65 percent lower when starch was the carbohydrate source than when either glucose or sucrose was given. The insulin in blood was about 20 percent higher after the sucrose drink than after the glucose drink.

I see many diabetics in my counseling, and most of them say that diabetes runs in their family. Recently I counseled a youthful 50-year-old diabetic patient. He was lean, wiry, an athlete, eager to change his diet any way that would keep him from having the usual complications of the disease, and especially to keep him from having to take insulin. The first thing he told me was that his mother is diabetic, "if that means anything." I realized that he wasn't convinced he had it because she did. He also said that he had recently lost 30 pounds, which left him at what seemed to be his perfect weight. He admitted, however, that when he was a teenager he "ate like an idiot," just as too many teenagers do—sweets, junk-food fats, too much beef and beer, doughnuts and cigarettes. He had taken himself off all that and even off the rich sauces so commonly served at every meal. He was determined to stay off insulin and not have his disease get worse. His mother had progressed from too much sucrose to high dosages of insulin and a miserable life marked by threats of blindness, amputations and heart attacks, the three most common complications of our third killer disease.

As he left my office, I watched him walk to his car. His step was light, his waistline was slim, his tummy was flat and I knew whatever booze or sweets he had to give up, he would give them up gladly to live the life he appreciated. He was on his way to the airport to fly to Europe. He had realized he had to go only the day before. But there was no stress because of the short notice. I know that he will handle his illness the way he handles the rest of his life—without adverse reactions!

As I watched him, I thought of the teenagers who, right now, are eating themselves into diabetes. Their families may understand the importance of no junk food, but the teenagers usually won't listen. They believe they can withstand all the insults to their bodies of white sugar, white flour and other junk foods. The sad thing is that when the diagnosis of diabetes comes, they can't turn back the clock. However, they can live normal lives on this food program if they will eat correctly. Even if everybody in their family has diabetes, if they haven't already developed it, they should never hear the dreaded diagnosis—diabetes.

Diabetes and Obesity

Diabetes and obesity have a very close relationship to each other. An American male who has diabetes and is obese has a greater risk of dying than one who is not obese. For example, a diabetic who is 20 percent above average weight has a 350 percent greater mortality risk (Cheraskin, 1968). Diabetes is the disease with the highest correlation with obesity. When patients reduce their weight, both their blood sugar and insulin often return to normal.

It has been noted that diabetes is closely associated with chronic, degenerative disease, and people with such a disease are unable to use carbohydrates well because of a deficiency of B-complex vitamins and other nutrients. As we know, empty-calorie foods (refined sugars, refined starches and alcohols) have had B vitamins processed out. Such deficiencies lead to high triglycerides, gout, atherosclerosis (fatty deposits in blood vessels), obesity and diabetes.

Weiss (1976) says that he insists that all obese patients who have diabetes reduce their weight. He also tests obese patients and finds many who have diabetes but didn't know it. Therefore, he says that diabetes and obesity are two facets of the same disease. These comments do not apply to juvenile and thin diabetics.

Weiss also says that diabetics do not have a shortage of insulin as previously thought, but they produce an insulin antagonist that cancels out some of the insulin they produce. Thus it is "bound" and can't be used. But if the pancreas can produce enough insulin to make up for the bound part, the patient doesn't have symptoms of diabetes.

This explains why pathologists have not understood why obese diabetics, on autopsy, have no damage to the islets of Langerhans where insulin is produced. The other two groups, thin and juvenile diabetics, have damaged islets of Langerhans and a complete absence of insulin.

Diabetes and Cancer

Blond (1960) said he thought it would be found that cancer is a nutritional deficiency disease, and diabetes is a precancerous syndrome.

These two diseases are often found in the same person. It may be that a disorder of the liver may cause both ailments. The veins that flow out of the liver can be locked by damaged cells. As a result, the waste products that collect irritate the pancreas. It is possible that some people never develop cancer because they die of diabetes first.

One of every five cancers, in a study of 256 diabetic patients, originated in the pancreas or in the gall bladder drainage system. Ninety-eight percent of the cases occurred in organs drained by the portal vein (the vein that drains blood from the intestines into the liver) or in organs connected with it; thus liver damage can cause diabetes (Blond, 1960).

Diabetes and Birth Defects

Although most investigators agree that mothers who are diabetic and prediabetic give birth to more babies who are malformed, nothing was known of diabetic and prediabetic fathers.

After a study of 102 fathers of babies born with severe birth defects and of 128 fathers of normal infants, the investigators found that there was no significant difference in the offspring of diabetic and normal fathers.

Diabetes and Heart Disease

Diabetics suffer from coronary heart disease more often than nondiabetics. More than 80 percent of adult-onset diabetics have vascular disease, and 50 percent of the diabetics die of myocardial infarction (heart attack). Five times more diabetics have atherosclerosis than those in the average population. It is difficult if not impossible to identify genetic factors in most patients who die of cardiovascular disease or of diabetes (Drash, 1973).

Usually more men than women have cardiovascular disease (CVD), but in women with diabetes, the deaths from CVD are at least as common as in men.

Diabetes is called a double disease (Weiss, 1976), and the major cause of death in diabetes is degeneration of the blood vessels, which continues even if the blood sugar is controlled. This is another instance of how drugs can mask symptoms of disease. When diabetics take insulin, their blood sugar levels are controlled, but the killer disease of the blood vessels gets worse.

Diseases of the large blood vessels damage the heart, vessels at a distance from the heart and vessels of the brain (causing strokes). Diseases of the small blood vessels damage the retina, nerves and kidneys and cause gangrene in the feet. Small-vessel diseases also cause thickening of tissue under the skin, which leads to rapid aging.

If you are already a diabetic, you can check the condition of your feet often to see if you may be developing gangrene. Gangrene is caused by poor circulation of the blood. Watch for the following signs:

1. Weak pulses in the feet and legs.
2. Cold, dry, pale skin on feet and legs.

3. No hair growing on toes.
4. Toes that turn reddish when you're sitting or standing.

Have Drugs Helped?

"In diabetics, oral drugs cause reactions which are so frightening that the drugs should be discouraged" (Fredericks, 1974). Now the danger is recognized, and the FDA requires a warning on labels that there is an increase of heart disease as a result of their use. Many physicians still prescribe them. People who have chronic illnesses such as diabetes and take drugs such as insulin need more vitamins and minerals than the average person. Drugs can decrease the appetite, keep the vitamins and minerals that are eaten from being absorbed and knock out the particular mechanism the body must use to benefit from vitamins and minerals (Passwater, 1975).

The medical profession uses drugs and a disease-producing diet to try to combat diabetes. After 10 to 15 years of this treatment, even in the very young, blood vessel disease is so severe that "nearly 80 percent of diabetics die of some form of blood vessel disease" (Robbins, 1974).

Investigators are now realizing that these problems are caused by the diet of high protein and high animal fat, with deficiencies of nutrients. More than 15 years ago, one wrote, "There will be many more diabetics in the years ahead. The average number of diabetic patients per physician will probably double or triple in the future. If this course is continued, more than half the American population will be diabetic" (Owen, 1972).

Fifty years after insulin was introduced as a drug for diabetes, physicians admit that there are still many questions they can't answer about the treatment. Many diabetics control their blood sugar quite well, but that doesn't mean that they won't have the severe complications of the disease.

We know that to avoid diabetic complications, patients will have to live on excellent food. But some patients may prefer junk food and a machine called a fuel cell that will monitor the patient's blood sugar and inject insulin when needed. It will be implanted in the body. It will be about the year 2000 before it is known how well the fuel cell works. We can change our diets and start getting better today.

Many of the several million maturity-onset diabetics have a mild disease. But often these diseases are the ones that suddenly cause severe heart disease. The patients probably had disease of the blood vessels first. Owen says physicians should probably realize that all diabetics will have heart disease sooner than nondiabetics.

The priority in treatment might be not to worry about controlling blood sugar, but to treat the victim as a heart patient. Diabetes and atherosclerosis tend to lead to high blood pressure, and high blood pressure leads to coronary disease, stroke and congestive heart failure, all killers. In the past, investigators passively watched the killer heart diseases develop in diabetics (Owen, 1972).

"It's time for a change," says Owen. "Perhaps there is an answer to the diabetes controversy if we are ready at last to accept it." The answer, of course, is nutritious food.

Old and New Diets

It is now thought by many researchers and physicians that the diet given diabetics since the discovery of insulin was the cause of most of the tragic complications of diabetes.

The old diet recommended by physicians included as calories:

40 percent carbohydrate
40 percent fat
20 percent protein

The new diet includes, for both diabetics and hypoglycemics:

75 percent *complex* carbohydrate
(no white sugar, no white flour)
10 percent fat
15 percent protein

Complex carbohydrates are whole grains of all kinds, vegetables both steamed and raw, and whole fruits (no fruit juice). Proteins are from dairy products, poultry and fish, with very little red muscle meat. The red meat and poultry should be organically raised—no pesticides, growth hormone or antibiotics. Plant proteins are emphasized, always combined with each other or with dairy products or animal proteins. Good combinations of plant proteins are whole grains and legumes (beans, peas and peanuts), with twice as much grains as beans.

This diet helps people lose weight or maintain a low weight. This is especially important with diabetics because overweight patients need increased insulin, and that's hard on the pancreas.

This new type of diet has been used since the 1930s, when a group of physicians gave their patients 65 percent of calories as complex carbohydrates. Levels of cholesterol and triglycerides were reduced.

Many studies prove the value of this program. Nathan Pritikin (1976), who directed the Longevity Research Institute in Santa Barbara, California, used a similar formula, and diabetic patients could walk six miles a day after six months on this diet. In a study in the *American Journal of Clinical Nutrition* reported by Kiehm (1976), the diet of 75 percent of calories as carbohydrates was well tolerated by the patients. Insulin and oral drugs were both stopped in nine of the 13 patients, and cholesterol and triglycerides were significantly lower.

Of great importance was the use of natural foods. Other subjects using a formula diet (not fresh, natural carbohydrates) didn't improve. A previous study had shown that unprocessed wheat bran helped lower the cholesterol and triglyceride levels. In this study, patients who needed more than 40 units of insulin were not able to do without insulin.

But in another study, Pritikin (1976) fed a group of four diabetic men—average age 60—a diet of 80 percent complex carbohydrates. They were off insulin in six weeks. Two had been taking insulin for 10 to 15 years. One of those had been taking 80 units a day.

A total of 38 men with varying ailments was reported on. In all, blood cholesterol dropped an average of 30 percent. One triglyceride level dropped from 360 to 85 percent. After five weeks, the treadmill activity increased 800 percent.

Dr. John M. Douglass (1975), an internist with the Southern California Permanente Medical Group in Los Angeles, puts his diabetic patients on a raw food diet with emphasis on nuts and salads. Insulin for some was reduced from 60 units to 15 units per day. Others completely discontinued medication.

The Carbohydrate Question

The large amount of carbohydrates suggested for this diet is all *complex*—no white sugar and no white flour, which are empty-calorie foods.

The average American eats about 285 pounds of empty-calorie foods a year (Pritikin, 1976):

> 130 pounds sugar
> 53 pounds refined fats and oils
> 88 pounds white flour
> 14 pounds corn sugar

The amount of corn sugar is increasing rapidly. More and more manufacturers are using corn sugar in manufactured foods.

What Kind of Sugar, if Any? Almost everyone thought the sugar problem was solved when aspartame (Nutra-Sweet) was developed. But the problem may now be worse than it was before.

What does Nutra-Sweet do to us or for us? For each molecule of Nutra-Sweet we put into our mouths, we release into the blood one molecule of wood alcohol, also called methanol. During Prohibi-

tion, when the alcoholics couldn't get their usual drink, they drank wood alcohol. Some of them died and some of them went blind. In the body, wood alcohol is oxidized to formaldehyde, a known carcinogen, and it produces squamous cell carcinomas in experimental animals when they inhale it. It can cause mutations and birth defects in laboratory animals. Other symptoms include confusion, leg cramps, severe headaches and loss of vision. Reports are now in newspapers and journals that Nutra-Sweet may cause changes in brain chemicals and behavior. That should be enough to get rid of those sweeteners forever.

Table sugar is called sucrose, which is half glucose and half fructose. Glucose goes directly into the blood, then to the liver, where some of it is stored as glycogen. The rest is released to the blood, and as it goes through the pancreas, insulin is released from the pancreas and it transports glucose to the cells. Fructose (fruit sugar) goes to the liver, where some of it is changed into glucose and then sent to the cells for energy. Some of it can be changed into fats (triglycerides). So if we eat too much fructose (as when we drink a glass of fruit juice containing four to seven teaspoons of sugar), our blood fats go up. It is now known that blood fats go up more when we eat fructose than sucrose (Reiser, 1983). When we eat whole fruit, we are getting fructose, but not an excessive amount as we do in concentrated fruit juice. So whole fruits are excellent foods and don't contain excessive sugar (Bland, 1981).

How about honey? It is really not any better than sucrose. It is still almost half glucose and half fructose, like table sugar, and honey must have insulin to get it to the cells.

What else is bad about fructose? It has "extremely adverse effects" (Fredericks, 1976), such as raising the fasting blood levels of insulin, cortisone, uric acid, cholesterol and triglycerides. Also, it makes the blood platelets stick together more than usual, which causes the blood to clot. The pancreas shrinks, and the liver and adrenal glands enlarge, which shows that the sugar is a stress on the body. These conditions are found in both animals and humans.

Thus excessive fructose as well as sucrose can cause gout, heart attacks, strokes, hardening of the arteries and gastric ulcers. The best thing about honey is that people would probably not eat 130 pounds of it a year, but it's obviously easy to eat that much white sugar a year since that's the average American intake.

Fructose is used more and more in manufactured products such as soft drinks. Soft drinks manufacturers can use fructose and put on the label "no sugar." This is legal because the nutritional literature defines sugar as sucrose—table sugar. Candy and many other products sweetened with fructose are appearing on the market and are called "sugarless" (Bland, 1981).

"Hidden" sugars are one of the big problems, especially those in soft drinks, which amount to an average of 30 pounds of sugar per person per year. Sugars have many other adverse effects. In adults with psychiatric problems and in children with learning and behavior problems, sugar causes disturbances in both mind and body. No doubt everyone accepts the fact that sugar causes tooth decay, but it is also one of the main causes of periodontal disease that can cause loss of teeth in more than 80 percent of Americans over the age of 35.

Sugar also increases the need for B vitamins, and it supplies none. Sugar contains only calories—no vitamins, no minerals. We've talked about the need for chromium to stabilize blood sugar in both hypoglycemics and diabetics. When the body takes on a load of sugar (which has no chromium in it), the tissues lose stores of chromium—a double reason to not eat sugar.

Studies show that if girls and women eat less sugar, they have less premenstrual tension and similar problems. Sugar also contributes to endometriosis, cystic mastitis, breast cancer, fibroid tumors of the uterus and perhaps to cancer of the uterus.

Although sugar is bad, starch is good, so in our high-carbohydrate diet we'll eat a lot of starch. Starch is digested and assimilated slowly, and it gets to the cells slowly, so our blood sugar stays level, without swings that are too high and too low. The worse your blood sugar problems are, the better will be your reaction to the high-carbohydrate diet. We've been told for 25 years or so to eat a high-protein, low-carbohydrate diet, but now I'm saying a moderate-protein, low-fat, high-carbohydrate diet and not one grain of white sugar or white flour. Those nonfoods do not contain the vitamins and minerals needed to turn white sugar and starch into substances our bodies can use.

All our cells need blood sugar—not to much and not too little, but the brain cells react more quickly than most other cells if they don't get enough blood sugar. If the brain needs food, it signals to other tissues and blood. The signals may be headaches, depression, fatigue, shaking or dizziness. We may perspire suddenly. Investigators have fed diabetic animals high-starch or high-sugar diets, and the high-sugar diets cause weight gain and fatty deposits, both signs of diabetes. The levels of both insulin and sugar are higher on a high-sugar diet than on a high-starch diet. An abundance of research shows that people with blood sugar problems do well on a high complex carbohydrate (starch) diet (Bland, 1981).

Starch is different from sugar also, because it contains no fructose. Thus it will not cause the "extremely adverse effects" that we've mentioned.

Now that we know we want to eliminate white sugar and white flour from our foods and eat more starch, what will our intake of food be?

Dr. James Anderson suggests a diet of 75 percent complex carbohydrates, 16 percent protein and 9 percent fat, with plenty of fiber. His studies showed that many patients on his diet could get off insulin or reduce the amount they take. Their blood sugar and blood fats both decreased. Other investigators found that some diabetics on insulin could stay off it even if they had taken as much as 80 units a day.

Good sources of fiber are dried beans and peas, whole-grain cereals (especially oats), raw and steamed vegetables and whole fruits.

DIET FOR BLOOD SUGAR PROBLEMS

The diet for low and high blood sugar has changed in the last few years. Formerly physicians recommended high animal protein and almost no carbohydrates, usually in six small meals a day (Vance, 1975).

The suggestion about six small meals is still good, but a high-protein, low-carbohydrate diet taxes the adrenal glands and makes them break down. That diet helps for a while, but makes the disease worse in the long run. It can lead to kidney damage, osteoporosis, atherosclerosis, pyorrhea, heart disease, arthritis and cancer, and can use deficiency symptoms of calcium, magnesium and vitamins A, B3 and B6 (Airola, 1977).

For protein, we need moderate amounts of fish, poultry (from health food stores), eggs and dairy products, with large amounts of plant proteins from whole grains and legume combinations—such as brown rice and red beans, lentil soup and wheat germ muffins or millet soufflé (whole grains combined with milk, eggs and cheese). These foods are good sources of both protein and starch, which will be digested slowly, allowing glucose to flow evenly to the body over several hours, so our blood sugar will stay level. Other carbohydrates are vegetables both cooked and raw, and whole fruits—no fruit juice. Whole fruit intake must be adjusted to what each individual can tolerate. Avocados do not call out an insulin response, so they are healthful for hypoglycemics (Fredericks, 1974). Carbohydrates will be about 70 percent of calories.

We should eat very little red meat (muscle meat—steaks, roasts, chops and hamburger—especially beef and beef fat). These foods can cause kidney and heart problems. Proteins will be only about 15 to 20 percent of our calories. We need small amounts of fat—half saturated (butter, cream and eggs are best) and half unsaturated (nuts and seeds are best). Fats will be about 10 percent of calories.

We need to eat more complex carbohydrates than anything else, especially whole grains and legumes. This emphasis on grain and legume combinations follows precisely the diet suggested by major nutritionists.

We eliminate all white sugar and white flour and everything made from them. This includes all commercial ice cream, pastries, cookies, candy, white bread and cereals. All of the above foods can be eaten in very small amounts if they are made at home of whole grains and natural foods. We use a little dark brown sugar, dates and raisins for sweetening. Hypoglycemics and diabetics may not be able to tolerate any sweets, no matter how small an amount, at this time. Later, they may find they can handle a little bit. These patients seem to lose their sweet tooth, anyway, and they will really enjoy whole-grain bread.

Foods that are *emphasized* are:

> *Grains,* especially millet, buckwheat and oats.
> *Seeds,* especially sesame, sunflower and pumpkin.
> *Nuts,* especially almonds, peanuts and walnuts (eat nuts raw except peanuts—always roast peanuts).
> *Soured milks* such as yogurt, kefir and buttermilk. Vary them. We eat butter, we never use margarine or hard white shortening; we cook with butter and use it as a spread on bread.
> *Vegetables,* especially onions, garlic and avocados.
>> Raw: Eat a raw vegetable salad every day.
>> Cooked: potatoes, squash, green beans, spinach, rhubarb, asparagus, cauliflower, cabbage, green leafy vegetables (most concentrated source of vitamins and minerals). Eat a steamed green or yellow vegetable at least once a day. Cook all legumes (beans, peas and peanuts). Don't eat them raw. Do eat vegetables raw, at least once a day. Choose a wide variety of vegetables for your lifetime diet.
> *Fruits,* especially sour fruits and berries; no fruit juice even if you squeeze it yourself. Eat fruits whole, raw and ripe, combined with nuts and seeds for slower digestion.

Severe complications of diabetes have been re-versed with this diet. A young woman had been diabetic for 17 of her 24 years and had been nearly blind for six months because of degeneration of the retina. She gradually phased out the drugs she had been on, and she took food supplements plus the high complex carbohydrate diet. She regained her sight and returned to her job in a bank.

Vitamin and Mineral Supplements

Vitamin and mineral supplements should be given to everyone with a blood sugar problem to keep all cells healthy, especially liver cells. If a substance that poisons the liver is given to test animals, they get diabetes. Also, the liver has a very important role in how carbohydrates are used in the body, although this fact is not always realized.

One of the best ways to get the needed nutrients is by eating liver. Back in the early 1930s, investigators gave diabetics six ounces of raw liver a day, which controlled their blood glucose levels. Also, they worked out a plan to replace so many units of insulin with so many ounces of raw liver. Patients with pernicious anemia later voted to die, however, rather than eat raw liver, so people must be given food that is palatable. Patients can tolerate desiccated liver dissolved in tomato or other vegetable juice. As Carlton Fredericks says (1974), the time to eat liver is before illness is diagnosed.

Deficiencies of B-complex vitamins are common in blood sugar problems. Following are some early symptoms of B deficiencies. If you have them you might want to do something about them now to avoid sugar problems later.

1. Inflammation of the tongue
2. Splitting of fingernails in layers
3. Pain over the heart
4. Oily skin around the nose and lips
5. Clouding of consciousness
6. Insomnia
7. Stomach and intestinal disturbances
8. Cracks in lips and corners of mouth
9. Nervousness
10. Inflammation of many nerves at once
11. Keratosis (a horny growth of the lower eyelid)
12. Inability to remember recent events

B vitamins influence blood sugar levels and estrogen activity. Too much estrogen is dangerous, but signs of excess are often seen in both men and women who have either hypoglycemia or diabetes. One sign is lack of sexual desire in men. This may be because, with a deficiency of B vitamins and protein, the liver isn't healthy enough to degrade estrogen, which must be broken down to less dangerous substances. The nutrients will often restore the desire. Deficiency of vitamins and protein are related to both menstrual disturbances and blood sugar problems.

Minerals are of great importance in blood sugar ailments. All minerals are needed by diabetics and hypoglycemics.

Brewer's yeast is one of the best foods for these patients because it is a good source of chromium, part of the Glucose Tolerance Factor (GTF). Chromium can be absorbed up to 25 percent from yeast grown on chromium-rich compounds. One of my friends was severely hypoglycemic. She began to take brewer's yeast at the rate of one-eighth teaspoon a day because that was all she could tolerate. The microorganisms in the intestines feed on the yeast, and that causes abdominal cramps if the person's digestive tract isn't in excellent condition. Later, she could take one heaping tablespoon three times a day, and she said she thought that helped her more than anything else she had done.

As early as 1959, it was found that chromium can be used as a treatment for diabetes, but until recently it was not well absorbed except from yeast. Now supplement tablets that are well absorbed are available in health food stores. These tablets are called the Glucose Tolerance Factor (GTF), which is a combination of nutrients needed to allow glucose to enter the cells so the blood sugar won't be too high. The main ingredient is chromium; others are vitamin B3 plus the amino acids—glutamic acid, glycine and cysteine. This factor was discovered in the late 1950s by Walter Mertz. He fed rats a diet deficient in chromium, and they developed the same signs of disease that people with diabetes had. Then Mertz gave the same rats a supplement of chromium and they got well. He realized that chromium is needed to help insulin put blood sugar into the cells.

The GTF combination is found in organ meats and brewer's yeast (not torula yeast). GTF is absorbed much better than any other form of chromium, which is not often found in maximum amounts in the average American diet. Good sources of chromium include wheat germ, the bran of grains and brewer's yeast. Since most people don't eat much of those foods, they may need the GTF because the nutrients it is made of work together better than if each nutrient is taken individually, at least in some people.

Diabetics who have been taking large amounts of insulin should take small amounts of yeast or GTF to start with—one to three teaspoons a day of yeast and go up gradually. Otherwise, a sudden overdose might make the symptoms worse. Chromium given in amounts as small as 40 mcg a day or up to 200 mcg, according to several researchers, eliminated the signs of diabetes and glucose tolerance became normal (Bland, 1981). The suggested amount of GTF needed per day is about 500 mcg; the estimated amount in food is about one-third that amount. One thousand mcg a day may be needed in cases of illness. Toxicity is less likely with chromium than with most other minerals, but more than 1,000 mcg is not needed (Quillin, 1982).

Food supplements that are especially important for low and high blood sugar patients are:

- Brewer's yeast (high in protein, B vitamins, zinc and trace minerals, especially chromium). Start with one-fourth teaspoon and work up to one or two tablespoons a day in divided doses.
- Desiccated liver (high in the same nutrients as brewer's yeast, probably even higher). Same dosage—vary the liver and yeast.
- All vitamins and minerals in supplement form. Don't leave even one out—we need the whole team of nutrients. Check the chart in Lesson 1.

Don't overlook the importance of minerals. They activate enzyme systems and help us use glucose correctly.

Moderate amounts of all food supplements are suggested, with large amounts of a few:

- Choline: 300 mg three times a day.
- Folic acid: 800 mcg three times a day.
- Vitamin A (as beta-carotene): 25,000 IU three times a day.
- Glucose Tolerance Factor (GTF). Go by the dosage on the label.
- Methionine, an amino acid needed to make adrenal hormones. Go by the dosage on the label.

Start with small amounts of these supplements, go up gradually, then taper down for maintenance.

Of great importance for both ailments:

Hydrochloric acid (as betaine hydrochloride with pepsin). Begin with one tablet each main meal, increase to two, three or four at three-day intervals, according to what your body tells you. If you get better fast, you must be taking the right amount. Without HCl, we can't digest protein, and amino acids aren't available to make hormones, enzymes and organs that help keep our blood sugar level.

Eliminate processed foods (canned, packaged, bagged, etc.), coffee, tea, cigarettes, booze, commercial ice cream and soft drinks, with sugar or without—they all increase blood sugar (sugar-free soft drinks are dangerous because of artificial flavors and colors, phosphates and strong acids).

Eliminate rancid fats—they cause holes to form in cell membranes (Miller, *JIAPM*, 1974). Reminders:

Don't overeat.

Don't get too hungry.

Exercise moderately.

FOOD AND SUPPLEMENT SUMMARY

Let's review the specifics of diet and food supplements for blood sugar diseases.

The following suggestions for foods and food supplements are not intended as medical advice but only as a guide when working with your nutrition-minded medical doctor. If you are now taking prescription medicine, your medication requirements may change when you switch to a natural food diet. Check with your doctor.

The diet will be the same as outlined in Lesson 1. This is the new diet suggested for both high and low blood sugar. It is a diet that repairs tissues by furnishing every nutrient needed for the health of all cells. The liver will be repaired, the pancreas will function again and the adrenal glands will make their hormones and direct the metabolism (use of foods) in the body.

The food supplements will be almost the same as in the chart in Lesson 1. Special supplements for blood sugar problems are in the previous section in this lesson.

Remember to start your new food program slowly, especially if you're seriously ill. You may have to switch slowly to the high complex carbohydrate, high-fiber diet. You may have a bad day now and then, but when you get into the entire program, you'll have all good days. Until you get every nutrient needed by every cell, you cannot expect to get well. The length of time for recovery depends on your condition now and on your dedication to your own well-being.

The joyous news is that, given all nutrients, the body will heal itself. All cells can be repaired. Almost all organs can be rejuvenated. So let's get our sick cells working again.

LETTERS FROM READERS

When I counsel and speak about nutrition, I receive many letters from people who have had hypoglycemia or diabetes and who have written to me to tell about their experiences with the new food program. Here are a few excerpts from some of those letters.

"My hypoglycemia improved after switching to this diet; especially important was the snack with a small amount of protein and whole fruit at night."

"I believe the best thing I am doing is omitting the white sugar from my diet."

"I feel 100 percent better since giving up junk foods. Now I know why I had so many headaches—too much fat and not enough fiber."

"I have been feeling a lot better with your nutrition diet. I like the natural foods, I get plenty of food to choose from and it is filling. Low blood sugar doesn't seem to bother me any more."

"My general health can be surmised from the fact that I have not spent five cents for any kind of medication since my first consultation several years ago. I have not even taken an aspirin."

"I feel much, much better than I ever have before. Taking vitamins, eating good food and cutting out 90 percent of the junk in my former diet have made 100 percent improvement in my energy level. One visit to you opened up a whole new world to me, and I will always owe you my thanks for that."

"I am still trying the natural food way of living, and I am finding that I am desiring the more wholesome foods."

"The changeover in eating has changed our whole family. We all feel better and enjoy our new eating habits. I have become very much interested in your books and have read most of them. I bought a set for my parents, and I have passed on my new-found knowledge to anyone who will listen."

"For six months, I have been on your program, including all vitamin and mineral supplements. I have made exceptional progress since our visit in March. I am totally satisfied with the natural food way of life. I believe it's the only possible way good health can be achieved. I will never return to my old ways. My entire family of four now feels the same way."

"This 'New Way of Life' has changed my life for the better, so much so that I'll never go back to preservatives, refined sugar and flour or processed foods again. I now know that they were a poison to my system. P.S. I've purchased several extra of your Volume 1's and given them to members of my family and to friends. Hopefully, at least some of them will gain from it as I have."

"After our visit with you, my husband and I started out to change our eating habits and to take the recommended supplements. I began to get my strength back, and in three weeks, I was doing yard work. It was easy for me to go into this new program of cooking because my husband bought me the cooking utensils you recommended in your cookbook, *Switchover*, such as the steamer and food processor, plus the yogurt maker. He also ate what I ate and did not complain. I plan on making this my life's pattern for preparing food. My husband still feels he needs meat with his main meal, and I must admit I also like meat, but a small portion satisfies me. I am also faithful in taking the vitamins and minerals, and I give them to my husband as well. I have been able to help several of my friends with some of their health problems or at least have told them what they need to take and what changes they need to make in their diet. I can truly say that I'm living proof that it works. I thank my Lord that He is using you to help those who want help."

"I am a firm believer in the natural food way of life. Nothing could persuade me to go back to eating the Standard American Diet. My mental and physical well-being are the most important things in my life, because without them, I am no good to anyone else."

"I feel like a million dollars. I will never go off the natural foods diet. If I had had someone to guide me in my adolescent years, I would not have the health problems I have today. But still, there are people worse off than I am. What I am striving for in my good diet is to avoid senility 30 years from now. Also, I want to be able to walk and see

until the day I leave this earth. My 93-year-old mother sits in a wheelchair in a nursing home. My sister and I go to visit her every week. We come home heartbroken from what we see with the old folks. My sister is a hypoglycemic and wanted me to tell you that with the advice you gave her, she has gained seven pounds already and hopes to gain more weight. She now weighs 93 pounds."

"I find that the hardest thing to 'give up' is sugar, especially ice cream. Getting off alcohol and caffeine was much easier, but sugar is a real problem. I wonder if my past hypoglycemic state has something to do with it? As far as my total well-being, there is no question that I have much more energy and a brighter outlook on life. I especially noticed an increased ability to concentrate and remember!"

The answer to all disease is natural food with all its nutrients intact. Low and high blood sugar can be prevented and treated, so they will no longer cause poor health. The time to change from junk food to good food is now, in order to be energetic and slim and to enjoy vibrant health.

QUESTIONS

TRUE/FALSE

1. White table sugar (sucrose) has no vitamins and no minerals, nothing except calories.

2. The ideal way to get energy is from starch stored in a healthy liver and released into the blood when our blood sugar gets low.

3. The first symptoms of low blood sugar usually pertain to the brain—depression, headaches, irritability and inability to concentrate.

4. The glucose tolerance test is not being used as often as formerly because it has adverse reactions on the body.

5. It is claimed that more than 95 percent of alcoholics have low blood sugar.

6. The diet for alcoholism is the same as for hypoglycemia.

7. Schauss says, "One of the easiest measures for preventing crime would be to eliminate all non-essential sources of sugar in the diet."

8. The blood sugar of laboratory rats given a lot of sucrose or glucose was much higher than in rats given complex carbohydrates.

9. Although every other person in our family may have diabetes, we won't develop it if we stay on a natural food diet.

10. Cancer and diabetes often are found in the same person, possibly because waste products irritate the pancreas.

11. People who have diabetes (and other chronic diseases) and take insulin (and other drugs) need more vitamins and minerals than the average person.

12. Diabetics need high complex carbohydrates and moderate fat and protein from natural foods.

13. One of the best ways to get vitamins and minerals needed is by eating liver.

14. Chromium as a supplement is an excellent new remedy for diabetes.

MULTIPLE CHOICE

1. In diabetes, the following conditions may be found: (a) body cells are surrounded by sugar that can't get into the cells, (b) cells break down protein and fat for energy, (c) water and minerals leak out of cells, (d) kidneys are overworked and diseased.

2. Complications of severe diabetes are: (a) amputation of feet, (b) kidney failure, (c) blindness, (d) infections.

3. Tragic statistics are quoted for diabetics: (a) more than 80 percent of adult-onset diabetics have blood vessel diseases, (b) five times more diabetics have atherosclerosis than those in the average population.

4. Choose the best carbohydrate for diabetics: (a) sucrose, (b) honey, (c) fructose, (d) complex carbohydrates.

5. The more sugar women eat, the more likely they are to develop: (a) premenstrual syndrome, (b) cystic mastitis, (c) fibroid tumors of the uterus, (d) breast cancer.

6. Choose the items best for a diabetic to eat: (a) whole grains, (b) white sugar, (c) fruit juice, (d) dried beans.

7. A diabetic should not eat: (a) white sugar and flour, (b) white flour pastries, (c) fruit juice, (d) whole fruit.

ANSWERS

True/False

1. T 2. T 3. T 4. T 5. T 6. T 7. T 8. T 9. T
10. T 11. T 12. T 13. T 14. T

Multiple Choice

1. a,b,c,d 2. a,b,c,d 3. a,b 4. d 5. a,b,c,d 6. a,d
7. a,b,c

REFERENCES

Airola, P. *Hypoglycemia, A Better Approach.* Phoenix: Health Plus, 1977.

Ballentine, R. *Diet and Nutrition, A Holistic Approach.* Honesdale, PA: Himalayan International Institute, 1978.

Bierman, J. and Toohey, B. *The Diabetic's Book.* New York: Houghton Mifflin, 1981.

Bland, J. *Your Health Under Seige.* Brattleboro, VT: Stephen Greene Press, 1981.

Blond, K. *The Liver, Porta Malorum.* Bristol: John Wright, 1960.

Cheraskin, E. et al. *Diet and Disease.* New Canaan, CT: Keats, 1968.

Cohen, A.M. *New Dynamics of Preventive Medicine.* Vol. 2, 1975.

Colby-Morley, E. The Reflection of Hypoglycemia and Alcoholism on Personality: Nutrition as a Mode of Treatment. *J. Ortho Psych.,* 11(2):132–139, 1982.

Douglass, J.M. *Ann. of In. Med.,* Jan. 1975.

Drash, A. Influence of the Level of Nutrition on Diabetes Mellitus. In: *Endocrine Aspects of Malnutrition,* Gardner, L.F. and Amacher, P. (eds.) KROC Foundation Symposia #1; Santa Ynez, CA, KROC Foundation, 1973.

Fredericks, C. *JIAPM* 1:146–52, 1974.

———. *Dr. Carlton Fredericks' New and Complete Nutrition Handbook.* Canoga Park, CA: 1976.

Goldman, J.A. and Israel, *J. Med. Sci.,* 10:698–701, July 1974.

Goldwag, W.J. Hypoglycemia: Multi-Faceted Disorder. *Bestways,* Aug. 1981.

Harrell, Ruth F. et al. Can Nutritional Supplements Help Mentally Retarded Children? *Proc. Nat. Acad. Sci. U.S.A.:* Medical Sciences 78(1):574–578, 1981.

Hawley, C. and Buckley, R. Sensitivity to Food Dyes in Hyperkinetic children. *J. Appl. Nutr.* 26(4):57–61, 1974.

Hoffer, A. and Walker, M. *Orthomolecular Nutrition,* New Canaan, CT: Keats, 1978.

Horrobin, D.F. *An Introduction to Human Physiology.* Davis, 1973.

Ibarra, J.D. Jr. Hypoglycemia. *Postgrad. Med.* 51:88–93, 1972.

Kiehm, et al. *Am. J. Clin. Nutr.* 29:895–897, Aug. 1976.

Levinson, A. and Bigler, J. D. Mental Retardation in Infants and Children. Chicago: Yearbook Publishers, 1960, p. 29.

Lyle, W.H. Jr. Hypoglycemia Diet in the Emotionally Disturbed. *J.Appl. Nutr.* 33:1, Spring 1981.

Miller, J.J. Hypoglycemia: A New View of an Old Disease. *J. Appl. Nutr.* 26:7–10, 1974.

Moriarty, J. D. *J. Appl. Nutr.* 26(3):27–35, 1974.

Owen, J. Jr. *Virginia Medical Monthly,* 99:1180–84, 1972.

Passwater, R. *Supernutrition: Megavitamin Revolution.* New York: Pocket Books, 1976.

Paterson, E.T. Aspects of Hypoglycemia. *J. Ortho. Psych.,* 11(3): 151–55, 1982.

Pauling, L. *How to Live Longer and Feel Better.* New York: W. H. Freeman, 1986.

Pritikin, N. *Live Longer Now.* New York: Grosset and Dunlap, 1976.

Quillin, P. Energy? Spell It Chrome. *Bestways,* May 1982, pp. 80+.

Reed, B. Diet Related to Killer Diseases V; *Nutrition and Mental Health.* Washington, DC: Government Printing Office, 1977.

Reiser, S. Physical Differences Between Starches and Sugars. In: *Medical Applications of Clinical Nutrition.* Ed. J. Bland. New Canaan, CT: Keats, 1983.

Robbins, S.L. *Pathologic Basis of Disease.* Philadelphia: Saunders, 1974.

Ross, H. Hypoglycemia. Leaflet. New York: Huxley Institute, 1975.

Salzer, H.M. *JAMA,* 58:12, Jan. 1966.

Schauss, A.G. *Orthomolecular Treatment of Criminal Offenders.* Olympia, Wash., 1978.

———. *Nutrition and Behavior.* New Canaan, Conn.: Keats, 1985.

Vance, R.B. Hypoglycemia. New Dynamics of Preventive Medicine, Vol. 3, *Practical Preventive Medicine.* New York: Stratton International, Continental Medical Book Corp., 1975.

Walczak, M. *JICAN* 31(1–2):2–3, 1979.

Weiss, H. New Dynamics of Preventive Medicine. Vol. 4, *Tomorrow's Medicine Today,* 101–114, International Academy of Preventive Medicine, Houston, 1976.

Williams, R.J. *The Prevention of Alcoholism Through Nutrition.* New York: Bantam, 1981.

——— and Kalita, D.K. Hypoglycemia, The End of Your Sweet Life. In: *A Physician's Handbook on Orthomolecular Medicine.* New Canaan, CT: Keats, 1977.

Lesson 11

CHILDREN'S PROBLEMS,
LEARNING, BEHAVIOR AND NUTRITION

LESSON 11—CHILDREN'S PROBLEMS, LEARNING, BEHAVIOR AND NUTRITION

THE HARRELL STUDY

PUT YOURSELF in this picture: Your first-born son is now seven years old. Not once in seven years has he said "Mama" or "Daddy." Not once has he gone to school with the other children. Why? Because he can't talk. What is going on in his brain? What will happen to him in this fast-moving world? What chance does he have for a normal life? Although his outlook seemed hopeless, G.S. (we'll call him) did have a chance, because someone said, "Let's try nutrition."

We all deserve good brains. Children, especially, deserve to develop their brains to their highest potential. It is now possible to improve our ability to think, whether we're five years old or 95 years old. How? By eating all of the nutrients in maximum amounts that are needed by the brain. For years, the brain was called the "Last Great Frontier." Now that frontier is being explored, and more has

been discovered about the brain in the last 15 years than has been known in all of history before that time.

A group of researchers studied severely mentally retarded children ages 5 to 15, to see if massive amounts of some nutrients, especially the B vitamins, would allow a retarded child to increase his IQ (Harrell, 1981).

The researchers were headed by Dr. Ruth Harrell, who has been studying learning-disabled children for many years; by her daughter, Dr. Ruth Harrell Capp; and by three other colleagues who published their results in January 1981. They were testing the hypothesis that mental retardation can be caused by not getting enough of one or all 50 of the essential nutrients that we must eat. There are about 20 vitamins, 20 minerals, eight amino acids (which are building blocks of protein), plus carbohydrates, fats and water. We all get some of the essential nutrients or we would die. That's what we mean by essential—essential for life itself. But many people need more than the average person does. If they get that amount, they will be healthy.

If they need more, the amount is determined by their genes. Thus, if someone says he inherits a disease, he inherits not the disease but the requirement for a larger amount of some nutrient. If he gets the larger amount, he doesn't get the disease. These diseases are called "genetotrophic" diseases. We all know what "gene" means—the pattern our cells are made by. "Trophis" means "nutrition." Thus, if the genes don't get good enough nutrition, they will not be able to make correct patterns for our cells. Thus there is illness.

IQs Improved

The researchers assembled a group of 16 retarded children with IQs of 17 to 70. They were all told to consume less sugary foods and soft drinks and to eat fruits and vegetables and to drink milk freely. They were divided into two groups, matched mostly by IQ. For four months, in a double-blind study, Group 1 was given moderate amounts of all vitamins and minerals, with relatively large doses of the B vitamins. Group 2 was given placebos. The first group increased their IQs from five to 10 points. The placebo group stayed about the same as when they entered the program. During the next four months, the two groups switched. The second experimental group increased their IQs by 10.2 points on the average. Five of the children stayed on the vitamins and minerals for the entire eight months, and their IQs came up 16 points.

Three of the four were Down's syndrome children who increased their IQs between 10 and 25 points and also improved physically. For example, Down's children have puffy tissues and their eyes are abnormal. Both of these conditions improved toward normal during the study.

One of the most thrilling cases was the seven-year-old boy we're calling G.S. He was severely retarded. At the beginning of the study, G.S. was still in diapers, couldn't dress himself, couldn't talk and had an estimated IQ of 25 to 30. After a few weeks on the program, he began to talk. After a few more weeks, he began to read and write, and at the age of nine, he was reading and writing on the elementary school level. He was moderately advanced in arithmetic, could ride a skateboard and a bicycle, play a flute and he had an IQ of about 90.

Just think of the first seven years of that child's life and how tragic it would have been if someone had not said, "Let's try nutrition." Even after seven years of malnutrition, he was able to dramatically improve when he got good food with the extra nutrients he needed.

Eyesight Improved

The eyesight of several of the children improved surprisingly. Some of the children would take their glasses off when they needed to see something more clearly. Two others who had worn glasses for years were told by their ophthalmologist that they didn't need to wear them anymore.

Other exciting changes came about. At the beginning of the study, one boy about six years old said only single words such as "Mama" and "Bye-bye" but after eight months, he could recite, without being prompted, the Pledge of Allegiance to the Flag. Two others were transferred, on their teachers' recommendations, from classes for the mentally retarded to regular classes.

There were no unfavorable side effects, but there were very favorable fringe benefits—improved texture of skin, hair and fingernails, and what their parents and teachers appreciated the most—no more hyperactivity.

A specific supplement formula was designed for this study. Ask your nutrition-minded physician about it. It is marketed by Bronson Pharmaceutical, a firm located in La Canada, California. The supplement is sold under the name "GTC." First, the tablets were made medium size, for a dosage of six a day, but some of the small children couldn't swallow tablets that big. Then they were made half size, for a dosage of 12 a day. Some of the children could take powder better, so now there are three choices. The powder in the pull-apart capsule is easier for small children to take with milk, yogurt, pureed fruit or whatever they prefer.

I met Dr. Capp at a convention and she said to begin with one tablet and work up to six or 12. There are 1,500 mg of vitamin C in the day's supply, and that may cause gas or diarrhea, so each child will take what he can handle without getting gas or diarrhea, according to Dr. Capp.

This is one of the most thrilling breakthroughs in brain research; let's tell any parents who need this information that it is available. Most health food stores carry GTC. If they don't, they will order it for you; or you can order direct from Bronson. I have told parents about this formula whenever I have met someone who might be interested because of Down's syndrome, schizophrenia, manic depression or learning disability. I have also suggested it to parents of two children who fell in swimming pools at their homes and nearly drowned. The mothers were well pleased with the results.

When this study was published in January 1981, a reporter from the *Houston Chronicle* called the

Children's Nutrition Center in the Texas Medical Center. He asked the authorities there if they intended to treat children with methods used by Dr. Capp and her colleagues. The authority answered, "Oh, no, after all, it hasn't really been verified. We'll wait until additional studies are done. If there is more research, we may test it out." Think of the seven-year-olds like G.S. who are living useless, tragic lives while someone waits to "test it out" when it has been well tested already.

Children Are Helped

Several children have got over their mental problems with the help of my natural food program. A 7-year-old boy came for counseling with his mother. The boy had been going to a psychologist for a year with no help. He was slightly autistic—he walked around the room talking to the walls; he wouldn't talk to or play with other children; he had a motor problem too and he couldn't skip or jump. When the psychologist was ready to leave for a months' vacation, she told the mother she could not help the boy any further, and for her to bring him to me for counseling. She came, and I put the boy on a natural food diet with moderate amounts of all nutrients, in supplement form and large amounts of B complex. When the psychologist went back to work a month later, she was astonished at the boy's improvement. She called me and told me this whole story. I had not realized he had been referred by a psychologist. She told me that the boy no longer talked to the walls, he played nicely with the other children and he could skip and jump. She said over and over, "He is a normal boy, he is a normal boy . . . and it's just been one month."

A more recent contact I had with a schizophrenic was when a woman brought her 22-year-old daughter to see me. The daughter was rather distraught; she walked from one room to another, she couldn't concentrate, couldn't or wouldn't talk to her mother and me, and if I asked her a question, her mother had to answer.

Just last week, her mother called me and said the girl was very cooperative about staying on the food program. At first, the mother had to get the vitamins out of the bottles and hand them to her, but now, she was taking them in the right amounts and keeping track of how many to take. She didn't eat any junk food. She stayed on the program of natural foods and food supplements. She looked alert, her eyes were bright and, when anyone asked her a question, she quickly answered before her mother did. Her mother also said that before she started the new diet, the daughter had spoken in short, bullet sentences—one thought at a time. Now she speaks in complex sentences; she is able to distin-

guish between main and subordinate thoughts. She responded well to the food program, as have other schizophrenics on my natural food programs.

Recently a 28-year-old man (I'll call him Dick) came to me because he had been on hard drugs when he was in high school, and since then he had been in and out of mental hospitals. He was trying to work, but was not able to cope with a regular job and keep regular hours. He said several other members of his family had had mental problems, and he just figured he had inherited the condition and could do nothing about it.

Dick has called me about every two weeks. With every call, he sounds better, is more encouraged by his diet and is now working. He is also faithful about taking his supplements and eating natural foods. He knows now that he doesn't have to be sick because his parents were sick. He enjoys taking the responsibility for his own health.

A man I'll call Oscar called me one January to tell me about his son. Oscar said that he had been at my Nutrition Education Conference the preceding April and heard Dr. Roger J. Williams talk about a good diet with moderate amounts of all supplements plus L-glutamine as a brain food. L-glutamine is a derivative of the amino acid, glutamic acid. Oscar said that he had gone home from the conference and given his 18-year-old mentally retarded soon L-glutamine and as good a food program as he could. Then in January, the son had been given another IQ test. His IQ had gone up 25 points, and he was no longer called mentally retarded—he was called a "slow learner." Think of the tragedy of the first 18 years that young man had lived through!

STATISTICS ARE DISHEARTENING

Estimates run from five to 10 million mentally retarded children in the United States. In percentages, this would be 12.5 to 25 percent of young people under 18 years of age. That means 126,000 or more babies born each year will be retarded (Cheraskin et al., 1968; Levinson and Bigler, 1960).

One infant in four is born not living, not normal or not healthy. Five percent of all births are premature. Good nutrition reduces the prematurity problem by 80 percent. Premature children and low-birth-weight babies have a greater risk of having learning disabilities than normal-weight babies (Fredericks, 1976). Children who have trouble sleeping, learning and sitting still are said to number 5 percent of all schoolchildren (Lublin, 1977). We have 20 million children who are either schizophrenic, autistic, learning disabled or retarded (Cott, 1973).

One of every seven Americans needs some form

of mental health care. One of every 35 Americans is mentally retarded. Symptoms of depression are common, affecting as many as 20 percent of the population at any one time. That's 50,000,000 people. Other emotional problems affect as many as 25 percent more at any one time. These statistics are from the report of the President's Commission on Mental Health, 1978.

We may suffer from mental disease and not realize it. It is estimated that 4.7 percent of the general population has some mental illness such as anxiety neuroses. That's about one in 20 people (Williams, 1971).

A group of scientists from the University of California reported that more than a million American infants and young children have suffered stunting of their brains or they risk brain damage because of malnutrition. A University of Texas study showed that one adult in five is unable to read well enough to get through the routine chores of modern city life (*Houston Post,* 1975).

One in a Thousand

Are you one in a thousand? This is the number of people believed to be well nourished according to a survey made by the Foundation for Nutrition and Stress Research at Pennsylvania State College (Cott, 1973). If your children have the problems mentioned in this lesson, they may be among the 999 who are not well nourished.

Another study in 1965–66, conducted by the U.S. Department of Agriculture, reported that the nutrients most lacking in the American diet were vitamins A and C and the mineral calcium. These nutrients were low in 25 to 30 percent of all diets.

Dr. Cott says that of every 100 children he ran a hair analysis on, 95 had lower than normal levels of three or more essential minerals. Also, levels of two toxic minerals (lead and mercury) were high in 85 and at near toxic levels in 10 (Cott, 1973).

Analysts note that a similar percentage of children having learning and behavior problems in school or adults having difficulty in life can blame their problems on brain damage from malnutrition before and after birth.

NUTRITIONAL THERAPY

Nutritional therapy is helpful in hyperactivity, minimal brain dysfunction, autism and childhood schizophrenia. Some cases of epilepsy respond to vitamin B6. (Drugs should not be taken at the same time.) B6 is helpful in alcoholism and drug addiction, possibly also with criminals. Also responding to nutrition therapy are fatigue, mild depression, insomnia, anxiety, tension and phobias, as well as

poisoning from pollutants such as heavy metals, pesticides, preservatives and food additives (Lesser, 1977).

Criminals' Diets

Many studies of adults who are criminals show that their diets are high in coffee, chocolate and cola drinks (Schellhardt, 1977), as well as in sweets, which obviously cause low blood sugar and lack of energy in the brain. When criminals' diets are improved, and sugar largely removed, their aggressive behavior improves. Parents should see that their children eat a natural food diet as we've been talking about.

Today's Living, February 1977, reported that sugar is the most dangerous item of diet, and causes most children's difficulties with learning, hyperactivity and emotional problems. Many of these problems could be eliminated by simply eliminating sugar.

Peer pressure to eat sugar is so great ("Let's have a soda") that the sugar habit is hard to break, especially after the child starts to school.

Dr. Weston Price

Dr. Weston Price studied peoples around the world and found that those who ate processed food had severe dental problems such as decayed teeth, malformed dental arches and crowding of teeth. They also had deformities of facial bones. All of these ailments were correlated with lower IQs and personality disturbances. The incidence of birth defects was high (Ballentine, 1978). No such defects and other problems were found in peoples on a native diet.

Dr. Carolyn Brown

Dr. Carolyn Brown, who has three schools for hyperactive and learning-disabled (LD) children in California, reported to the McGovern Committee on her work (Brown, 1977).

Dr. Brown says that much of the learning disability they see in children is caused by a deficiency of nutrients in the diet. The food Americans eat is getting less nutritious; chemicals in the food are increasing, as is synthetic food; radiation from nuclear testing and from physicians' X-rays is widespread. All of these conditions have happened during the last 25 years, and, during that time, six times as many children have been arrested, suspected of murder, nonnegligent manslaughter, aggravated assault and rape. There has been a decline for the last 14 years in the scores of gifted children on the Scholastic Aptitude Test. During the years from 1958 to 1966, the number of children with chronic disease rose to 24.6 percent.

Dr. Brown reports that some LD and hyperactive

children in her schools show dramatic improvement after changes in their diet. She notes that the diet should be free of chemicals and synthetic food, low in refined carbohydrates (white sugar and white flour) and it should be supplemented with vitamins and minerals.

Dr. Michael Lesser

In his report to the McGovern Committee of the United States Senate on Nutrition and Human Needs, Dr. Michael Lesser, of the University of California at Berkeley, says that nutrient therapy has a lot of advantages over drugs. For one thing, nutrients are less expensive, and they are safer because they are natural substances normally present in the body. The main reason they are better than drugs is that they get at the cause of the problem and don't just mask the symptoms as drugs do.

But drugs can be patented, and the profits from sales pay for research on more drugs. Thus, tranquilizers and such drugs as Ritalin are widely used.

People who are used to the instant response that drugs usually give may have to wait longer for help from foods. However, some food responses are dramatic, and there are no dangerous side effects from foods as there are from drugs. (Lesser, 1977).

Dr. Allan Cott

Dr. Allan Cott reports on pangamic acid, also called dimethyl-glycine, and its use with children who have severe disorders of learning, behavior and communication. One report on children who took 20 mg of pangamic acid three times a day declared that 12 to 15 improved considerably in speech development. The general mental state and intellectual activity of the children improved.

One child, age seven, could use only five or six words. About eight months later, after treatment with 200 mg of pangamic acid daily, his mother wrote, "It's the most exciting thing I have ever experienced. Jimmy speaks, asks questions and smiles."

Other case histories list success in treatment of allergies, asthma, emotional disturbances, disagreeable behavior, lack of cooperation and even cerebral palsy. One patient was described thusly: "Since the addition of pangamic acid to the megavitamins, the whole picture seems to be even more improved" (Cott, 1977).

Dr. Richard Passwater

L-glutamine is a brain fuel that is getting a lot of attention. It is an amino acid. Our major concern with it here is that tests show it improves intelligence (Passwater, 1976). Also it helps heal ulcers,

us up when we're tired and helps us avoid alcohol, sweets and even schizophrenia.

Very few substances can get to the brain. Usually we hear that glucose is the only substance that can be used as brain food. This is because if the brain cells were too permeable, they could be damaged by foreign invaders.

But glutamic acid really isn't an invader. It is one of the amino acids, although not one of the eight essentials. If we eat more protein to get more glutamic acid, it may not cross the blood-brain barrier, but if we eat a different form of glutamic acid (L-glutamine), it does cross the barrier, and it quickly changes to glutamic acid in the brain.

The two things glutamic acid does are furnish fuel for the brain and eliminate ammonia. We don't want ammonia in our cells because it is poisonous. It must be changed by the liver into urea, which is excreted in the urine. L-glutamine also helps form energy in the citric acid cycle.

Dr. Lorene Rogers of the University of Texas discovered that L-glutamine improved the IQs of mentally deficient children. Dr. Abram Hoffer also uses L-glutamine with other nutrients to improve schizophrenia and mental retardation.

Recommended amounts according to Roger J. Williams are 1,000 to 4,000 mg a day for an adult (age 13 or over). At our rate of one-half that for six- to 12-year-olds, 500 to 2,000 mg would be suggested. For a child one to six, 250 to 1,000 mg a day would be recommended.

Dr. Passwater suggests that adults start with one 500-mg capsule twice a day the first week, one three times a day the second week and two twice a day for the first part of the third week. He says this method will use up a bottle of 50 capsules, and by then people will be able to tell how much benefit they're getting. For children, remember the reduced doses and start slowly and build up gradually while observing the results.

Dr. Bernard Rimland

Vitamins in rather large amounts can be taken without danger, except for vitamins A and D, which are oil-soluble (Rimland, 1974). Now beta-carotene, a provitamin A, is usually used, and it is not changed to vitamin A until the body needs it. Therefore, it is almost impossible to get a toxic level of beta-carotene. It is rare to find reports of adverse symptoms, even when oil-soluble vitamin A is given. In any case, vitamins are much, much safer than the drugs regularly given to children. With the water-soluble vitamins, the body excretes what it doesn't need.

A popular fallacy is that everybody gets all the

needed vitamins if he eats a "well-balanced diet." This, says Rimland, is "sheer nonsense."

We are all individuals and some of us need 20 times as much as others, according to Roger J. Williams (1956).

Mental problems have recently been studied and reported on in hundreds of medical journal articles. Reports show that nutritional deficiencies are often the cause of mental and behavior problems.

Cott (1973) says: "In the treatment of mental problems, the future is here." Many physicians are using orthomolecular therapy, which means providing the right amounts of all substances normally present in the brain. In mental problems, there are usually low amounts of B1, B3, B6, B12, biotin, ascorbic acid and folic acid.

Drugs cure nothing. They mask symptoms and cause nerve damage (Feingold, 1973). A nutritious diet has no risk, and the sooner the diet is improved, the better chance the child has to recover completely. If he reaches puberty without good nutrition, he may not be cooperative in changing his eating habits and he may go on to delinquency.

Let's Get the Message Out

Exciting things do happen when we eat good food and take food supplements. The problem is how to get this message to the many people who need it. Through the years, I have occasionally spoken to parents of learning-disabled children. When I mention food, they pay no attention to me. They have been so programmed that food has nothing to do with their children's mental problems that they do not open their minds and even give it a try. About six months ago, I was asked to speak at a meeting of adults with cerebral palsy. They were so excited about their prospects of improvement by changing their diets to natural foods that that was all they could talk about the rest of the day. The director of the cerebral palsy group asked me to send in a proposal to the national office to begin a program of excellent nutrition for the group. I sent it in, but I never heard anything from either office. Finally, I called and the director made excuses about needing housing and transportation; they didn't have time to help the people walk and talk better. We had even figured a way to try to pay for the food supplements they would need. Perhaps the reason the director vetoed the idea is that he and others who are employed to run the program would be out of a job if the patients improved.

THE BRAIN

To talk about learning disabilities, we need to know a little about the brain. Let's first review what we said in Lesson 2. The brain has 100 billion cells. Ten billion are neurons, which are thinking cells. Ninety billion are glial cells, which hold the neurons together. "Glial" derives from the Greek word for glue.

The brain is really the boss of the body (Rosenfeld and Klivington, 1975). Although it weighs only 2 percent of the total weight of the body, the brain grabs 20 percent of the blood—first! Thus the brain is protected from harm, especially from the harm of nutritional deficiencies. In case of malnutrition, muscles and other tissues are broken down to feed the brain, so it is the last to starve.

It is said that we have two brains—one the analytical; the other the emotional, which also governs appetite, sexuality, aggression and the output of the glands that produce hormones. The components of the brain are very finely connected to each other. And the brain is where the mind and spirit are. A famous maxim says, "No twisted thought without a twisted molecule."

However, if a neuron dies, we never make another one to take its place. A neuron can obviously get sick and not function well. When it gets the nutrients it needs, it recovers, just like cells in the rest of the body. Some of us eat so poorly that we kill off our thinking cells at about 10,000 a day. At that rate we may become senile at 50! Others possibly kill off only about 1,000 a day. At that rate, we would have enough thinking cells to last 125 years, if we live that long. Of course, our brain cells need all of the nutrients to stay healthy.

The section of the brain where growth is the fastest, because cells divide fast, is the hippocampus, the place where most of the damage occurs. It determines emotions, even epileptic seizures and hallucinations. A person can't learn well without a healthy hippocampus. And he will not have normal sense of sight, sound, touch, taste and smell (Goodhart and Shils, 1973).

When there is something wrong with the brain cells and their food supply, there is mental illness. The brain cells can't get what they need unless we eat the right kind of food.

Probably all mental disease has a biochemical basis (Williams, 1971). Nerves are damaged by nutritional deficiencies. Mild deficiencies of B1 cause irritability, loss of memory and loss of appetite. Deficiencies of pantothenic acid and B2 cause severe nerve lesions, as do B12 deficiencies. Without enough thyroid hormone, children become idiots; iodine is essential for the production of thyroid hormone. Even mild deficiencies of all these nutrients can lead to severe mental illness. Niacin deficiency causes a severe psychosis.

Our individual genetic requirements may be extra high in particular nutrients. Without that high amount, we get sick. If a young person gets the right amounts he needs, he can prevent mental illness. Our bodies can be trained to utilize good food, but malnutrition can cause a variety of health problems.

Three hundred thousand mentally retarded children are born each year. Most of them would profit from glutamic acid or L-glutamine, an amino acid (protein) and all other nutrients. This is true of schizophrenics also. Another nutrient, vitamin C, is burned up about 10 times faster in schizophrenics than in normal people.

Sodas, potato chips and sweets, eaten so much by children and teenagers, erode brain cells. Anyone under stress needs large amounts of pantothenic acid. B6 helps psychotic children.

Nutrients especially needed by depressed people are B1, B2, biotin and folic acid. The absence of any one of these vitamins can cause hallucinations, severe agitation, manic behavior, inability to concentrate, groundless panic, memory loss, sensitivity to noise and withdrawal states. All other vitamins and minerals must be taken at the same time.

The vast majority of children whose nutrition is neglected would profit from good food and food supplements (Williams, 1971).

The earliest symptom of nerve damage is in the brain and spinal cord, causing a nerve disease marked by chronic, abnormal fatigue; feelings of inadequacy; insomnia; lack of attention; failure to concentrate and irritability. I often think of schoolchildren who are told, "Behave yourself," "Get your head on straight" or "Be a good boy and pay attention in school." There's no way a child can be good and pay attention when he's missing B vitamins and other nutrients. When the missing vitamins are added, the changes are usually sudden and very dramatic.

Dr. Lendon Smith, the "baby doctor," who often appears on the "Tonight Show," gives injections of B's and C to children with behavior problems the first day they come to his office. He calls the mother the next day. Usually the children are much better—no longer hyperactive but very cooperative. They feel good, and, of course, the mother feels good. After that, Dr. Smith gives the vitamins by mouth (Smith, 1976).

Brain Studies

Linus Pauling has done a great deal of research into nutrition and the brain. One of his papers was published in *Science*, April 19, 1968. He emphasizes that most bodily processes work with the help of enzymes, which are substances that make reactions happen fast. Thus, an egg we eat for breakfast can be used to repair our brain cells and all other tis-

sues if we have enough enzymes and if they work fast enough. Enzymes are made out of amino acids from the food we eat, with the help of vitamins and minerals we have eaten. If we have ailments of any kind, we obviously haven't been making enough enzymes to react fast enough to make the nutrients needed for our cells.

If we take vitamin and mineral supplements, we have a good chance of getting maximum amounts of enzymes and of the nutrients needed to make them work. The reaction rate of the enzymes increases a great deal with the increase of nutrients, thus the cells get everything they need. Every tissue and every organ will then be healthy and we will be healthy.

Our brains are so sensitive to the food provided through the blood that they need an even larger concentration of the essential nutrients than other tissues, because the reactions have to take place faster. If we miss getting a tiny amount of one of the B vitamins, the brain will react and we may not make an "A" on a test. If a fraction of the magnesium that we need is missing because we ate a white-bread sandwich instead of making our own whole-grain bread, we may not be able to think well enough to learn our lessons at school.

A deficiency of B12 can cause brain problems, and there are many reasons why we can have a deficiency. If we're taking any doctors' drugs, they may have destroyed some of the B12 needed to save our sanity. A severe deficiency of B12 leads to insanity, and mental problems show up long before physical problems do. B12 deficiency can also be caused by undigested protein, which results from lack of hydrochloric acid in the stomach.

The undigested protein becomes encrusted around the walls of the colon. Tremendous colonies of poisonous bacteria live year after year on the vitamins and minerals in that crust, causing a terrible odor from the stools. But that's not the worst. The bacteria use up so much of the B12 that there's not enough left to keep our brains healthy. Therefore, if we don't make enough hydrochloric acid to digest protein, we can go insane. Usually the change from sanity to insanity is gradual. Consider your friends and relatives. Maybe even the teenagers at home are gradually changing. Have they become more difficult to be with? There may be a very real reason: a gradual deterioration of the brain, hardly noticeable at first, but a very common result of a high-sugar diet and other junk foods, especially bottled and canned drinks. There are many other symptoms and signs of unhealthy brains—inability to concentrate, anxiety, lack of attention, irritability, aggression and others.

Recently I counseled a young mother who was so

upset by her two-year-old daughter's irritability that she kept putting her head in her hands and wailing about the "obnoxious child." When I discussed the poisonous bacteria that live in the colon and make the feces smell bad, she suddenly cried out, "That's what's wrong with my daughter. Her stools smell terrible."

Obviously, all nutrients are needed for the brain. Some are especially important, such as B3, which is niacin or niacinamide, and L-glutamine, which one study showed has raised IQs from five to 20 points in many children with mental deficiencies.

Although people are slow to believe in nutritious food for health, let's tell them about it every time we get a chance. If they hear it often enough, they might be curious enough to try it.

LEARNING PROBLEMS

The first thing to do for children with learning or behavior problems is to get them off white sugar, white flour and soft drinks, and give supplements of the entire B complex, plus vitamin C and all other nutrients (Cott, 1973).

Drs. Knobloch and Pasamanik say that often the only way to prove that vitamin and mineral deficiencies are causing mental and behavior problems is to provide the nutrients and observe the results (1968). Sometimes the children have other aches and pains that might not seem to be connected to learning and behavior problems. Dr. R. G. Green (1970) reports on a 10-year-old girl who had abdominal pains, pains in her leg, sore throat and several other complaints. She was getting poor grades in school. With the diet and vitamin-mineral therapy, her physical as well as mental problems cleared up. She then returned to the top third of her class.

We can quote the authors of *Biochemistry and Behavior* (Eiduson et al., 1964): "We cannot conceive of even a thought occurring without bodily processes making the thought happen." The processes pertaining to thoughts are in the brain. The brain depends on proteins, carbohydrates, fats, vitamins, minerals and water for its cells to function well enough to make a thought occur.

Symptoms of Learning Disability

Symptoms of learning disability are commonly found in many children. The children range from near-normal to above-average intelligence with mild to severe learning disabilities (LD). The most common sign of LD is hyperactivity. Other signs are perceptual and motor problems, severe personality and emotional disturbances, impulsive behavior, lack of coordination (sometimes severe), inability to concentrate, short attention span, speech disorders, slow learning, diabetes and hypoglycemia.

Sometimes these signs are not noticed until children start to school. Then they can have reading disabilities, they can't use their hands well, they have emotional and psychological problems. Some of these children are really not mentally retarded; their average IQ is about the same as in the general population.

Some of the problems are due to vitamin or mineral *dependency*—that is, an inherited need for larger than usual amounts of one or more vitamins or minerals. Most of the problems are due to vitamin or mineral *deficiencies*. People simply don't eat enough nutrients because they eat too much junk food in which the nutrients have been processed out.

Most of the children treated with diet and food supplements improve without the use of drugs. Often the first sign of improvement is increased attention span, better learning ability and cooperation with parents and teachers.

No serious side effects have ever been found in hundreds of children treated with nutrients. The only mild symptoms found are if the dosage is too high, which causes increased frequency of bowel movements and urination. These symptoms subside when the dose is reduced.

The complete team of nutrients must be provided: about 20 vitamins, 20 minerals, eight amino acids, carbohydrates, fats and water. Without any one of these, we die, but we usually won't die quickly. It is very likely that we'll have brain, nerve and behavior problems—or worse, drug or alcohol addiction, which leads to a pitiful, wasted life. Physical problems are also caused by eating food that does not furnish the vitamins and minerals we need, and that leads to heart disease and cancer, our two greatest killer diseases.

Studies of Children

One of my favorite studies was conducted by an elementary school teacher who was interested in nutrition. At the beginning of a semester, he was given permission to give half the children in his class supplements of vitamins and minerals. The other half were given candy. The vitamin group had only 12 absences that semester; the candy group, 58; the vitamin group had seven tardies, the candy group 22; the vitamin group disrupted the class 36 times, the candy group, 65. How about their mental ability? The vitamin group gained 4.82 points in IQ; the candy group went down 1.88 points. That means the vitamin child had a relative gain of 6.70 IQ points in one semester.

Last spring, I taught nutrition to a group of women who had one or more children with LD. The children attended a private school for LD children, and the director of the school asked me to teach the course. All the mothers had either hypoglycemia or allergies, thus their diets had been poor for years, and their children had been malnourished from conception.

This group of young mothers became the most excited people I've taught, after they changed their diets and their children's diets. One of the women had an 11-year-old daughter who had been on Ritalin for five years. After a few weeks of good, nutritious food and moderate amounts of supplements, the child went off Ritalin with no problems. Every other mother reported similar improvement with learning disabilities and with allergies.

Several investigators have studied high- and low-IQ children and their nutrition. Hardy and Hoefer (1968) found that of all the children they studied with IQs of 130 and above, not one was bottle-fed. They compared intelligence, education, performance and the age when the children began to talk, and found that the bottle-fed children showed lower scores than the breast-fed children.

Another study showed that children with chronic malnutrition had low scores on behavior and on anything relating to the brain and nerves. With lack of protein and calories for energy, the IQs were lower. Also, with a deficiency of vitamin C, the IQ of normal students was lower.

The B-complex group of vitamins must be present in large amounts for the central nervous system (CNS, the brain and spinal cord) to develop. If there is an early deficiency in B's in experimental animals, the animals can't learn well. Likewise, if the fetus doesn't get around B's or if the baby animal doesn't get enough before it is weaned, the learning ability is worse than if the deficiency started later—at any age after being weaned (Cheraskin et al., 1968).

Dr. Hoffer (1963) tells us, "If all the vitamin B3 were removed from our food, everyone would become psychotic with one year. Most of the victims would recover if the B3 were replaced in their diet. But many would be so severely damaged that they would have to take massive doses of B3 for life." This is what happens to 1 or 2 percent of our population. These are generally the schizophrenics.

LD children have been studied and their diets were shown to be high in refined carbohydrate foods and sweets. Dr. Cott found deficiencies of trace minerals. He analyzed the patients' hair and found lead present in 85 of 100 children (as high as 45 ppm in 10 children), and mercury in near-toxic levels in 10. Children who have low amounts of calcium in their diet absorb more lead.

Cadmium is another dangerous mineral that causes brain problems. One of the reasons is that cadmium and zinc (a protective mineral) compete for absorption in our cells, and when we eat white bread, we are six times more likely to get cadmium than zinc. When we eat whole-wheat bread, we are six times more likely to get zinc than cadmium (Cott, 1973).

Variety of Nutrients

In reviewing reports of some controlled studies and some double-blind studies on humans, we find the following definitely encouraging results:

1. A good diet significantly increased the IQ in normal and retarded children.
2. Vitamin C, B1, B2, B3 and iron brought a significant increase in IQ in each of a battery of mental tests in normal children.
3. Vitamin C brought a significant gain in IQ if enough was given.
4. Glutamine led to increased IQ in all ages of mentally retarded.
5. Lecithin and B1 brought a significant improvement in movements required in writing and in arithmetic performance in normal high school seniors. (This was a double-blind study with placebo-treated controls. "Double-blind" means that neither the parents nor the doctors knew which person was getting the nutrients.) Improvement was noted by the end of the first day of supplements.
6. Vitamin B3 brought improvement in memory and in cases of mental retardation in all ages.
7. Vitamin B1 led to significantly improved mental performance in children.
8. Vitamin E brought improvement of subnormal mentality in children and mental improvement of mongoloid children (Cheraskin, 1968).

A study was done on three- and four-year-old children whose mothers had added nutritional supplements to their own diets rather late in pregnancy, but even so, there was a significant difference in IQs of the children whose mothers received vitamins and those whose mothers received placebos.

In still another study, when both retarded and mentally normal children took nutritional supplements there was an increase of 10 points in IQ for the retarded and 18 points for the normal children.

Dr. Ruth F. Harrell of Columbia University, in a double-blind study, gave vitamin supplements to a group of normal children for one year, and no supplements to the control group. The group getting the supplements improved from 25 percent to 3,200 percent. Thus, it seems that children who are presumably normal can profit from dietary supplements.

A variety of nutrients used alone or in combination can help our brains stay healthy, but let's remember—we need the entire team of 50 nutrients plus a good diet.

BEHAVIOR PROBLEMS

Let's zero in on behavior and review published studies related to behavior problems. Here are some findings from *Diet and Disease* (Cheraskin et al., 1987).

Variety of Nutrients

1. Low absorption of vitamin B12 led to confusion and even paranoia.
2. Retention of sodium brought about psychotic depression.
3. Low vitamin C absorption led to disorders of the senses: sight, sound, touch, taste, smell.
4. Low blood sugar resulted in depression, schizophrenia, anxiety, irritability, fatigue, mental confusion and uncontrolled emotional outbursts. (There are about 100 recognized symptoms of low blood sugar.)
5. Deficiencies of magnesium in the blood led to disorientation; severe deficiency caused delirium.

Many other studies can be mentioned that show abnormal behavior patterns. Among the most important are lack of enough B vitamins to metabolize carbohydrates.

1. Vitamin B1 deficiency causes agitation, confusion, depression and anxiety.
2. Vitamin B2 deficiency leads to depression.
3. Vitamin B3 deficiency brings about confusion, depression and/or psychosis.
4. Vitamin B6 deficiency leads to extreme nervousness and confusion.
5. Pantothenic acid deficiency causes depression and sullenness.
6. Iodine deficiency causes dullness and apathy in adults (Cheraskin et al., 1987).

Supplementing diets with various nutrients helped a wide variety of behavior problems.

1. Removing white sugar and white flour and supplying adequate protein and fats led to recovery from depression, violent temper, fatigue and irritability.

2. Vitamins and minerals in supplement form and supplements of glutamate led to behavior improvement in elderly schizophrenics.
3. Supplements of L-methionine or L-tryptophan (both are amino acids—eggs are good sources) led to significant improvement in schizophrenics.

You may think, "My child is not schizophrenic," and you're probably right. But behavior problems in school are often the forerunner of schizophrenia. If nothing is done about the behavior problems by the time a child is a teenager, he may become schizophrenic. And the only help is from food and supplements.

4. Vitamin C supplements brought improvement in depression and paranoid symptoms plus overall personality improvement.
5. Intramuscular B12 injections brought complete recovery from severe depression, anxiety and paranoia.

In addition, a high bromide intake causes apathy, delirium and memory loss. Bromide is found in soft drinks and in drugs. In large amounts it causes severe mental illness.

You may be thinking that different nutrients clear up the same problems. That's true, and you don't know which one will apply to your child, or which nutrients you'll need to give your high school senior to improve his arithmetic performance. The answer is—give all nutrients. Dr. Roger J. Williams says that we need the whole team. All the nutrients work together, so we can never take just one or even a few and expect good results.

Rimland (1974) conducted a study of 191 children with behavior disorders. They were given a potent B complex and several grams of vitamin C. After two weeks, B3 and B6 were added in dosages several hundred times the usual (which is 1 to 2 mg). Later, large amounts of pantothenic acid were added. Doses were based on the child's weight.

A few of the children became irritable, hyperactive and sensitive to sounds, and they wet the bed. Rimland got a phone call from Adelle Davis, who had helped him work out the diet. She asked if he were giving magnesium, which he was not. She told him the symptoms he would see without magnesium, and they were exactly the ones he had observed: hyperactivity, irritability, sensitivity to sound and bed-wetting.

Rimland said that in future studies he would use minerals with the vitamins. This study was reported in 1974.

Results showed that with the high dosages of vitamins, 66.5 percent were definitely helped.

Some of the comments of the parents given a few weeks after the study:

"Frustration level extremely high without the vitamins. Much yelling and irritability. Changes were evident after three days of no vitamins and grew worse each following day."

"Without the vitamins, he no longer showed the lively interest in the world around him that had marked the previous month."

"With vitamins, he improved in every area on the checklist. Without the vitamins, he is agitated and crying practically all the time."

Hyperactivity

The medical textbooks have no definite cause for hyperactivity. They say it may be due to brain damage: probably from birth injuries, infections, premature birth, difficult labor, small-at-birth babies or maybe from lack of oxygen at delivery (Thurston, 1976).

Some investigators think the difficulty is caused by lead poisoning. *Lancet*, a British medical journal, proved that more lead is in the tissues, especially of the brain, than in normal children. It's possible to get rid of lead from the system by eating kelp or amino acid–chelated calcium. Both substances attract lead and carry it out of the body. Calcium, iron and zinc are especially important in eliminating lead. These healthful minerals are found in natural foods, especially whole grains, vegetables and whole fruits.

The symptoms are different in different children. The children may be restless, impulsive and even destructive at times. They resent being corrected or restrained. They are easily excited and have a short attention span. They can seem to be interested in something, then all of a sudden go off on a tangent. They may be quarrelsome, and may have problems with muscular coordination. They may rock back and forth or sometimes knock their heads against the floor or wall. As they get older, they usually have problems in school (Thurston, 1976).

Ritalin Is Dangerous

The medical treatment often used is Ritalin. Ritalin is a stimulant for adults, but it also calms children down. These treatments have sometimes been disastrous, but, nevertheless, 243 million Ritalin tablets were sold in 1970. Two million persons took the drug and 50 percent of total sales were used for hyperactivity. A 10-year-old boy was treated with 5 mg a day of Ritalin; every week, the dosage was increased by 5 mg a day. At 15 mg a day, the boy had grand mal seizures. Other children treated with Ritalin had growth retardation (Feingold, 1973).

Drugs are not effective in most cases. Even if they calm the child and help other symptoms, they never cure, because they don't get to the cause of the trouble (Cott, 1973).

But nutritionists have had outstanding success with diet and vitamin therapy. It is well known that Dr. Ben Feingold's diet for hyperactivity—eliminating artificial colors and flavors—has helped many children. But Dr. Feingold's original theories did not go far enough. He allowed white sugar and white flour. His diet calmed children down, but it did not keep them well. Toward the end of his life, he realized that sugar is often a problem.

Some of my nutrition students have been teachers who have taught children with hyperactivity. One fourth-grade teacher in an affluent school said that about half of her students were on Ritalin. The usual procedure is that, if a child doesn't stay in his seat and keep quiet, his parents are told he is hyperactive, and he should be given drugs. The school counselor "cooperates," doctors prescribe drugs and the treatment begins. The child may become a zombie; he may never be normal. It may never be known what the child is really like when he isn't drugged.

According to Dr. Michael Lesser of the University of California at Berkeley (1977), "When children are given drugs to control behavior problems, we are setting a time bomb that eventually is going to explode in tremendous numbers of schizophrenics, psychotics and mentally ill people who will be ill for life."

The drug keeps the child quiet in school so that he doesn't disturb the teacher and the other students, but it doesn't help what has caused the problem.

A NEW DIET NEEDED

What these children need is a new diet. Here are some guidelines.

Protein: Fish, poultry (from the health food store), no more than two glasses of milk, eggs, cheese, red meat (muscle meat—steaks, roasts, chops, hamburgers, only in small amounts, 2 to 4 ounces at one serving). Plenty of plant proteins—whole grains combined with legumes (beans, peas and peanuts—always cooked).

Fats: In moderate amounts, some saturated from animals (butter, cheese and eggs are the best) and some unsaturated from vegetables (nuts and seeds are the best).

Carbohydrates: No refined carbohydrates such as white sugar and white flour and products made from them are allowed. Complex carbohydrates in large amounts—beans, whole grains, vegetables and whole raw fruits; no fruit juice.

Multivitamins and minerals: Emphasis on vitamin C, B complex and especially pantothenic acid (Moriarty, 1974).

Hazards to the body from overeating moderate amounts of protein are nil, but the effects of deficiency are severe. B6 is needed for practically every step in protein metabolism. If we don't have enough B6, we can't benefit from protein even if we eat enough. It's hard to get enough B6 because the whole grains aren't good sources—animal foods are the best sources. Also, B6 is not returned to white flour as "enrichment."

We have many children with hyperactivity and psychological problems because of the greater use of sugar and white flour. But we can immediately begin to change these diets without a lengthy series of tests. They need all nutrients—about 20 vitamins, 20 minerals, 8 amino acids, carbohydrates, fats and water. Also, we need to absorb what we take in. Thus, digestive enzymes may be necessary for a short while (Smith, 1976).

B6 Helps Protein

Vitamin B6 helps metabolize almost all nutrients. Severe deficiencies may lead to convulsions. If a person is twitchy, jumpy, restless, a worrier or has insomnia, he may need B6. All nutrients should be given with it. If the B complex is unbalanced, deficiencies of some of the B's may show up. For example, if too much B6 is given, a deficiency of B2 may appear. One sign of the deficiency is cracks in the corners of the mouth.

Hyperactivity is related to low serotonin levels. Serotonin is a neurotransmitter that helps impulses travel along the nerves in the brain. B6 helps increase the levels of serotonin. All the other B vitamins are needed to metabolize carbohydrates so that the brain and all other cells will have energy (Smith, 1976).

B3 helps lower the levels in the brain of harmful chemicals that are related to schizophrenia.

Vitamin D helps absorb calcium. Calcium and magnesium have a calming effect on hyperactive children. Sometimes children need one or the other or both. The amount usually taken, however, is about one-half as much magnesium as calcium.

Vitamin E protects cells from pollutants and affects many enzyme systems, especially in the liver. Exercise reduces the level of vitamin E, so people who exercise heavily may need more E. E helps reduce muscle cramps as do vitamin D and calcium. Dr. Lendon Smith says that 100 to 400 units daily of vitamin E seems like a good idea for anyone who is "breathing, eating or drinking." He says start with 100 and work up.

There are cautions with vitamin E. If you've ever had congestive heart failure or rheumatic heart disease, then don't take E without your physician's permission. If you now have high blood pressure or diabetes, start with 30 units and go up 30 each month. At the end of a year, you'll be taking 360 a day. (Passwater, 1976). See the chart in Lesson 1 for more information about vitamin E.

Eliminate Fruit Juice

Many children are drinking too much sugar when they drink fruit juice. We have two special factors to consider about fruit juice.

1. How much hydrochloric acid is in the stomach.
2. How fast we metabolize or use our foods—that is, the Basic Metabolic Rate.

If these two are functioning, the body can break down the organic acids from fruits and vegetables, otherwise the body will be too acid. Acidosis is a dangerous ailment.

Also, the sugar in fruit juices is too concentrated for children or others to drink. We get one teaspoon of natural sugar in one apple. If we press the apples and drink a glass of apple juice, we get about four teaspoons of sugar, which is too much at one time. We would never eat four apples at one time. It is better to eat fruits whole, raw and ripe.

The Feingold Association is famous all over the country for relieving some cases of hyperactivity by eliminating artificial colors and flavors. A certain percentage of the children respond well to this treatment, as anyone would think, since many foods that have artificial colors and flavors are also foods that have white sugar and white flour and are certainly not whole, natural foods.

The Feingold Association reported on a study of 32 children who went on the Feingold diet. Eleven had an "excellent response," eight were judged as "probably improved" and 13 "had no response."

Possibly with the elimination of white sugar and white flour from the diet, the percentage of "excellent responses" would have been higher.

Physicians may not know how dangerous sugar can be. A young mother told me on the phone one day, "My 19-month-old son was born with a heart defect—a hole between the two lower chambers of the heart. He has not eaten well and now he is so thin that I asked my doctor how I could fatten him up." The doctor said, "Sprinkle sugar on everything he eats—he'll gain weight." (Of course, this is just the opposite of what should be done.)

Megavitamin Therapy

Megavitamin and orthomolecular therapy have helped very disturbed and hyperactive children. Megavitamin therapy means getting extra amounts of certain nutrients, whereas orthomolecular therapy means getting the right amount of any substance normally found in the body.

B6 is often in short supply, but it is used in five of the twelve known disorders involving genetic vitamin dependency. Vitamin "dependency" means that the person inherited a need for a high amount of a certain vitamin. Vitamin "deficiency" means a person needs just an average amount, but he isn't getting it.

These are newly discovered diseases, and the amount of vitamins used is much higher than the usual vitamin needs. When children need and get larger amounts, they are less hyperactive, and they can concentrate better and pay attention longer. Therefore they learn better and are eager to learn.

With orthomolecular therapy, sometimes results are quick and dramatic. But sometimes it takes two to six months to notice a difference. The hyperactivity subsides slowly. But with drugs, the hyperactivity may or may not be controlled.

Nutrients for Children and Family

The children should keep to the diet; in fact, the whole family should be on the diet and on moderate amounts of all nutrients in supplement form. The problem children may need larger than usual doses of the B's.

Other nutrients used are vitamin E, folic acid, glutamic acid and pangamic acid (B15). The latter two have been shown to raise IQs in both mentally retarded and normal children.

Some people seem to convert harmless nutrients—for example, wheat—to harmful substances. Celiac disease and learning disabilities occur in the same people more often than not, and they have many common features. Mild malnutrition can cause children to be "picky eaters." They sometimes gag on certain foods. Sometimes they swallow the foods then vomit.

There are many fringe benefits of a low-sugar diet. When kids are taken off sugar, their teeth don't decay as much, they aren't sick as much and they get better grades in school. Often parents of such children insist they are being well fed. It is always a pleasant surprise when these children improve so much.

ALLERGIES

Many investigators are describing food allergies that cause behavior problems as "cerebral allergies" (Hawley and Buckley, 1974). This subject has been discussed fully in Lesson 4. Let's review it here.

Children with allergies may have mental symptoms such as disinterest in learning and thus be called "learning disabled." Often the symptoms are called "minimal brain dysfunction," but if the allergies improve, the brain dysfunction is gone.

Here are the most common signs of such allergies:

1. Not reading at their age level, poor spelling, difficulty with arithmetic, poor visual-motor coordination.
2. Poor painting, writing or drawing; inability to copy simple designs.
3. Clumsiness or awkwardness.
4. Hyperactivity, talkativeness, disorganized thinking.
5. Impulsiveness, antisocial behavior, nonconforming in school.
6. Quick temper, irritability and aggressiveness.
7. Short attention span.
8. Poor finger coordination, slow speech development.
9. Abnormal brain-wave test.

We actually get allergies because we can't digest our food. Proteins should be broken down into amino acids, carbohydrates to simple sugars and fats to fatty acids. Then these small molecules go into the bloodstream and circulate through the blood to every cell in the body. There, they build up the special kinds of proteins, carbohydrates and fats that make up our bodies—hair, muscles, eyes, bone, nerves, brain cells and all others (Tintera, 1958).

Enzymes Needed

If we don't have enough enzymes to break down the large molecules, they get into our bloodstream and go to our cells. These are foreign invaders, whether from food we've eaten and haven't digested or from something we've breathed in, such as pollen, dust or chemicals. Any time we have allergies, it's because some substance got into our tissues that didn't belong there, and our immune system was too weak to get rid of it. Roast beef is good food, but it doesn't belong in our cells. The amino acids broken down from the roast beef do belong in our cells.

We also breathe in foreign substances that get in the bloodstream and tissues. An inflammatory response is set up to get rid of the foreign particles. The response starts with the adrenal glands, which send hormones into the blood to make antibodies and other defensive substances that then go to the allergen and attack it. An allergic reaction won't take place because the allergen is destroyed by antibodies.

If anybody has unhealthy adrenal glands and there aren't any hormones to call out antibodies, the allergens will not be destroyed. The person has no protection from chemicals and other allergens. He is allergic.

While all this is going on, histamines are released into the blood. They are always released when a cell is damaged, whether by a foreign invader, by injury or by bacteria or viruses. At first the histamines are good; they are one of the defensive substances that help the inflammatory reaction by walling off the invaders and keeping them from scattering all over the body. But when histamines go through the liver they should be destroyed by an enzyme called histaminase. If our livers are not healthy, the enzyme is not manufactured and we keep piling up histamines in the bloodstream. Too many histamines irritate tissues. If you've ever had to take antihistamine drugs, it's because your own liver did not make enough histaminase to detoxify the histamines in your body.

The excess histamines cause allergic reactions, including cerebral allergies, which means that brain cells have an allergic reaction and this can lead to behavior problems.

Vitamins and minerals help us avoid allergies. Vitamin A helps keep our skin inside and outside the body in good condition. If the skin is sick, allergens can burrow into the tissues. Then the inflammatory reaction starts. We're like doughnuts; if something gets into the tube that goes from mouth to anus and is excreted, it doesn't harm our tissues. If our cells are healthy, the allergen is washed through the excretory systems by the mucus from the mucous membranes that line all the body cavities.

All of these so-called allergies are caused by unhealthy tissue in the body. If we eat well, we won't have allergies because our tissues will all be healthy. It is tragic for people to suffer from allergies for weeks or years when good food would make their immune systems so healthy that they would destroy the allergens.

Antioxidants Needed

Another important group of nutrients is called the antioxidants. They are vitamins E and C; selenium, a mineral; and methionine, an amino acid. These antioxidants keep oxygen from making our cells rancid. Holes appear in rancid cells, and allergens go right through those holes into the tissues. Anyone who doesn't eat enough antioxidants to stop the rancidity will have allergies.

White blood cells that get rid of the allergens cannot function without vitamin C.

Also, C keeps a lot of the poisonous substances out of the cells, and it destroys the substances that do get in. Both vitamin C and vitamin A build

healthy cells, especially mucous membranes, which will wash away the allergens.

We can build healthy adrenal glands if we feed them all 50 nutrients, plus lecithin and acidophilus or yogurt.

Importance of Digestion

Most nutritionists agree that people with allergies should take hydrochloric acid in the form of betaine hydrochloride with pepsin. This enzyme digests protein in the stomach and helps break it down to peptides. If the undigested protein goes on through the stomach and gets into the small intestine, it cannot be broken down to amino acids there because there aren't enough enzymes to break down proteins. There are just enzymes to break down peptides, but we didn't change the proteins to peptides!

Since small children can't swallow tablets, they won't be able to take hydrochloric acid. It is dangerous to hold the tablets in the mouth because they can burn the tongue. The child will begin to make his own digestive enzymes again when he has been on this food program long enough to make and repair all tissues. Until then, the child may have allergies or other ailments.

Our intestines can't be healthy unless they have more friendly bacteria than unfriendly. The unfriendly bacteria will be kept under control when we take acidophilus. It comes in powder, tablets or liquid. It doesn't take much, but some form of acidophilus should be taken almost daily until our stools are healthy. Healthy stools will be light colored, big around yet soft, they will float and they won't have a bad odor. If they're the opposite— that is, dark colored, hard and smelly—poisonous bacteria are plastered around the walls of the colon. They are picked up by the blood and deposited in any cell, causing disease anywhere in the body. Inspect your children's stools; feed them acidophilus and help them to get better fast.

Yogurt also helps clean out the bad bacteria. Get the "live culture" yogurt—that means the milk is pasteurized first, then cultured. Otherwise, if the culture is put in first, the heat of pasteurization kills the culture. Health food stores have live-culture yogurt. Better still, make your own!

A good diet and moderate amounts of nutrients in supplement form usually bring dramatic improvement quickly.

This entire therapy, says Dr. Michael Lesser (1977), will improve most sick people, and studies show that it has been used successfully in large groups of incorrigible teenagers, formerly treated unsuccessfully by psychiatric therapy.

Natural Foods

The diet of natural foods to clear up allergies is advocated by John Tintera (1958), who says allergies are signs of exhausted adrenal glands, and the glands must be rebuilt before allergies can be eliminated, whether they're cerebral or any other kind.

This rebuilding may take several months because sometimes adrenal glands contain scar tissue that must be replaced by healthy cells.

Livingston, writing in *Herald of Health* (March 1971), emphasizes that inadequate nutrition is the major cause of all types of allergies. Overeating refined carbohydrates; stimulants, such as coffee, tea and chocolate milk; and lack of protective nutrients (vitamins and minerals) cause foods not to be digested, poisons to get in the blood and mucous membranes to be so damaged that they can't wash away the allergens.

Dr. Lendon Smith says, "An allergist should refuse to treat patients if they eat white sugar and white flour. Sugar should not be in any home. Children should nibble on protein. All school candy machines should be axed down. Protein snacks should be in all classrooms. Criminals and alcoholics should all have five-hour glucose tolerance tests. Pregnant girls should be forced to nibble on protein and should have been given extra vitamins, minerals and glutamic acid for years before conception.

"If a child is moody, irritable, depressed or violent, is upset by crowds and cries more than he laughs, his diet should be changed" (Smith, 1976).

LOW BLOOD SUGAR

Low blood sugar causes mental and learning disabilities. The subject is discussed at length in Lesson 10.

The brain feeds on a kind of sugar called glucose. It has been estimated that a child needs about twice as much blood sugar as an adult needs.

The blood sugar can fall fast—from 150 to 60 in an hour or two. With a level of 60, a child can't think, because the brain doesn't have enough energy (fuel, glucose) for nerves to send messages.

The adrenal glands pour out hormones to raise blood sugar. Then there's so much for a while that the child may be hyperactive. But soon, the insulin from the pancreas takes sugar out of the blood, and the blood sugar drops. Again, the brain doesn't have enough energy for nerves to send messages. The child goes from too active to dull, nervous or irritable.

Headaches are common. Often a child is hyperactive, hyperexcitable or extra hungry before a headache. Sometimes children vomit when they live on fats, which cause acidosis.

Blood Sugar Seesaw

After days or weeks of this blood sugar seesaw, the children's adrenal glands are damaged, and they don't make enough hormones. Then there are real behavior problems. Their personalities change, they're crabby, they're always tired.

These changes are caused by too little sugar in the brain. But if the children eat sugar or white flour, they get worse. They need good sources of protein, but very little red (muscle) meat. Best proteins are chicken and eggs from the health food store, fish, dairy products and combinations of plant proteins such as whole grains and legumes. Many good combinations can be found: brown rice and red beans, lentil soup and wheat germ muffins, peanuts combined with whole-wheat crackers or with other nuts. Eggs and all dairy products go with both grains and legumes.

The Brain Suffers

When the blood sugar drops too low, the brain suffers because it doesn't get sufficient food. That's similar to when a diabetic gets an overdose of insulin, all the sugar enters the cells, and since there's none left in the blood, the person goes into a coma.

Hypoglycemics usually don't have such a drastic drop, but when blood sugar gets low, the adrenal glands secrete adrenaline, which pulls stored glucose from the liver and puts it into the blood. It also sets off a general alarm, and the body prepares for stress.

We feel apprehensive and shaky and our hearts beat fast. Our hands may be cold and clammy, and our breathing may be shallow.

We don't always have such severe responses; that depends on how low the blood sugar drops and how drastic the adrenal glands' response is.

The response can be determined by measuring breakdown products of adrenaline in the urine. If the products are there, it means a more or less continual stress situation with wear and tear on the adrenals and more exhaustion of the glands. This causes mental and emotional problems, increased irritability and difficulty in working with others. If this condition continues, it can cause ulcers, headache and general exhaustion.

The answer is not to eat refined carbohydrates, to get plenty of B vitamins and all minerals, especially chromium, which is part of the Glucose Tolerance Factor. Cream is a good source of chromium, so if anyone drinks milk, he should drink whole milk.

Fretful Children

Many irritable, fretful children suffer from hypoglycemia, but their parents don't realize it. When they finally do find out what's wrong, that junk food is causing the problem, they switch the children to natural foods and the fretfulness is gone.

Some mothers I talk with don't really understand why many of our foods are junk foods. They believe that one popular white, cooked cereal is fit to eat just because it has a lot of iron added to it. But there's nothing natural about it—almost everything good was removed in processing the whole grain to white cereal, and the iron put back in is not in a form that the body can use well. It's in a form that doesn't damage the machines that process the cereal.

Others think that gelatin desserts are healthful because gelatin has a lot of protein in it. But gelatin has such a high content of the amino acid glycine that it makes the rest of the amino acids deficient. Then there's all that sugar—much too much.

Here's the way hypoglycemia may affect an infant. Dr. Lendon Smith (1976) explains that a baby may get a cramp from something he ate or from not eating on time. He cries, and the stress of crying uses up more blood sugar; the adrenal glands pour out adrenaline, which sends more sugar from the liver to the blood. Usually this is enough, but he may be too exhausted to eat enough to replace his blood sugar, and he may not have enough stored.

Then he wakes up and cries again. If his parents don't feed him, his adrenals become more and more exhausted. If he is given sweet foods or fruit juice, or cola drinks in a bottle, the extra sugar aggravates the pancreas and may exhaust the insulin-producing cells. Older children also exhaust their pancreases by eating junk foods.

Children who wet the bed past age four, for example, don't get the message in their brains that they need to get up and go to the bathroom. Parents may think it is laziness or that the child has played so hard all day that he sleeps too soundly to get up. The next morning Mother fusses, but the part of the brain that hears Mother didn't know anything about the bed-wetting.

If the child has eaten sugar in the evening, his blood sugar level may fall so low in the night that his nerves can't carry the messages to the brain. Protein snacks are recommended before bed to keep the blood sugar level normal.

An exciting or worry-filled day may use up so much blood sugar that the level is very low, and the child's nerves don't carry messages. These children can even steal if they see candy in the supermarket; the nerves to their consciences don't work well enough to say, "Don't steal." Later, they may not even know what they did, because the brain may not have enough energy to remember things.

Thus our adrenal glands determine whether we are pleasant or unpleasant, calm or jittery, energetic or always tired. Even more important, they regulate our personalities and our ability to think. If they do a good job, it's because we feed them well.

The root of the trouble is sugar and white flour. If you would like to improve your child's personality and eliminate blood sugar problems, try feeding him only natural foods—no junk.

Babies and Chromium

Jeffrey Bland (1982) reports on a study of pregnant women whose hair chromium content was measured during several pregnancies. The hair was found to contain less and less chromium in succeeding pregnancies. This makes us realize the possibility of children being born with a blood sugar problem, since chromium is an important nutrient for the body's ability to tolerate glucose. For a child to be born with a normal ability to use glucose for brain fuel, the mother must have a normal glucose tolerance, which depends on the amount of chromium available to her cells.

AUTISM, HEAVY METAL POISONING AND SUICIDES

Learning and behavior problems may be mild or so severe that they lead to death.

Autism

Autism is a serious problem but it's relatively rare. Only three or four in 10,000 children are autistic (Cott, 1973). An autistic child may not speak, learning is impaired, behavior is bizarre and ritualistic.

Treatment with food supplements has dramatic results in many children. Sometimes it takes three to six months, but in many instances parents report a "miracle" response within one or two weeks.

Heavy Metal Poisoning

Children with minimal brain dysfunction, autism, hyperactivity, fatigue, depression, insomnia, anxiety, tension and phobias may have brain poisoning from pollutants such as lead, mercury or cadmium. A nervous illness is often the first sign of such poisoning (Lesser, 1977).

Lead poisoning can produce permanent damage, nervous disorders, hyperactivity, speech impairment, high blood pressure and even death (Pfeiffer, 1975).

Street dust that we breathe while riding in cars contains poisonous metals. The only defense is to eat foods high in calcium, magnesium and iron, which will help crowd out the dangerous metals.

One of the best sources of useful minerals is beans. They're excellent protein too, so be sure to encourage children to eat beans. Also excellent are whole grains such as wheat, rye, triticale (combination of wheat and rye), brown rice, corn, bulgur, buckwheat, oats and millet.

The best way to eat whole grains is as cereals from the health food store and in bread, crackers and muffins that you make yourself.

The brain may be damaged by the aluminum we eat as additives in processed foods. Patients with senile dementia have amounts of aluminum equal to the amounts in experimental animals given injections of aluminum (Pfeiffer, 1975).

Aluminum is added to processed cheese and to table salt to keep it from caking. One of the bleaching agents used to whiten flour is an aluminum compound. One more reason not to eat white flour!

Cott (1973) reports that school lunches were studied in 300 schools. The lunches should have provided one-third of the daily allowances of vitamins and minerals, but 14 percent of the children were deficient in calcium, 60 percent in magnesium and 20 percent of boys and 90 percent of girls in iron. They were marginal or deficient in chromium, copper and manganese.

He also notes that high levels of lead may cause mental deficiency. At a clinic in London, investigators found that half of the mentally retarded children had much more lead in their blood than the highest levels of a group of normal children. Most of the lead we take in is from auto exhaust, canned foods and water (Cott, 1973).

Animals that received lead in their drinking water absorbed four times as much lead when their diets were deficient in calcium as those with a normal intake of calcium.

Some investigators suggest the following nutrients to help rid the body of lead:

2,000 mg of vitamin C, morning and evening
30 mg zinc, morning and evening.

This is not a massive dose, and both of those nutrients are in short supply in many diets.

Suicide

Although this lesson is about young children, it is interesting to note an article in the *Houston Chronicle,* January 22, 1978, about adolescent suicides. Suicide is the second leading killer of young people. These adolescents were young children just a few years ago, and many of them were suffering then from stress and behavior problems that later led to suicide.

The pressures the children have to endure are the usual family, school and play problems, and drugs prescribed by doctors, especially antibiotics.

all of which damage the liver, causing sick cells anywhere in the body including the brain.

Specific signs of possible suicides in young people aged 10 to 19 are listed:

1. Mental depression
2. Sleeplessness
3. Loss of appetite
4. Weight loss
5. Headache and general aches and pains
6. Psychological symptoms such as lethargy, crying, apathy and inability to concentrate

These symptoms are identical to those of a vitamin B-complex deficiency. Thus, a child who is deficient in B vitamins and other nutrients may become a teenage suicide if the deficiency continues. It is so easy to try nutrition for these problems that it seems criminal not to try. Even if the child will eat nothing but cookies and other sweets, try sweets made with whole grains, butter, eggs, whole milk, carob rather than chocolate, and fortify them with wheat germ, bran, soy powder and plenty of nuts of all kinds for extra protein and vitamins. Other tasty treats are toasted sunflower, pumpkin and sesame seeds. Not many teenagers will turn down those excellent snacks. If he will not take supplements, sneak them into these foods also.

NUTRITIONAL TREATMENT

Let's review the foods we need to rebuild health. First, we eliminate all white sugar and white flour. No sugar is healthful, but almost any sugar can be used in moderation to make food palatable. When you get all the excellent food value in a cookie that I described in the preceding paragraph, the small amount of sugar in each bite will not detract too much from the healthful ingredients. It is a good idea to use date sugar or whole fruit as your major sweetener, but add the least amount possible of dark brown sugar if you have to, at first. Later, their tastes will change and they won't crave sugar. Many people say, "I'll never quit craving sugar." But they do.

You'll find excellent breads and dessert recipes in my cookbook, *Switchover!* or other health food cookbooks. Many of my counselees ask, "What can I give my family to replace the junk we've been eating?" Just browse through the cookbooks; you'll find something to appeal to everyone. They'll probably never want to go back to their old way of eating.

Proteins are of first importance. We should not eat much muscle meat (red meat—steaks, roasts, chops and hamburger). The amount suggested for adults is no more than four ounces four times a week. Adjust your child's protein intake according to his size. He should have plenty of protein because he's growing, and he uses protein for growth as well as for repair.

Here are some excellent protein choices: fish several times a week, one or two eggs a day—cook with extra eggs (the cholesterol scare is over); chickens and turkey from the health food store; cheese (light-colored and natural); whole milk—no more than ½ glass twice a day, and not really required; and combinations of whole grains, nuts, seeds and legumes (beans, peas and peanuts). No processed meat, especially bacon.

Carbohydrates include whole grains, vegetables both cooked and raw, and whole fruits—no fruit juice. Our major fats should be real butter, nuts and seeds.

As for vitamin and mineral supplements, those given in Lesson 1 in this course are recommended by the most respected nutritionists in this country.

Some children may need larger amounts of some nutrients. Ask a nutrition-minded physician to work with you. Some children will respond greatly when they eliminate all white sugar, white flour and bottled drinks.

In any case, drugs are dangerous; food is the answer. Food supplements provide nutrients that we can't get from our too-processed, too-refined food. We have to choose the food we put into our bodies carefully. But when we see the new way of life—mentally, physically and emotionally in our precious children and grandchildren—we know where our priorities will be from now on for the rest of our lives.

QUESTIONS

TRUE/FALSE

1. In Dr. Harrell's experimental study, supplements of vitamins and minerals were given, especially large amounts of B complex.

2. Symptoms of depression affect as many as 20 percent of the population at any one time.

3. L-glutamine has helped increase the IQs of learning-disabled children.

4. A child's diet should be changed to good food as soon as possible, because if he doesn't improve by his mid-teens, he may go on to delinquency.

5. Some people need 20 times as many vitamins and minerals as others.

6. When there is something wrong with the brain cells and their food supply, there is mental illness, because the brain cells can't get what they need unless we eat the right kind of food.

7. Our bodies can be trained to utilize good food, but malnutrition can cause a variety of health problems.

8. Often the first signs of improved brain power are increased attention span, better learning ability and cooperation with parents and teachers.

9. In a controlled study, vitamin supplements improved the condition of normal children from 25 percent to 3,200 percent.

10. In a study, B12 in muscular injections brought complete recovery from severe depression, anxiety and paranoia.

11. There are no hazards in overeating moderate amounts of protein, but the effects of deficiency are severe.

12. To reduce muscle cramps, take vitamin E, vitamin D and calcium.

13. Friendly bacteria in the intestines are more plentiful if we eat yogurt almost daily.

MULTIPLE CHOICE

1. List the items needed to improve the brains of slow learners: (a) B complex, (b) sugary foods, (c) no more than two glasses of milk a day, (d) whole fruits.

2. Note the improvements made by the boy on Dr. Harrell's program: (a) ability to talk, (b) ability to read and write, (c) advancement in arithmetic, (d) IQ increased to 90.

3. List the nutrients found to be the most deficient in a study done by the Department of Agriculture: (a) vitamin A, (b) vitamin C, (c) calcium, (d) vitamin B6.

4. List the disorders that respond to nutritional therapy: (a) fatigue, (b) mild depression, (c) insomnia, (d) poisoning from food additives.

5. List the requirements of a diet for learning-disabled and hyperactive children: (a) man-made chemicals, (b) refined carbohydrates, (c) supplements of vitamins and minerals.

6. Food and food supplements have helped children improve their ailments such as: (a) allergies, (b) asthma, (c) disagreeable behavior, (d) cerebral palsy.

7. List the nutrients especially needed by depressed people: (a) vitamin B1, (b) vitamin B2, (c) biotin, (d) folic acid.

8. The following supplements brought improvement to learning-disabled children: (a) vitamin C, (b) L-glutamine, (c) lecithin and B1, (d) vitamin B3 and vitamin E.

9. List the signs of hyperactivity in children: (a) restlessness, (b) impulsiveness, (c) short attention span, (d) quarrelsomeness.

10. B6 deficiencies may be present if a person is: (a) twitchy, (b) jumpy, (c) a worrier or (d) has insomnia.

11. Fringe benefits of a low sugar diet include: (a) less tooth decay, (b) fewer illnesses, (c) better grades in school.

12. List valid blood sugar conditions: (a) at a blood sugar level of 60, a child can't think, (b) the brain feeds on glucose, (c) too little sugar in the brain causes personality changes.

ANSWERS

True/False

1. T 2. T 3. T 4. T 5. T 6. T 7. T 8. T
9. T 10. T 11. T 12. T 13. T

Multiple Choice

1. a,c,d 2. a,b,c,d 3. a,b,c 4. a,b,c,d 5. c 6. a,b,c,d
7. a,b,c,d 8. a,b,c,d 9. a,b,c,d 10. a,b,c,d 11. a,b,c
12. a,b,c

REFERENCES

Ballentine, R. *Diet and Nutrition, A Holistic Approach.* Honesdale, PA: The Himalayan International Institute, 1978.

Bland, J. JIAPM 34(2), Fall 1982.

Brown, C. (in) *Diet Related to Killer Diseases V, Nutrition and Mental Health.* Washington, DC: U.S. Gov't. Printing Office, 1977.

Cheraskin, E., Ringsdorf, W.M. and Clark, J.W. *Diet and Disease.* New Canaan, CT: Keats, 1987.

Cott, A. *J. of Appl. Nutr.,* 25 (1,2):15–24, 1973.

———. Pangamic Acid: B15. (in) *A Physician's Handbook on Orthomolecular Medicine.* New York: Pergamon Press, 1977.

Eiduson, S., Geller, E., Yuwiler, A. and Eiduson, B.T. *Biochemistry and Behavior.* Princeton: D. Van Nostrand, 1964.

Feingold, B. Food Additives and Hyperactivity in Children. *Congressional Record,* Oct. 30, 1973.

Goodhart, R.S. and Shils, M.E. *Modern Nutrition in Health and Disease.* Philadelphia: Lea and Febiger, 1973.

Green, R.G. *Doctors Speak.* New York: Huxley Institute for Biosocial Research, 1970.

Hardy, M.C. and Hoefer, C. (in) *Diet and Disease* by Cheraskin, E. et al. New Canaan, CT: Keats, 1968.

Hoffer, A. Nutrition and Behavior. (in) *Medical Applications of Clinical Nutrition,* J. Bland (Ed.). New Canaan, CT: Keats, 1983.

Houston Post, Section 2B, Wednesday, Nov. 12, 1975.

Hunter, B.T. *The Great Nutrition Robbery.* New York: Scribner's, 1978.

Knobloch, H. and Pasamanik, B. (in) *Diet and Disease* by Cheraskin, E. et al. New Canaan, CT: Keats, 1968.

Lesser, M. (in) Diet Related to Killer Diseases V, *Nutrition and Mental Health.* Washington, DC: U.S. Gov't. Printing Office, 1977.

Lublin, J.S. Food for Work or Sex? (in) Diet Related to Killer Diseases V, *Nutrition and Mental Health.* Washington, DC: U.S. Gov't. Printing Office, 1977.

Passwater, R. Solgar (3). Lynbrook, NY 11563.

Pfeiffer, Carl C. *Mental and Elemental Nutrients.* New Canaan, CT: Keats, 1975.

President's Commission on Mental Health. *Washington Post,* A-22, Apr. 28, 1978.

Rimland, B. An Orthomolecular Study of Psychotic Children. *Ortho. Psy.,* 3(4):371–77, 1974.

Rosenfeld, A. and Klivington, K.W. Inside the Brain, The Last Great Frontier. *Saturday Review,* Aug. 9, 1975.

Schellhardt, T.D. Can Chocolate Turn You Into a Criminal? (in) Diet Related to Killer Diseases V, *Nutrition and Mental Health.* Washington, DC: U.S. Gov't. Printing Office, 1977.

Smith, L. *Improving Your Child's Behavior Chemistry.* Englewood Cliffs, NJ: Prentice Hall, 1976.

Thurston, E.W. *Nutrition for Tots to Teens.* New Canaan, Conn.: Keats, 1979.

Tintera, J. What You Should Know About Your Glands and Allergies. *Woman's Day,* Feb. 1958.

Williams, R.J. *Biochemical Individuality.* New York: John Wiley and Sons, 1956.

———. *Nutrition Against Disease.* New York: Pitman, 1971.

Lesson 12

WEIGHT CONTROL AND NUTRITION

LESSON 12—WEIGHT CONTROL AND NUTRITION

WE GET LETTERS

"ONE REMARKABLE result of my new diet and food supplement program is the cessation of my constant hunger—this is really remarkable to me. I am satisfied with less food, but feeling satisfied is a new situation for me. I used to feel constant hunger, even when full. Thank you for your great advice."

If you were a nutritionist with a weight-loss/good-health program, how would you feel if you got a letter like that? Just the way I felt—delighted!

One woman who had been sick (and fat) for years wrote, "I've been on your diet only eight days. I've felt better than I have since I was 11 years old (now about 40). The first night on the diet, I kept waking my husband saying, 'I feel good.' Besides, I've already lost five pounds, and I haven't been hungry. The food is so satisfying and tastes so good, it's a pleasure to be on this food program."

Another letter: "I am very happy with the way the diet is making me feel. I am almost down to my former weight, I don't ache all over, and I am not so tired all the time."

Still another: "I feel good with more energy. I have been taking the food and vitamin supplements for six weeks now and have lost 10 pounds. In previous attempts at dieting I would feel so tired that I would have to either go to bed, which was impossible with children to take care of, or eat, which is what I did. Now I am feeling good, eating about 1,500 calories per day, and losing weight slowly."

A WEIGHT-LOSS PROGRAM

With such reports of this weight-loss program, I'm convinced of its value, and I'm sure you will be too, when you try it. It's really strange that many fat people eat less than their thin friends, but surveys show that it's true (Goodhart and Shils, 1973). Garrow says that the mechanism that maintains energy balance is not understood. The explanation given by Roger J. Williams (1971) may not be "understood" by everyone, probably because they haven't read it, but it makes such good sense to me, and it works for so many people, judging by the letters I get and by what people tell me, that I think if Williams' research were more widely publicized, many more fat folks would turn into the slender, lithe people they dream of becoming.

Do you ever starve yourself, trying to lose weight, then step on the scale and find that you've gained a pound or two? Williams (1971) explains what happens in a case like that. It's because the water content of the body varies. A 150-pound man's body contains about 93 pounds of water and 57 pounds of dry material—protein, carbohydrate, fat and minerals. The next time he weighs, the water may weigh 100 pounds, and he has gained weight. The water content of individuals varies from about 45 percent to 70 percent. Men's bodies contain about 10 percent more water than women's bodies. Our 150-pound man may contain from 81 pounds of solids down to 45 pounds.

When a fat person begins to feel better than he ever has before, he is energetic, active and eager all at the same time—eager to eat the good food that has done so much for him. Then he becomes more active—it's impossible to sit still or lie around all day when you're energetic. The new way of life becomes a happy cycle of small, delicious meals and active work and play.

This is no ordinary diet like those you've tried before and couldn't stay on because it took so much self-discipline that neither you nor anyone else could be happy on it. When you cut calories too much, you suffer from mental depression and finally you think, "It isn't worth it." Then you go on a binge and eat more than you should, mostly junk food. To make up for that, you go without eating until you again say, "It isn't worth it." So you eat, and this vicious cycle continues.

HOW FAT STARTS

Fat cells are always being formed and replaced. Excess glucose is changed to fat, and refined carbo-hydrates and alcohol are changed to triglycerides. Then these fats are broken down for energy. But fat people use less energy, so not as much fat is used as is deposited (Schauf, 1976).

Very few studies have been done with humans on how often food is fed. But several have been done with rats. When rats are fed one meal a day, they store much more fat than when they eat several meals. When the rats are allowed to nibble (the way humans on my program do when they eat six small meals and snacks a day) they use their food for energy, and they don't store it as fat.

Some people eat little or no breakfast and lunch, and eat a big meal at night. They probably complain often and loudly: "Everything I eat turns to fat."

The rats fed one meal a day gained much fat and also lost almost 50 percent of lean tissues. This is explained this way: When the rats eat their entire ration at one meal, the liver can't store that much sugar, and it goes on into the blood. It then calls out insulin, which takes the sugar out of the blood so we won't have diabetes, and puts it into the fat cells in the tissues.

Hormones and Nerves Help Use Fats

Hormones and nerves pull fats out of fat cells. Adrenaline, noradrenaline, growth hormone, thyroid hormone, cortisone and ACTH all help mobilize fat. Physical exertion also helps. But if all the nutrients needed to make those hormones aren't in the diet, there's no chance to get the fat out of the fat cells. Often obese people are tired and don't have the energy to exercise. If they would just eat the nutrients to make the hormones, they would immediately feel so much peppier that they would exercise more. This would lead to fat stores being reduced. Adelle Davis always said, "Just improve the diet, and weight will take care of itself."

When we eat refined carbohydrates (white sugar and white flour), we increase fat stores; when we eat complex carbohydrates (green leafy vegetables, whole fruits, whole grains and legumes) plus proteins from dairy products, fish and poultry from the health food store, we get so many nutrients that our energy is high and we decrease our fat stores.

When fat is being stored in the fat cells, obesity is being produced; when it is leaving fat cells and being burned as energy for all our cells, obesity is diminished.

About 80 million people in this country are overweight (Fox, 1983). No doubt all 80 million long to be slim. Most of them go on weight-loss diets and lose a few pounds, but 96 percent will gain all their weight back within one year. Then they try another diet, lose a little, gain it back and continue that yo-yo lifestyle, maybe for years.

Many people decide they will lose weight quickly, and they exercise a lot and try to sweat off their weight. That's pretty easy to do, but it's even easier to put it back on. It may take two or three days, but everyone must drink water, and when the water is replaced, the weight returns. Taking weight off and putting it on jeopardizes the health of the body, because minerals needed by every cell are lost for a few days until the water builds back up and replaces the minerals (Fox, 1983).

Complex Carbohydrates Are Important

Another way to lose weight advocated by people not interested in good health is to cut down on the amount of carbohydrate you eat. We've heard that we should eat low-carbohydrate diets, but we should really eat *high-complex* carbohydrate diets and *low-refined* carbohydrate diets. We give up white sugar and white flour completely, and eat a high-fiber diet of whole grains, legumes (beans, peas and peanuts), vegetables and whole fruits. Without sufficient carbohydrate, the body doesn't have enough energy, and it begins to lose water. Minerals are lost at the same time, and without sodium, magnesium, potassium and other minerals, muscles can't contract. Since the heart is a muscle, the heart will quit beating if the condition becomes severe. This is actually how about 20 percent of our heart attacks happen—deficiency of minerals because we eat a lot of junk food that has had the minerals processed out.

The fat stored around the body must be burned off if the weight loss program succeeds without damage. This is a slow but safe way to lose. If you eat natural foods and exercise sensibly, you'll lose slowly; but you'll feel good, and you'll keep the weight off if you follow the diet.

Fox (1983) suggests that his patients carry a plastic bag full of fresh raw vegetables to tide them over between meals.

CHANGING THE DIET

Some people may think that eating quality food will be "hard." I often hear this from my counselees. What I think is "hard" is to be sick—or fat! To be slim and healthy is easy. It means giving up junk food, which is easy if you want to. It means making your own baked goods—brads, crackers, muffins, biscuits, even cookies—which is easy. About 70 percent of the average American diet is refined sugar, white flour and fat. And too much of the other 30 percent is canned vegetables, too-sweet fruit juice and canned fruit with very little food value. Giving up these nonfoods is easy because you lose weight and feel good doing it.

Proteins

Although protein foods are of first importance—that's what the word "protein" means—we can't live on protein. The more protein we eat, the more calcium, magnesium and other nutrients we need. Dieters don't often eat high-mineral foods such as whole-grain breads and cereals, fresh vegetables and nuts and seeds. They usually think the carbohydrate foods, nuts and seeds are fattening. But in small amounts they're essential; for one thing, they contain magnesium. A deficiency of magnesium makes people nervous. We can't afford to ruin our nerves!

When we don't eat enough carbohydrates, fat isn't completely burned in the body. Ketone bodies are formed. The ketones must be excreted by the kidneys, but if the kidneys are overloaded, the ketones accumulate in the blood. This causes acidosis, an unbalanced acid condition of the body that is dangerous if it continues.

This problem occurs in starvation, fasting or crashing dieting, or in a high-fat diet. In these conditions, we don't eat enough carbohydrate to burn fat. It also happens in diabetes, when there is not enough insulin to put sugar into the tissues.

The major effect of acidosis on the body is depression of the central nervous system. An individual first becomes disoriented then later goes into a coma. The best remedy for this problem is to eat moderate amounts of carbohydrate in a diet containing all nutrients (Guyton, 1976).

Fats

We have to cut down on fat—way down. The best animal fats are butter, cream and egg yolk. We eat these in moderation. We eat one or two eggs a day.

We eat very little fat from meat because we eat very little red meat (steaks, roasts, chops and hamburger). The average American intake of fat is about 42 percent of calories. It should be 10 to 20 percent of calories.

We eat nuts and seeds that are polyunsaturated fats and contain linoleic acid, an essential fatty acid (we can't live without it). The average adult needs from three to six small measures of nuts and seeds. A small measure is two teaspoons of pumpkin, sunflower or sesame seeds; two walnut halves; four pecan halves; six almonds or 12 peanuts. We use fat for energy from the neck down and glucose (a kind of sugar) from the neck up. If you need larger amounts of fat than the average, you can gradually increase those amounts until you get the amount that is right for you. (See Lesson 1.) Let's remember that moderation is important in all things. Fat will burn fat if we eat it in small amounts throughout the day.

Food Supplements

People who diet to lose weight should take food supplements. Fat people are overfed but undernourished; they aren't active enough to burn off the calories they eat. In fact, about all they get in their food is empty calories. Many vitamins and minerals are missing. Even so, when they diet to lose weight, the few vitamins and minerals are almost completely eliminated. So they must take vitamin and mineral supplements, as we all do, because so much of the food value is processed out of our food.

We'll discuss the diet and food supplements in detail at the end of the lesson.

Fiber

Eating a high-fiber diet is not only helpful but also a most pleasant way to lose weight. High-fiber foods are whole grains, legumes, vegetables and whole fruits. All these foods are complex carbohydrates, and they should make up 60 to 80 percent of our calories, whether we're fat or thin.

If we need to gain weight, we eat more high-starch vegetables such as potatoes, both sweet and white, plus a little more fat. Other high-fiber foods such as grains and beans don't add many calories. They do add food value, as they are first broken down by enzymes; then the fiber is somewhat broken down by bacteria in the intestines (Monte and Vaughan, 1982).

We have about three pounds of microorganisms in our intestines. If we eat fibrous foods, which are easily and quickly passed through the body, we will have more friendly bacteria, which will help get rid of the unfriendly, poisonous bacteria. If we eat no fiber, if our diet consists of white sugar and flour, corn and potato chips, processed meats, soft drinks, candy bars and milk, we will build up the colonies of poisonous bacteria, and the friendly bacteria will be crowded out. In that case, gas builds up, with bloating and a too-full feeling after meals. Many people complain of this condition. Some of them tell me they can't even drink water without getting gas.

High-fiber foods are filling, and we have to chew them more, so we don't eat so much. Also, chewing causes secretion of more saliva and gastric juice, which makes us feel more satisfied with less food. With high-fiber foods, we don't absorb nutrients in the intestines so fast, but we do get the food value; we must absorb the nutrients more slowly.

I've always said, "Don't drink fruit juice," and Monte (1981) quotes a study in which animals were given either apple sauce (high fiber, low sugar) or apple juice (no fiber, high sugar). The animals receiving apple juice showed a much lower level of blood sugar an hour after the meal. This is because the high content of sugar in the juice causes the pancreas to overreact and secrete so much insulin that too much sugar is taken out of the blood. The resulting low blood sugar leads to depression and fatigue that say "EAT." Gorging often follows; the body is trying to counteract those symptoms and about 98 others that may go with low blood sugar.

It isn't enough just to put food into our mouths, we must assimilate it. Our protein and fat will be well digested if we eat moderate amounts of fiber at the same time. If we don't eat any carbohydrate, we will always lose protein (nitrogen) from the body (Monte, 1981). However, an experiment in which humans were given five to seven oranges a day showed a significant loss of protein and fat. Obviously, those two nutrients were swept out of the body too fast for digestion. But we know better than to eat five to seven oranges a day. Our middle name is "moderation," and that is *not* a moderate amount of oranges.

When six humans were given from 86 to 100 percent of their food as whole-wheat bread, they couldn't easily digest the oil in the grain. Also, one person had tetany (muscle twitchings and cramps) because of the low level of calcium in the diet. Other grains cause the same problem if we eat too much. That's why we need to be moderate and why we should stay on this natural food program as it is written. A high-fiber diet does not cause loss of vitamins; in fact, just the reverse seems to be true.

When we change our diet to one that keeps us healthy, energetic and slim, we will gradually lose weight while we recover from fatigue, depression and overweight—all caused by a junk food diet.

Three Special Suggestions

Bland (1982) notes that maintaining proper weight is related to: (1) appetite, (2) the use of brown fat and (3) the amount of nutrients in our food, compared to the number of calories we eat.

Our ideal weight is determined mainly by the amount of oxygen we have in our tissues, which is determined by the amount of exercise we get and the amount of good food we eat. Almost everyone thinks that our ideal weight increases as we get older, but it is not so. With good food and exercise, we will weigh less and have less fat and water stored in our cells.

A way to measure the correct amount of exercise is to maintain the exercise pulse rate of about 180 beats a minute minus the age in years of the individual. This pulse should be maintained for between 10 and 15 minutes at a fairly constant rate. Any kind of exercise is good: bicycling, trampolining, rowing, jumping rope, dancing, swimming and racket sports. If you haven't been doing these exercises regularly, you could probably work up to the required pulse rate just by walking fast on level ground.

The second way to maintain proper weight is to "use" brown fat. Brown fat burns fat to help the body produce heat to keep us at a temperature of 98.6 degrees F. Thyroid hormone helps activate brown fat, as do vitamin C, zinc and copper. However, sodium inactivates brown fat and causes water and triglycerides to accumulate in the tissues. If we can exercise and keep our thyroid and adrenal glands working well and add some sunflower and sesame seeds to our diets, the brown fat will burn extra fat and we will not gain weight.

Third, people who are very much overweight will lose weight faster if they have small amounts of an excellent high-protein drink, such as the Super Health drink in Lesson 1, plus plenty of vitamins and minerals in supplement form. Then we add large amounts of vegetables, either steamed, made into soup, or raw, plus whole fruit but never fruit juice. This food program would be all you need for a few days to begin your new way of life. You will feel better, and you will not be hungry. Later, you can add a moderate amount of all vitamins and minerals. The diet in Lesson 1 will be your diet for the rest of your long, healthy, slim life.

Fish body oils that contain eicosapentaenoic acid (EPA) help keep weight off (and protect the heart while they're doing it), especially in people who have high triglycerides (caused primarily by eating white sugar and white flour). We can eat fish or take supplements of EPA, available at health food stores. This not only can help maintain our weight without gaining, but also it keeps the platelets in the blood from sticking together and causing fatty plaques that lead to heart attacks and strokes. Bland says that this program will help us stay young in body and healthy in mind and we'll be energetic and slim.

STATISTICS ON OBESITY

Anyone who is 20 pounds over his ideal weight is called obese. By this measurement, 25 percent of men over 30, and 40 percent of women over 40 are obese. The same figures are found in adolescents.

Overweight people have chronic diseases in pairs more often than people with normal weight. High blood pressure, for example, is found in normal-weight people with arthritis 1.47 times more than expected, but in overweight people, it is found 2.28 times more than expected. In adult diabetics, at least 80 percent are now or have been obese. When diabetics lose weight, sometimes both blood sugar and insulin levels become normal.

American men who weigh 20 percent above the normal amount have a 350 percent greater risk of dying (Cheraskin, 1987). About three percent of children in Great Britain are obese, and, in New York 10 percent of schoolboys are overweight. This is the same number of overweight 18-year-olds who signed up for the draft. Only half that many were underweight. Mild overweight doesn't seem to cause severe illness, but when a person gets to be 20 percent over his normal weight, there is a greater increase in later life of diabetes, hardening of the arteries, high blood pressure and kidney disease (Mann, 1974).

Do fat children grow up to be fat adults? Statistics show that 80 to 90 percent of them do. Also, three-fourths of overweight children have at least one overweight parent. The fatter the children, the fatter they usually are as adults, and the harder it is to lose weight.

Fat teenagers seem to be less active than those with normal weight. It is difficult for physicians who specialize in treating the obese to treat these children because drugs to reduce their appetites are useless. They must have food because they're growing. If they fast, ketosis sets in, and that's dangerous. Physicians suggest exercise to get rid of fat. In fact, since physicians have had so little success in reducing children's weight, the Committee on Nutrition of the American Academy of Pediatrics says, "... our ignorance" concerning the cause, disease state and treatment of obesity "is remarkable."

THE HYPOTHALAMUS REGION OF THE BRAIN

Probably the most helpful information about weight loss is understanding the function of a region in the brain called the hypothalamus. This region sets our appetite, and we will be able to lose weight easily and keep it off if our hypothalamus works. It sends a message through our nervous system when to eat and when to stop eating. Researchers know that the hypothalamus does this, and to test it, they assembled two groups of rats and put food in front of both of them. Then they cut the nerves on one side of the hypothalamus in the rats in Group A. The rats starved to death with food in front of them because they didn't get the message to eat. Then they cut the nerves on the other side of the hypothalamus in the rats in Group B. Those rats gorged themselves to death because they didn't get the message to stop eating.

No one cuts the nerve cells in the hypothalamus in humans, but some people don't get the message to eat and they become anorexic. Others don't get the message to stop eating, and they become obese or bulimic. Why didn't they get the messages? It was because the nerve cells were damaged by lack of nutrients and they couldn't make healthy cells.

Neurotransmitters

How do the messages flow from one nerve cell (neuron) to another so everybody will get the message and not be too thin or too fat? Messages travel on neurotransmitters, which are chemicals manufactured in the axon of one neuron and sent to a receptor on another neuron. The receptor either accelerates the nerve to "eat" or inhibits the nerve to "not eat," whichever is needed at the time.

When all our neurotransmitters receive the nutrients they need, our weight stays within bounds, so we are neither too thin nor too fat. But we know many people do not have their weight under control, and they need to gain or lose. What has happened to the messages that should say "eat" or "stop eating"?

The neurons could not manufacture the neurotransmitters because the ingredients needed to make them were not available. Those ingredients are not provided by the brain itself; they are in the blood that flows through the capillaries in the brain. There is no way for the brain cells to get the nutrients they need to make neurotransmitters except from the food we eat at each meal, which then goes to the blood and to each cell in the brain.

Ingredients for Neurotransmitters

1. *Enzymes* are catalysts that make all reactions happen fast. They are made of amino acids, which are the breakdown products of the protein we eat.

2. *Vitamins* are coenzymes. B vitamins are especially important to make healthy brain cells. What are the major food sources of B vitamins? Brewer's yeast, wheat germ, lecithin and liver. Not many people in the general population eat these foods. Usually, it's only those people who read books like this one and try to keep well.

Tests show that some canned vegetables have lost 50 to 70 percent of the B vitamins in the processing; frozen vegetables, from 30 to 50 percent.

3. *Vitamin C* is found in a certain concentration in blood vessels all over the body. In the brain and spinal cord, there is a tenfold greater concentration; in the neurons, a hundredfold concentration. Why is there 100 times more vitamin C in the neurons than in any blood vessel in the body? Because vitamin C is needed in large amounts to make neurotransmitters. If we don't eat good sources of vitamin C or take food supplements, we won't have enough of the vitamin to make the neurotransmitter messengers.

4. *Glucose* is brain fuel. We need tremendous amounts of glucose to furnish the energy to first

manufacture the neurotransmitters, and then to ship them to the 12 billion neurons that use them every second of every hour of every day. Many people have low blood sugar, and they know well that if their blood sugar is low, they can't think well, and they can't get a message that says "eat" or "stop eating." Many of the 100 symptoms of low blood sugar have to do with the brain.

5. *Minerals* activate enzyme systems. Even if the enzyme, coenzyme and glucose are present, if the mineral is not there to activate the system, the message can't flow.

6. We have one more nutrient needed before the neurotransmitter will tell us to eat or to stop eating. It is a precursor of a neurotransmitter. Many precursors have been discovered and more are being found all the time. Most of the precursors are *amino acids,* which we have in our blood if we eat and assimilate the protein our brain cells need. You probably have read about them if you've ever read magazines and books from the health food stores. Some names of precursors that may be familiar to you are "tryptophan" and "tyrosine." The neurotransmitters they work with are serotonin and the catecholamines, including dopamine, well known for its influence on Parkinson's disease. Another precursor is a vitamin B cousin named "choline." It is a precursor of acetylcholine. We get choline from lecithin, available at all health food stores. Choline helps us think, remember and not be depressed. It also helps our hearts by keeping the blood at the right consistency—not too thick and not too thin.

Healthy Brain Cells

If we eat all the nutrients we need to make healthy brain cells, we will make the neurotransmitters that will turn our appetites on and off so we won't fight the battle of the bulge or refuse to eat altogether.

Some people are always hungry and they usually become obese. Their neurotransmitters never say "stop eating." Why doesn't the hypothalamus turn off the appetite before they become too fat? Because the junk food that people eat doesn't have enough nutrients to make healthy cells. If a lot of junk food is eaten, the fractions of nutrients in some junk foods (none in white sugar) may furnish enough food value to keep someone alive one more day, but he would probably be sick. All systems in our bodies are designed to keep us alive at all costs.

A 13-year-old boy was brought to me for nutrition counseling. His father told me earlier that the boy was eating 24 candy bars a day. Then he said, "His grades have dropped. Do you suppose there's any connection between the candy bars and his poor grades?"

Yes, the poor grades are 100 percent caused by

excess sugar. But the hypothalamus didn't tell him to stop eating because if there's a peanut or two in the candy bar, there might be enough food value in the peanuts in 24 candy bars to keep him going for a while.

This is evidence that humans who have healthy hypothalamuses will be able to count on them to determine their intake of food—not too much, not too little. Some of the faults in the way the hypothalamus works are caused by lack of exercise. At least some exercise is needed to keep the appetite working.

Another way to damage the hypothalamus seems to be with cigarette smoke. This assumption is based on the fact that people tend to gain weight when they stop smoking. To regain a healthy hypothalamus, laboratory mice have been given vitamin B1 when they wouldn't eat. The animals bounced back immediately with a good appetite (Williams, 1971).

Animals that are given a choice of food, with definite amounts of protein and carbohydrate, can regulate their own diets (Wurtman, 1983). If an animal eats a lot of carbohydrate, it will crave protein, and vice versa. Humans choose similar foods in similar circumstances. Thus the brain cells will regulate our appetite so we will eat a varied diet if the brain cells are healthy. High-protein, low-refined-carbohydrate meals are often found on weight-loss diets, but such diets cause the dieter to crave carbohydrates. If we get the right messages from healthy brain cells, we will eat the right amount of both protein and carbohydrate so that we will not be too thin or too fat.

Ross Hume Hall (1978) reviewed the function of the hypothalamus. A healthy gland regulates our desire for food. Other mechanisms regulate stomach contractions, blood sugar levels, type of food in the stomach and other reactions of hormones and nerves. These are "internal cues" that our bodies use to make us want to eat or stop eating.

Then we're also "invited" to eat by external cues—the sight of a juicy homemade hamburger on a whole-wheat bun, a crisp apple or a fresh carrot salad. Fat folks react mainly to the sight of food—an external cue—and their internal cues are suppressed. If there are no appealing but unhealthful snack foods around the house, the overweights won't be so easily tempted.

HOW TO GAIN WEIGHT

Anyone who has tried to gain weight will probably tell you it's harder to gain than to lose. It is easier to gain on this natural food program than on any other you've tried, and you'll feel better too.

High-Protein Foods

First, eat the diet outlined in the weight-gain section of this lesson. Next, add a little more fat and a lot more starch. How do we do that? Butter, nuts and seeds are the main fats we eat, so every time you eat a good starch such as a fluffy muffin or biscuit you made of whole grains, add about double the amount of butter you used to add. Eat more baked white or sweet potatoes with more butter on them. Add butter to servings of brown rice, millet, cracked wheat and corn grits, all excellent starches you've prepared for main meal dishes. Don't forget to combine these delicious whole grains with legumes (beans, peas and peanuts). On a weight-maintaining diet, we should eat about twice as much grains as legumes for the correct complete protein ratio. But to gain weight, eat about the same amount of each, since legumes have more calories than grains. You may need to add a little animal protein to make the ratios correct. You can do that with the special high-protein drink in Lesson 1.

Some excellent combinations are brown rice and red beans, black-eyed peas and cornbread, millet and garbanzo beans. When I cook that combination, I serve it mixed together (or separate) with a little "pep" added as chunks of zucchini, yellow squash or broccoli—or all three. Add your favorite condiments, maybe toasted peanuts or sesame seeds, a little sliced roast chicken from the health food store or your favorite cheese.

The next time the dish is served, which is about four days later, since we follow Rule 4, "Vary Your Diet," add a beaten egg or two with a little whole-grain flour and wheat germ made into patties and frizzled in butter. Nothing better! If I have enough for another meal, I often make soup with a base of brown and white sauce seasoned with vegetable salt or soup seasoning from the health food store. I sometimes toast the patties and cut them in bite-size pieces and add them to the soup. There are so many ways to prepare these foods, you'll never get tired of them.

Grains and Beans

A new combination of grains and legumes is available at most health food stores. It is bulgar and soy, already mixed in the package. Besides tasting good it is a complete protein. You might like some Eastern condiments with this dish. Try toasted peanuts with coconut, raisins or currants (go easy, you don't want it too sweet) and bits of roast chicken, scrambled egg and cheese.

The list of such combinations is endless. Each one is better than the other. As you gain weight, you'll be learning a new way of eating, and you'll feel better than ever before. The most important thing is to make sure the hypothalamus becomes healthy.

High-Protein Drinks

One more healthful hint. The high-protein drink we mentioned is all natural food, no processed, canned protein extracted by man from soy or milk. We prefer whole food. I call it a Super Health Drink.

The recipe is easy—1 cup of whole milk or nut milk (¼ cup nuts, ground dry in a blender, plus about 1 cup water), one raw egg, one teaspoon to one tablespoon of lecithin and from ¼ teaspoon to 1 tablespoon of brewer's yeast. If you haven't eaten yeast before, you should start slowly with ¼ teaspoon and go up gradually to 1 teaspoon.

Make up one cup a day, and drink about ⅓ cup *after* each snack. Satisfy your appetite, and then add a little more of this high-protein, energizing drink. This is an excellent bodybuilder. It not only adds weight, but when taken at the end of a meal, it also adds energy. If you've tried to gain by just adding any old calories, you'll be delighted with this program of natural food that builds health with every bite.

EXERCISE HELPS

Yes, of course, we must exercise to be well, so we should exercise whether we are trying to gain or lose. The important thing about exercise is to make sure all nutrients that every cell needs are in the blood. Then, when you exercise, the nutrients will flow through the bloodstream fast and will reach every cell and bring health. If we exercise without having all nutrients in the blood, the blood will flow faster to the cells, of course, but it won't build health because the needed nutrients are not in the blood.

What kind of exercise? Mild! At first, anyway. One of the best ways to exercise is to jump on a mini-trampoline. The surface of the trampoline is resilient, which means you don't jar your bones on a hard surface, as when you run. Running can cause shin splints and severe damage to bones. You must eat plenty of calcium and other minerals needed for healthy bones before you begin to run or jog. Many experts say "don't run at all."

On a television program not long ago, Dr. Michael DeBakey, the noted heart specialist, said he was tired of being called out of bed at 6 A.M. to take care of a jogger who had had a heart attack. Try out the mini-trampoline, you might like it.

You may have said at some time or heard someone else say, "I'm going to walk around the block to walk off the big meal I just ate." I've heard that often, but I still can't believe people don't know how dangerous it is to exercise after meals. We should never perform strenuous exercise just after eating a big meal because the blood will go to our arms, legs and brain to feed those cells, when it is needed in the stomach and intestines to digest our food.

Suggestions for Exercising

Kugler (1978) gives us several other warnings about weight loss and exercise.

1. Don't overdo exercising.
2. Don't sit or lie down immediately after exercising. Keep moving mildly for at least 10 minutes.
3. Don't use rubber suits, rubber belts, steam or sauna baths. You'll be dehydrated; you won't burn excess body fat.
4. Don't use rollers or vibrators. They won't get rid of fat or increase muscle tone, and they can be dangerous when used for massage.

Maybe some people will appreciate those hints. Maybe they didn't want to knock themselves out with hard exercise anyway. We should be moderate in everything. Kugler's *Newsletter* published some interesting comments for weight-conscious people. If we eat 3,600 more calories a day than we need, we gain one pound. To exercise this off, we would have to exercise 90 minutes at a time, three times a week. Long walks are a good exercise to burn the extra calories.

If you're the first one to reach for a sweater, your sodium-potassium pumps—required for good health in general, plus heart problems and weight control in particular—are not working well. You need more exercise to keep the pumps working. If you don't exercise, you probably don't need many calories, and you probably overeat often. Don't eat sweets; eat more vegetables and whole grains. Those foods will fill your stomach faster, and you will feel comfortably full soon, without eating so much that you gain weight.

Fitness, Especially for Women, But Men Can Listen Too

Men's bodies contain more water than women's. Women have a much harder time developing muscles than men (Boyd, 1983). Women who are bodybuilders must work intensely at lifting weights or other exercise because of the action of female hormones. In fact, women sometimes take male sex hormones to balance their female hormones and make weight gain easier.

All of these conditions may cause some women to have different and untrue ideas about weight gain or loss. But whatever food they eat from the three major food categories—protein, carbohydrate or fat—ends up as body fat, unless it is burned for energy, used to make tissue or exercised off.

The older people get, the slower their tissues and

organs work, and the fewer nutrients are absorbed, but the more fat is accumulated. However, we need just as much protein as we needed in younger years. If we don't get it, we accumulate more fat and lose lean muscle. Remember that the heart is a muscle. We literally cannot make muscle without protein. Some of the muscles we make and repair all through our lives, in addition to our hearts, are in the walls of the intestines, the stomach, lungs and arteries.

We don't use protein to enlarge muscles unless we have plenty of protein to repair tissues first. If you aren't very active, you don't need a great amount of protein; active people need more. If a person who is inactive eats a lot of protein, then he or she won't make muscles out of the protein and it turns into fat.

You can tell if you have too much stored fat or if your weight is muscle mass. Test yourself in front of a full-length mirror. Pinch yourself here and there and you'll feel the difference in fat and muscle tissue.

If you go on a crash diet to lose weight, you can whittle down the fat deposits, but you'll also lose similar amounts of muscle mass, so that the ratio of fat to lean stays about the same. Don't think you have to eliminate all fat from your diet. We must have fat. People who do not eat fat cannot assimilate fat-soluble vitamins or make sex hormones. But fat should be kept in normal bounds by exercise and diet. Otherwise it can stack up on top of muscles and change the shape of the body to the opposite of what the program was planned to do.

It would be nice if we could reduce in spots, but weight experts say that it is not possible (McArdle and Magel, 1983). Exercise gets rid of fat deposits just about equally all over the body. Thus if an area has more fat deposits, more fat will be removed from those areas. But there is no evidence that fat is released from fat pads directly over a muscle that is being exercised.

To determine this, researchers compared the arms of tennis players. The playing arm was larger, but the extra size was due to extra muscle, not to extra fat. Of course, regular exercise helps reduce total body fat, and more fat will be reduced in areas where more fat is deposited. So we should continue with moderate exercise and get rid of fat all over.

Aerobic exercise is especially good for removing body fat and for being able to use your muscles longer without tiring, both of which we need (Boyd, 1983). When aerobic exercise is continued for a while, the carbohydrate stores are exhausted, and fatty tissues are broken down and used as fuel for long-term exercise.

Sometimes it seems that we get fat overnight. When "fat" is deposited that fast, it is usually wa-ter, because fat takes a long time to build up. Also, it takes a long time for fat to be removed. The water deposits might be caused by taking the Pill, but the body can get rid of the water fairly easily by eating less salt and taking more vitamin B6 in tablet form.

FAD METHODS OF LOSING WEIGHT

With the amazing number of diet books on the market, it would seem that the answer to obesity would have already been found. Everyone seems to be looking for the magic bullet—a quick, easy way to lose.

One-Food Diets

Many diets concentrate on one food—i.e., fat meat, bananas or grapefruit. The dieter can eat all he wants of the one food if he doesn't eat any of another list of foods. After a few days of gorging on one food, the dieter gets tired of the food and eats less (Mann, 1974). But, of course, none of these diets is complete. None builds health. None provides the energy the fat person hopes for.

One of the most important reasons for all the diet books is that the authors and publishers will make money with them.

Low-Carbohydrate Diets

Many fad diets allow unlimited intake of proteins and fats, but they severely limit the amount of carbohydrate to 60 grams or less. This is explained by saying that, in obese people, carbohydrate is changed to fat tissue rather than being used for energy, whereas calories from fat and protein are burned up by the body and are not stored as body fat. This is simply not true. What does seem to be true is that excess calories from all sources are not easily used in fat people, and they're more easily stored (Fineberg, 1972).

When people start on a low-carbohydrate diet, they usually lose water, not fat. People don't realize this, and it has probably caused more confusion in the treatment of obesity than any other single factor. If the patient eats a low-calorie diet containing carbohydrate, he loses fat, then he begins to retain water, and that counterbalances the fat loss. The scales may show no change. The patient is hungry, but he is storing water and is discouraged because he isn't losing weight. Then his physician gives him a diuretic, which causes loss of water and minerals and upsets the entire metabolism. The merry-go-round continues.

Group Therapy

We've all heard of groups of fat people who get together to share problems. Some are "Weight

Watchers" and "TOPS" (Take Off Pounds Sensibly). They seem to do more good than the physicians and their drugs, but they mostly stress willpower. And they don't usually have specific answers about good nutrition—the only answer for good health.

Ileal Bypass

Several famous people have had ileal bypass surgery to lose weight, and have received a lot of publicity about it. This means that a section of their intestines is cut out; there is so little digestive surface remaining that they can't assimilate food. The food goes right through and doesn't furnish nutrients for their bodies. They have such poor absorption that they develop diarrhea. Most of the patients lose weight steadily for 12 to 18 months. They finally reach a plateau and are still obese, but not as bad as before.

These patients want to avoid diarrhea, so they eat less. The short section of the small intestine that was left tends to get bigger after a time, and the patients absorb more food. They they stop losing weight.

One complication of this treatment is that the wound where the intestines were sewed together may split open. Also liver disease is common in these people. As is often the case, physicians don't know why the liver is diseased. They say "cause unknown." But with any illness, the cause is poor nutrition (Mann, 1974).

I received a letter from a sorrowful woman who had submitted to an ileal bypass operation to lose weight. Here's what she wrote:

> Dear Dr. Long: I need help. I had the bypass operation for weight loss and I'm in trouble. I have severe loss of hair, severe hemorrhoids, gallstones and who knows what else. Should I have the operation reversed? I read recently that I would have liver problems.
>
> I was never told by my doctor about the awful side effects. The reason I had the operation—I was 5 feet 3 inches tall, weighed 247, blood pressure of 170/120. My age is 58. I was on medication but was unable to bring my pressure down one point. I only wish I had known of your work before I had the operation. I feel that this operation should be outlawed, and I will work to see that it is.
>
> Can you help me? I want to learn all about your program. I have severe loss of memory, but I will study hard and try to understand.

Liquid Protein

The liquid-protein diet that had such tragic consequences in 1977 or 1978 was an example of why

not to take up every new crash diet that comes along.

The protein in some of these diets is made of predigested pigskin. The inexpensive skins are boiled in acid, then neutralized with lye; all of this destroys vitamins and minerals. Next they are broken down with enzymes and dried to almost a solid. The major protein of pigskin is collagen, which is tough and stringy; but the worst thing about it is that it is deficient in some essential amino acids. One, tryptophan, is completely absent. Thus the protein value of collagen is zero, which means it can't be used to build tissue if it's the only protein eaten.

What about the people who lost so much weight on that diet—did they keep it off? Seventy-five percent did not—they bounced back to their previous weight (Hall, 1978).

Protein Drinks

Popular "diet" drinks have very few nutrients for the calories. Most of the calories are from sugar and refined oil. The added vitamins and minerals can't match those found in a fresh peach or even in a piece of watermelon.

A popular diet is having one or two meals a day of a high-protein drink, and another meal of the average American diet. These are not healthful for a long period. They do not have enough of the needed nutrients. Liver and wheat germ oil, for example, contain antifatigue nutrients. When those foods were given to animals, the animals could exercise 300 percent longer. A nutrient factor in carrots reduces the body's need for oxygen. These nutrients aren't found in a liquid diet formula.

Fox (1983) says that one popular high-protein, weight-loss diet is "essentially a starvation diet, likely to send you to the hospital." People need more for their health than a certain number of calories they get when they follow such a diet according to directions. That diet is man-made. It contains no completely natural food, thus there may be nutrients missing.

"Light" Foods

You may think that if you eat the foods on the market called "light" you'll get light! What are they? They're foods that have been tampered with and filled with nondigestible material. Refined wood pulp is a favorite with manufacturers; it's also called methylcellulose. Some breads have 15 percent of this substance. It's advertised as having 30 percent fewer calories and five times the fiber of 100 percent whole-wheat bread.

We need fiber, but do we need tree fiber? Some of the methylcellulose is absorbed into our bloodstream and goes to the kidneys to be excreted. No one knows how long the kidneys will last if they have to handle this unnatural substance (Hall, 1978).

Fructose

One "light" food is fructose—widely advertised and touted as being perfect for people with blood sugar problems, because it doesn't call out an insulin response. Fructose is almost twice as sweet as sucrose (white table sugar). High-fructose corn syrup is a popular item. The high-fructose syrup was introduced in 1972, but since then the use of all sugars has increased about 8 percent per person. Refined sugars now amount to an average of one-fourth to one-third of the daily calories—that's about 684 calories a day for each baby, child and adult in North America (Hall, 1978).

The major problem of fructose is that most people think it's all right to eat a lot because it doesn't call out insulin. But there are many reasons why fructose is bad. Many studies show that if animals are given high-fat diets with starch, they do not develop heart disease. But if they're given high-fat diets with fructose, they quickly develop severe fatty plagues in the arteries, which lead to heart attack.

For hundreds of thousands of years, humans used daily about 300 grams of glucose mainly from starch, and only about eight grams of fructose from fruits and honey. Now in the wealthy nations, the intake of fructose has increased tenfold, to an average of about 90 grams a day. The increase is partly due to the use of corn sweeteners, which are fructose. Pauling (1972) says, "There is little doubt that this great intake of fructose," which humans aren't used to, "is the cause of many of our ills."

It is known that fructose formed in the digestion of sucrose undergoes changes in the body that lead to acetate, which is then in part converted to cholesterol. Obviously, fructose in such large amounts would cause more acetate, and therefore more cholesterol.

So let's look into the fads such as fructose and not get fooled by a half-truth—that it doesn't call out insulin. What it does is even worse—it calls out cholesterol (Pauling, 1986).

Fasting

Fasting is the greatest crash diet of all time. I don't approve of it for anyone; the following information about fasting may help you decide not to fast. Total fasting allows only noncaloric liquids and, of course, no protein. An adequate protein intake is absolutely required for health.

To quickly estimate your required protein intake, divide your weight in pounds by two. The figure will be approximate, but close enough. If you weigh 100 pounds, you need about 50 grams of protein a day; at 125, you need about 62 grams; at 150, 75 grams. This figure is a little on the high side, but it's better to have a little more than a little less, if it's protein. If you don't get the protein you need, your own muscles will be broken down to supply protein for repair of tissue. Some organ tissue is also broken down for protein. Can you do without part of your heart or kidneys?

When you lose lean body tissue, you regain your weight quickly when you start eating again, even if you're on a low-calorie diet, as long as it includes protein. This is because you replace the protein so fast. For every pound of protein replaced, there will be an increase of four pounds of body weight; apparently three pounds of water are incorporated into the cells with each pound of protein mass. So the dieter continues to gain weight until the protein has been completely restored (Fineberg, 1972).

This is why you hear so many fat people say, "I lost 40 pounds, but when I went off my diet, I put it all right back on." Most people are dieting this way. It's really yo-yo dieting.

Total fasting should be done in a hospital because it is so dangerous. It's even dangerous in a hospital because it deprives the body of lean body tissue and important minerals. These changes cause severe alterations in mood and physiology, including abnormal heart rhythms.

In 1965, a study showed that after fasting for 10 days, healthy sailors lost 20 pounds, 13 of which was lean tissue and only 7 of which was fat (Schauf, 1976).

When people go without food, they think they're going to lose a lot of weight quickly. They probably will, but they may not realize what happens in the body that doesn't maintain itself with food (Horrobin, 1973).

1. Glycogen stores are used up within the first two days. Glycogen is starch that is stored in the liver and can be changed to glucose immediately when needed. Remember, glucose is the sugar that the brain feeds on.

2. Fat is burned for energy. But fat cannot be completely burned without carbohydrates. Without carbohydrates, ketone bodies are formed and cause acidosis, as we've already explained.

Protein is broken down slowly along with the fat. Muscles lose bulk. When the fat deposits are finally used up, protein (lean body tissue) is the only food left, and it is then broken down rapidly.

Fluid accumulates in the legs and abdomen, probably because the heart is too weak to pump the blood around, and because there is less protein concentrated in the blood plasma. Fluid escapes from the capillaries into the tissues.

Urea (the breakdown product of protein) is produced and excreted rapidly. This is called the "pre-mortal" period, because if the fast continues, death soon follows (Horrobin, 1973).

Hypnotism

Some physicians treat obesity with hypnotism. Usually a group of people are hypnotized together. The diet contains only 500 calories a day. With or without hypnotism, that small number of calories would make anyone lose. If the patient is hypnotized enough, he may imagine he isn't hungry on the 500 calories.

Nevertheless, he is probably losing lean body mass (muscle and tissue) and he will probably go right back to his higher weight when he gets off the diet and stops being hypnotized.

Drugs to Lose Weight

In the 1930s, patients who took certain drugs refused to eat. These drugs, then, were used to keep fat people from eating. The drugs were "aggressively promoted and not often evaluated." Finally, after long use, tests showed that the drugs were not helpful. About one-third of the subjects showed no response at all; another third stayed away from food not only on the drug but also on the placebo. The last third were helped, but they were young and only moderately obese (Mann, 1974).

Let's remember that, even for young and moderately obese patients, all drugs have adverse reactions. My plan calls for excellent health and energy while we're losing weight.

The FDA says that all drugs to lose weight are potentially habit-forming and should be used with extreme care. They are for short-term use, and the diet should be restricted while the drugs are used. The total effect of drug-induced weight loss is "potentially dangerous," but most physicians still like to use them (Mann, 1974).

Most over-the-counter pills are worthless; some are dangerous. Some contain ammonium chloride, which we've learned (Lesson 7) is dangerous and can cause kidney damage. Don't use them.

Amphetamines may reduce hunger, but they can have side effects. They can cause dry mouth, restlessness, irritability, insomnia and sometimes constipation. They're even worse for heart patients—the heart rate may be increased, and there may be abnormal rhythms of the heart (Goodhart and Shils, 1973).

Smoking and Obesity

Usually people who stop smoking gain weight. In fact, people tend to gain weight as they age, but those who stop smoking gain about four pounds more in 10 years than the average nonsmoker. This study was the same with 20-year-olds up to 55-year-olds (Mann, 1974).

The Grapefruit Diet

It's a myth that grapefruit burns up fat in the body. Grapefruit is low in calories, but every calorie more than we need will be turned into fat (Seddon and Burrow, 1977).

Other Diets

Other diets that have been popular in the past are the "all-meat diet" and a low-protein diet called the "Rockefeller diet," which emphasized vegetables, fruits, concentrated carbohydrates and fats. The "Rice diet" consisted of rice and low-calorie fruits. Both of the latter didn't have enough protein to keep a person healthy. They are semi-starvation diets.

Many of the diets emphasize low carbohydrates. They are high in protein, and many do not restrict fat. One is called the "Mayo Clinic diet" but it has nothing to do with the Mayo Clinic. Then there's the "Air Force diet," which has no connection with the Air Force. The "Drinking Man's diet" allows martinis. Dr. Taller's "Calories-don't-count diet" calls for safflower oil to burn calories. Dr. Stillman's "Quick-weight-reduction diet" allows no carbohydrates except the 2.8 percent in cottage cheese. Dr. Atkins' "Diet Revolution" begins with no carbohydrate and goes to about 40 grams a day.

All these low-carbohydrate diets produce ketosis and can be dangerous (Sherman, 1973).

ILLNESSES PERTAINING TO WEIGHT

Obesity is said to be one of the most common diseases. It causes many ailments, but we can change our diet easily and feel better than we ever have before. Get started on your new diet now. You'll no doubt feel so good—and look so good—you'll never want to change back to junk food.

Anorexia Nervosa

Anorexia nervosa is a psychophysiological disease that causes loss of appetite. Doctors say the victims dream about food, feel hunger and are often obsessed with food. Most of the victims are young women. The symptoms are dramatic and unusual. Some of them are:

1. Excessive weight loss because of willful starvation.
2. Total lack of menstruation.

3. Distorted body image. The victim can't realize she has a severe physical condition. Many patients see themselves in the mirror—skin and bones—and still think they are over-weight.

4. Compulsive eating in spells, with days of starvation.

5. Muscle-wasting. This is a disease of the body feeding on itself. Muscles are broken down to make energy and to keep the heart beating.

6. Constipation. This is common, so patients take large amounts of laxatives.

7. Obsession with food. Many times, the patients prepare food for friends and family, but don't eat any themselves.

Although anorexics seem to be deliberately trying to starve themselves to death, starvation is not the main problem. The real reason for going against nature is that they have personality problems.

One of the victims explains her feelings. "It's like there are two of me," says Janie (not her real name). "One of me knows all about nutrition so I know what I should eat, but the other me is emotional and will not let me eat." Janie wouldn't allow herself to weigh more than 70 pounds. But this is a dangerous level, and she was put in a hospital and fed intravenously; otherwise, she might have died.

Janie says she realizes she may die, and she knows that if she takes cold, she will probably get pneumonia and die. "But," she says, "I can't eat more." In fact, Janie prepares her one meal of the day after the rest of the family has gone to bed so no one will add even one calorie to the total of 776 ⅓, which is all she'll eat. Her meal consists of dry cottage cheese, low-calorie rice patties, eggplant, one apple, a dietetic gelatin product, low-calorie coffee and herb tea. Janie even measures the water for tea, and if she has drawn more than she thinks she needs, she throws it out.

There are many opinions about what causes anorexia nervosa. Some think it's strictly emotional, some say the young women refuse to grow up. Many patients first become ill when they go away to school for the first time or leave home to go to work (*Houston Chronicle*, 1978).

I have known and worked with two anorexia patients. One, a woman about 35, came out of her problems quickly on the diet advocated in this lesson. About two months after her visit with me, I saw her at a party and didn't recognize her. She had gained weight and she felt good. The other was a college girl who fits into the "Janie" category. She was very much interested in nutrition and knew what to eat. But she couldn't make herself eat nor-mally. When she was at home during the summer, she would sometimes eat a half-gallon of ice cream at one time, then not eat again for days. Finally she went to a hospital and now has been discharged and is back at school.

Probably the most famous person who had anorexia and lived to tell about it was Cherry Boone, singer, and daughter of Pat and Shirley Boone. She weighed 140 pounds at age 16 and was 5 feet 7 inches tall. She began to lose weight and got down to 92 pounds (Tuber, 1982).

Cherry also had bulimia, which is a combination of eating and vomiting. These people go on binges and eat so much they're miserable, and they vomit or use laxatives so that the food can be eliminated without putting on any weight.

Cherry said she conformed to the usual pattern for anorexics. Her parents were successful and protective, the family was close-knit and she was a perfectionist. About 80 percent recover from the disease. Cherry said that many women are under the pressure of working, keeping house, taking care of children and trying to be perfect in all those fields. Then they stop eating, which they subconsciously think will keep them from maturing and having to perform well.

In spite of the varied opinions about the cause of anorexia nervosa, it seems logical to me that it is a condition caused by lack of nutritious food. When the point is reached in semi-starvation that the hypothalamus region in the brain does not get the nutrients it needs, it doesn't work well, and all the symptoms mentioned can become evident. The only way to get over the condition is to finally get enough nutrients to feed the brain so the hypothalamus will recover.

When an animal's hypothalamus is destroyed, it will not eat. Thus, it is possible that the hypothalamus in anorexics is damaged. Another reaction to a damaged hypothalamus is a deficiency of hormones usually released by the hypothalamus that should stimulate the ovaries to produce estrogen. Without estrogen, ovulation fails and there is no menstrual period. All of this can be returned to normal when the patient eats essential nutrients. Weight gain follows. Of course, it is best to start good food early in life so the person does not gain in the first place. Then she (most patients are girls) will not want to lose weight and her life will be normal. There is a support group called Help Anorexia, Inc. for these half-million people, with headquarters in Los Angeles. They report that from 5,000 to 6,000 people die of this ailment every year.

Bulimia

Bulimia is similar to anorexia. It is starvation,

but it begins with overeating and continues to purging (induced vomiting). The brain is affected first, because, without food, brain cells do not function normally, and the patient has mental and emotional problems.

Girls make up 95 to 98 percent of the patients. Usually they are only a little overweight, but they go on a strict diet to lose weight. Then they gorge by eating an average of 4,800 calories at one time. After that, they vomit and soon they overeat again. Usually this cycle starts when girls are stressed emotionally or physically, and they sometime have 11 episodes of bingeing and purging a week.

The patients usually lose weight, they have no energy and they become depressed. They then eat more to gain comfort from food.

Several reactions follow the bulimia: tooth and gum decay, potassium deficiency, which may cause muscle cramps, irregular heartbeat and a heart attack. When people vomit excessively, they lose the hydrochloric acid they need to digest protein and they have alkalosis. Sometimes bulimics take from 50 to 100 laxatives a day, which can cause rectal bleeding, rupture of the stomach and abnormal heart rhythms. Sometimes the girls eat normally with their families, but get up and eat and purge after everyone else has gone to bed, and their families don't know they're sick. One woman hid her illness this way for 20 years (Williams, 1982).

Suggested diets for these people exclude white sugar, white flour and white rice, plus processed foods and chemical additives. They should eat all natural foods and take all food supplements, especially vitamin C, B complex and pantothenic acid. These foods are all emphasized in my food program. The bulimic should feed her hypothalamus, which means all vitamins and all minerals in a natural food diet, so she will gain clear-headedness and be able to handle her intake of foods.

Diabetes

It is well known that many obese people have poor glucose tolerance. This means that they have diabetes more often than slender people. Obese subjects are more resistant to insulin, which may be why adult-onset diabetics have less severe disease when they lose weight. Fat people given a glucose load have more insulin in their blood than normal. If they lose weight, the amount of insulin in their blood goes down (Mann, 1974).

Dieting and Mental Disease

Crash dieting causes many ailments: heart disease, arthritis, kidney failure, gallbladder disease, even cancer. But mental and emotional problems are the most common results of crash dieting

(Cheraskin, 1974). Some researchers in Israel studied 10 dieters who went on a rapid weight-loss diet. Those who lost the most weight the fastest also had severe mental problems.

When we don't eat enough of all the essential nutrients, both the body and brain have to draw on reserves to function. At first we can handle our needs, but before long, we get nervous, can't make decisions and are easily upset. We may grind our teeth while we sleep. This is because on a diet without any one of the 50 needed nutrients—fats, proteins, vitamins, minerals and carbohydrates—our brain cells degenerate rapidly. Then our emotions and intelligence are upset.

How sick was the dieter before he began his diet? Studies show that people only 10 pounds overweight had more dandruff, more hemorrhoids, more flat feet, more varicose veins and more dental decay than people of normal weight. Their nails and hair didn't grow as fast. But worst of all, they had psychological problems.

It is obvious that most obese people are not metabolically normal, which is probably the result of their overweight caused by years of eating processed, junk foods. Thirty-six men of normal weight were on a 1,500-calorie diet for six months. None of them became physically ill, but they all suffered from mental problems. They became weak, irritable, apathetic and antisocial. Many of them lost interest in women; they thought about food so much they couldn't think of anything else.

Someone else did a similar study of normal-weight women on a low-calorie diet. They lived together, and before three months were over, they began to quarrel constantly, they were anxious and hostile and felt persecuted. They couldn't remember things, they became clumsy and couldn't pay attention to their work. Brain cells depend on a steady supply of nutrients (Cheraskin, 1974).

Cholesterol

If your looks as an overweight person haven't shocked you into losing weight, hear what Mann (1974) says about obesity (which is often related to cholesterol). He reports that it predicts angina pectoris and sudden death. However, age makes a difference, and we realize that older men tend to be obese and to have more heart attacks than younger men.

Obese people have slightly higher cholesterol levels in their blood than people with normal weight. They also manufacture more cholesterol—20 mg per kg body weight, probably because they have more fat cells than normal-weight people, who manufacture only 12 mg per kg body weight. Cholesterol is made in the fat cells, the liver and the intestines. When we lose weight, we make less cholesterol and have less in the blood (Mann, 1974).

THE NEW NUTRITION WEIGHT-LOSS PLAN

Most Americans eat too much. Their meals at dinner often look like this:

Animal protein (usually red meat)
Starch (potatoes or white rice)
Vegetable (often canned peas or canned corn— which is a grain, not a vegetable)
Raw vegetable salad (white iceberg lettuce—a no-no—not enough food value—use green leaf lettuce)
Bread or roll (made with white flour—doesn't deserve any space in the stomach)
Dessert (apple pie made with chemicals or commercial ice cream made with similar chemicals— not good)

We've been so programmed to this type of meal that we expect it, but we don't need all this food at one time. And we don't need processed food ever.

Lunch is often anything anyone can grab quickly, possibly a white bread and lunch-ham sandwich or a soft drink and potato chips. All these items are really nonfoods—off-limits to everyone, not just to people who want to lose weight.

What to Eat for Good Health and Weight Loss

Eat three small meals at regular mealtimes and three smaller snacks between meals. This is Rule 1 of my food program for everybody for good health (see Lesson 1). It helps us lose weight healthfully, because when we eat small amounts at a time, we can digest and assimilate the food well. The food is satisfying and we won't overeat. Many studies show that animals that gorge will live only half as long as those that nibble. We should nibble to lose weight and to prolong our healthy years.

Breakfast. One soft-cooked egg and one-half cup or less of whole-grain cereal. Buy your cereal at the health food store, either dry (as granola without sweetener) or to be cooked, (as oatmeal, seven-grain or four-grain cereal, cracked wheat or triticale flakes). Add a few raisins or any fresh fruit for sweetening. If you're rushed in the morning, cook your cereal overnight in a thermos. Put one cup of boiling water in a wide-mouth thermos with a plastic liner. Pour in one-half cup of any good breakfast cereal, put the top on tight, swish it around a little and let it sit on the counter all night. In the morning, it will be cooked and ready to eat, and it only cost you 30 seconds in time. Eat bread if you wish or a muffin, biscuit or cracker you made yourself.

Don't eat too much; you'll be eating a snack in 2½ hours.

Snacks. Midmorning, midafternoon and evening snacks are all similar but different. They're all fresh fruit and nibbles of protein such as two or three bites of cottage cheese, yogurt, kefir, buttermilk or hard cheese, a graham cracker you made with peanut butter from the health food store or a few nuts and seeds combined with a few peanuts.

Here are some suggestions:

¼ to ½ apple and 6 almonds
or ¼ banana and ¼ cup yogurt
or ½ peach, 1 walnut,
 and 1 whole-wheat cracker you made
or 1 plum, ½ wheat-germ muffin,
 and 2 or 3 bites of yogurt
or 8 grapes and 1 whole-grain cracker
 with peanut butter

Lunch and dinner. Our two main meals consist of a moderate amount of protein—four ounces or so of red meat (steak, roast, chops or hamburger). Don't eat meat more than four times a week; you don't have to eat any. You may eat about six ounces of fresh or frozen fish that you poach, broil or bake. We never fry anything. "Fry" means a hot skillet with oil. We "frizzle" foods, which means we cook them in a moderate skillet with butter or with butter and a little water. We also eat moderate amounts of dairy products such as eggs (one or two a day) and natural, light-colored cheese. We can eat poultry if we buy it at health food stores.

Grain and bean combinations are ideal protein dishes. Two old Southern favorites are black-eyed peas and cornbread and, especially from Louisiana, brown rice and red beans. A good combination comes in one package from the health food store. It is bulgar and soy flakes combined, which makes a complete protein cooked and served as you serve rice. Many other combinations are listed in my cookbook, *Switchover!*

We eat steamed green or yellow vegetables (a big helping of one or more seasoned with a little butter—no margarine) OR a big raw vegetable salad (green leaf lettuce) OR small servings of both cooked and raw vegetables.

If everybody in the family eats their salad at noon, everybody will be ready for steamed vegetables for the evening meal.

Six times a day we eat a small serving of unsalted nuts or seeds: two teaspoons of sesame, sunflower or pumpkin seeds, two walnut halves, four pecan halves, six almonds or 12 peanuts. You can eat all nuts and seeds raw except peanuts. Be sure to roast peanuts and cook all other legumes (peas and beans).

Any time a big person at your house doesn't get

enough to eat with these moderate servings of proteins plus large amounts of raw and steamed vegetables, he or she can have whole-grain bread—a muffin, biscuit, cracker or pancake—made at home—to round out the meal.

This is the strict weight-loss diet. If you're a big man and just can't make it to the next meal or midmeal on these amounts, then eat more. You can have a larger serving of the protein dish and a little more butter on your vegetables. At snack time, eat a whole piece of fruit if you can't last until the next meal. Adjust your food intake to your size and activity. But *don't overeat.* You'll be able to regulate your food intake so you won't be hungry, but you will lose weight, up to two pounds a week.

You'll probably be surprised to find how satisfying good food is. Two or three bites of real, natural food will keep you from being hungry. Just don't overdo it.

I'm not telling you how much to eat. You may be six feet four or four feet ten. Just don't overeat.

The importance of the butter with vegetables at lunch and supper, and of the nuts and seeds at snacks is to eat nibbles of fat in its best form, because fat is digested very slowly, and you won't be hungry again so soon.

One of my counselees, a man of about 40, called me about a week after he had been to see me. He said he had always bragged about his cooking, with lots of fancy sauces on the vegetables. But now he eats steamed vegetables with only a little butter as seasoning, and he said he has never tasted anything better.

When I say nibbles of fat in its best form, I'm talking about nuts and seeds. We don't use bottled oils, but we should eat the equivalent of one teaspoon of oil six times a day to help burn fat. Equivalents of one teaspoon are two teaspoons of sesame, sunflower or pumpkin seeds, or two walnut halves, four pecan halves, six almonds or 12 peanuts. On a reducing diet, don't exceed these amounts; don't go under, either. We need small amounts of fat so our skin won't get wrinkled—inside or out—and so we'll have plenty of energy.

Do's and Don'ts of Weight Loss

1. Don't drink water with meals. This is a rule for everyone, so your whole family will be doing this along with you. The reason is that if we drink water with meals, we dilute the hydrochloric acid in our stomachs that our enzymes need to break down protein to amino acids. The only way to repair tissue is with amino acids from protein. We use protein also for several hundred jobs in the body. Another one is to pick up waste water; thus we won't need diuretics that withdraw minerals

from the cells while they're getting rid of the water. No more puffy eyelids in the morning, no more tight rings because of swollen fingers and no more oversize ankles caused by accumulation of fluids when we stand a while. So, to get all the amino acids we need, let's drink our water 30 minutes before meals or two hours after, which will be 30 minutes before the next meal or snack.

This way, our reducing diet will be healthful, and while we're slowly losing weight, we'll be feeling peppier than we've ever felt before. Crash diets often make us tired and crabby. How nice it will be to lose weight and feel better than ever.

2. Eat small bites at a time, chew till the food is water and then swallow. We should eat slowly because it takes about 20 minutes for the message that we have had enough to eat to reach the brain.

3. Drink *no* coffee, tea, cola, cocoa, bottled or canned drinks—or fruit juice. Drink *only* water, whole milk, herb tea, organically grown vegetable juices and soup. Milk and soup can be drunk with meals. If you drink vegetable juices or herb tea, drink them instead of water, 30 minutes before eating. Don't drink vegetable juices unless you can get organically grown vegetables. There are so many poison sprays on commercial vegetables that they may poison our bodies if we consume enough vegetables to make a glass of juice.

4. Never overeat. Eat small amounts only. When you get through eating, you should not feel stuffed.

5. Don't drink any fruit juice. It's too sweet with natural sugar, even if you don't add any sugar.

6. You've been told all your life, "Clean your plate." Now we say, halfway through the meal, ask yourself, "Can I last two and a half hours if I stop eating now?" If so, get up and walk off.

If you prepare more food than you want, don't think you have to eat it to keep it from wasting. Keep a soup jar in the freezer and put any leftovers in it. I find some mighty strange combinations of food in my soup jar, but they all taste good. If I especially like the soup and wanted to have it again, I couldn't do it; I'd never get that combination again. One time I had a little leftover tamale pie, made with cornmeal mush and pinto beans seasoned with chili, plus many bits and pieces of many other meals. That was really super soup.

7. Put your fork or spoon down on your plate between bites. Don't rush. You want to finish your meal about the same time your companions finish theirs. They may not know the best way to eat, and they may be skinny so they aren't eating as carefully as you are.

8. When I have people come in for counseling, I tell them to bring a list of the food they've eaten,

drunk and snacked on for three days before our visit. They often tell me when they get here that they were startled at how much junk food they were eating. So list the food you eat for a week or so. You may be surprised not only at how much junk food you're eating, but also at how much total food you're eating.

9. Your grocery shopping list should not have any junk food on it because the calories and ailments come from junk food. You'll be buying some foods from health food stores, especially all whole grains, including flours, breakfast cereals and brown rice, millet and other grains used for lunch and dinner dishes. We buy eggs, chickens, turkeys, cheese and yogurt there. You will be making most of your bread, but in an emergency you can buy a loaf at the health food store. Also, buy vegetables and fruits there if you can get them organically grown. Also buy raw milk there if it is available.

At the supermarket, buy dried beans and peas, fresh fruits and vegetables if your health food store doesn't stock them. It's difficult to get raw milk; if you can't, get pasteurized, homogenized milk from the supermarket. But don't drink more than one glass a day—too much food value is lost in the processing. You can eat one glass of yogurt a day. Food supplements are taken with yogurt during meals.

People occasionally tell me, "I can't manage all those snacks because I work, and it would take all day to get my food ready for the next day." How about these ideas (they work for me and maybe you'll like them too):

I keep a little jar of almonds or mixed nuts in my purse. They'll also keep in a desk drawer. Several of each with a small whole peach or apple or half a banana make a good snack. It's really no trouble to split a muffin and spread a little peanut butter on it. It fits well in a purse or briefcase. You can get fancier if you wish. I like "travel bars" also, and they're easy to carry, whether you're traveling around town or around Europe. Use any cookie recipe such as oatmeal cookies or carob brownies, and add plenty of coconut, soy powder, non-instant powdered milk and chopped nuts. Use half the amount of dark brown sugar the recipe calls for or use raisins. Press the dough into a pan about 9″ × 9″ × 1″ and cut it into bars after it's done. Wrap in plastic. It's very easy to carry.

When you eat your between-meal snacks, you might think you'll never stop with six almonds or four pecan halves. Don't sit at the table and make a "meal" of your snack. Walk around if you've been sitting; sit and chat with a friend at work if you've been standing. In either case, get away from the source of supply so you won't be able to get more nuts. When you finish, you can resume your work or play.

I spoke at a TOPS group once. Those poor fat girls were living on coffee. Do you know what coffee does to your stomach? Besides the damage from caffeine, it makes your stomach churn, and your food gets digested faster. That makes you hungrier.

We haven't mentioned vitamin and mineral supplements, but the subject is pretty well covered in Lesson 1. Food supplements are extremely important. Most fat people are malnourished, so supplements are especially important for them. Don't overlook hydrochloric acid and other digestive enzymes to help get the most value from food.

If you're trying to lose weight, eating less salt might help a lot. Salt makes our tissues store water, and many fat people have edema (retention of fluid). Many people are given diuretics, but if they're taken over a long period of time they can cause kidney damage.

Physical exercise is important, but don't overdo it. If you've lost lean body mass, you might collapse. Remember the heart is a muscle and it might have been broken down to carbohydrate to furnish energy for the cells. You don't want to have a heart attack, which could happen before you get your muscles built up with good food. Other organs might not be in good condition either, especially bones. Jogging may cause bone problems.

When we talk about diet, we emphasize all fresh natural foods. The green vegetables should be fresh. If you're lucky enough to live where you can buy organically grown vegetables (without poisonous sprays or chemical fertilizers), buy those or grow your own. They're even better. There is a tremendous difference in canned green beans, for example, and in fresh. The canned beans have had too much salt added, and many of the nutrients are destroyed in the processing.

We should eat grains that are whole, not refined to a fraction of their food value. There will be much more food value than in processed grains.

Some of the most helpful and healthful foods are brewer's yeast and desiccated liver, wheat germ and lecithin. All should be included in a weight-loss diet. Desiccated liver, although it tastes awful, can give you such pep and energy that you won't care what it tastes like. Try it for your afternoon snack. You won't have that let-down feeling that hits you around four o'clock. Really, it doesn't taste so bad, either, in tomato juice or V-8. A friend of mine got so used to taking desiccated liver in tomato juice that she thought the tomato juice without the liver just didn't taste right.

Complete information on these supplements is in Lesson 1.

This way of life includes moderate amounts of vitamins and minerals in supplement form. As we've said before, fat folks are deficient in nutrients or they probably wouldn't be fat. So they should take all vitamins and minerals. Sometimes a terribly deficient person cannot tolerate large amounts of food supplements to start with. In that case, take small amounts and build up to the amounts that give you the pep and energy and the feel-good you're looking for and that you deserve. Instructions that precede the chart in Lesson 1 will tell you just how to start and how to determine what *you* need of each supplement.

Some of my counselees have severe allergies and can't start out with even moderate amounts of cer-tain foods or food supplements. In that case, I suggest they grind up the hard supplement pills they intend to take at one time, and take a few grains of the powder every hour or so. In that way there won't be enough at any one time to cause nausea or allergy. Take any new food in tiny amounts, and build up gradually. All this is explained at length in Lesson 4, "Allergies and Nutrition."

You may feel like writing me a letter like the ones at the beginning of this lesson when you get into this new diet. I hope you will. Many fat people say, "I'm me—what difference does it make that I'm fat? Can't people accept me as I am?" Yes, but all the time the fat folks long to be thin.

We can be. We can be anything we want to be with the help of natural foods. We can be healthy, energetic and slim.

QUESTIONS

TRUE/FALSE

1. When rats are on nibble diets (like ours), they use their food for energy; they don't store it as fat.

2. A good weight-loss diet includes high amounts of complex carbohydrates.

3. The more proteins we eat, the more calcium, magnesium and other nutrients we need.

4. If we don't eat enough carbohydrates, we can't burn fat; the central nervous system may be depressed and a person may go into a coma.

5. The average American intake of fat is 42 percent of calories; that amount should be reduced to 10 to 20 percent.

6. If our nerve cells are healthy, we will get the messages: "start" or "stop" eating.

7. Vitamin C is required in large amounts to make and send messages to eat or not to eat.

8. Exercise is important, because when all nutrients are in the blood, exercise will make the blood flow fast, and the nutrients will go to every cell.

9. Most of the calories in diet drinks are from sugar and refined oil.

10. Pauling says, "This great intake of fructose is the cause of many of our ills."

MULTIPLE CHOICE

1. Bland says that our weight depends on our: (a) appetite, (b) use of brown fat (c) the amount of nutrients in our food compared to the number of calories we eat.

2. Weight statistics show: (a) adult diabetics are now or have been obese, (b) American men who weigh 20 percent above the normal amount have a 350 percent greater risk of dying, (c) fat children usually grow up to be fat adults.

3. Ingredients to make neurotransmitters include: (a) enzymes, (b) coenzymes, (c) vitamin C, (d) glucose.

4. Tips for exercisers: (a) don't overdo exercising, (b) don't use rubber suits, (c) don't use rollers or vibrators.

5. All the food we eat ends up as body fat unless it is: (a) burned for energy, (b) used to make tissue, (c) exercised off.

6. Certain muscles should be carefully fed all through our lives: (a) heart, (b) intestinal walls, (c) stomach, (d) arteries.

7. A low-carbohydrate diet can cause: (a) loss of fat (b) retention of water, which causes weight gain.

8. When we fast, we have certain reactions: (a) stored starch is used up in two days, (b) fat is burned for energy, (c) protein is broken down.

9. List the signs of anorexia nervosa: (a) excessive weight loss, (b) total lack of menstruation, (c) muscle-wasting, (d) constipation.

10. Women on a strict diet developed the following conditions: (a) hostility, (b) persecution complex, (c) lack of memory, (d) lack of attention to work.

11. Rules of weight loss include: (a) don't drink liquids with meals, (b) eat small bites at a time, (c) chew well.

12. More rules for weight loss: (a) never overeat, (b) don't drink fruit juice, (c) put your fork down between bites, (d) occasionally list the food you eat for a week.

ANSWERS

True/False

1. T 2. T 3. T 4. T 5. T 6. T 7. T 8. T 9. T
10. T

Multiple Choice

1. a,b,c 2. a,b,c 3. a,b,c,d 4. a,b,c 5. a,b,c
6. a,b,c,d 7. a,b 8. a,b,c 9. a,b,c,d 10. a,b,c,d
11. a,b,c 12. a,b,c,d

REFERENCES

Bland, J. *J. Appl. Nutr.*, 34(2):91–102, Fall 1982.

Boyd, J. Women and Fitness. *Health Express*, July 1983.

Cheraskin, E. et al. *Diet and Disease.* New Canaan, CT: Keats 1987.

———*Psychodietetics.* New York: Bantam, 1974.

Fineberg, S.K. The Realities of Obesity and Fad Diets. *Nutr. Today*, July/Aug. 1972.

Fox, A. *Let's Live.* July 1982.

———The Lifestyle Diet. *Let's Live.* March 1983.

Fredericks, C. *Nutrition Handbook.* Canoga Park, CA: Major Books, 1976.

Garrow, J.S. Diet and Obesity. *Proc. R. Soc. Med.*, 66:642–44, July 1973.

Goodhart and Shils. *Modern Nutrition in Health and Disease.* Philadelphia: Lea and Febiger, 1973.

Guyton, A. C. *Textbook of Medical Physiology.* Philadelphia: W.B. Saunders, 1976.

Hall, R.H. Overweight: Clue to Decline in Quality of Nourishment. Entrophy Institute, Vol. 1(5), July/August 1978.

Horrobin, D.F. *An Introduction to Human Physiology.* Davis, 1973.

Houston Chronicle, page 9, section 4. Monday, May 29, 1978.

Kugler, H.J. *Seven Keys to a Longer Life.* New York: Stein and Day, 1978.

Mann, G.V. The Influence of Obesity on Health, Part II. *N. E. J. Med.*, 291(5):226–31, 1974.

McArdle, W.D. and Magel, J.R. Weight Management and Exercise. (in) *Medical Applications of Clinical Nutrition*, J. Bland (Ed.), New Canaan, CT: Keats, 1983.

Monte, W. C. Fiber: Its Nutritional Aspect. *J. Appl. Nutr.* 33(1):63–103, 1981.

——— and Vaughan, L.A. *J. Appl. Nutr.* 34(1):46–62, 1982.

Passwater, R.A. *Supernutrition.* New York: Pocket Books, 1976.

Pauling, L. Sugar: Sweet and Dangerous. *Executive Health* 9(1):1–4, 1972.

Schauf, G.E., *JIAPM*, 3(2):33–41, Dec. 1976.

Seddon, G. and Burrow, J. *The Natural Food Book.* New York: Rand McNally, 1977.

Sherman, W.C. Obesity. *Food and Nutrition News*, National Livestock and Meat Board, 45(1):3, Nov. 1973.

Tuber, K. Anorexia. *Let's Live.* July 1982.

Williams, M.E. Bulimia. *Let's Live.* July 1982.

Williams, R.J. *Nutrition Against Disease.* New York: Pitman, 1971.

Wurtman, R.J. Behavioral Effects of Nutrients. *Lancet*, May 21, 1983.

INDEX

INDEX

STRETCHING IN THE 21ST CENTURY
40TH ANNIVERSARY EDITION

Stretching is one of the most popular fitness books of all time. It has sold 3¾ million copies worldwide and is in 23 languages.

Stretching has been updated in this revised 40th anniversary edition, with:

• New stretching routines for smartphone users
• Suggestions for dealing with the conditions known as "tech neck" and "text neck"
• Tips on improving posture

* * * *

Stretching is a simple, gentle activity that can be done by anyone, anywhere, at any time.

This 40th Anniversary Edition of *Stretching* contains:

• 150 stretches with simple instructions for each stretch
• One- or two-page graphic stretching routines, including:

  • 17 routines for everyday activities
  • 10 routines for computer users and office workers
  • 37 routines for different sports

• Graphic index of all 150 stretches — useful for doctors, medical professionals, and body workers in prescribing stretches for patients

• Body tools

• Caring for your back

• PNF stretching

You can make photocopies of different routines for easy reference. Just the one page will give you a series of stretches tailored to your individual needs. Keep in a desk drawer or put on the wall or floor when stretching.

If you stretch in the right way (no bouncing, no pain), you'll feel better. It's that simple.

–Bob and Jean Anderson

STRETCHING

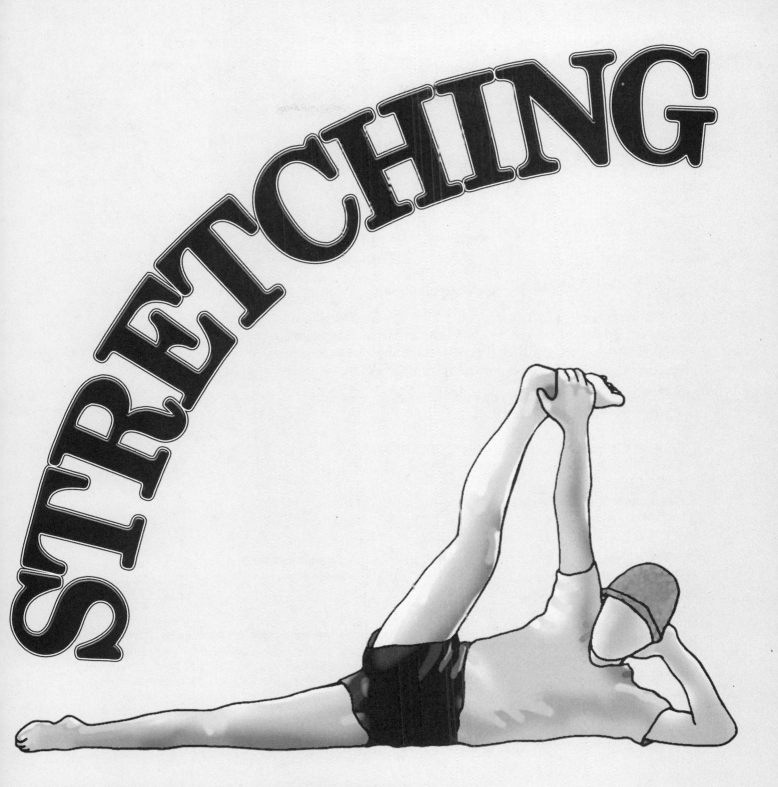

40th Anniversary Edition

BOB ANDERSON
Illustrated by JEAN ANDERSON

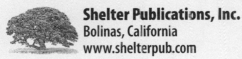

Shelter Publications, Inc.
Bolinas, California
www.shelterpub.com

Distributed in the United States by Publishers Group West and in Canada by Publishers Group Canada

Library of Congress Control Number: 2020941173

5 4 3 — 23 22 21
(Lowest digits indicate number and year of latest printing.)

Printed in Canada

This book is printed on FSC®-certified paper, contains post-consumer fiber and other controlled sources, is manufactured using renewable energy — Biogas and processed chlorine free.

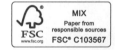

MIX
Paper from
responsible sources
FSC® C103567

Shelter Publications, Inc.
P.O. Box 279
Bolinas, California 94924
415-868-0280
Email: shelter@shelterpub.com

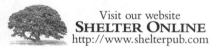

Visit our website
SHELTER ONLINE
http://www.shelterpub.com

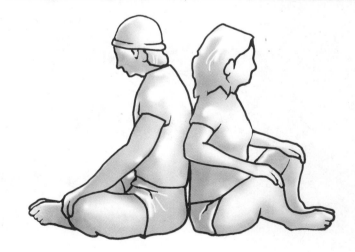

CONTENTS

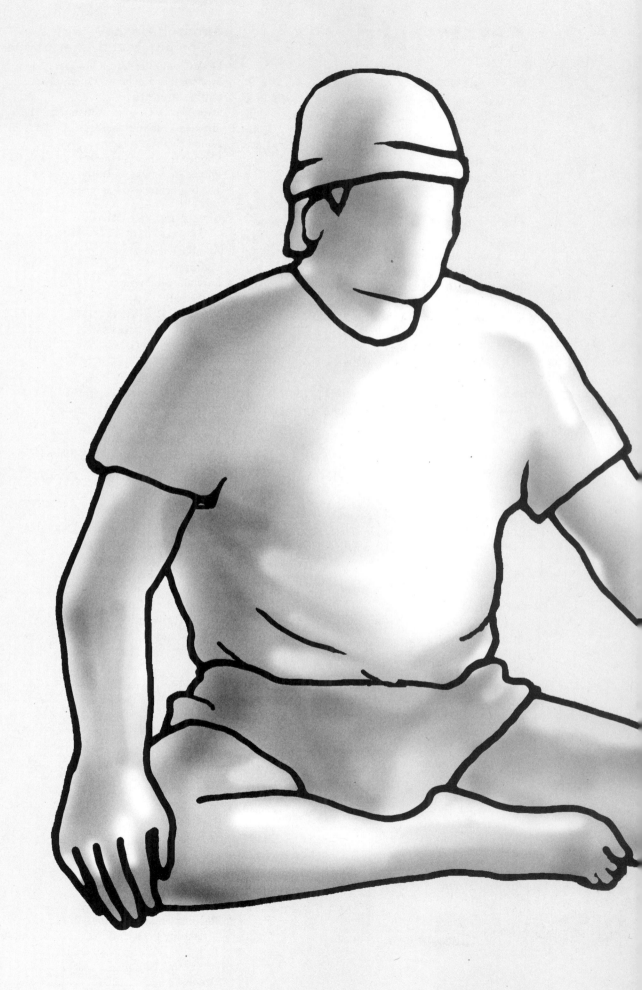

GETTING STARTED

This first section is an introduction to stretching. It is very important to read pages 12–13, "How to Stretch," so you will understand how to co the stretches in the rest of the book. Then, if you are new to stretching, the section "Getting Started," on pages 15–21, will take you through a series of simple stretches.

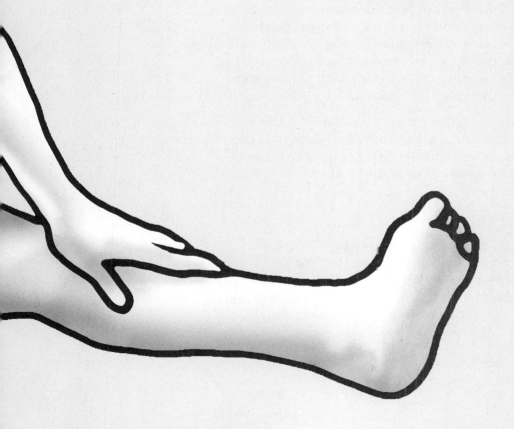

INTRODUCTION

Today millions of people have discovered the benefits of movement. Everywhere you look they are out, running, cycling, skating, playing tennis, or swimming. What do they hope to accomplish? Why this relatively sudden interest in physical fitness?

Many recent studies have shown that active people lead fuller lives. They have more stamina, resist illness, and stay trim. They have more self-confidence, are less depressed, and often, even late in life, are still working energetically on new projects.

Medical research has shown that a great deal of ill health is directly related to lack of physical activity. Awareness of this fact, along with fuller knowledge of health care, is changing lifestyles. The current enthusiasm for movement is not a fad. We now realize that the only way to prevent the diseases of inactivity is to remain active — not for a month, or a year, but for a lifetime.

* * * *

Our ancestors did not have the problems that go with a sedentary life; they had to work hard to survive. They stayed strong and healthy through continuous, vigorous outdoor work: chopping, digging, tilling, planting, hunting, and all their other daily activities. But with the advent of the Industrial Revolution, machines began to do the work once done by hand. As people became less active, they began to lose strength and the instinct for natural movement.

Machines have obviously made life easier, but they have also created serious problems. Instead of walking, we drive; rather than climb stairs, we use elevators; while once we were almost continuously active, we now spend much of our lives sitting. Computers have made us even more sedentary. Without daily physical exertion, our bodies become storehouses of unreleased tensions. With no natural outlets for our tensions, our muscles become weak and tight, and we lose touch with our physical nature, with life's energies.

But times have changed. We have found that health is something we can control, that we can prevent poor health and disease. We are no longer content to sit and stagnate. Now we are moving, rediscovering the joys of an active, healthy life. What's more, we can resume a more healthy and rewarding existence at any age.

* * * *

The body's capacity for recovery is phenomenal. For example, a surgeon makes an incision, removes or corrects the problem, then sews you back up. At this point, the body takes over and heals itself. Nature finishes the surgeon's job. All of us have this seemingly miraculous capacity for regaining health, whether it's from something as drastic as surgery, or from poor physical condition caused by lack of activity and bad diet.

What does stretching have to do with all this? It is the important link between the sedentary life and the active life. It keeps the muscles supple, prepares you for movement, and helps you make the daily transition from inactivity to vigorous activity without undue strain. It is especially important if you run, cycle, play tennis, or engage in other strenuous exercises, because activities like these promote tightness and inflexibility. Stretching before and after you work out will keep you flexible and may prevent common injuries such as knee problems from running and sore shoulders or elbows from tennis.

With the tremendous number of people exercising now, the need for correct information is vital. Stretching is easy, but when it is done incorrectly, it can actually do more harm than good. For this reason it is essential to understand the right techniques.

* * * *

Over the past three decades I have worked with amateur and professional athletic teams and have participated in various sports medicine clinics throughout the country. I have been able to teach athletes that stretching is a simple, painless way of getting ready for movement. They have found it enjoyable and easy to do. And when they have stretched regularly and correctly, it has helped them avoid injuries and perform to the best of their abilities.

Stretching feels good when done correctly. You do not have to push limits or attempt to go further each day. It should not be a personal contest to see how far you can stretch. Stretching should be tailored to your particular muscular structure, flexibility, and varying tension levels. The key is regularity and relaxation. The object is to reduce muscular tension, thereby promoting freer movement — not to concentrate on attaining extreme flexibility, which often leads to overstretching and injury.

We can learn a lot by observing animals. Watch a cat. It instinctively knows how to stretch. It does so spontaneously, never overstretching, continually and naturally tuning up muscles it will have to use.

* * * *

Stretching is not stressful. It is peaceful, relaxing, and noncompetitive. The subtle, invigorating feelings of stretching allow you to get in touch with your muscles. It is completely adjustable to the individual. You do not have to conform to any unyielding discipline; stretching gives you the freedom to be yourself and enjoy being yourself.

Anyone can be fit, with the right approach. You don't need to be a great athlete. But you do need to take it slowly, especially in the beginning. Give your body and mind time to adjust to the stresses of physical activity. Start easily and be regular. There is no way to get into shape in a day.

When you are stretching regularly and exercising frequently, you will learn to enjoy movement. Remember that each one of us is a unique physical and mental being with our own comfortable and enjoyable rhythms. We are all different in strength, endurance, flexibility, and temperament. If you learn about your body and its needs, you will be able to develop your own personal potential and gradually build a foundation of fitness that will last a lifetime.

WHO SHOULD STRETCH

Everyone can learn to stretch, regardless of age or flexibility. You do not need to be in top physical condition or have specific athletic skills. Whether you sit at a desk all day, dig ditches, do housework, stand at an assembly line, drive a truck, or exercise regularly, the same techniques of stretching apply. The methods are gentle and easy, conforming to individual differences in muscle tension and flexibility. So, if you are healthy, without any specific physical problems, you can learn how to stretch safely and enjoyably.

> **Note:** If you have had any recent physical problems or surgery, particularly of the joints and muscles, or if you have been inactive or sedentary for some time, please consult your health care professional before you start a stretching or exercise program.

WHEN TO STRETCH

Stretching can be done any time you feel like it: at work, in a car, waiting for a bus, walking down the road, under a nice shady tree after a hike, or at the beach. Stretch before and after physical activity, but also stretch at various times of the day when you can. Here are some examples:

- In the morning before the start of the day.
- At work to release nervous tension.
- After sitting or standing for a long time.
- When you feel stiff.
- At odd times during the day, as for instance, when watching TV, listening to music, reading, or sitting and talking.

WHY STRETCH

Stretching, because it relaxes your mind and tunes up your body, should be part of your daily life. You will find that regular stretching will do the following things:

- Reduce muscle tension and make the body feel more relaxed
- Help coordination by allowing for freer and easier movement
- Increase range of motion
- Help prevent injuries such as muscle strains. (A strong, flexible, pre-stretched muscle resists stress better than a strong, stiff, unstretched muscle.)
- Make strenuous activities like running, skiing, tennis, swimming, and cycling easier because it prepares you for activity; it's a way of signaling the muscles that they are about to be used.
- Helps maintain your current level of flexibility, so as time passes you do not become stiffer and stiffer
- Develop body awareness; as you stretch various parts of the body, you focus on them and get in touch with them; you get to know yourself.
- Help loosen the mind's control of the body so that the body moves for "its own sake" rather than for competition or ego
- Feel good

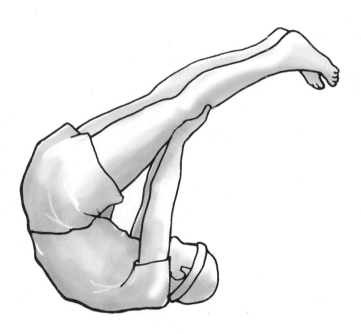

HOW TO STRETCH

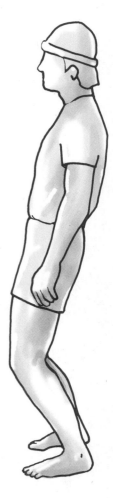

Stretching is easy to learn. But there is a right way and a wrong way to stretch. The right way is a relaxed, sustained stretch with your attention focused on the muscles being stretched. The wrong way (unfortunately practiced by many people) is to bounce up and down or to stretch to the point of pain: these methods can actually do more harm than good.

If you stretch correctly and regularly, you will find that every movement you make becomes easier. It will take time to loosen up tight muscles or muscle groups, but time is quickly forgotten when you start to feel good.

The Easy Stretch

When you begin a stretch, spend 5–15 seconds in the *easy stretch*. No bouncing! Go to the point where you feel a *mild tension,* and relax as you hold the stretch. The feeling of tension should subside as you hold the position. If it does not, ease off slightly and find a degree of tension that is comfortable. You should be able to say, "I feel the stretch, but it is not painful." The easy stretch reduces muscular tightness and tension and readies the tissues for the developmental stretch.

The Developmental Stretch

After the easy stretch, move slowly into the *developmental stretch*. Again, no bouncing. Move a fraction of an inch further until you again feel a mild tension and hold for 5–15 seconds. Be in control. Again, the tension should diminish; if not, ease off slightly. Remember: If the stretch tension increases as the stretch is held and/or it becomes painful, you are stretching too far! The developmental stretch fine-tunes the muscles and increases flexibility.

Breathing

Your breathing should be slow, rhythmical, and under control. If you are bending forward to do a stretch, exhale as you bend forward and then breathe slowly as you hold the stretch. Do not hold your breath while stretching. If a stretch position inhibits your natural breathing pattern, then you are obviously not relaxed. Just ease up on the stretch so you can breathe naturally.

Counting

At first, silently count the seconds for each stretch; this will insure that you hold the proper tension for a long enough time. After a while, you will be stretching by the way it feels, without the distraction of counting.

The Stretch Reflex

Your muscles are protected by a mechanism called the *stretch reflex*. Any time you stretch the muscle fibers too far (either by bouncing or over-stretching), a nerve reflex responds by sending a signal to the muscles to contract; this keeps the muscles from being injured. Thus, stretching too far tightens the very muscles you are trying to stretch! (You get a similar involuntary muscle reaction when you accidentally touch something hot; before you can think about it, your body jerks away from the heat.)

Pushing a stretch too far or bouncing up and down strains the muscles and activates the stretch reflex. This causes pain, as well as physical damage due to the microscopic tearing of muscle fibers. This in turn leads to the formation of scar tissue in the muscles, with a gradual loss of elasticity. The muscles become stiff and sore. It's hard to get enthused about daily stretching and exercise when you're pushing it to the point of pain!

No Gain *with* Pain

Many of us were conditioned in high school to the idea of "no gain without pain." We learned to associate pain with physical improvement, and were taught that "... the more it hurts, the more you get out of it." Don't be fooled. Stretching, when done correctly, is not painful. Learn to pay attention to your body, for pain is an indication that something is *wrong*.

The easy and developmental stretches, as described on the previous page, do not overactivate the stretch reflex and do not cause pain.

This Diagram Will Give You an Idea of a "Good Stretch"

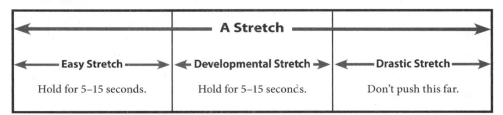

← Easy Stretch →	← Developmental Stretch →	← Drastic Stretch →
Hold for 5–15 seconds.	Hold for 5–15 seconds.	Don't push this far.

The straight-line diagram represents the stretch that is possible with your muscles and their connective tissue. You will find that your flexibility will naturally increase when you stretch, first in the easy, then in the developmental phase. By stretching regularly and staying relaxed, you will be able to go beyond your present limits and come closer to your personal potential.

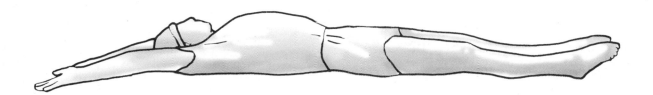

WARMING UP AND COOLING DOWN

Warming Up

There has been some controversy in recent years about stretching before you warm up. If you are going to stretch, will you get injured if you stretch without specifically warming up first? No — if you stretch comfortably and not strenuously. However, I suggest that you do several minutes of general movement (walking and swinging arms, etc.) to warm the muscles and related soft tissue before you stretch. This will get the blood moving. You still have to stretch correctly whether you are warmed up or not.

Some runners have reported they are more likely to get injured if they don't warm up before stretching. It is possible to get hurt stretching if:

• you are in too much of a hurry (not relaxed)

• you push too far, too soon (overstretching a cold muscle)

• you are not paying attention to the feeling of the stretch

You will not get hurt stretching if you stretch correctly (see pp. 12–13). You will sense how far to stretch if you are paying attention to how the stretch feels; tune into your body.

Here's my advice if you are engaging in an activity such as running or cycling or whatever: Warm up by doing the activity you are about to do, but at a lower intensity. For example, if you are about to run — walk or jog for 2–5 minutes or until you break a light sweat. (Walking and jogging provide a good, basic warm-up for many activities. This will increase muscle and blood temperature and raise total body temperature to provide an effective warm-up.) Then stretch. After you have stretched, continue to warm up for another 5 minutes or so to complete a full warm-up.

Cooling Down

Conversely, you should cool down after exercise by doing a scaled-down version of the main workout. Get your heart rate back down towards a resting rate. Then stretch to prevent muscle soreness and stiffness.

GETTING STARTED

Here we will walk you through nine stretches that will help you to understand the phrase "Go with the *feel* of the stretch." Once you understand this technique, it will be easy to learn and use the stretches in this book.

Note: Blue shaded areas indicate the parts of the body in which you will probably feel the stretch, but because no two people are the same, it is possible that you may feel a stretch in an area other than those marked.

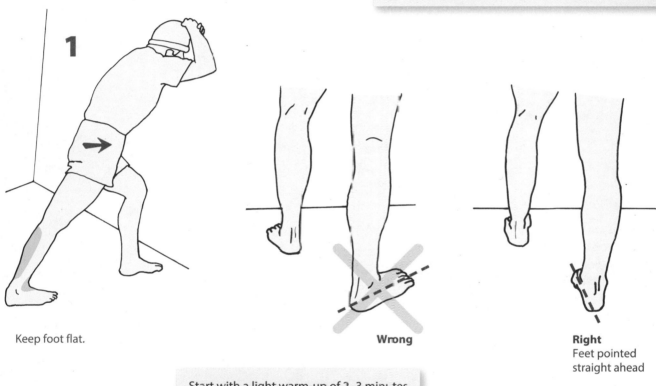

Keep foot flat.

Wrong

Right
Feet pointed straight ahead

Start with a light warm-up of 2–3 minutes (walking in place while moving your arms back and forth across your upper body).

First we'll do a calf stretch. Lean on your forearms, using a wall, or something else for support. Rest your forehead on the back of your hands. Bend one knee and bring it toward the support. The back leg should be straight, with the foot flat and pointed straight ahead or slightly toed-in.

Now, without changing the position of your feet, slowly move your hips forward as you keep the back leg straight and your *foot flat*. Create an *easy feeling* of stretch in your calf muscle.

Hold an easy stretch for 5–10 seconds, then move slightly further into a developmental stretch for 10 seconds. Don't overstretch.

Now stretch the other calf. Does one leg feel different from the other? Is one leg more flexible than the other?

Sitting Groin Stretch: Next, sit on the floor. Clasp the soles of your feet together with your hands as shown. Gently lean forward *from the hips* until you feel an easy stretch in your groin. Contract your abdominal muscles mildly as you go into the stretch. Hold an easy stretch for 5–15 seconds. If you are doing it right, it will feel good; the longer you hold the stretch, the less you should feel it. If possible, without strain, keep your elbows on the outside of your lower legs. This will help give you stability and balance.

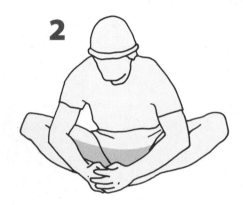

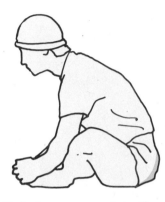

Exhale as you go into the stretch. Breathe slowly and rhythmically as you hold it. Relax your jaw and shoulders.

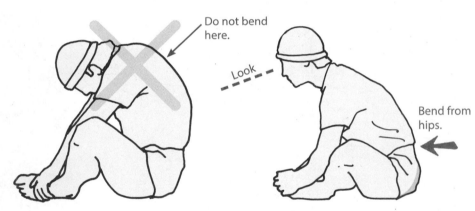

Do not bend here.

Look

Bend from hips.

Do not bend forward from your head and shoulders. This rounds the shoulders and puts pressure on lower back.

Concentrate on making the initial move forward from your hips. Keep your lower back flat. Look out in front of you.

After you feel the tension diminish slightly, increase the stretch by gently pulling yourself a little further into the stretch feeling. Now it should feel a bit more intense *but not painful.* Hold for about 15 seconds. The feeling of tension should decrease slightly the longer the stretch is held. Slowly come out of the stretch. Please, no jerky, quick, bouncing movements!

Stretch by the *feel* of the stretch, not by how *far* you can stretch.

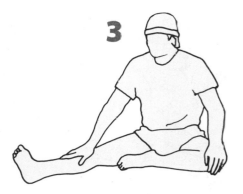

3

Next, straighten the right leg as you keep the left leg bent. The sole of the left foot should be facing the inside of the right upper leg. Do not keep the knee of the straight leg "locked." You are in a straight-leg, bent-knee position.

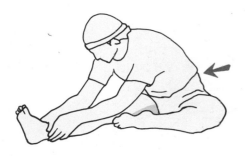

Now, to stretch the hamstrings and left side of the lower back (some will feel a stretch in the lower back, others won't), bend forward *from your hips* as you exhale until you feel a very slight stretch. Hold for 5–15 seconds. Breathe slowly and rhythmically. Touch the quadriceps of your right thigh to make sure that these muscles are relaxed. They should be soft, not tight.

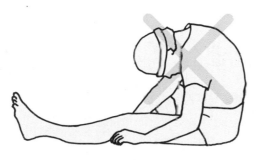

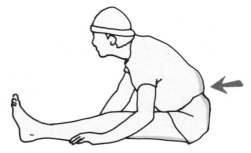

Don't make the initial movement with your head and shoulders. Don't try to touch your forehead to your knee. This will only round your shoulders.

Do initiate the stretch from the hips. Keep your chin in a neutral position. Keep your shoulders and arms relaxed.

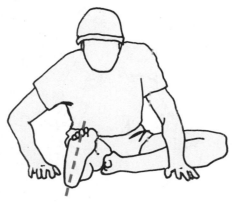

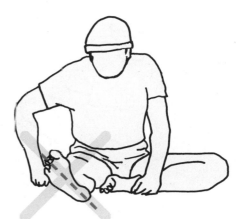

Be sure the foot of the leg being stretched is upright, with the ankle and toes relaxed. This will keep you aligned through the ankle, knee, and hip.

Do not let your leg turn to the outside because this causes misalignment of the leg and hip.

If you are not very flexible, use a towel around the bottom of your foot to do this stretch.

After the feeling of the easy stretch has subsided, slowly go into the developmental stretch for 5–15 seconds. You may only have to bend forward a fraction of an inch. Do not worry about how far you can go. Remember, we are all different.

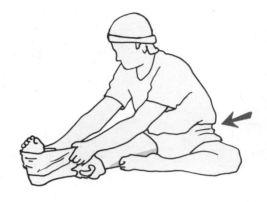

Slowly come out of the stretch. Do the same stretch on the other side. Keep the front of your thigh relaxed and your foot upright, with ankle and toes relaxed. Do an easy stretch for 15 seconds, and then slowly find the developmental phase of the stretch and hold for 5–15 seconds.

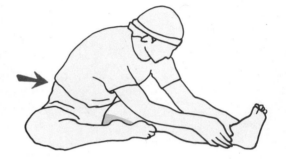

It takes time and sensitivity to stretch properly.

Develop your ability to stretch by how you feel and not by how far you can stretch.

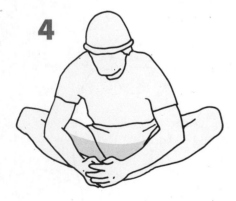

4

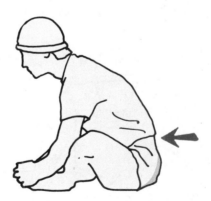

Repeat the sitting groin stretch. How does this feel as compared to the first time you did it? Any change at all?

A number of things are more important than concentrating solely on increasing flexibility:

1. Relaxation of tense areas such as feet, hands, wrists, shoulders, and jaw when stretching

2. Learning how to find and control the right amount of tension in each stretch

3. Awareness of lower back, head and shoulders, and leg alignment during the stretch

4. Adjusting to daily changes, for every day the body feels slightly different

5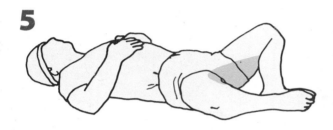

Lying Groin Stretch: Now lie on your back with the soles of your feet together. Let your knees fall apart. Relax your hips and let gravity give you a very mild stretch in your groin. Stay in this very relaxed position for 40 seconds. Breathe deeply.

Let go of any tension. The stretch feeling here will be subtle.

6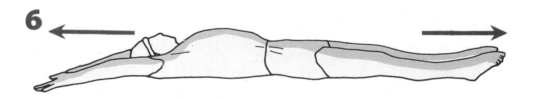

Elongation Stretch: Slowly straighten both legs. With your arms overhead, reach out with your hands while pointing your toes. Hold for 5 seconds, then relax. Repeat 3 times. Each time you stretch, gently pull in your abdominal muscles to make the middle of your body thin. This feels really good. It stretches arms, shoulders, spine, abdominals, as well as muscles of the rib cage, feet, and ankles. This is a great stretch to do first thing in the morning while still in bed.

7

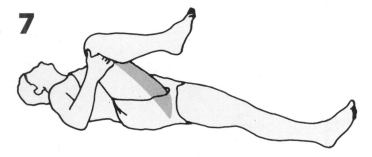

Next, bend one knee and gently pull it toward your chest until you feel an easy stretch. Hold for 30 seconds. You may feel a stretch in your lower back and back of the upper leg. If you do not feel any stretch, don't worry about it. This is an excellent position for the entire body, good for the lower back and very relaxing whether you feel a stretch or not. Do both sides and compare. Do not hold your breath.

> Gradually get to know yourself.

8

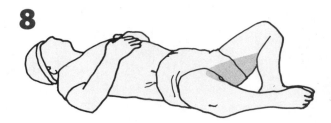

Repeat the lying groin stretch and relax for 30 seconds. Let go of any tension in your feet, hands, and shoulders. You may want to do this stretch with your eyes closed.

How to Sit Up from a Lying Position

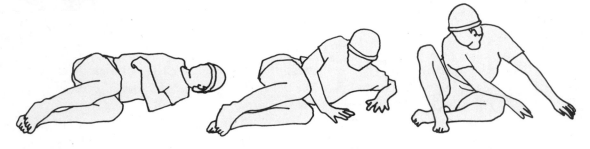

Bend both knees and roll over onto one side. While resting on your side, use your hands to push yourself up into a sitting position. By using your hands and arms this way, you take the pressure or stress off the back.

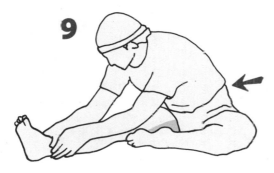

9 Now repeat the stretches for your hamstrings. Have you changed at all? Do you feel more limber and less tense than before stretching?

SUMMARY

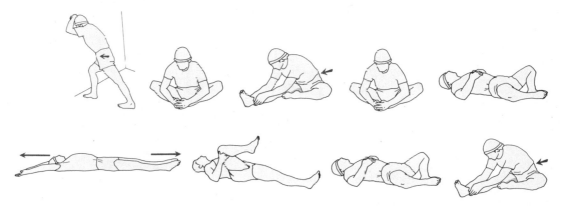

These are just a few stretches to get you started. I want you to understand that stretching is not a contest in flexibility. Your flexibility will naturally improve with proper stretching. Stretch with feelings you can enjoy.

After a while the amount of time (20–30 seconds) you hold stretches will vary. Sometimes you may want to hold a stretch longer because you are extra tight that day, or you are just enjoying the stretch. Or you may not want to hold a stretch as long when your body already feels fairly limber; this would generally be when you hold a stretch for 5–15 seconds. *Remember that no two days are the same* so you must gauge your stretching by how you feel at the moment.

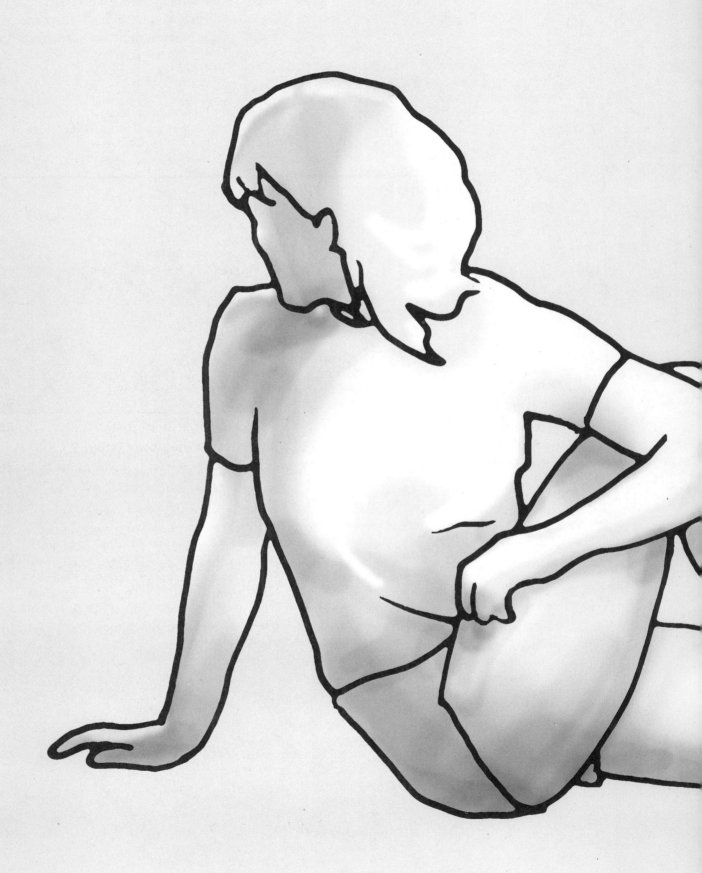

THE STRETCHES

In the following section (*pp. 26–103*) are all the stretches in the book, with instructions for each position. They are grouped according to body parts and presented as a series, but any of them may be done separately without doing the entire routine.

Note: You need not stretch as far as the drawings indicate. Stretch by how you feel without trying to imitate the figure in the drawings. Adjust each stretch to your own personal flexibility, which will vary daily.

Learn stretches for the various parts of the body, at first concentrating on the areas of greatest tension or tightness. On the next two pages is a guide to various muscles and body parts, with reference to the page where each may be found in the book.

Stretching Guide

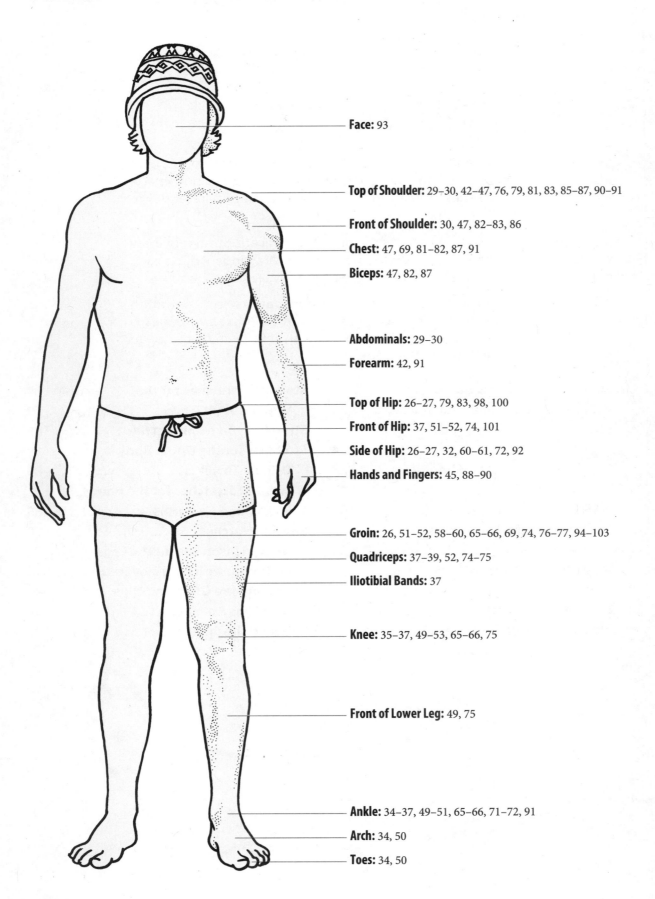

Face: 93

Top of Shoulder: 29–30, 42–47, 76, 79, 81, 83, 85–87, 90–91

Front of Shoulder: 30, 47, 82–83, 86

Chest: 47, 69, 81–82, 87, 91

Biceps: 47, 82, 87

Abdominals: 29–30

Forearm: 42, 91

Top of Hip: 26–27, 79, 83, 98, 100

Front of Hip: 37, 51–52, 74, 101

Side of Hip: 26–27, 32, 60–61, 72, 92

Hands and Fingers: 45, 88–90

Groin: 26, 51–52, 58–60, 65–66, 69, 74, 76–77, 94–103

Quadriceps: 37–39, 52, 74–75

Iliotibial Bands: 37

Knee: 35–37, 49–53, 65–66, 75

Front of Lower Leg: 49, 75

Ankle: 34–37, 49–51, 65–66, 71–72, 91

Arch: 34, 50

Toes: 34, 50

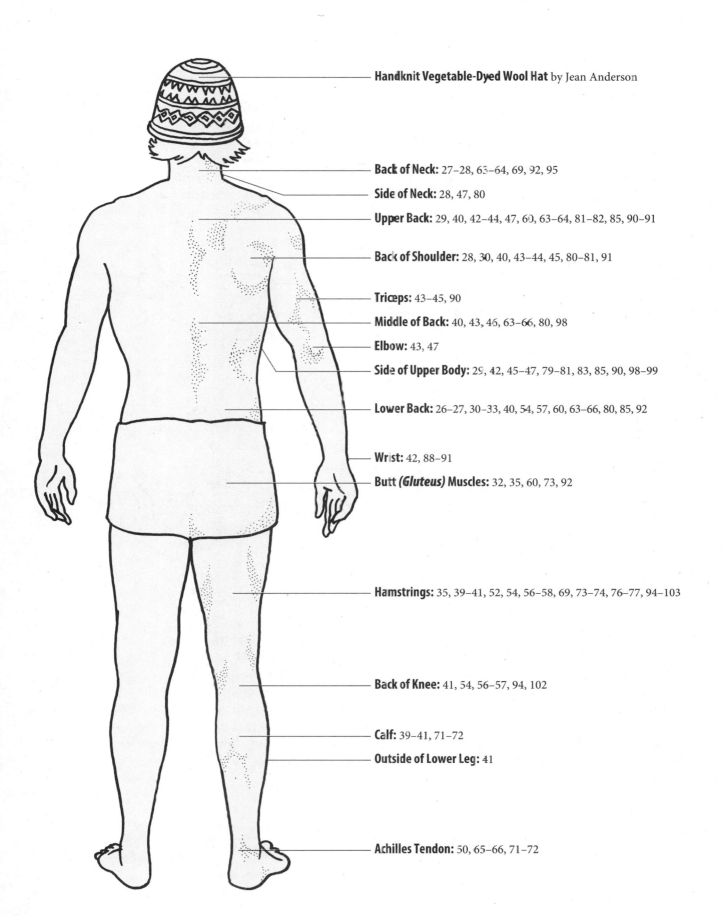

Handknit Vegetable-Dyed Wool Hat by Jean Anderson

Back of Neck: 27–28, 63–64, 69, 92, 95

Side of Neck: 28, 47, 80

Upper Back: 29, 40, 42–44, 47, 60, 63–64, 81–82, 85, 90–91

Back of Shoulder: 28, 30, 40, 43–44, 45, 80–81, 91

Triceps: 43–45, 90

Middle of Back: 40, 43, 46, 63–66, 80, 98

Elbow: 43, 47

Side of Upper Body: 29, 42, 45–47, 79–81, 83, 85, 90, 98–99

Lower Back: 26–27, 30–33, 40, 54, 57, 60, 63–66, 80, 85, 92

Wrist: 42, 88–91

Butt (*Gluteus*) Muscles: 32, 35, 60, 73, 92

Hamstrings: 35, 39–41, 52, 54, 56–58, 69, 73–74, 76–77, 94–103

Back of Knee: 41, 54, 56–57, 94, 102

Calf: 39–41, 71–72

Outside of Lower Leg: 41

Achilles Tendon: 50, 65–66, 71–72

Relaxing Stretches for Your Back

This is a series of very easy stretches that you can do lying on your back. This series is beneficial because each position stretches a body area that is generally hard to relax. You can use this routine for mild stretching and relaxation.

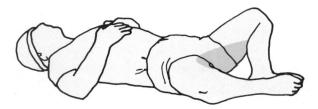

Relax, with knees bent and soles of your feet together. This comfortable position will stretch your groin. Hold for 30 seconds. Let the pull of gravity do the stretching. You may want to put a small pillow behind your head for comfort.

Variation: From this lying groin stretch, gently rock your legs as one unit *(see dotted lines)* back and forth about 10–12 times. These are real easy movements of no more than one inch in either direction. Initiate movements from top of your hips. This will gently limber up your groin and hips.

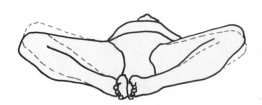

A Stretch for the Lower Back, Side, and Top of Hip

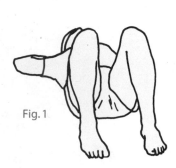

Fig. 1

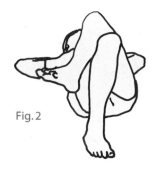

Fig. 2

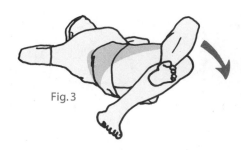

Fig. 3

Bring your knees together and rest your feet on the floor. Interlace your fingers behind your head with your arms on the floor *(fig. 1)*. Now lift the left leg over the right leg *(fig. 2)*. From here, use your left leg to pull your right leg toward the floor *(fig. 3)* until you feel a good stretch along the side of the hip or in the lower back. Relax. Keep the upper back, back of head, shoulders, and elbows flat on the floor. Hold for 10–20 seconds. *The idea is not to touch the floor with your right knee, but to stretch within **your** limits.* Repeat the stretch for the other side, crossing the right over the left leg and pulling down to the right. Exhale as you go into the stretch, then breath rhythmically as you stretch.

- Do not hold your breath.
- Breathe rhythmically.
- Relax.

If you have sciatic* problems of the lower back, this stretch can help. But *be careful*. Hold only stretch tensions that feel good. Never stretch to the point of pain.

PNF Technique: *Contract — Relax — Stretch. (See pp. 222–225.)*

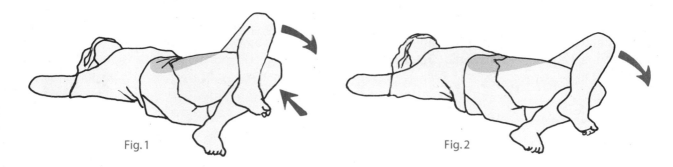

Fig. 1   Fig. 2

To do this, hold down the right leg with the left leg, as you try to pull the right leg back to an upright position. This contracts the muscles of the hip area (*fig. 1*). Hold the contraction for 5 seconds, then relax and do the previous stretch (*fig. 2*). This technique is good for people who are tight.

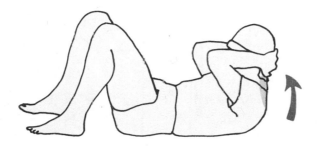

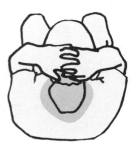

To reduce tension in the neck: While still lying on the floor, you can stretch your upper spine and neck. Interlace your fingers behind your head at about ear level. Slowly pull your head forward until you feel a slight stretch in the back of the neck. Hold for 3–5 seconds, then slowly return to the original starting position. Do this 3–4 times to loosen up the upper spine and neck gradually. Keep your jaw relaxed (back teeth slightly separated) and keep breathing.

---

*The sciatic nerve is the longest and largest nerve of the body. It originates in the lumbar portion of the spine (lower back) and travels down the entire length of both legs and out to the great toe.

PNF Technique: *Contract — Relax — Stretch.* From a bent-knee position, interlace your fingers behind your head (not your neck). Before stretching the back of your neck, gently lift your head upward and forward off the floor. Then move the back of your head downward toward the floor as you resist this movement with your hands and arms. Hold this isometric contraction for 3–4 seconds. Relax for 1–2 seconds, then gently pull your head forward (as in the previous stretch), with your chin going toward your navel until you feel a mild, comfortable stretch. Hold for 3–5 seconds. Do 2–3 times.

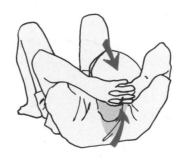

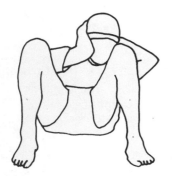

Gently pull your head and chin toward your left knee. Hold for 3–5 seconds. Relax and lower your head back down to the floor, then pull your head gently toward your right knee. Repeat 2–3 times.

With the back of your head on the floor, turn your chin toward your shoulder (as you keep your head resting on the floor). Turn your chin only as far as needed to get an easy stretch in the side of your neck. Hold for 3–5 seconds, then stretch to the other side. Repeat 2–3 times. Keep your jaw relaxed and don't hold your breath.

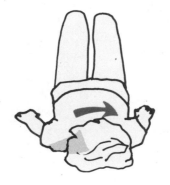

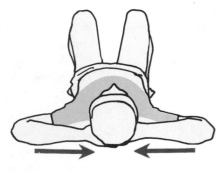

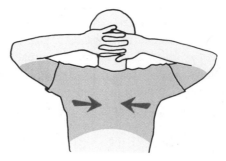

Shoulder Blade Pinch: Interlace your fingers behind your head and pull your shoulder blades together to create tension in the upper back area. (As you do this your chest should move upward.) Hold for 4–5 seconds, then relax and gently pull your head forward as shown on p. 27. This will also release tension in the neck.

Think of creating tension in the neck and shoulders, relaxing the same area, then stretching the back of the neck to help keep the muscles of the neck free to move without tightness. Repeat 3–4 times.

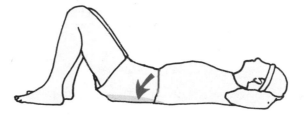

Lower Back Flattener: To relieve tension in your lower back, tighten your butt (*gluteus*) muscles and, at the same time, tighten your abdominal muscles to flatten your lower back. Hold this tension for 5–8 seconds, then relax. Repeat 2–3 times. Concentrate on maintaining constant muscle contraction. This pelvic tilting exercise will strengthen the butt (*gluteus*) and abdominal muscles so that you are able to sit and stand with good posture.

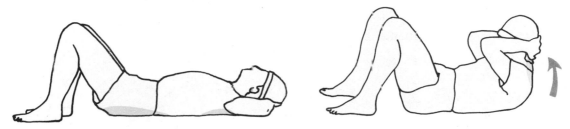

Shoulder Blade Pinch and Gluteus Tightener: Now, simultaneously do the shoulder blade pinch, flatten your lower back, and tighten your butt muscles. Hold contraction for 5 seconds, then relax and pull your head forward to stretch the back of your neck and upper back. Repeat 3–4 times. This feels great.

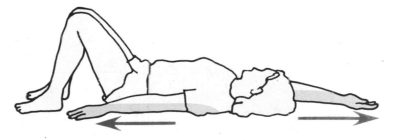

Now put one arm above your head (palm up) and the other arm down along your side (palm down). Reach in opposite directions at the same time to stretch your shoulders and back. Hold stretch for 6–8 seconds. Do both sides at least twice. Keep your lower back relaxed and flat. Keep your jaw relaxed.

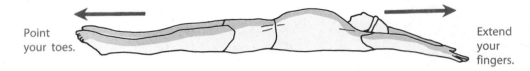

Point your toes.

Extend your fingers.

Elongation Stretches: Extend your arms overhead and straighten out your legs. Now reach as far as is comfortable in an opposite direction with your arms and legs. Stretch for 5 seconds, then relax.

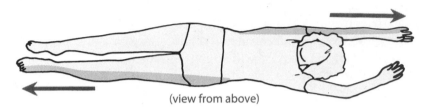

(view from above)

Now stretch diagonally. Point the toes of your left foot as you extend your right arm. Stretch as far as is comfortable. Hold for 5 seconds, then relax. Stretch the right leg and the left arm the same way. Hold each stretch for at least 5 seconds, then relax.

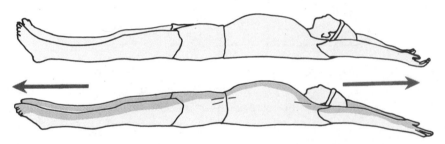

Now, at the same time, stretch both arms and both legs again. Hold for 5 seconds, then relax. This is a good stretch for the muscles of the rib cage, abdominals, spine, shoulders, arms, ankles, and feet.

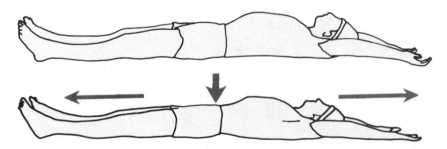

As a variation of this stretch, pull in with the abdominal muscles as you stretch. This will make you feel slim, and is a great exercise for your internal organs.

Doing these elongation stretches three times will reduce tension and tightness and relax your spine and entire body. They help reduce overall body tension quickly. You could do these just before sleeping.

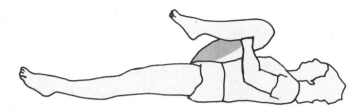

Pull your right leg toward your chest with hands behind the knee. For this stretch keep the back of your head on the floor or mat if possible, but don't strain. Hold an easy stretch for 5–15 seconds. Repeat, pulling your left leg toward your chest. Be sure to keep your lower back flat. If no real stretch is felt, don't worry. If the position feels good, use it. This is a very good position for the legs, feet, and back.

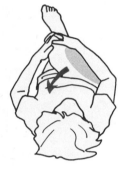
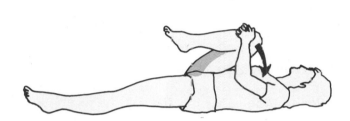

Variation: Pull your knee to your chest, then pull the knee and leg across your body toward your opposite shoulder to create a stretch on the outside of your right hip. Hold an easy stretch for 5–15 seconds. Do both sides.

Variation: From a lying position, gently pull your right knee toward the outside of the right shoulder. Your hands should be placed on the back of your leg, just above your knee. Hold for 10–20 seconds. Breathe continuously and deeply. Repeat for the other leg.

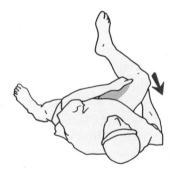

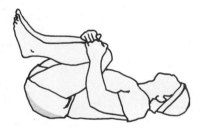
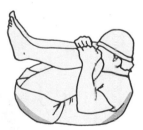

After pulling one leg at a time to your chest, pull both legs to your chest. This time concentrate on keeping the back of your head down and then curling your head up toward your knees.

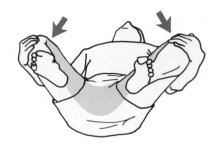

Lie on your back with your knees flexed toward your chest. Place your hands on your lower legs just below your knees. To stretch the insides of your upper legs and groin area, slowly pull your legs out and down until you feel a mild stretch. Hold for 10 seconds. The back of your head can be flat on the floor, resting on a small pillow or up off the floor so that you can look between your legs.

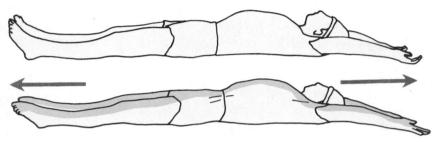

Straighten out both legs again. Stretch and then relax.

A Stretch for the Lower Back and Side of Hip

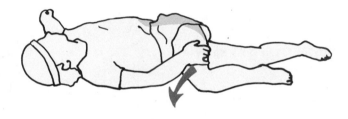

Bend your left knee at 90° and, with your right hand, pull that bent leg up and over your other leg as shown above. Turn your head to look toward the hand of the left arm that is straight out from the shoulder (head should be resting on floor, not held up). Now, using the right hand on your left thigh (resting just above knee) pull your bent (left) leg down toward the floor until you get a mild stretch feeling in your lower back and side of hip. Relax your feet and ankles and keep the back of your shoulders flat on the floor. Hold an easy stretch for 5–15 seconds, each side.

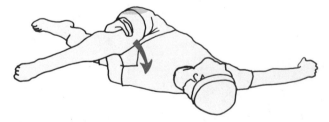

To increase the stretch in your buttocks, reach under your right leg and behind your knee. Slowly pull your right knee toward your opposite shoulder until you get a mild stretch. Keep both shoulders flat on the floor. Hold for 5–15 seconds. Do both legs.

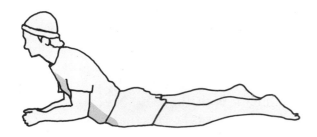

Back Extension: Starting from a prone position (lying on your stomach), place your elbows beneath your shoulders. A mild tension should be felt in the middle to lower back area. Keep the front of the hips on the floor. Hold for 5–10 seconds. Repeat 2–3 times.

You can end a series of stretches for your back by lying in the fetal position. Lie on your side with your legs curled up and your head resting on your hands. Relax.

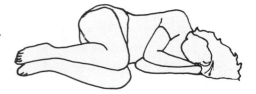

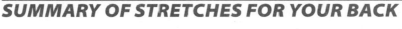

SUMMARY OF STRETCHES FOR YOUR BACK

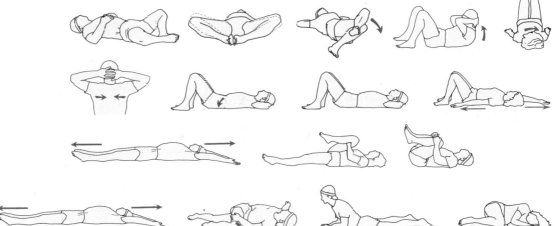

Do these stretches, in this order, to relax your back.

Learn to listen to your body. If the stretch builds or you feel pain, your body is trying to let you know that something is wrong, that there is a problem. If this happens, ease off gradually until the stretch feels right.

Stretches for the Legs, Feet, and Ankles

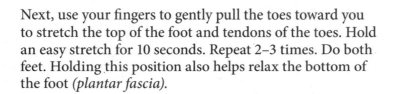

Rotate your ankle clockwise and counterclockwise through a complete range of motion with slight resistance provided by your hand. This rotary motion helps to gently stretch out tight ankle ligaments. Repeat 10–20 times in each direction. Do with both ankles and feel if there is any difference between ankles in terms of tightness and range of motion. Sometimes an ankle that has been sprained will feel a bit weaker and tighter. This difference may go unnoticed until you work each ankle separately and make a comparison.

Next, use your fingers to gently pull the toes toward you to stretch the top of the foot and tendons of the toes. Hold an easy stretch for 10 seconds. Repeat 2–3 times. Do both feet. Holding this position also helps relax the bottom of the foot (*plantar fascia*).

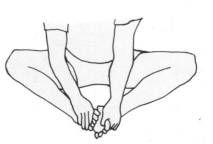

Place your thumbs at the base of your large toes (bottom of feet where toes come out of the foot), index fingers slightly bent, and placed over the nails of your large toes. Use your fingers and thumbs to move your large toes back and forth for 15–20 seconds, then rotate your large toes in a circular motion both clockwise and counterclockwise for 10–15 seconds. Concentrate on increasing the range of motion of your toes as you manipulate this area. A great way to improve or maintain the flexibility and circulation of this area.

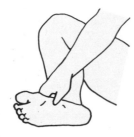

With your thumbs, massage up and down the longitudinal arch of your foot. Use circular motions with a good amount of pressure to loosen tissues. Do both feet. This should help reduce the tension and tightness in the feet.

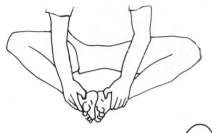

Variation: Massage the arches of your feet with your thumbs. Move up and down the arches, working out sore areas with circular massage. This is good to do while watching TV or just before going to sleep. Massage with pressure that feels good.

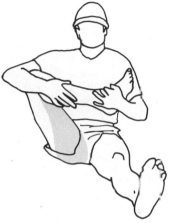

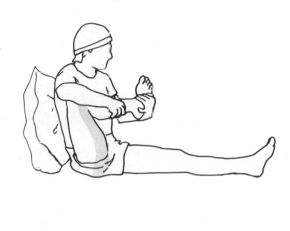

To stretch the upper hamstrings and hip, hold onto the outside of your ankle with one hand, with your other hand and forearm around your bent knee. Gently pull the leg *as one unit* toward your chest until you feel an easy stretch in the back of the upper leg. You may want to rest your back against something for support. Hold for 5–15 seconds. Make sure the leg is pulled as one unit so that stress is not felt in the knee. Slightly increase the stretch by pulling the leg a little closer to your chest. Hold this developmental stretch for 10 seconds. Do both sides. Is one leg more flexible than the other?

For some of you, this position will not provide a stretch. If that is the case, do the stretch shown below.

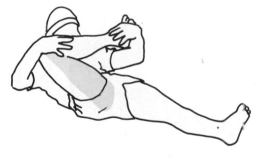

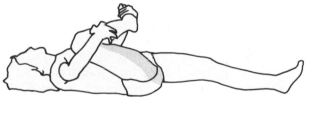

Begin by lying down, then lean forward to hold onto your leg as described in the previous stretch. Gently pull your leg as one unit toward your chest until you feel an easy stretch in the butt and upper hamstring. Hold for 5–15 seconds. Doing this stretch in a lying position will increase the stretch in the hamstrings for people who are relatively flexible in this area. Do both legs and compare.

Experiment: See the difference in the stretch when your head is forward and when the back of your head is on the floor. Always keep every stretch within a personal comfort range. You can place a small pillow behind your head for comfort.

Lie on your back. Bend your right knee and put the outside of your right lower leg just above your opposite knee. With your hands just below your left knee, gently pull your leg toward your chest until a stretch is felt in your buttocks area *(piriformis)*. Hold for 10–20 seconds. Stretch both legs. Lift the back of your head off the floor and look straight ahead as you stretch. Breathe slowly and deeply.

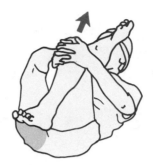

PNF Technique: *Contract — Relax — Stretch.* Another way to stretch the buttocks is to use the contract-relax-stretch technique. Starting from the previous position, move your left leg downward as you resist movement (contraction) for 4–5 seconds. Then relax and stretch for 10–20 seconds as previously described. A really good stretch for the *piriformis*.

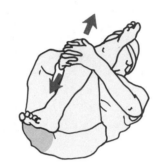

Lie on your left side and rest the side of your head in the palm of your left hand. Hold the top of your right foot with your right hand between the toes and ankle joint. Gently pull the right heel toward the right buttock to stretch the ankle and quadriceps (front of thigh). Hold an easy stretch for 10 seconds.

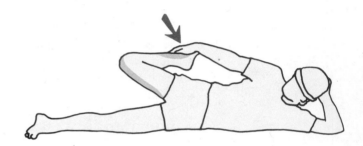

Never stretch the knee to the point of pain. Always be in control.

Now move the front of your right hip forward by contracting the right thigh *(quadriceps)* muscles as you push your right foot into your right hand. This should stretch the front of your thigh and relax your hamstrings. Hold an easy stretch for 10 seconds. Keep the body in a straight line. Now stretch the left leg in the same way. (You may also get a good stretch in the front of the shoulder.) At first it may be hard to hold this for very long. Just work on the proper way to stretch without worrying about flexibility or how you look. Stretching regularly will create a positive change. I like to follow this stretch with the hamstrings stretch at the top of page 58.

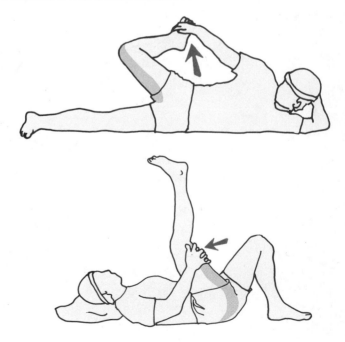

Stretching Your Iliotibial Bands

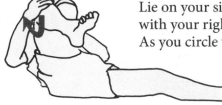

Lie on your side while holding the front of your lower leg from the outside with your right hand. Circle your leg in front of you, then lightly behind you. As you circle your leg, move your right hand to the top of your right ankle.

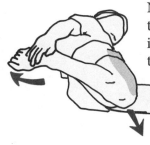

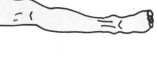

Now you should be on your side as in the figure to the left. To stretch the iliotibial band, gently pull your right heel toward your buttocks as you move the inside of your knee downward toward the floor. You should feel a stretch on the outside of your upper leg. Hold for 10–15 seconds. Do both legs.

> If you experience any knee pain with these stretches, don't do them. Instead, use the opposite-hand-to-opposite-foot technique of stretching the knee (p. 75).

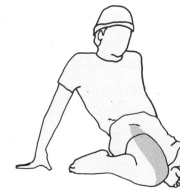

A Sitting Stretch for the Quadriceps: First sit with your right leg bent, with your right heel just outside your right hip. The left leg is bent and the sole of your left foot is next to the inside of your upper right leg. (You can also do this stretch with your left leg straight out in front of you.)

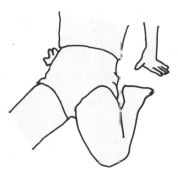

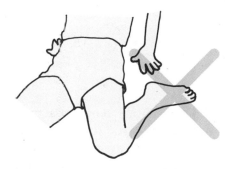

Your foot should be extended back with the ankle flexed. If your ankle is too tight, move your foot just enough to the side to lessen the tension in your ankle.

Do not let your foot flare out to the side in this position. By keeping your foot pointed straight back, you take the stress off the inside of your knee. The more your foot flares to the side, the more stress there is on your knee.

Now, slowly lean *straight back* until you feel an easy stretch. Use your hands for balance and support. Hold this easy stretch for 5–15 seconds.

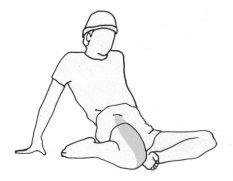

Some people will have to lean back a lot further than others to find the right stretch tension. And some people may feel the right stretch without leaning back at all. Be aware of how you feel and forget about how far you can go. Stretch to where you are comfortable and don't worry about anyone else.

Do not let your knee lift off the floor or mat. If your knee comes up, you are leaning back too far and overstretching. Ease up on the stretch.

> Be sure to hold only stretches that are comfortable.
> **Be careful to not overstretch.**

Now slowly, and in complete control and comfort, increase into the developmental stretch. Hold for 10 seconds, then slowly come out of it. Switch sides and stretch the left thigh the same way.

Can you feel any difference in tension? Is one side more limber than the other? Are you more flexible on one side?

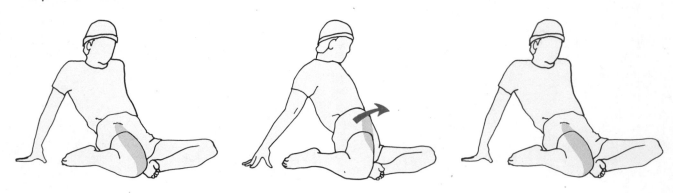

After stretching your quads, practice tightening the buttocks on the side of the bent leg as you turn the hip over. This will help stretch the front of your hip *(iliopsoas)* and give a better overall stretch to upper thigh area. After contracting the butt *(gluteus)* muscles for 5–8 seconds, let the buttocks relax. Drop your hip down and continue to stretch the quads for another 10–15 seconds. Practice to eventually get both sides of the buttocks to touch the floor at the same time during this stretch. Now do the other side.

Note: Stretching the quads first, then turning the hip over as the buttocks contract will help change the stretch feeling when you return to the original quads stretch.

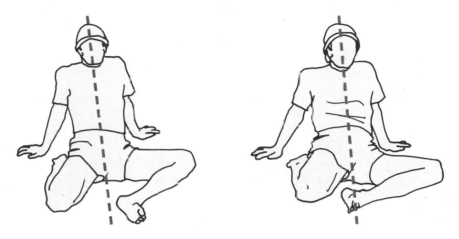

If this produces pain in the knee, move the knee of the leg being stretched closer to the midline of your body until it's more comfortable. Moving this way may take the stress off the knee, but if there is continuing pain, stop doing this stretch.

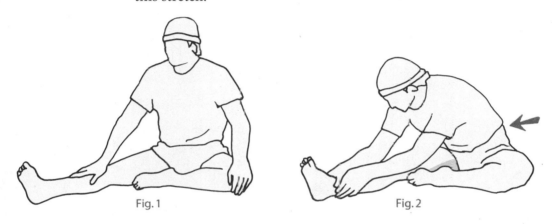

Fig. 1   Fig. 2

To stretch the hamstrings of the same leg that was bent (see previous page), straighten the right leg with the sole of your left foot slightly touching the inside of your right thigh. You are now in the straight-leg, bent-knee position (*fig. 1*). Slowly bend forward from the hips toward the foot of the straight leg (*fig. 2*) until you create the slightest feeling of stretch tension. Hold for 5–15 seconds. After the stretch tension has diminished, bend forward from the hips a bit more. Exhale as you hold this developmental stretch for 10 seconds, breathing rhythmically. Then switch sides and stretch the left leg in the same manner.

During this stretch, keep the foot of the straight leg upright, with the ankle and toes relaxed. Be sure the quadriceps are soft to the touch (relaxed). Do not dip your head forward when initiating the stretch.

I have found that it is best to stretch your quads first, then the hamstrings of the same leg. It is easier to stretch the hamstrings after the quadriceps have been stretched.

Use a towel or elastic cord to help you stretch if you cannot *easily* reach your foot.

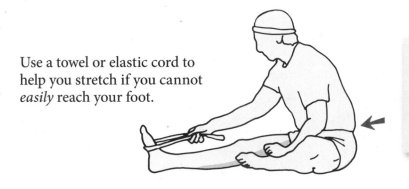

Get used to doing variations of basic stretches. In each variation you will use your body in a different way. You will become more aware of all the stretch possibilities when you change the angles of the stretch tension, even if the angle changes are very slight.

Variations of the Straight-leg, Bent-knee Position

Reach across your body with your left arm to the outside of your right leg. Place your right hand out to the side for balance. This will stretch the muscles of the upper back and spine and the side of the lower back, as well as the hamstrings. To change the stretch, look over your right shoulder as you turn the front of your left hip slightly to the inside. This will stretch the lower back and in between the shoulder blades. Breathe easily. Do not hold your breath. Hold for 10–15 seconds.

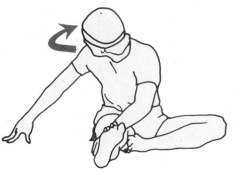

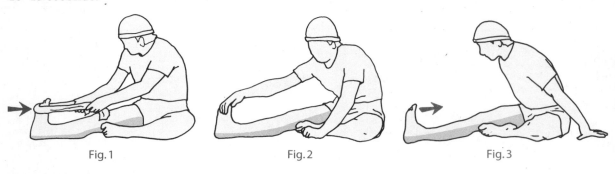

| Fig. 1 | Fig. 2 | Fig. 3 |

To stretch the back of the lower leg (calf and *soleus* muscles), use a towel around the ball of your foot to pull your toes toward your knee (*fig. 1*) or if you are more flexible, use your hand to pull your toes toward your knee (*fig. 2*). Or pull your foot toward your knee (dorsiflexion) without using your hand, and hold, then lean slightly forward to stretch your calf (*fig. 3*). Hold for 10–20 seconds.

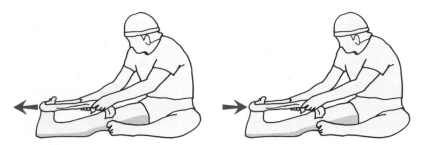

PNF Technique: *Contract — Relax — Stretch.* Another way to stretch the back of your lower leg is to first contract this area by pushing your foot downward as you resist with a towel for 4 to 5 seconds. Then relax. Now use the towel to pull your foot toward your knee. Hold for 5–15 seconds.

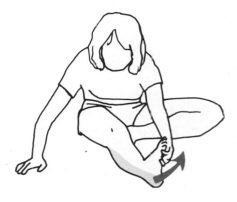

To stretch the outside of your lower leg, reach down with your opposite hand and hold onto the outside border of your foot (*see drawing*). Now, gently turn the outside of your foot to the inside to feel a stretch on the outside of your lower leg. This stretch can be done with a straight leg, or it can be done with your leg flexed at your knee if you are unable to *easily* hold onto the outside border of your foot with your leg straight. In the straight-leg position the quadriceps should be soft and relaxed. Hold an easy stretch for 10 seconds.

Never lock your knees when doing sitting stretches. Be sure to keep the front of your thigh (*quadriceps*) relaxed in all positions using a straight leg. You can't stretch the hamstrings correctly when the opposing set of muscles (the quadriceps) are not relaxed.

SUMMARY OF STRETCHES FOR THE LEGS, FEET, AND ANKLES

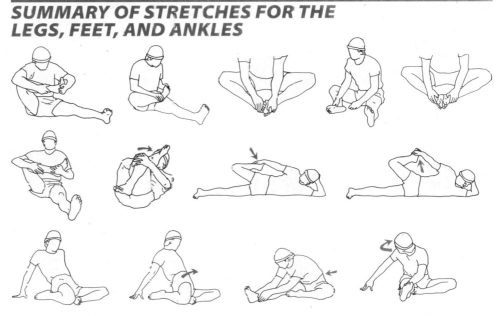

Do these stretches, in this order, as a routine.

Bouncing while stretching can actually make you tighter, rather than more flexible. For example, if you bounce four or five times while touching your toes, then bend over again several minutes later, you'll probably find that you are farther away from your toes than when you started! Each bouncing movement activates the stretch reflex, tightening the very muscles you are trying to stretch.

Stretches for the Back, Shoulders, and Arms

There are many stretches that can reduce tension and increase flexibility in the upper body. Most of the sitting or standing stretches can be done anywhere.

Many people suffer from tension in the upper body because of stress in their lives. Quite a few muscular athletes are stiff in the upper body because of not stretching that area.

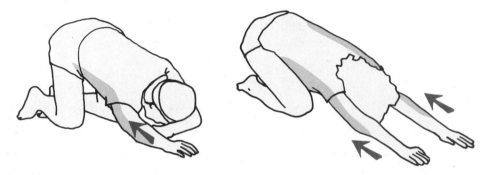

With legs bent under you, reach forward with your hands, then pull back with straight arms while you press down slightly with your palms.

You can do this stretch one arm at a time or both at the same time. Pulling with just one arm provides more control and isolates the stretch on either side. You should feel this in your shoulders, arms, lats (*latissimus dorsi*) or sides, upper back, and even your lower back. When you do this for the first time, you may feel it only in the shoulders and arms, but as you do it more you will learn to stretch other areas; by slightly moving your hips in either direction, you can increase or decrease the stretch. Don't strain. Be relaxed. Hold for 15 seconds.

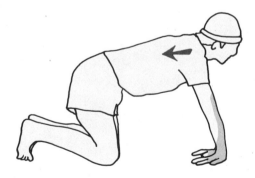

A Forearm and Wrist Stretch: Support yourself on your hands and knees. Thumbs should be pointed to the outside, with fingers pointed toward knees. Keep palms flat as you lean back to stretch the front part of your forearms. Hold an easy stretch for 5–15 seconds. Relax, then stretch again. You may find you are very tight in this area.

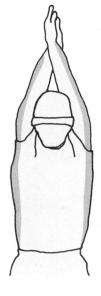

Keep your knees slightly flexed during standing upper-body stretches.

With arms extended overhead and palms together as drawing shows, stretch your arms upward and slightly backward. Breathe in as you stretch upward. Hold for 5–8 seconds, as you breathe easily.

This is a great stretch for the muscles of the outer portions of the arms, shoulders, and ribs. It can be done any time and any place to relieve tension and create a feeling of relaxation and well-being.

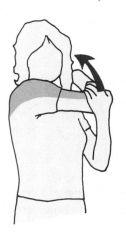

Remember: Keep your jaw relaxed and breathe deeply as you stretch.

To stretch your shoulder and the middle of your upper back, gently pull your elbow across your chest toward your opposite shoulder. Hold for 10 seconds.

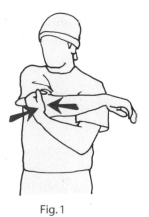

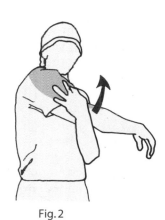

Fig. 1   Fig. 2

PNF Technique: *Contract — Relax — Stretch.* Stand with knees slightly flexed. With your left hand, hold the outside of your right arm just above your elbow. Move your right arm away from your body as you resist with your left hand. Hold an isometric contraction for 3–4 seconds (*fig. 1*). After relaxing a moment, gently pull your right arm across your body toward your shoulder until you feel a comfortable stretch in the outside of your shoulder and upper arm (*fig. 2*). Hold for 10 seconds, then repeat to other side.

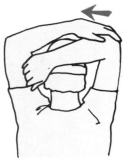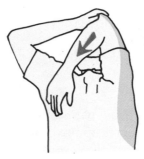

Here is a simple stretch for your triceps and the top of your shoulders. With arms overhead, hold the elbow of one arm with the hand of the other arm. Gently pull the elbow behind your head, creating a stretch. Do it slowly. Hold for 15 seconds. Do not hold your breath.

Stretch both sides. Does it feel as if one side is a lot tighter than the other side? This is a good way to begin loosening up your arms and shoulders. You can do this stretch while walking.

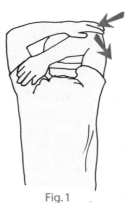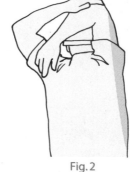

Fig. 1   Fig. 2

PNF Technique: *Contract — Relax — Stretch*. Stand with your knees slightly flexed and your feet about shoulder-width apart. Hold your right elbow with your left hand. Move your right elbow downward as you resist this movement with your left hand (isometric contraction) for 3–4 seconds (*fig. 1*). After relaxing a moment, gently pull your elbow over, behind your head until you feel a mild stretch in the back of your upper arm as in the previous stretch (*fig. 2*). Hold for 5–15 seconds. Repeat to other side.

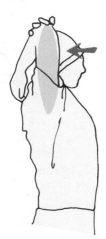

Start in a standing position with your knees slightly flexed. Bend your right elbow and put your arm behind your head. Hold onto your right elbow with your left hand. To stretch the armpit area and shoulder move the back of your head back against your right arm, until a mild stretch is felt. Hold for 10–15 seconds. Do both sides.

Variation: From a standing position, with your knees slightly bent (1 inch), gently pull your elbow behind your head as you bend from your hips to the side. Hold an easy stretch for 10 seconds. Do both sides. *Keep your knees slightly bent for better balance.* Do not hold your breath.

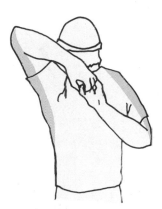

Another Shoulder Stretch: Reach behind your head and down as far as you can with your left hand and, if you are able, grab your right hand coming up, palm out. Grab your fingers and hold for 5–10 seconds. If your hands do not meet, try one of the following:

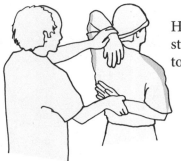

Have someone pull your hands slowly toward each other until you get an easy stretch and hold it. Do not stretch too far. You may get a great stretch without touching your fingers. Stretch within *your* limits.

Or drop a towel behind your head. With your upper arm bent, reach up with your other arm to hold onto the end of the towel. Gradually move your hand up on the towel, pulling your upper arm downwards.

Work a little on it every day and get a good stretch. After a while you will be able to do this stretch without help. It reduces tension and increases flexibility. It also acts as an upper body revitalizer when you are tired.

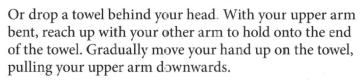

Interlace your fingers out in front of you at shoulder height. Turn your palms outward as you extend your arms forward to feel a stretch in your shoulders, middle of upper back, arms, hands, fingers, and wrists. Hold an easy stretch for 15 seconds, then relax and repeat.

Single Shoulder Shrug: Start with your shoulders relaxed downward. Bring your left shoulder up toward your left ear lobe. Hold for 3–5 seconds. Relax your shoulder downward and repeat on other side. This stretch is excellent for shoulder tension.

PNF Technique: Contract — Relax — Stretch.

Shoulder Shrug: First, raise the top of your shoulders toward your ears until you feel a slight tension in your neck and shoulders. Hold for 5 seconds. Then relax shoulders downward. Think: "Shoulders hang, shoulders down."

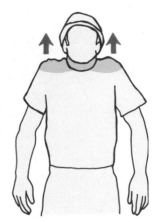

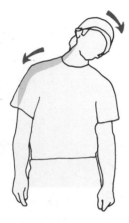

Then gently lower your right shoulder downward as you lean your head, with your ear toward your left shoulder. Hold a comfortable stretch for 5 seconds, then repeat on your other side.

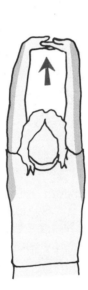

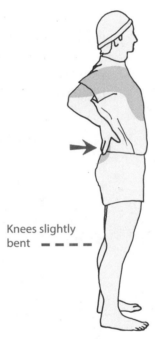

Knees slightly bent

Now interlace your fingers above your head and, with your palms facing upward, push your arms slightly back and up. Feel the stretch in your arms, shoulders, and upper back. Hold for 15 seconds. Do not hold your breath. This stretch is good to do anywhere, anytime, and is excellent for slumping shoulders. Breathe deeply.

Standing with your knees slightly bent, place your palms on your lower back just above your hips, fingers pointing downward. Gently push your palms forward to create an extension in the lower back. Hold for 10 seconds. Repeat twice. Use this stretch after sitting for an extended period of time. Do not hold your breath.

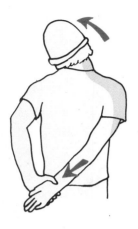

To stretch the side of your neck, lean your head sideways toward your left shoulder as your left hand pulls your right arm down and across, behind your back. Hold an easy stretch for 5–10 seconds. Do both sides.

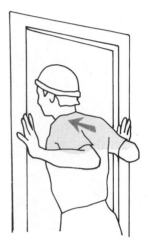

Stand in a doorway and place your hands at about shoulder-height on either side of the doorway. Move your upper body forward until you feel a comfortable stretch in your arms and chest. Keep your chest and head up and knees slightly bent while doing this stretch. Hold for 15 seconds.

The next stretches are done with your fingers interlaced behind your back.

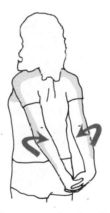

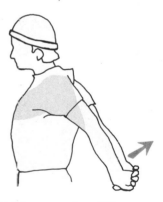

For the first stretch, slowly turn your elbows inward while straightening your arms. This stretches the shoulders, arms, and chest. Hold for 5–10 seconds.

If that is fairly easy, then lift your arms up behind you until you feel a stretch in the arms, shoulders, or chest. Hold an easy stretch for 5–10 seconds. This is good to do when you find yourself slumping forward from the shoulders. Keep your chest out and chin in. This stretch can be done any time.

SUMMARY OF STRETCHES FOR
BACK, SHOULDERS, AND ARMS

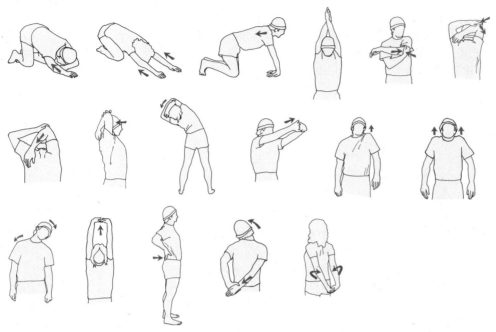

You can do these stretches, in this order, as a routine.

It is better to understretch than to overstretch. Always be at a point where you can stretch further, and never at a point where you have gone as far as you can go.

A Series of Stretches for the Legs

Toe Pointer: This is another good stretch for the legs. You can do a series of stretches for the legs, feet, and groin from the toe pointer position.

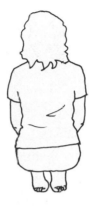

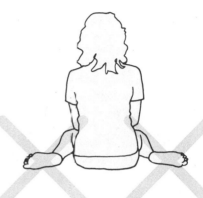

This position helps stretch the knees, ankles, and quadriceps. The toe pointer will also help relax the calves so they may be stretched more easily.

Do not let your feet flare out to the sides when doing this stretch. A flared-out position of the lower legs and feet may cause overstretching of the inside (medial collateral) ligaments of the knee.

Caution: If you have or have had knee problems, be very careful bending the knees underneath you. Do it slowly and under control. If there is any pain, discontinue the stretch.

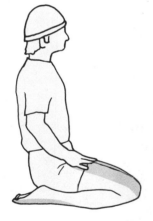

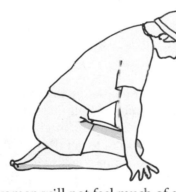

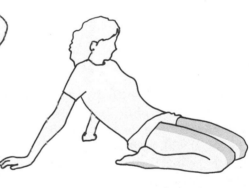

Most women will not feel much of a stretch in this position. But for tight people, especially men, this position lets you know if you have tight ankles. If there is a strain, place your hands on the outside of your legs for support as you balance yourself slightly forward. Find a position you can hold for 10–30 seconds.

If you are tight, do not overstretch. Regularity in stretching creates positive change. There will be noticeable improvement in ankle flexibility within several weeks.

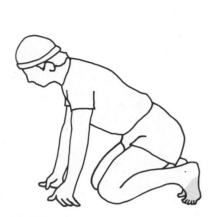 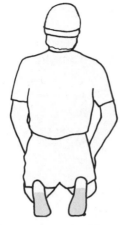

Variation: To stretch your toes and the bottom of your foot *(plantar fascia)*, sit with your toes underneath you *(see above).* Put your hands in front of you for balance and control. If you want to stretch further, slowly lean backwards until it feels right. Hold only stretches that feel good and you can control. Stretch easily for 5–10 seconds. Be careful. There may be a lot of tension in this part of the foot and toes. Be patient. Gradually get your body used to changing by stretching regularly. Return to toe pointer after doing this stretch.

To Stretch the Achilles Tendon Area and Ankles

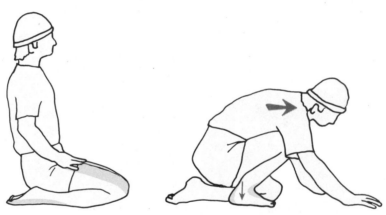

Bring the toes of one foot almost even with or parallel to the knee of the other leg. Let the heel of the bent leg come off the ground one-half inch or so. Lower your heel toward the ground while leaning forward on your thigh (just above the knee) with your chest and shoulder. The idea is not to get the heel flat, but to use the forward pressure from your shoulder on your thigh to gently stretch the Achilles tendon area. Be careful. The Achilles tendon area needs only a *very slight stretch.* Hold for 5–10 seconds.

This stretch is great for tight ankles and arches. Be sure to work both sides. Here again, you will probably find that one side is more flexible than the other.

> As we get older or go through periods of inactivity and then are active again, there is a lot of stress and strain on the lower legs, ankles, and arches. One way to reduce or eliminate the pain and soreness of new activity is to stretch before and after exercise.

Be careful if you have had knee problems. Do not stretch with any feeling of actual pain. Use control so you find the proper stretch feeling.

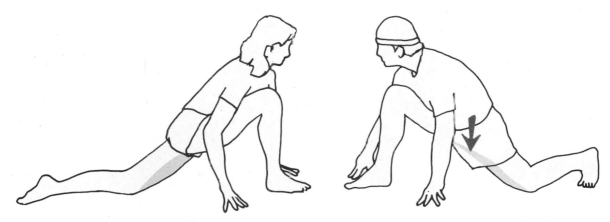

To stretch the muscles in the front of the hip *(iliopsoas)*, move one leg forward until the knee of the forward leg is directly over the ankle. Your other knee should be resting on the floor. Now, without changing the position of the knee on the floor or the forward foot, lower the front of your hip downward to create an easy stretch. Hold for 10–20 seconds. You should feel this stretch in the front of the hip and possibly in the hamstrings and groin.

Stretching for 10–20 minutes in the evening is a good way to keep your muscles well tuned, so you feel good the next morning. If you have any tight areas, or soreness, stretch these areas before retiring (or while watching TV) and feel for yourself the difference the next morning.

Do not have your knee forward of the ankle. This will hinder the proper stretching of the hip and legs. The greater distance there is between the back knee and the heel of the front foot, the easier it is to stretch the hips and legs.

Variations: Turn the left hip slowly to the inside to change the area of the stretch. By only slightly changing angles, you are able to stretch many different, adjacent areas of the body. Hold an easy stretch for 5–15 seconds. Stretch both legs. This is excellent for the hips, lower back, and groin. You can look over your shoulder, behind you, to stretch your neck and upper back.

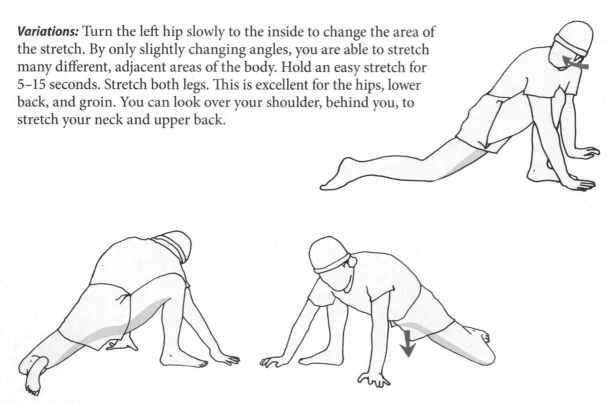

From the previous hip stretch you can isolate a stretch for the inside of the upper leg. Bend your rear knee and move your rear foot to the inside. This will make a 90° angle at the knee joint. Now move your shoulders off your knee and put your hands to the inside of your body for support. Move your hips downward to stretch the inside of your upper leg (groin). Do not move your back knee or front foot. Be sure that your front knee is directly above your ankle. Hold an easy stretch for 5–15 seconds. Try on the other side. Stretch both legs.

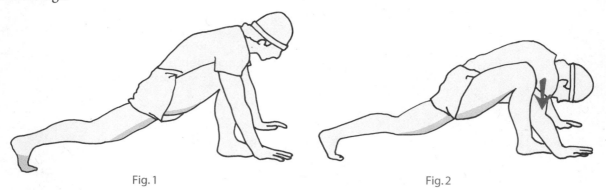

Fig. 1   Fig. 2

An excellent stretch for hip flexibility: With your front knee directly above your ankle, shift your weight up onto the toes and ball of your back foot (*fig. 1*). Now hold an easy stretch with a fairly straight back leg for 15–20 seconds. Think of the front of your hip going down to create the right stretch tension. Use your hands for balance. This stretches the groin, hamstrings, and hip, and possibly behind the knee of the back leg. Do both legs.

Another variation is to change the stretch by gently lowering your upper body to the inside of the knee of the forward leg (*fig. 2*). Hold a comfortable stretch for 10–15 seconds.

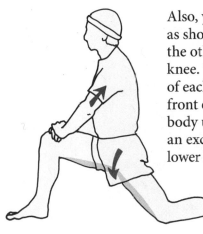

Also, you can stretch your pelvic area with your upper body upright as shown in the next two stretches. Start with one leg in front of the other, with the ankle of your front leg directly below your front knee. The other knee is resting on the floor. Place your hands on top of each other on your thigh, just above your knee. To stretch the front of your hip and thigh, straighten your arms to keep your upper body upright, as you lower the front of your hip downward. This is an excellent stretch for the front of hip *(iliopsoas)* and good for your lower back area. Hold for 5–15 seconds. Repeat for other side.

Use the same technique as in the last stretch, except your back knee is off the floor and you are on the ball of your foot, making your back leg much straighter. This stretch further promotes flexibility in the pelvis/hip area. Hold for 5–15 seconds. Do both sides. This position will challenge you to balance and stretch at the same time. As in the previous stretch, lower the front of your hip downward as you keep your torso upright (vertical).

SUMMARY OF STRETCHES FOR LEGS

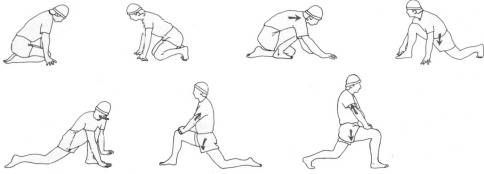

Do these leg stretches, in this order, as a routine.

Stretches for the Lower Back, Hips, Groin, and Hamstrings

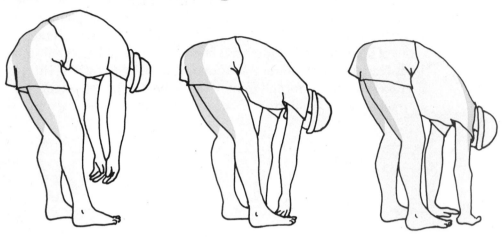

Start in a standing position with your feet about shoulder-width apart and pointed straight ahead. Slowly bend forward from the hips. *Keep your knees slightly bent* (1 inch) during the stretch so your lower back is not stressed. Let your neck and arms relax. Go to the point where you feel a slight stretch in the back of your legs. Stretch in this easy phase for 5–15 seconds, until you are relaxed. Let yourself relax physically by mentally concentrating on the area being stretched. Do not stretch with your knees locked, or bounce when you stretch. Simply hold an easy stretch.

> Stretch by how you *feel* and not by how *far* you can go.

When you do this stretch, you will feel it mostly in your hamstrings (back of thighs) and back of the knees. Your back will also be stretched, but you will feel this stretch mostly in the back of your legs.

Coming Back to an Upright Position

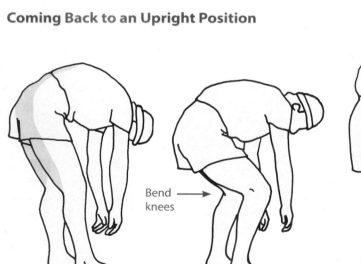

Bend knees →

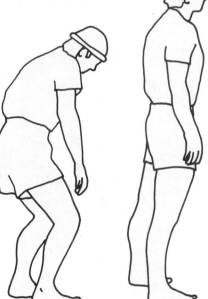

Important: Whenever you bend at the waist to stretch, remember to bend your knees slightly (1 inch or so). It takes the pressure off your lower back. Use the big muscles of the upper legs to stand up, instead of the small muscles of the lower back. Never bring yourself to an upright position with knees locked.

This principle is also important in lifting heavy objects off the ground (*see pp. 218–220, Caring for Your Back*).

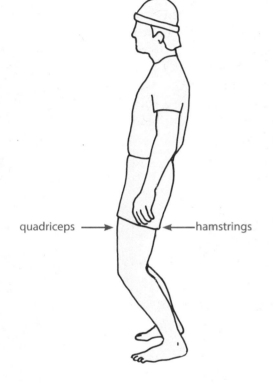

quadriceps → ← hamstrings

> Stretching is not competitive. You may well not be able to touch your toes. The point is for *you* to get more flexible, not to stretch as far as others.

PNF Technique: *Contract — Relax — Stretch.* Next, assume a bent-knee position with your heels flat, toes pointed straight ahead, and feet about shoulder-width apart. Hold for 30 seconds. In this bent-knee position, you are contracting the quadriceps and relaxing the hamstrings. The primary function of the quadriceps is to straighten the leg. The basic function of the hamstrings is to bend the knee. Because these muscles have opposing actions, contracting the quadriceps will relax the hamstrings.

As you hold this bent-knee position, feel the difference between the front and the back of your thigh. The quadriceps should feel hard and tight, while the hamstrings should feel soft and relaxed. It's easier to stretch the hamstrings if they are first relaxed.

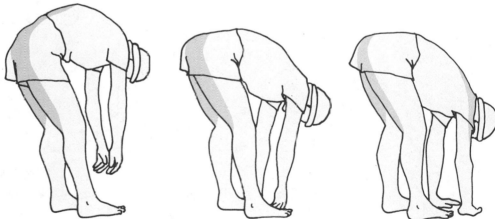

After holding the bent-knee position, stand up and then bend down again with knees slightly bent (1 inch). Don't bounce. You probably can go a little farther already. Hold about 5–15 seconds.

You must be in a comfortable and stable position when you stretch.

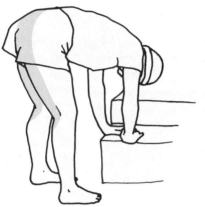

You will find it easier to hold this stretch if you can distribute your weight between your arms and legs. If you are unable to reach your toes (or ankles) with your knees slightly bent (many people cannot), then use a stair or curb, or a pile of books to rest your hands on. Find a balance between your hands and feet so you can relax.

Variation: With your hands, hold onto the back of your lower legs in the calf or ankle area. By pulling your upper body downward (gently!) with your hands, you will be able to increase the stretch in your legs and back, while you concentrate on relaxing in a very stable position. Do not go too far. Relax and stretch. Keep your knees slightly bent.

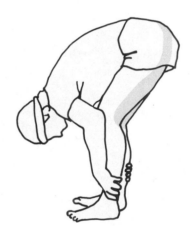

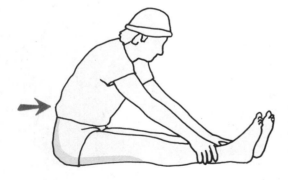

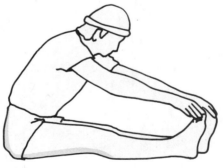

Next, sit down with your legs straight and feet upright, heels no more than six inches apart. Bend from the hips to get an easy stretch. Hold for 5–15 seconds. You will probably feel this just behind your knees and in the back of your upper legs. You may also feel a stretch in the lower back if your back is tight.

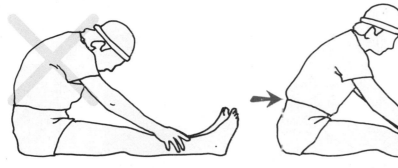

Do not dip your head forward as you begin this stretch. Try to keep your hips from rolling backwards.

Think of bending from your hips without rounding your upper back.

You may need to sit against a wall to keep your lower back flat. This position in itself may be enough of a stretch for you if you are extremely tight.

If you have trouble relaxing while doing this stretch, use a towel to help. Pull yourself forward (gently!) from the hips to where you can relax and still get a stretch. Use your hands and arms to pull yourself forward. Work your way down the towel with your fingers, until the stretch feels right. Be careful here. Do not overstretch.

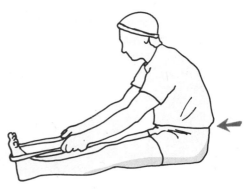

If this stretch seems to put pressure on your lower back, or you have had lower back problems, do the stretches shown on pages 39 and 58. These will feel more comfortable.

Be careful when you stretch with both legs in front of you or when bending forward at the hips in a standing position. You must not overstretch in these positions. Since the back of each leg probably differs in tightness and tension, don't stretch both legs at the same time if you have lower back problems. When one or both legs are extremely tight, it's difficult to stretch both legs at the same time and get the correct stretch for each leg. It is easier on your back to stretch each leg separately.

Lie on your back and lift your leg up toward a 90° angle at the thigh joint. Keep the lower back flat against the floor. Hold for 10–20 seconds. Repeat for other leg. If necessary, hold onto the back of your leg to create the stretch. Or put a towel or elastic cord around the bottom of your foot and pull gently. Only stretch as far as is comfortable. Also, you can place a pillow under your head for more comfort.

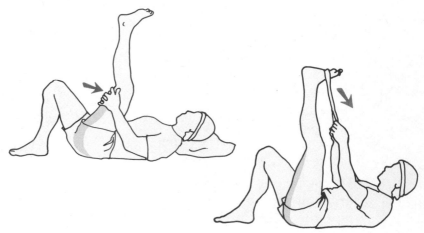

To Stretch the Groin Area

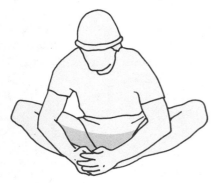 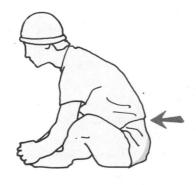

Put the soles of your feet together and hold onto your toes. Gently pull yourself forward, bending from the hips until you feel a good stretch in your groin. You may also feel a stretch in the back. Hold for 20 seconds. Do not make the initial movement for this stretch from your head and shoulders. Move from the hips (*see p. 16, Getting Started*). Try to get your elbows on the outside of your legs so you are stable and balanced. Contract your abdominal muscles mildly as you lean forward; this will increase your forward flexibility.

> Remember — no bouncing when you stretch. Find a place that is fairly comfortable, one that allows you to stretch and relax at the same time.

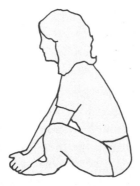 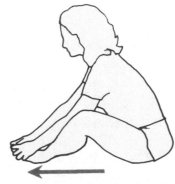

If you have any trouble bending forward, your heels may be too close to your groin area.

If so, move your feet farther out in front of you. This will allow you to move forward from your hips.

Variations If You Are Tight in the Groin Area

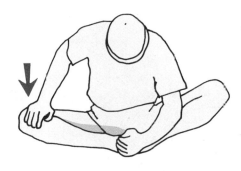

Hold onto your feet with one hand, with your elbow on the inside of the lower leg to hold down and stabilize the leg. Now, with your other hand on the inside of your leg *(not on the knee)*, gently push your leg downward to isolate and stretch this side of the groin. If you are tight in the groin area, this is a good isolation stretch that will limber up your groin and allow your knees to fall more naturally downward. Do both sides. Hold for 10–15 seconds.

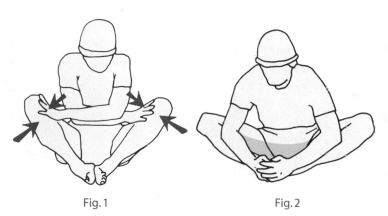

Fig. 1   Fig. 2

PNF Technique: *Contract — Relax — Stretch.* With your hands supplying slight resistance on the insides of opposite thighs, try to bring your knees together just enough to contract the muscles in the groin *(fig. 1).* Hold this stabilized tension for 4–5 seconds, then relax and stretch the groin as in the preceding stretches *(fig. 2).* This will help relax a tight groin area. This technique of contract-relax-stretch is valuable for athletes with groin problems.

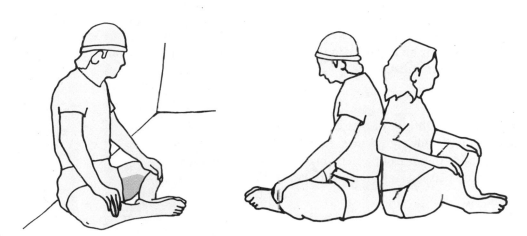

Another way to stretch tight groin muscles is to sit against a wall or sofa: something that will provide support. With your back straight and the soles of your feet together, use your hands to push gently down on the inside of your thighs (not *on* the knees, just above them). Push gently until you get a good, even stretch. Relax and hold for 20–30 seconds.

It is also possible to do this stretch with a partner. Sit back-to-back for stability.

If you have trouble sitting cross-legged, these groin stretches will start to make that position easier for you.

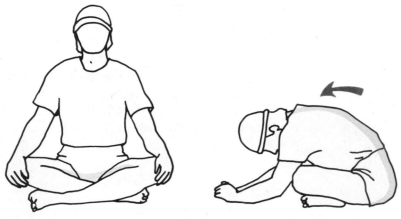

To stretch the back and inside of the legs, sit in a crossed-leg position and then lean forward until you feel a good comfortable stretch. Get your elbows out in front of you if you can. Hold and relax. This is a simple stretch for most people and really feels good in the lower back. Do not hold your breath. Stretch for 15–20 seconds.

Variation: Move your upper body over your knee instead of straight ahead. This is good for your hips. Think of bending from the hips.

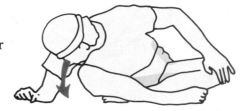

The Spinal Twist

The spinal twist is good for the upper back, lower back, side of hips, and rib cage. It will improve your ability to turn to the side or look behind you without having to turn your entire body.

Sit with your right leg straight. Bend your left leg, cross your left foot over and to the outside of your right knee. Then bend your right elbow and rest it on the outside of your upper left thigh just above the knee. Use your elbow to keep this leg stationary with controlled pressure to the inside.

Now, with your left hand resting behind you, exhale slowly and turn your head to look over your left shoulder; at the same time rotate your upper body toward your left hand and arm. As you turn your upper body, think of turning your hips in the same direction (though your hips won't move because your right elbow is keeping the left leg stationary). This should give you a stretch in your lower back and side of hip. Hold for 5–15 seconds. Do both sides.

Breathing:
• Deep
• Relaxed
• Rhythmic

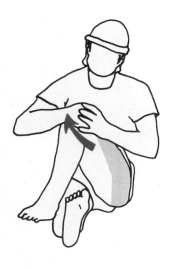

Variation: Pull your knee across your body toward your opposite shoulder until you feel an easy stretch on the side of the hip. Hold for 10–15 seconds. Do both sides.

People tend to spend more time on the first leg, arm, or area they stretch, and they usually will stretch their "easy" or more flexible side first. Thus more time is spent on the "good" side and less on the "bad" side. To remedy this, stretch your tight side first. This will help even out your overall flexibility.

SUMMARY OF STRETCHES FOR LOWER BACK, HIPS, GROIN, AND HAMSTRINGS

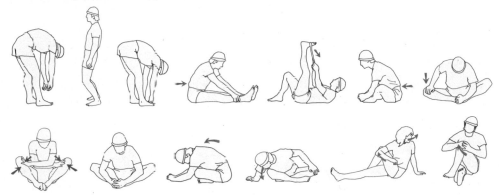

You can do these stretches, in this order, as a routine.

At this time let's go over some of the basic techniques of stretching:

• Don't stretch too far, especially in the beginning. Get a slight stretch and increase it after you feel yourself relax.

• Hold a stretch in a comfortable position; the stretch tension should subside as you hold it. No drastic static stretches.

• Breathe slowly, deeply, and naturally — exhale as you bend forward. Do not stretch to a point where you cannot breathe normally.

• Do not bounce. Bouncing tightens the very muscles you are trying to stretch.

• *Think about the area being stretched.* Feel the stretch. If the tension becomes greater as you stretch, you are overdoing it. Ease off into a more comfortable position.

• Don't focus on flexibility. Just learn to stretch properly and flexibility will come with time. (Flexibility is only one of the many by-products of stretching.)

Other things to be aware of:

• We are different every day. Some days we are tighter, other days looser.

• Drink plenty of water. Your muscles stretch more easily when your body is properly hydrated.

• You can control what you feel by what you do.

• Regularity is one of the most important factors in stretching. Stretch regularly and you will naturally want to become more active and fit.

• Don't compare yourself with others. Even if you are tight or inflexible, don't let this stop you from stretching and improving yourself.

• Proper stretching means stretching within your own limits, being relaxed, and not making comparisons with what other people can do.

• Stretching keeps your body ready for movement.

• Stretch whenever you feel like it. It will always make you feel good.

Stretches for the Back, Hips, and Legs

It's best to stretch on a firm but not hard surface, such as a soft rug or firm mat, when doing these stretches for the back. If the surface is too hard, you won't be able to relax as easily.

Lie on your back and pull your left leg toward your chest. Keep the back of your head on the mat if possible, but don't strain. If you can't do it with your head down, use a small pillow under your head. Keep the other leg as straight as possible, without locking your knee. Hold for 30 seconds. Do both sides. This will slowly loosen up the back muscles and hamstrings.

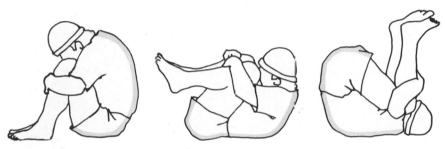

Spinal Roll: Don't do this stretch on a hard surface; use a mat or rug. In a sitting position hold your knees with your hands and pull them to your chest. Gently roll up and down your spine, keeping your chin down toward your chest. This will further stretch the muscles along the spine.

Try to roll evenly and with control. Roll back and forth 4–8 times or until you feel your back start to limber up. Do not rush.

Remember: If you have a neck problem, be very careful with these stretches.

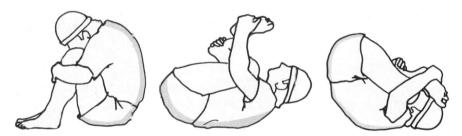

Spinal Roll with Crossed Legs: Next is the spinal roll with lower legs crossed. Begin your roll in the same sitting position as for the previous spinal roll. As you roll backwards, cross your lower legs and, at the same time, pull your feet (from the outside) toward your chest. Then, release your feet as you roll up to a sitting position with your feet together and uncrossed. (Always start each roll with the legs uncrossed.)

On each repetition, alternate the crossing of your lower legs so that, with the pull-down phase of the roll, the lower back will be stretched evenly on both sides. Do 6–8 repetitions.

Take your time in stretching your back. Do not rush through the stretches. Concentrate on relaxing in every stretch that you do. Find a stretch tension that feels good. Do not torture yourself.

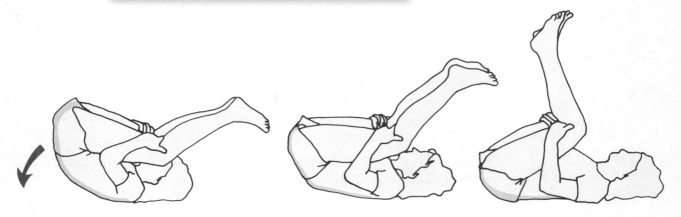

With legs in a moderate overhead position, roll down slowly, trying to roll on each vertebra, one at a time. At first you will probably come down fast, but if you practice, your back will limber up so you will be able to lower yourself slowly, vertebra after vertebra.

Put your hands directly behind your knees and *keep your knees bent* as you roll down. Use your arms and hands to hold your legs still. This will give you greater control of the speed at which you lower yourself. Keep your head on the floor. You may need to tilt your head slightly upward for balance as you roll downward.

Rolling out of the legs-overhead position slowly like this is a good way to find out exactly what part of your back is the tightest. The part or parts of your back that are the hardest to lower *slowly* are the tightest. But you can stretch the tightness and inflexibility out of the spine if you spend a little time working on it gently every day.

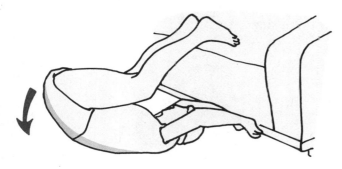

To gain more control over the stretch in your back when lowering your legs, place your arms over your head and hold onto something that is stable such as a heavy piece of furniture. Now, with a slight bend in your arms and bent knees, *slowly* lower yourself one vertebra at a time. By holding onto something with your hands you are able to stretch the back more fully. Do this slowly and under control.

Do not overdo things, but instead, *gradually* develop your physical well-being.

Stretching with legs in a moderate overhead position is good for stretching the back and helps in the circulation of blood from the lower limbs to the upper body.

The Squat: Many of us get tired in the lower back from hours of standing and sitting. One position that helps to reduce this tension is the squat.

Be careful: I believe that the squat is one of our most natural positions. However, due to particular knee problems, some people cannot and should not squat. Always check with a qualified professional if you have any concerns about what your body is capable of.

From a standing position, squat down with your feet flat and toes pointed out at approximately 15° angles. Your heels should be 4–12 inches apart, depending on how limber you are, or as you become familiar with stretching, depending on exactly what parts of your body you want to stretch. The squat stretches the knees, back, ankles, Achilles tendon areas, and deep groin. Keep your knees to the outside of your shoulders, directly above the big toes. Hold comfortably for 10–15 seconds. For many people this will be easy, for others very difficult.

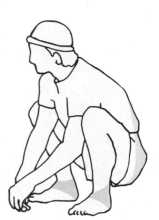

Variations: At first there may be a problem with balance, such as falling backwards because of tight ankles and tight Achilles tendons. If you are unable to squat as shown above, there are other ways to learn this position.

Try the squat on the downward slant of a driveway or hillside

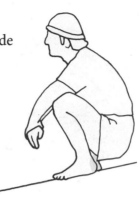

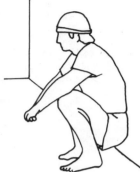

or by leaning your back
against a wall.

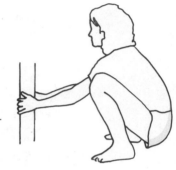

You can use a fence or pole for balance.

After you have done it for a while, the squat becomes a very comfortable position and helps relieve tightness in the lower back. Now return to a standing position as shown on the opposite page.

Variations: From a standing position, place your hands slightly to the inside of your upper legs, just above the knees. Your feet should be at least shoulder-width apart. Slowly lower your hips downward as you gently push your upper legs outward until you feel a mild stretch in the groin area. Hold for 15 seconds. This also stretches the ankles and Achilles tendon area. Don't let your hips drop below your knees.

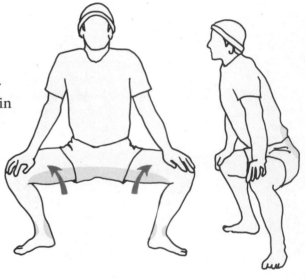

> Be careful if you have had any knee problems. If pain is present, discontinue this stretch.

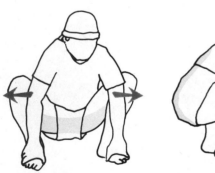

To increase the stretch in the groin from the squat position, put your elbows on the inside of your knees, gently push outward with both elbows as you bend slightly forward from your hips. Your thumbs should be on the inside of your feet, with your fingers along the outside of the feet. Hold for 15 seconds. Do not overstretch. If you have trouble balancing, elevate your heels slightly.

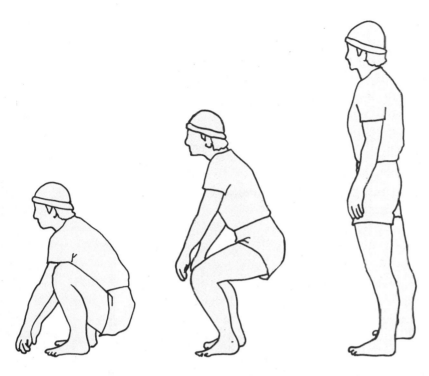

To stand up from the squat position, pull your chin in slightly and rise straight up *with your quadriceps doing all the work and your back straight*. Do not dip your head forward as you stand up; this puts too much pressure on your lower back and neck.

SUMMARY OF STRETCHES FOR THE BACK, HIPS, AND LEGS

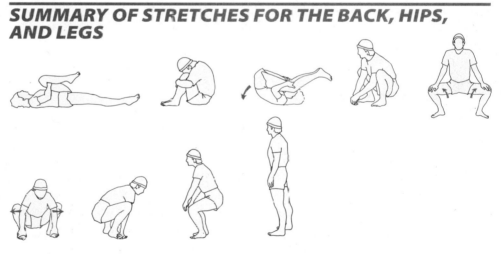

You can do these stretches, in this order, as a routine for your back.

Holding the right stretch tensions for a period of time allows the body to adapt to these new positions. Soon the area being stretched will adapt to the slight tension and your body will be able to assume the new positions without the tightness formerly felt.

Elevating Your Feet

Elevation of the feet before and after activity is a great way to revitalize your legs. It helps keep the legs light with plenty of consistent energy for everyday living and activity. It's a wonderful way to rest and relax tired feet, especially if you have been standing all day. It helps the entire body feel good. And it's a simple way to help prevent or relieve varicose veins. I recommend elevating the feet at least twice a day for 2–3 minutes or longer for revitalization and relaxation.

Lying on the floor and resting your feet against a wall is a simple way to elevate your feet. Keep your lower back flat. Your butt should be at least 3 inches from the wall If there isn't a wall close by, you can elevate your feet from the legs-overhead position or simply put a few pillows under your feet to raise them above your heart. At first, elevate your feet for only about one minute, gradually increasing the time. If your feet start to go to sleep, roll over on your side and then sit up. (See p. 20 for the proper way to sit up from this position.) *Don't get up quickly after elevating your feet* or you may get a light-headed feeling.

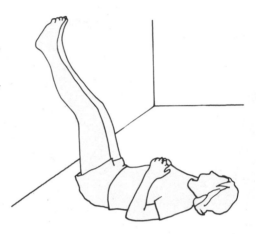

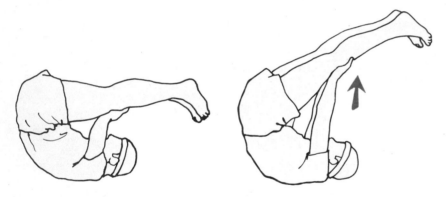

Put the palms of your hands on your knees with fingers pointed toward your toes. Straighten your arms. If you relax at the hips, your arms will take care of the weight of your legs. This is a very relaxing position. In hatha yoga it is called the "pose of tranquility." There is a balancing point, at the back of your head and the top of the spine when you are in this position. The balance is difficult to find but not as hard as it might seem at first. Give it at least 10–12 good tries. A little practice makes it simple.

Be careful doing this if you have any problem with your upper back or neck.

> We may know that stretching and regular exercising are beneficial, but knowledge alone is not enough. *Doing* is what is important, for what good is knowledge if we do not use it to live more fully?

The BodySlant®: A great way to elevate your feet and stretch is to lie on a BodySlant. Don't do any exercises on the BodySlant, just lie there and relax for about 5 minutes, gradually increasing the time to 15–20 minutes. Placing your hands on your chest or stomach will decrease the arch in your lower back.

This is a good position for pulling in your stomach and being thin. The internal organs will gradually fall back into a normal position. For people who want to look and feel thin, the BodySlant is excellent

When getting up from the BodySlant, sit up for 2–3 minutes before you stand. You should get up slowly from all positions with feet elevated so you don't become dizzy.

Stretching on the BodySlant

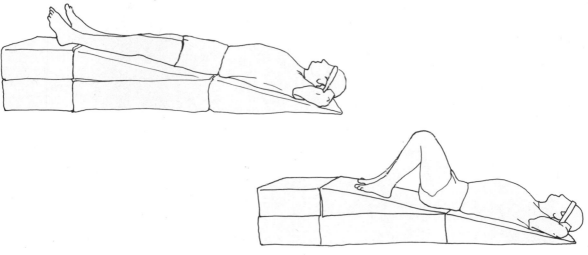

See p. 29.

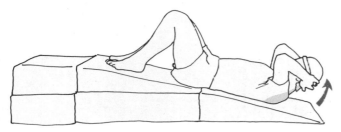

See p. 27.

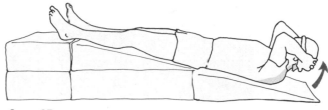

See p. 27.

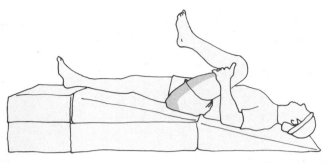

See p. 31.

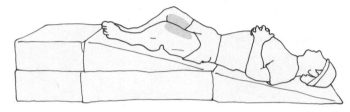

See p. 26.

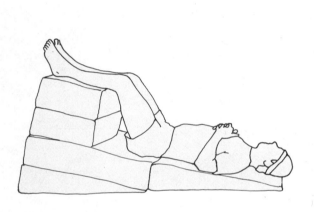

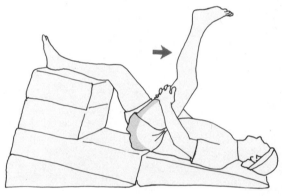

See p. 58.

SUMMARY OF STRETCHES FOR ELEVATING YOUR FEET

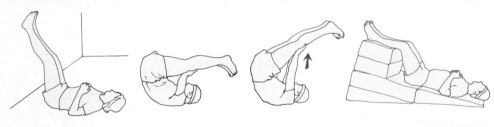

Standing Stretches for the Legs and Hips

This series of stretches will help your walking or running. It will give flexibility and energy to your legs. All these stretches can be done while standing.

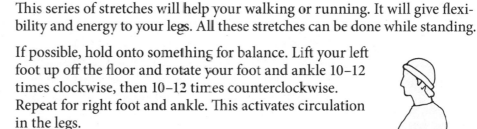

If possible, hold onto something for balance. Lift your left foot up off the floor and rotate your foot and ankle 10–12 times clockwise, then 10–12 times counterclockwise. Repeat for right foot and ankle. This activates circulation in the legs.

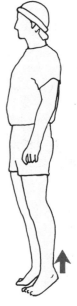

PNF Technique: *Contract — Relax — Stretch.* Before stretching your calves, stand on your toes for 3–4 seconds to contract your calves. Then use the following calf stretch. This should make it easier.

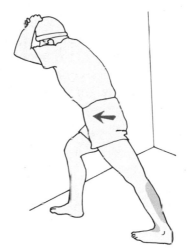

To stretch your calf, stand a little way from a solid support and lean on it with your forearms, head resting on hands. Bend one leg and place your foot on the ground in front of you, with the other leg straight behind. Slowly move your hips forward, keeping your lower back flat. Be sure to keep the heel of the straight leg on the ground, with toes pointed straight ahead or slightly turned in. Hold an easy stretch for 10–15 seconds. Do not bounce. Now stretch other leg. *Also see p. 15,* Getting Started.

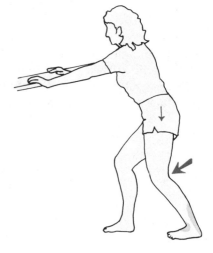

To create a stretch for the *soleus* and Achilles tendon area, lower your hips downward as you bend your knee slightly. Be sure to keep your back flat. Your back foot should be slightly toed-in or straight ahead during the stretch. Keep your heel down. This stretch is good for developing ankle flexibility. Hold for 10 seconds. The Achilles tendon area needs only a *slight feeling of stretch.*

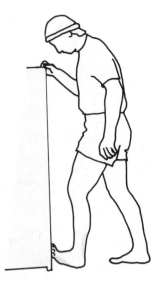

The Achilles tendon area and ankle may be stretched another way. Place your left foot against a wall, with your ankle flexed and toes up as shown in the illustration. Move your upper body forward until you feel a mild stretch tension in the Achilles tendon area. Hold for 8–10 seconds. This also stretches the bottom of your foot and toes.

To stretch the outside of the hip, start from the same position as in the calf stretch. Stretch the right side of your hip by turning your right hip slightly to the inside. Project the side of your right hip to the side as you lean your shoulders very slightly in the opposite direction of your hips. Hold an even stretch for 5–15 seconds. Do both sides. Keep the foot of your back leg pointed straight ahead with the heel flat on the ground.

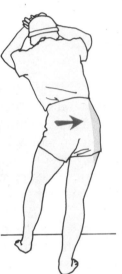

Lifelong Fitness Could Start in School

In the old days, high school students spent many hours in PE classes, learning only games and sports. If stretching was taught at all, it was the bouncing, "no pain—no gain" approach. These days a new generation of teachers has the opportunity to teach students how to take care of themselves: to stretch properly, to eat right, to make exercise a natural component of a healthy lifestyle. It would be great if kids could come out of school with a positive attitude toward staying healthy for the rest of their lives.

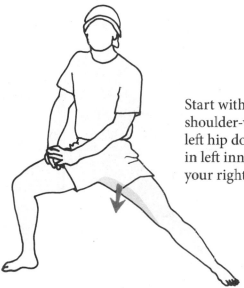

Start with your feet pointed straight ahead and a little more than shoulder-width apart. Bend your right knee slightly and move your left hip downward toward the right knee. This gives you a stretch in left inner thigh (left groin). Hold for 5–15 seconds and repeat for your right thigh.

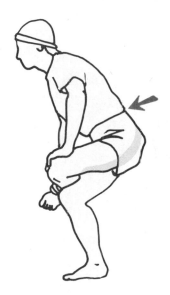

Stand on one foot with your knee slightly flexed and place the outside of the opposite leg just above your knee. Put one hand on the inside of your ankle and the other on your thigh. Now bend your knee a little more as you move your chest forward over the bent leg. This will test your balance. Hold a mild stretch for 5–10 seconds. Do both sides. This stretches the outside of the hip (*piriformis* area). Do not hold your breath.

Hold onto something and pull your knee toward your chest. Do not lean forward at the waist or hips. This gently stretches your upper hamstrings, butt, and hips. The foot on the ground should be pointed straight ahead, with the knee slightly bent (1 inch). Hold an easy stretch for 5–15 seconds. Do both legs.

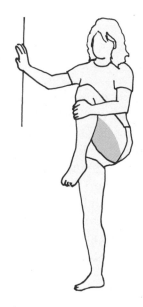

Place the ball of your foot up on a secure support of some kind (wall, fence, table). Keep the standing leg pointed straight ahead. Now bend the knee of the raised leg as you move your hips forward. This should stretch your groin, hamstrings, and front of hip. Hold for 10–15 seconds. Do both sides. If you can, for balance and control, use your hands to hold onto the support. This stretch will make it easier to lift your knees.

Variation: Instead of having the standing foot pointed straight ahead, turn it to the side (parallel to the support), and stretch the inside of the upper legs. Hold for 10–15 seconds.

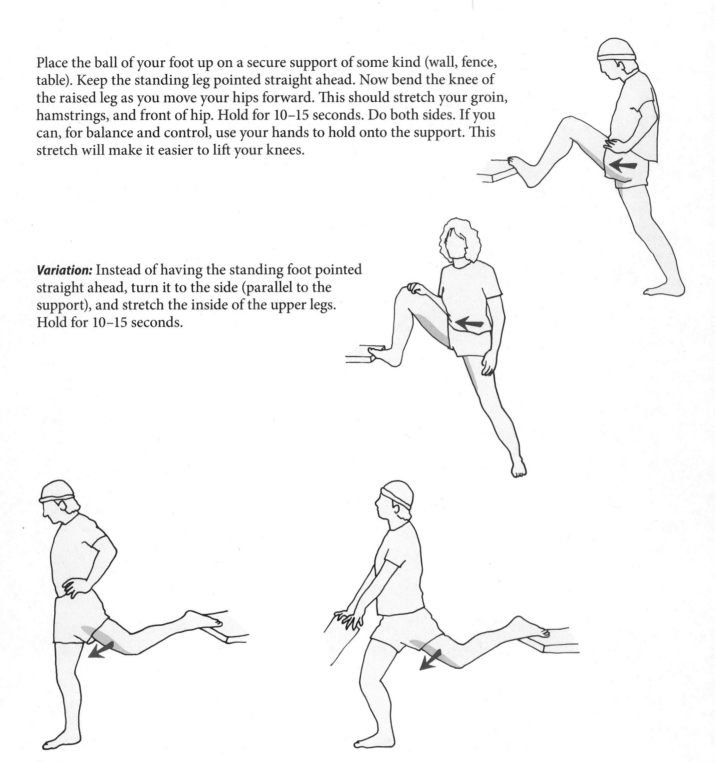

Extend your foot behind you, placing the top of your foot on a table, fence, or bar at a comfortable height. Think of pulling your leg through (moving your leg forward) from the front of your hip to create a stretch for the front of the hip and quadriceps. Flex your butt (*gluteus*) muscles as you do this stretch. Keep the standing knee slightly bent (1 inch) and the upper body vertical. The foot on the ground should be pointed straight ahead. You can change the stretch by slightly bending the knee of the supporting leg a little more. Hold an easy stretch for 5–15 seconds. Through relaxed practice, learn to feel balanced and comfortable in this stretch. Breathe. Use a chair or something for balance if necessary.

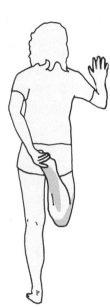

To stretch the quads and knee, hold the top of your *right* foot with your left hand and gently pull your heel toward your buttocks. The knee bends at a natural angle when you hold your foot with the opposite hand. This is good to use in knee rehabilitation and with problem knees. Hold up to 10–20 seconds for each leg.

Variation: This stretch can also be done lying on your stomach. Be sure to stretch without pain. Reach behind you with your hand and hold the top of your opposite foot between the ankle joint and toes. Gently pull your heel toward the middle of your buttocks. Hold for 5–15 seconds.

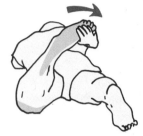

Important note: If you have knee problems, be very careful with these stretches.

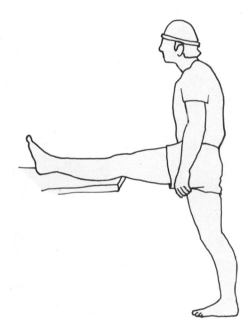

Remember to stretch under control. Start in a place that is fairly easy and go from there. Improvement will occur faster if you go from an easy stretch to a developmental stretch. Let yourself limber up slowly. Remember, straining will keep you from fully realizing the many benefits of stretching.

Place the back of your lower leg on a table or ledge that is about waist high or at a comfortable height. The leg on the ground should be slightly bent at the knee (1 inch), with your foot pointed forward as in a proper running or walking position.

Be careful to not overstretch in this position. Overstretching can put too much stress on the back of the knee, especially if the lower leg is not supported fully.

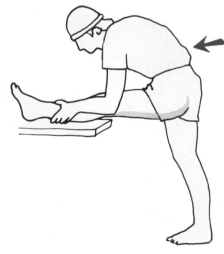

Now, while looking straight ahead, slowly bend forward at the hips until you feel a good stretch in the back of the raised leg. Hold for 5–15 seconds and relax. Find the easy stretch, relax, and then increase it slightly. This is very good for running or walking.

Keep your knees slightly flexed with all these leg-up stretches.

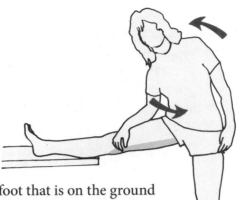

To stretch the inside of your raised leg, turn the foot that is on the ground so it is parallel to the support. Face your upper body in the same direction as your standing foot and turn your right hip slightly to the inside. Slowly bend sideways with your right shoulder going toward your right knee. This should stretch the inside of your upper right leg. Hold an easy stretch for 5–15 seconds. Be sure to keep the knee of the standing leg slightly bent. Repeat for the other leg.

Variation: To change the stretch, use your right hand to pull your left hand and arm up and over your head. This is good for the sides of your upper body and the inside of your raised leg. Keep the knee of the standing leg slightly bent. Hold an easy stretch for 5–15 seconds. Do both sides. Feel the difference in each side. To do this stretch you must be fairly flexible.

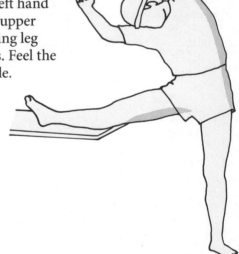

To change the stretch, bend at the waist toward the foot on the ground. The raised leg should remain straight but will turn to the inside as you bend over. This stretches the hamstrings of the supporting leg. The knee of that leg should be slightly bent (1 inch) during the stretch. Hold an easy stretch for 5–15 seconds. Do not hold your breath.

If you want to stretch the groin area of the raised leg, bend the knee of the supporting leg and keep the raised leg straight. If you can, rest your hands on the ground to give you added balance. Hold an easy stretch for 5–15 seconds.

SUMMARY OF STANDING STRETCHES FOR THE LEGS AND HIPS

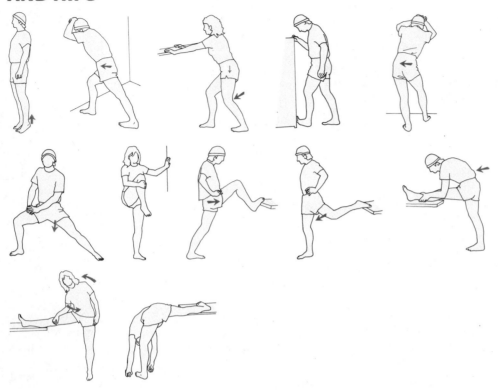

You can do these stretches, in this order, as a routine for the legs and hips.

Avoid creeping *rigor mortis*: It is important to maintain good flexibility throughout our lives, so that as we get older we can avoid the problems that go with stiff joints, tight muscles, and bad posture. One of the striking characteristics of aging is the loss of range of motion, and stretching is perhaps the single most important thing you can do to keep your body limber.

Standing Stretches for the Upper Body

These next two stretches are excellent for stretching the muscles along your side from your arm to your hips. They are done standing, so you can do them at any time, anywhere. Remember to keep your knees slightly bent (flexed) for better balance and to protect your lower back.

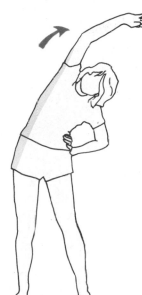

Stand with your feet about shoulder-width apart and toes pointed straight ahead. With knees slightly bent (1 inch), place one hand on your hip for support while you extend your other arm up and over your head. Now slowly bend at your waist to the side, toward the hand on your hip. Move slowly; feel a good stretch. Hold for 5–15 seconds and relax. Gradually increase the amount of time you are able to hold the stretch. Always come out of a stretch slowly and under control. No quick or jerky movements. Breathe and relax.

Instead of using your hand on your hip for support, extend both arms overhead. Grasp your right hand with your left hand and bend slowly to the left, using your left arm to gently pull the right arm over the head and down toward the ground.

By using one arm to pull the other you can increase the stretch along your sides and along the spine. *Do not overstretch.* Hold an easy stretch for 8–10 seconds.

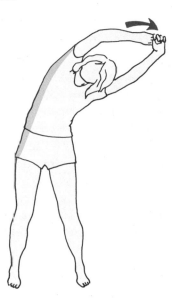

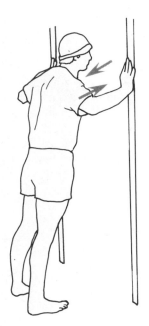
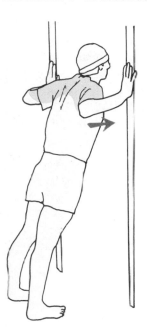

PNF Technique: *Contract — Relax — Stretch.* Stand behind a doorway. With your hands on the door jambs a little above shoulder height, with arms bent, push yourself back by straightening your arms, as in a push-up. Do 3–5 repetitions of this exercise, then relax and slowly let your upper body go toward the doorway to stretch the front of your shoulders and chest. Hold for 15–20 seconds at a comfortable tension.

This stretch for the upper body stretches the muscles laterally along the spine.

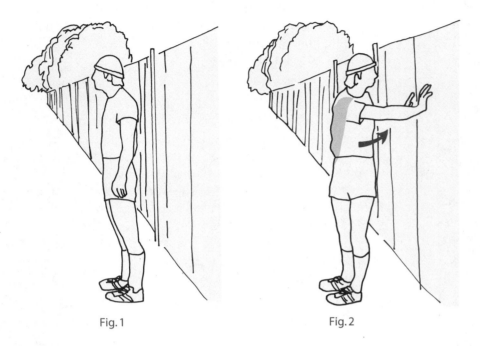

Fig. 1   Fig. 2

Stand about 12–24 inches away from a fence or wall with your back toward it (*fig. 1*). With your feet about shoulder-width apart and toes pointed straight ahead, slowly turn your upper body around until you can easily place your hands on the fence or wall at about shoulder height (*fig. 2*). Turn in one direction and touch the wall, return to the starting position, and then turn in the opposite direction and touch the wall. Do not force yourself to turn any farther than is fairly comfortable. If you have a knee problem, do this stretch very slowly and cautiously. Stop if there is pain. Be relaxed and do not overstretch. Hold for 5–15 seconds. Keep knees slightly bent (1 inch). Do not hold your breath. Stretch the other side.

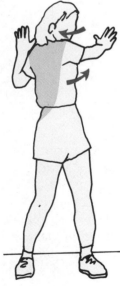

Variation: To change the stretch, turn your head and look over your right shoulder. Try to keep your hips facing forward and parallel to the fence. Hold an easy stretch for 5–15 seconds. Do both sides.

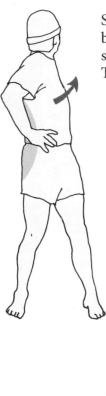

Start with your hands on your hips, feet pointed straight ahead, knees slightly bent. Rotate hips to the left as you look over your left shoulder. Hold an easy stretch for 10 seconds. Stretch each side twice. Be relaxed and breathe easily. This is a good stretch for lower back, hips, and upper body.

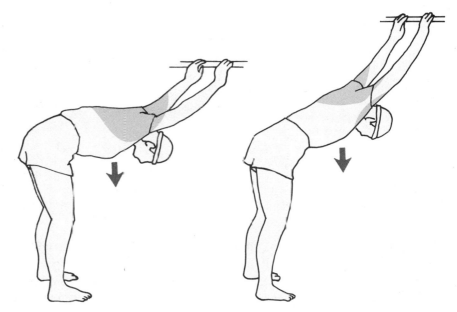

Another good upper body and back stretch is to place both hands shoulder-width apart on a fence or ledge (or the top of refrigerator or filing cabinet) and let your upper body drop down as you keep your knees slightly bent (1 inch). Your hips should be directly above your feet, your breathing rhythmical.

Now, bend your knees just a bit more and feel the stretch change. Place your hands at different heights to change the area of the stretch. After you become familiar with this stretch it is possible to really stretch the spine. Great to do if you have been slumping in the upper back and shoulders all day. This will take some of the kinks out of a tired upper back. Find a stretch that you can hold for at least 20 seconds. Bend your knees when coming out of this stretch.

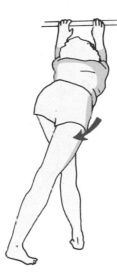

Variation: To increase and change the area of the stretch in another way, bring one leg behind and across the midline of your body as you lean in the opposite direction. This will stretch those hard-to-reach areas of the upper body. Hold for 10 seconds. Do both sides.

I find these arm and shoulder stretches to be very good before and after running. They allow for a relaxed upper body and a freer arm swing. They are also good to do during weight training workouts or as part of a warm-up for any upper body activity such as tennis, baseball, handball, etc.

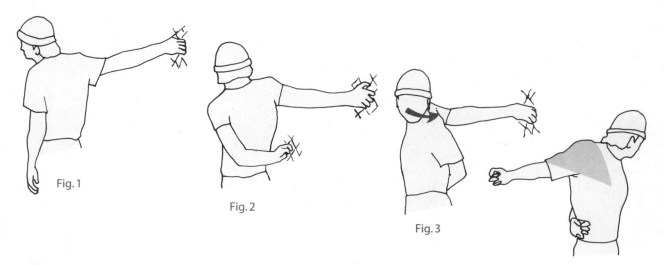

Fig. 1

Fig. 2

Fig. 3

View from the other side of the fence

This stretch is for the front of the shoulders and arms. You need a chain-linked fence, doorway, or wall. Face the wall or press against it with your right hand at shoulder level *(fig. 1)*. Next, bring your other arm around your back and grab the wall (or whatever you are using) as in fig. 2. Now, look over your left shoulder in the direction of your right hand. Keep your shoulder close to the wall as you slowly turn your head *(fig. 3)*. Trying to look at your right hand behind you gives you a stretch in the front of the shoulders.

Stretch the other side. Do it slowly and under control. The feeling of a good stretch is what is important, *not how far you can stretch*.

Variation: From the previous position, stretch your arm and shoulder at various angles. Each angle will stretch the arm and shoulder differently. Hold for 10 seconds.

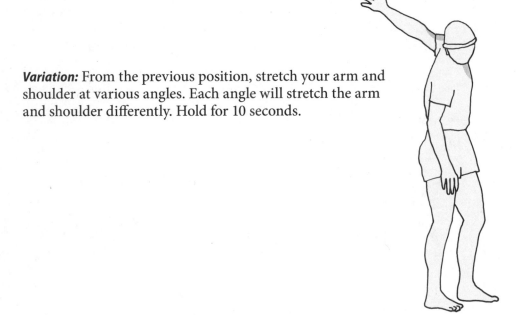

Here is another stretch you can do while using a chain-linked fence or wall for support and balance.

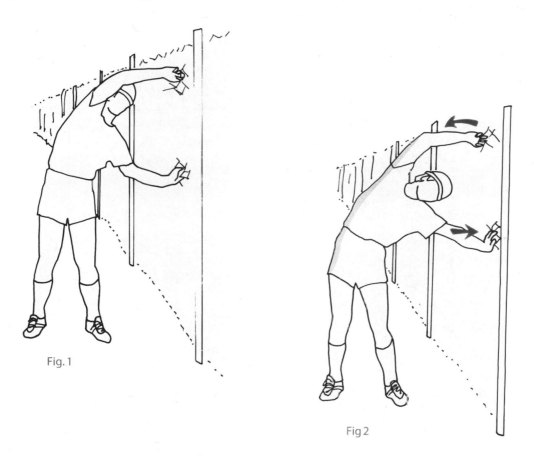

Fig. 1

Fig 2

Hold onto the fence at about waist-high with your left hand. Now reach over your head with your right arm and grab the fence with your right hand. Your left arm will be slightly bent with the right arm extended (*fig. 1*). Keep knees slightly bent (1 inch).

To stretch your waistline and sides, straighten your left arm and pull over with your (upper) right arm (*fig. 2*). Hold for 5–10 seconds. Do both sides.

Slowly go into each stretch and slowly come out of each stretch. Do not bob, jerk, or bounce. Keep your stretching fluid and under control.

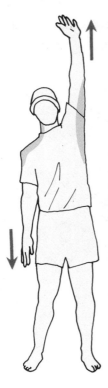

Reach in opposite directions with your arms while standing. Hold for 10 seconds each side. Keep your jaw relaxed and breathe rhythmically. This is an excellent stretch for upper body tension. It stretches the sides of the upper body, shoulders, and arms.

SUMMARY OF STANDING STRETCHES FOR THE UPPER BODY

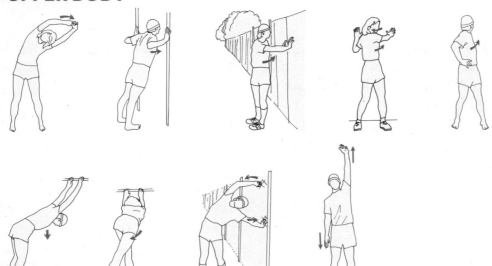

You can do these stretches, in this order, as a routine for the upper body.

Stretching on a Chin-up Bar

With the help of gravity, it is possible to get a fine stretch on a chin bar.

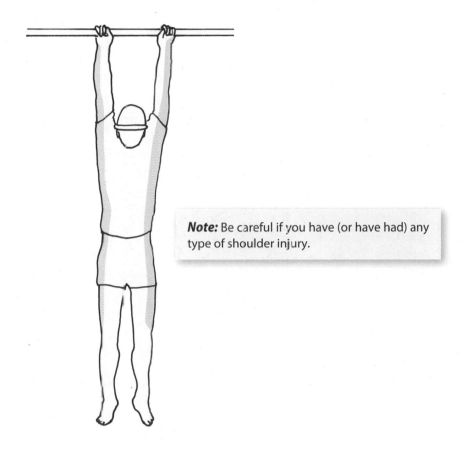

Note: Be careful if you have (or have had) any type of shoulder injury.

Hold onto the bar with both hands, relax your chin forward as you hang, with feet off the ground. A great stretch for the upper body. Begin holding for 5 seconds, gradually increasing to at least 30 seconds. A strong grip will make this stretch easier.

Enjoy stretching by the way it feels. If you torture yourself with drastic tensions in an attempt to get more flexible, you deprive yourself of the true benefits of stretching. If you stretch correctly, you'll find the more you stretch, the easier it becomes, and the easier you stretch, the more you will naturally enjoy it.

Stretches for the Upper Body Using a Towel

Most of us have a towel in our hands at least once a day. A towel or elastic cord can aid in stretching the arms, shoulders, and chest.

Hold the towel near both ends so that you can move it, with straight arms, up and over your head and down behind your back. Do not strain or force it. Your hands should be far enough apart to allow for relatively free movement up and over your head and down behind your back. Breathe slowly. Do not hold your breath.

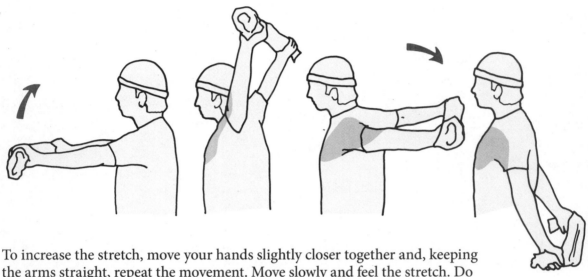

To increase the stretch, move your hands slightly closer together and, keeping the arms straight, repeat the movement. Move slowly and feel the stretch. Do not overstretch. If you are unable to go through the full movement of up, over, and behind while keeping your arms straight, then your hands are too close together. Move them farther apart.

You can hold the stretch at any place during this movement. This will isolate and add more of a stretch to the muscles of that particular area. For example, if your chest is tight and sore, it is possible to isolate the stretch there by holding the towel at shoulder level with arms straight behind you, as shown above. Hold for 5–15 seconds.

Stretching is not a contest. You needn't compare yourself with others, because we are all different. Moreover, each day we are different: some days we are more limber than others. Stretch comfortably, within your limits, and you will begin to feel the flow of energy that comes from proper stretching.

Here is another series of stretches using a towel.

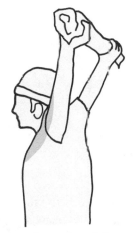

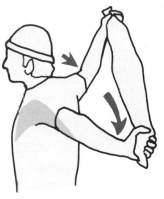

Bring the towel overhead, keeping your arms straight.

Lower the left arm back and behind you at shoulder level as your right arm bends to approximately a 90° angle.

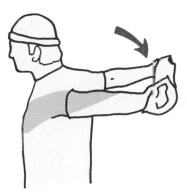

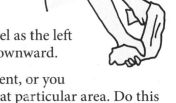

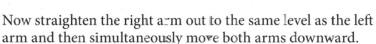

Now straighten the right arm out to the same level as the left arm and then simultaneously move both arms downward.

This can he done slowly, in one complete movement, or you can stop at any point to increase the stretch in that particular area. Do this completed movement toward the other side by lowering your right arm first.

As you become more flexible, you will be able to hold the towel with your hands closer together. But again, do not strain.

I think that limberness in the shoulders and arms really helps tennis, running, walking, and of course swimming (to name only a few activities for which you need this flexibility). Stretching the chest area reduces muscle tension and tightness and increases circulation and ease of breathing. It is actually very simple to stretch and keep the upper body limber, if you do it *regularly*.

> **Note:** Be careful if you have (or have had) any type of shoulder injury. Proceed slowly and discontinue if there is pain.

A Series of Stretches for Hands, Wrists, and Forearms (Sitting or Standing)

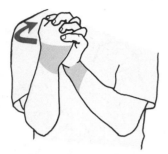

First, interlace your fingers in front of you and rotate your hands and wrists clockwise 10 times.

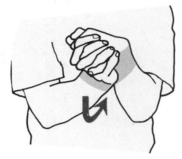

Repeat counterclockwise 10 times. This will improve the flexibility of your hands and wrists and provide a slight warm-up.

Then separate and straighten your fingers until the tension of a stretch is felt. Hold for 10 seconds, then relax.

Next, bend your fingers at the knuckles and hold for 10 seconds. Then relax.

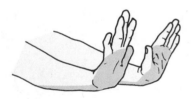

Now, with your arms straight out in front of you, bend your wrists with fingers pointing upwards. This will stretch the back of your forearms. Hold for 10–12 seconds. Do twice.

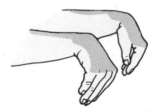

Then bend your wrist with your fingers pointing downwards to stretch the top of your forearms. Hold for 10–12 seconds. Do twice.

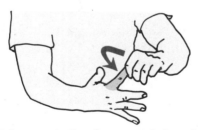

With your index finger and thumb gently hold a finger or the thumb of the opposite hand. Use your index finger and thumb to rotate each finger and thumb 5 times clockwise and counterclockwise.

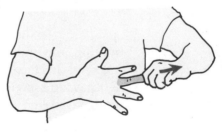

Next gently pull each finger and thumb straight out and hold for 2–3 seconds.

Now, shake your arms and hands at your sides for 10–12 seconds. Keep your jaw relaxed and let your shoulders hang downward as you shake out tension.

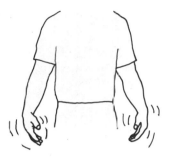

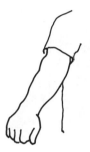 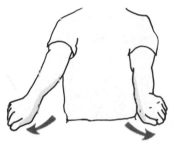

Start with your arms straight out in front of you. Slowly turn your hands to the outside (as you keep your arms straight) until a stretch is felt along the inside forearms and wrists. Hold for 5–10 seconds.

Place your hands palm-to-palm in front of you. Then, move your hands downward, keeping your palms together, until you feel a mild stretch. Keep your elbows up and even. Hold for 5–8 seconds.

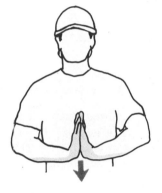

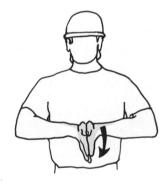

From the above stretch, rotate your palms around until they face more or less downward. Go until you feel a mild stretch. Keep your elbows up and even. Hold for 5–8 seconds.

Place your hands palm-to-palm in front of you. Push one hand gently to the side until you feel a mild stretch. Keep your elbows up and even. Hold for 5–8 seconds.

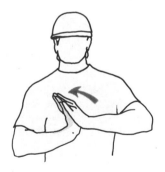

Use some or all of these stretches to counteract the problems that may come from repetitive movements, such as computer work. Use these daily, especially at work.

Sitting Stretches

A series of stretches you can do while sitting: These are good for people who work at office jobs. You can relieve tension and energize parts of your body that have become stiff from sitting.

Sitting stretches for upper body: Interlace your fingers, then straighten your arms out in front of you with palms facing out. Feel the stretch in arms and through upper part of back (shoulder blades). Hold stretch for 20 seconds. Do at least twice.

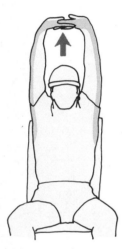

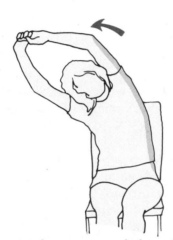

Interlace fingers, then turn palms upward above your head as you straighten your arms. Think of elongating your arms as you feel a stretch through your arms and upper sides of the rib cage. Hold only a stretch that feels good. Do three times. Hold for 10 seconds.

With arms extended overhead, hold onto the outside of your left hand with right hand and pull your left arm to the side. Keep arms as straight as comfortably possible. This will stretch the left arm and side of body and shoulder. Hold for 10 seconds. Do both sides.

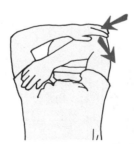

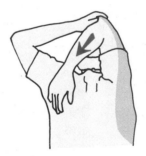

PNF Technique: *Contract — Relax — Stretch*. Hold your right elbow with your left hand. Move your right elbow downward as you resist this movement with your left hand (isometric contraction) for 3–4 seconds.

After relaxing a moment, gently pull your elbow over, behind your head until you feel a mild stretch in the back of your upper arm. Hold for 5–15 seconds. Repeat to other side.

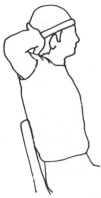

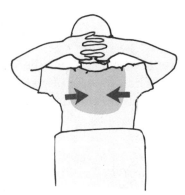

With your fingers interlaced behind your head, keep your elbows straight out to the side with your upper body in a good, aligned position. Now think of pulling your shoulder blades together to create a feeling of tension through the upper back and shoulder blades. Hold, with a feeling of releasing tension, for 4–5 seconds and then relax. Do several times. This is good to do when your shoulders and upper back are tense or tight. This is also good to do while standing.

With your left hand hold your right arm just above the elbow. Now gently pull your elbow toward your left shoulder as you look over your right shoulder. Hold stretch for 10 seconds. Do both sides.

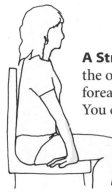

A Stretch for the Forearm: With the palm of your hand flat, thumb to the outside and fingers pointed backward, slowly lean back to stretch your forearm. Be sure to keep palms flat. Hold for 10 seconds. Do both sides. You can stretch both forearms at the same time, if you wish.

Sitting Stretches for Ankles, Side of Hip, and Lower Back

While sitting, rotate your ankles clockwise and then counterclockwise. Do one ankle at a time, 20–30 revolutions.

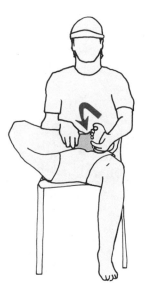

Hold onto your lower left leg just below the knee. Gently pull it toward your chest. To isolate a stretch in the side of your upper leg, use the left arm to pull the bent leg across and toward the opposite shoulder. Hold for 15 seconds at an easy stretch tension. Do both sides.

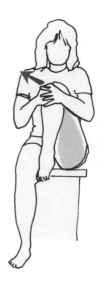

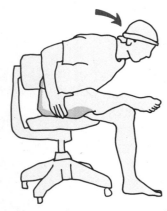

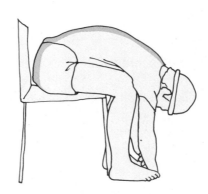

Cross you right leg over your left leg, right ankle and foot resting just to the outside of your left knee. To stretch the side of your right hip (*piriformis* area), slowly lean your upper body forward, bending from the hips until you feel a mild stretch. Hold for 5–15 seconds. Stay relaxed and breathe rhythmically. Repeat, crossing your left leg over your right leg.

Lean forward to stretch and take the pressure off your lower back. Even if you do not feel a stretch, it is still good for circulation. Hold for 15–20 seconds. Put your hands on your thighs to help push your body to an upright position.

Stretches for the Face and Neck

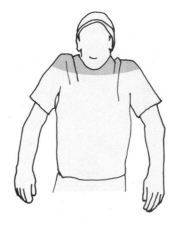

Raise the top of your shoulders toward your ears until you feel a slight tension in your neck and shoulder. Hold for 5 seconds, then relax shoulders downward into normal position. Do several times at the first sign of shoulder tension. It really works!

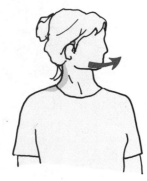

Turn your chin toward your left shoulder to create a stretch on the right side of your neck. Hold correct stretch tensions for 5–10 seconds. Stretch to each side twice. Keep your shoulders relaxed downward. Do not hold your breath.

This stretch may cause people around you to think you are a bit weird, but you often find a lot of tension in your face from frowning or squinting because of eye strain.

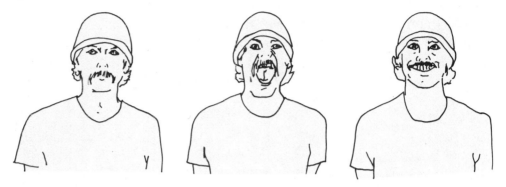

Raise your eyebrows and open your eyes as wide as possible. At the same time, open your mouth to stretch the muscles around your nose and chin and stick your tongue out. Hold this stretch for 5–10 seconds. Getting the tension out of the muscles in your face will make you smile. Do several times.

Caution: If you hear clicking or popping noises when opening your mouth, check with your dentist.

SUMMARY OF SITTING STRETCHES

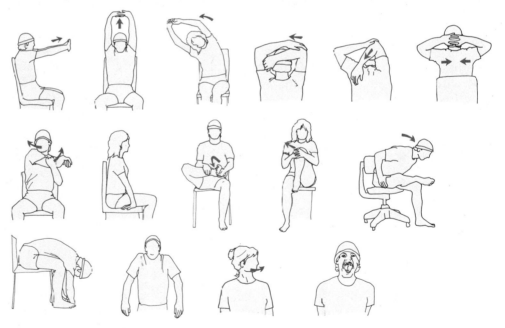

Do these sitting stretches, in this order, as a routine.

Advanced Stretches for the Legs and Groin with Feet Elevated

A wall or doorway can be useful for stretching the legs while you relax on your back. When doing these stretches think of the easy stretch, gradually increasing into the developmental stretch.

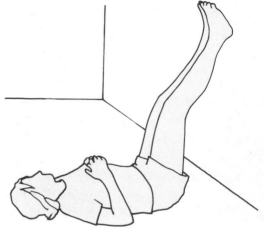

Start with your legs elevated and close together, with your butt about 3–5 inches away from the wall so that your lower back is flat and not arched or off the floor.

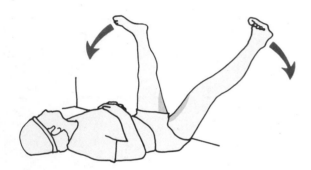

It's possible to stretch your groin from this position by slowly separating your legs, with your heels resting on the wall, until you feel an easy stretch. Hold for 30 seconds and relax. Breathe rhythmically.

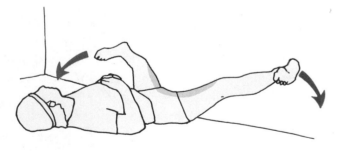

As this position becomes easier over time, you can gradually stretch further by lowering your legs. An advanced position is shown here. Do not try to copy this, but stretch within your limits. Do not strain. The wall makes it possible to hold these stretches longer in a relaxed, stable position.

Remember to keep your butt 3–5 inches from the wall. If you are too close to the wall you may feel tightness in your lower back.

Variation:

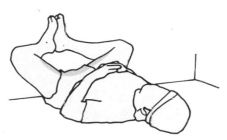

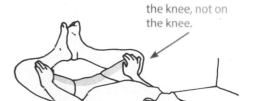

Push a little above the knee, not on the knee.

Put the soles of your feet together, resting them against the wall. Relax.

To increase the stretch, use your hands to gently push down on the inside of your thighs until you feel a good, easy stretch. Relax while you stretch. Hold for 10–15 seconds.

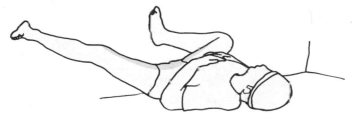

To isolate and increase the stretch in each side of the groin area, straighten one leg out. Hold each leg for 10–15 seconds.

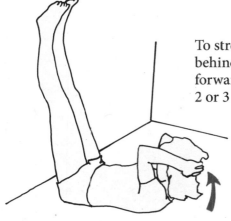

To stretch your neck from this position, interlace your fingers behind your head (at about ear level) and gently pull your head forward until you feel an easy stretch. Hold for 5 seconds. Repeat 2 or 3 times. *(See p. 27 for further information on neck stretches.)*

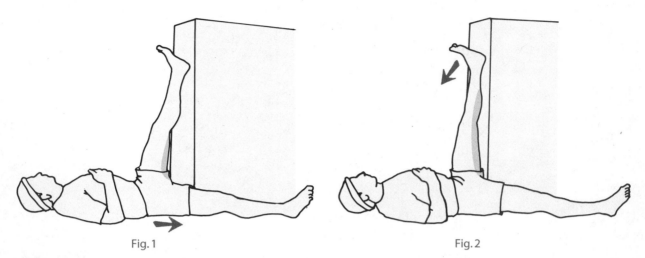

Fig. 1   Fig. 2

Here is an excellent way to stretch your hamstrings. Begin by lying on your back with your foot up on a doorway or wall and the other leg in a doorway or space where it can lie straight. To stretch the hamstrings of the leg up on the wall, move your body forward, toward the doorway, until a mild stretch is felt (*fig. 1*). Hold for 10–15 seconds. To stretch your calf and hamstrings from this position, bring your toes toward your shin until you feel a stretch in your calf (*fig. 2*). Hold for 10–15 seconds. Breathe easily.

SUMMARY OF ADVANCED STRETCHES FOR THE LEGS AND GROIN WITH FEET ELEVATED

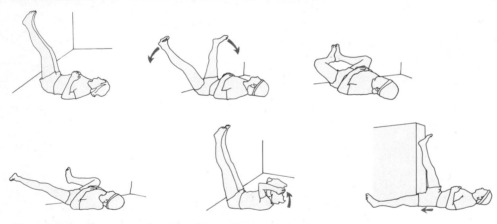

You can do these stretches, in this order, as a routine.

If you don't have much uninterrupted time available, use short periods of stretching (1–3 minutes) every three or four hours. This will help you to feel consistently good throughout the day.

Stretching the Groin and Hips with Legs Apart

The following stretches will make lateral movement easier, help maintain flexibility, and can prevent injuries. Gradually become accustomed to these stretches, which are primarily for the center of your body.

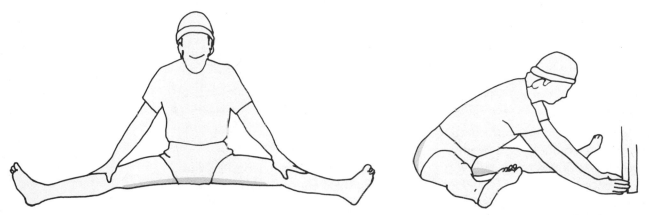

Sit with your feet a comfortable distance apart. To stretch the inside of your upper legs and hips, slowly lean forward from your hips. Be sure to keep your quadriceps relaxed and feet upright. Hold for 10–20 seconds. Keep your hands out in front of you for balance and stability or hold onto something for greater control. Breathe deeply.

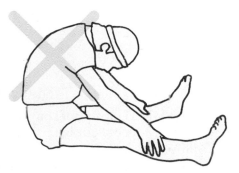

Do not lean forward with your head and shoulders. This will cause your upper back to round and put pressure on your lower back. If, when you lean forward, your lower back is rounded (causing your hips to tilt backward), it is because your hips, lower back, and hamstrings are tight. To bend from your hips correctly, you must keep your lower back straight (upright) so you can move forward from the hips (or thigh joints), and not by rounding your back.

Don't stretch to be flexible. Stretch to feel good.

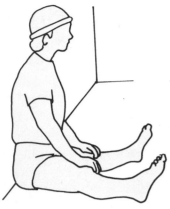 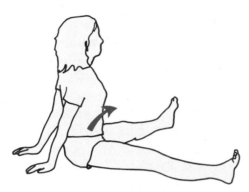

A good way to adapt your hips and lower back gradually to a proper, upright position is to sit with your lower back flat against a wall. Hold an easy stretch for 30 seconds.

Another way is to sit with your hands behind you. Using your arms as a support will help lengthen your spine as you concentrate on moving your hips slightly forward. Hold for 20 seconds.

Do not bend forward until you are able to feel comfortable doing the variations above. Get your body used to these positions before you try to stretch any further.

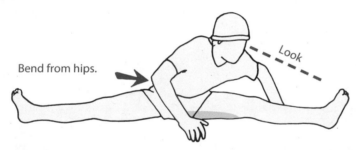

Bend from hips.

Look

Variation: To stretch your left hamstrings and the right side of your back, slowly bend forward from the hips, toward the foot of your left leg. Keep your chin in and your back straight. Hold a good stretch for 10–15 seconds. If necessary, use a towel. Don't look down. Look just over your toes. Stay relaxed and breathe easily.

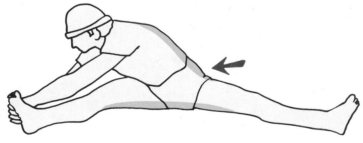

Another variation is to reach across your body with the left hand to the right foot, putting your right hand out to the right side for balance. This will increase the stretch in your hamstrings and in your back, as far up as the shoulder blades and as far down as the hips. Do this across-the-body stretch in both directions. This stretch requires good, overall flexibility. Hold for 5–15 seconds.

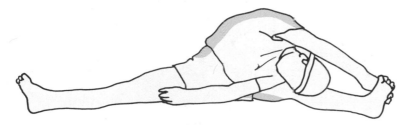

An Advanced Stretch: Reach overhead with your hand and grasp the opposite foot. Keep your other arm resting close to your body in front of you. This is a good lateral stretch for the back and legs. Hold for 5–15 seconds. Do both sides. Do not overstretch. Do not hold your breath.

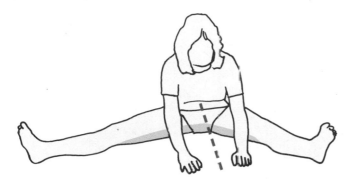

Learn to hold stretch tensions at various angles. Stretch forward, left, and right, then teach yourself to hold stretches at angles toward left of center and right of center. Use the same leg and upper body alignment as previously described. Hold for 5–15 seconds. Stretch with complete self-control.

If you feel and look tight doing these stretches, do not be discouraged. Stretch without worrying about flexibility. Then you can gradually adapt your body to these new angles with stretch tensions that feel right.

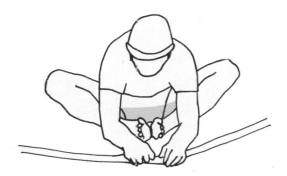

A More Advanced Groin Stretch: With the soles of your feet together, lean forward and hold onto something near the floor in front of you (this may be the edge of the mat, or the leg of a piece of furniture). Use this object to help you hold a comfortable stretch and to pull yourself forward to increase the stretch. Do not overstretch. Hold and relax for 10–20 seconds. Remember to contract your abdominals as you lean forward.

Holding onto something will stabilize your legs and make it easier to hold a stretch when you are sitting with legs apart.

Sitting on the corner of the mat, place your legs and feet along the outside edges. Find a position where it is easy to relax while you feel a slight stretch. Hold for 10–15 seconds. Use your hands behind you for balance and support.

Keep quads relaxed.

Keep toes and feet relaxed and upright.

Lean forward from hips.

Use hands for stability and support.

To increase the stretch, move your butt and hips forward, sliding your legs down along the sides of the mat. Keep toes and feet upright. Do not let your legs turn in or out. A good stretch for limbering up groin and hips.

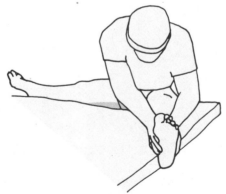

To stretch one leg at a time, sit on the corner of the mat in a comfortable position. Turn to face one foot and bend forward from the hips in that direction. Reach down with your hands and hold your leg at a point that gives you an easy stretch. Think of your chin going toward or just beyond your knee (even though it may not), as you look just above your toes. Relax. Sit up and stretch the other leg in the same way. Stretch your tightest leg first. If necessary, put a towel around the bottom of your foot to help you stretch. Hold an easy stretch for 5–15 seconds. No bouncing. This is a good stretch for the hamstrings, lower back, and hips. Breathe and relax.

Learning the Splits

This section is for a limited number of people. Unless you are training for gymnastics, dance, or need extreme flexibility (as does an ice hockey goalkeeper, or a first baseman, or a ballet dancer), the other sections in this book should handle most of your stretching needs. I'm not trying to discourage you, but for everyday living being able to do the splits is hardly necessary!

Note: Be sure to do an adequate warm-up prior to these stretches. Do some easier stretches and 5–6 minutes of aerobic activity.

Forward Splits

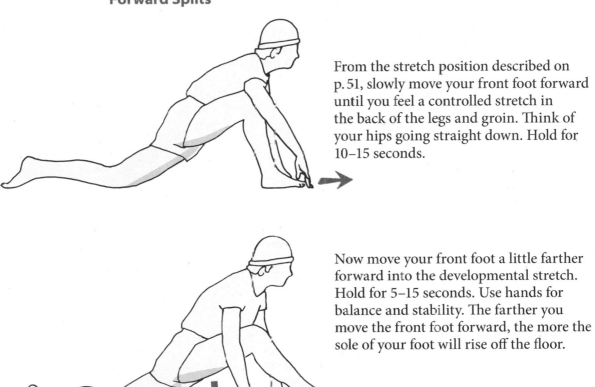

From the stretch position described on p. 51, slowly move your front foot forward until you feel a controlled stretch in the back of the legs and groin. Think of your hips going straight down. Hold for 10–15 seconds.

Now move your front foot a little farther forward into the developmental stretch. Hold for 5–15 seconds. Use hands for balance and stability. The farther you move the front foot forward, the more the sole of your foot will rise off the floor.

A good way to prepare for the splits is to do the stretches on pp. 94–100.

As you become more flexible, continue to move the front foot forward as you lower your hips. Keep your shoulders directly above your hips and your back vertical. Hold for 10–15 seconds. Repeat for the other side.

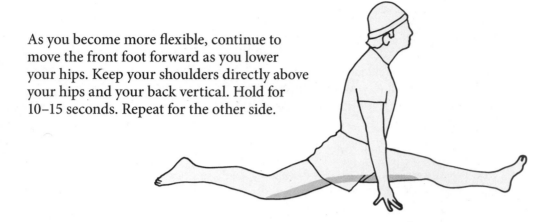

Learning to do the splits takes time and regular practice. Be sure not to overstretch. Let your body gradually adapt to the changes needed to accomplish the splits comfortably. Do not be in a rush and injure yourself.

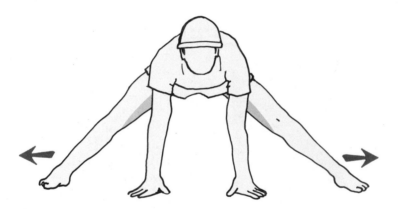

Side Splits

From a standing position, with feet pointed straight ahead, gradually spread your legs until you feel a stretch on the inside of your upper legs. Think of your hips going straight down. Use hands for balance. Hold an easy stretch for 5–15 seconds.

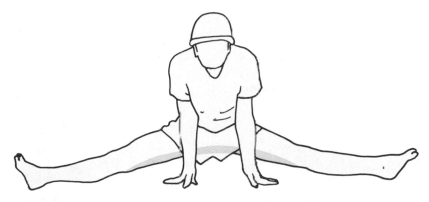

As you become more limber, keep moving your feet apart until the desired stretch is created. As you get lower in this stretch, keep your feet upright, with your heels on the floor: this will keep the stretch on the inside of the upper legs and the extreme tension off the ligaments of the knee. (If you keep your feet flat on the floor there is a possibility of overstretching the inside ligament of the knees.) Hold for 5–15 seconds. As your body gradually adapts, slowly increase the stretch by lowering your hips a bit further. *Be careful of overstretching.*

Doing the stretches below will help you in learning the splits.

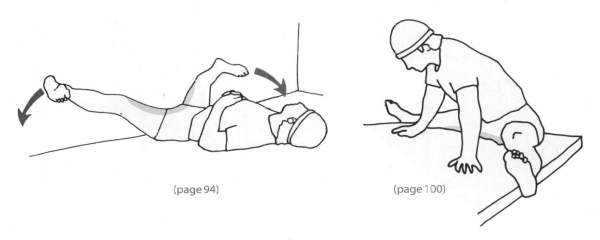

(page 94)   (page 100)

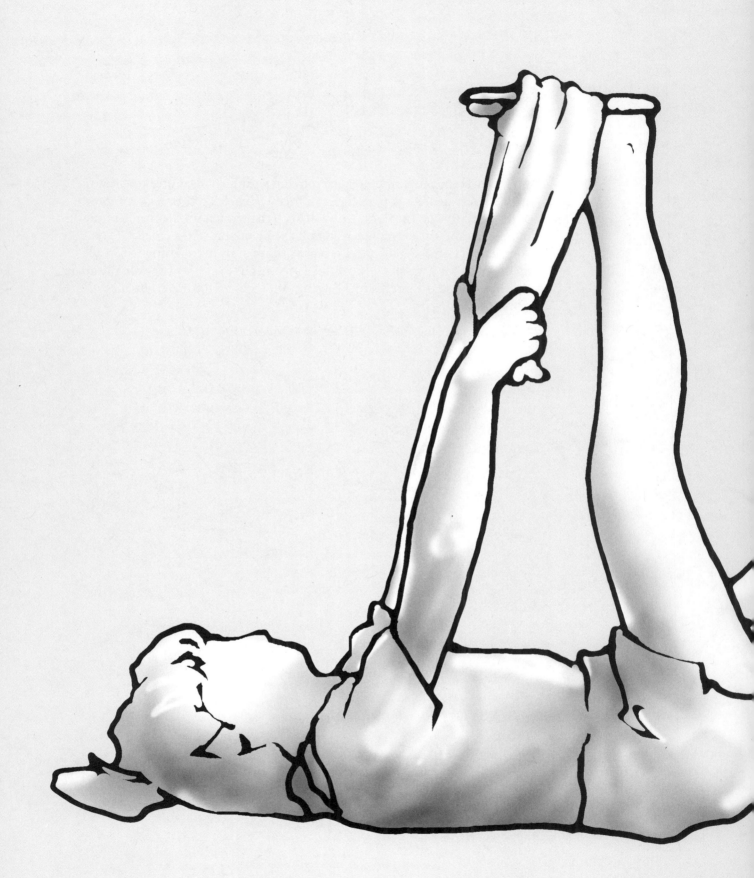

STRETCHING ROUTINES
Everyday Activities

These are stretching routines that can help you in dealing with the muscular tension and tightness of everyday life. There are routines for different age groups, different body parts, different occupations and activities, as well as stretches to do spontaneously at odd moments throughout the day. Once you learn how to stretch, you will be able to develop your own routines to suit your own particular needs.

When you first do the routines, you can look up the instructions for each stretch in the page numbers listed. After a while you will know how to stretch without looking at the instructions each time.

IN THE MORNING

APPROXIMATELY 4 MINUTES

Start the day with some relaxed stretches so your body can function more naturally. Tight and stiff muscles will feel good from comfortable stretching. The first four stretches can be done in bed before you get up. After arising and you've moved around a bit, do the next four stretches.

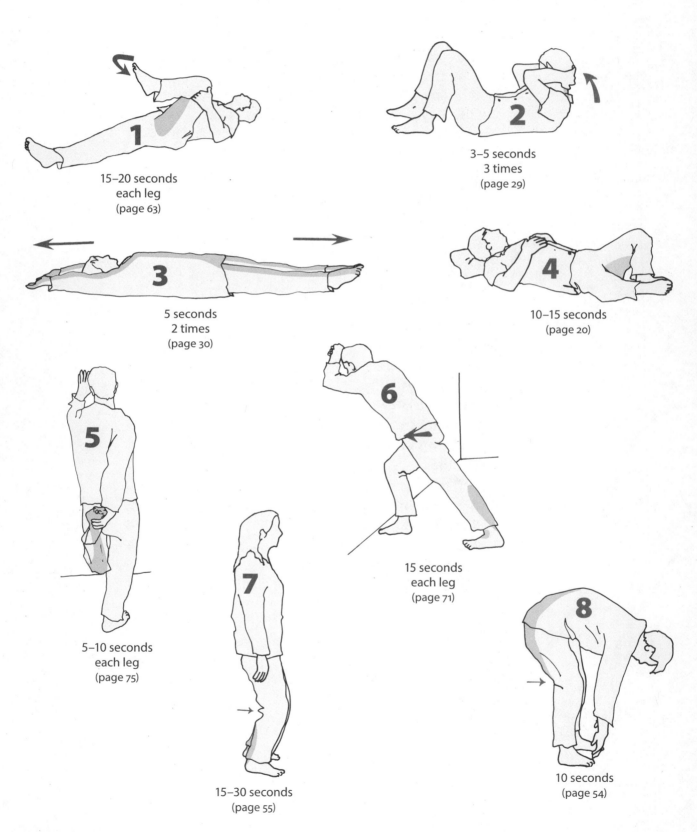

1
15–20 seconds
each leg
(page 63)

2
3–5 seconds
3 times
(page 29)

3
5 seconds
2 times
(page 30)

4
10–15 seconds
(page 20)

5
5–10 seconds
each leg
(page 75)

6
15 seconds
each leg
(page 71)

7
15–30 seconds
(page 55)

8
10 seconds
(page 54)

APPROXIMATELY 3 MINUTES

This is a great time to stretch every day. These stretches will relax your body and help you to sleep more soundly. Take your time, and *feel* the body parts being stretched. Stretch lightly, breathe deeply, and be relaxed.

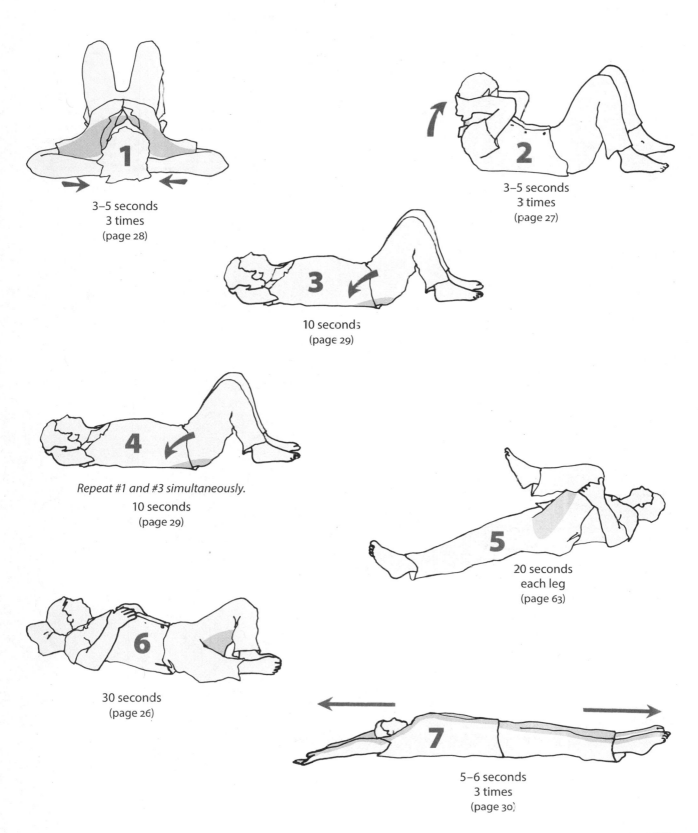

3–5 seconds
3 times
(page 28)

3–5 seconds
3 times
(page 27)

10 seconds
(page 29)

Repeat #1 and #3 simultaneously.
10 seconds
(page 29)

20 seconds
each leg
(page 63)

30 seconds
(page 26)

5–6 seconds
3 times
(page 30)

EVERYDAY STRETCHES

APPROXIMATELY 8 MINUTES

Start with several minutes of walking. Then use these everyday stretches to fine-tune your muscles. This is a general routine that emphasizes stretching and relaxing the muscles most frequently used during normal day-to-day activities.

In the simple tasks of everyday living, we often use our body in strained or awkward ways, creating stress and tension. A kind of muscular *rigor mortis* sets in. If you can set aside 10 minutes every day for stretching, you will offset this accumulated tension so you can use your body with greater ease.

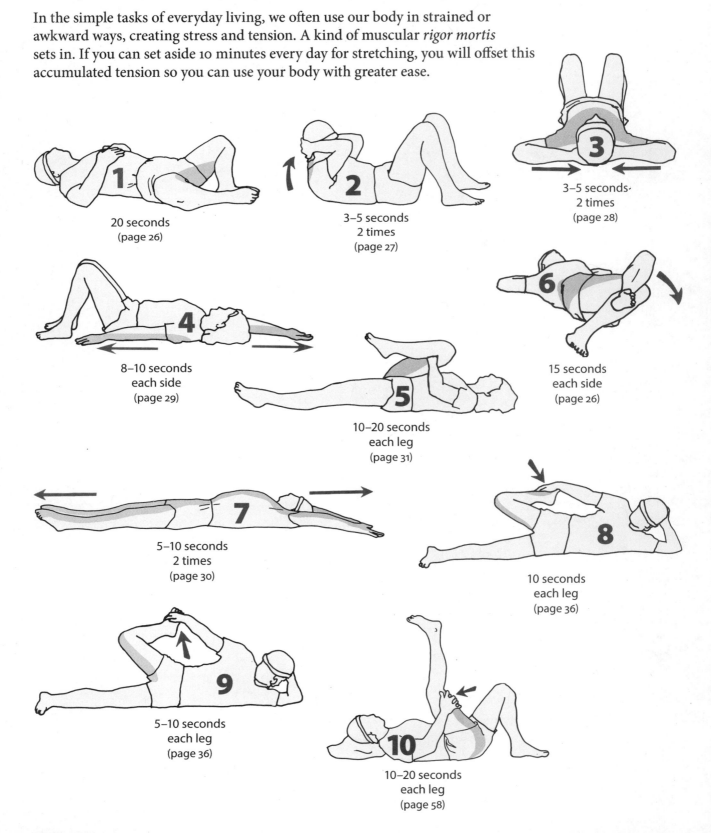

1
20 seconds
(page 26)

2
3–5 seconds
2 times
(page 27)

3
3–5 seconds
2 times
(page 28)

4
8–10 seconds
each side
(page 29)

5
10–20 seconds
each leg
(page 31)

6
15 seconds
each side
(page 26)

7
5–10 seconds
2 times
(page 30)

8
10 seconds
each leg
(page 36)

9
5–10 seconds
each leg
(page 36)

10
10–20 seconds
each leg
(page 58)

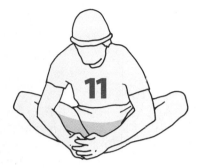
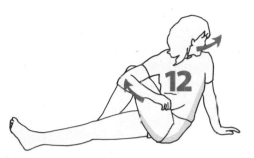
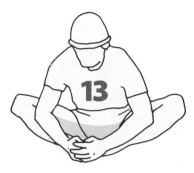

20–30 seconds
(page 58)

8–10 seconds
each side
(page 60)

10 seconds
Repeat stretch #11.
(page 58)

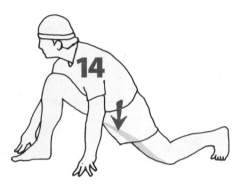
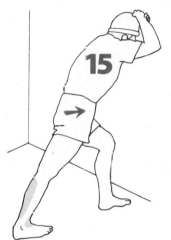
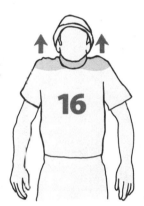

5–15 seconds
each leg
(page 51)

10–15 seconds
each leg
(page 71)

4–5 seconds
2 times
(page 46)

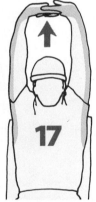
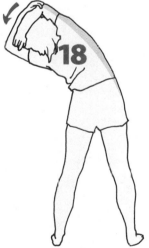

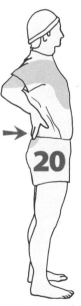

10–12 seconds
2 times
(page 90)

8–10 seconds
each side
(page 44)

20–30 seconds
(page 47)

10 seconds
2 times
(page 46)

HANDS, ARMS & SHOULDERS

APPROXIMATELY 4 MINUTES

This series of stretches works for repetitive stress problems in the hands and arms. Breathe naturally, stay comfortable, and be relaxed as you stretch.

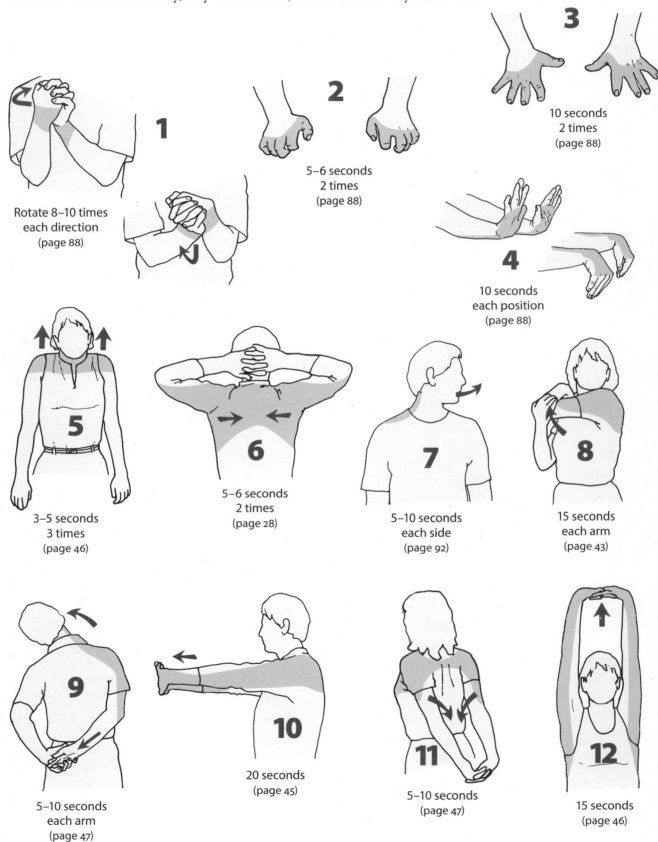

1 Rotate 8–10 times
each direction
(page 88)

2 5–6 seconds
2 times
(page 88)

3 10 seconds
2 times
(page 88)

4 10 seconds
each position
(page 88)

5 3–5 seconds
3 times
(page 46)

6 5–6 seconds
2 times
(page 28)

7 5–10 seconds
each side
(page 92)

8 15 seconds
each arm
(page 43)

9 5–10 seconds
each arm
(page 47)

10 20 seconds
(page 45)

11 5–10 seconds
(page 47)

12 15 seconds
(page 46)

NECK, SHOULDERS & ARMS

APPROXIMATELY 5 MINUTES

Many people carry stress in their neck and shoulder area. This stretching routine will help with that problem. Do these stretches throughout the day. Breathe deeply and relax.

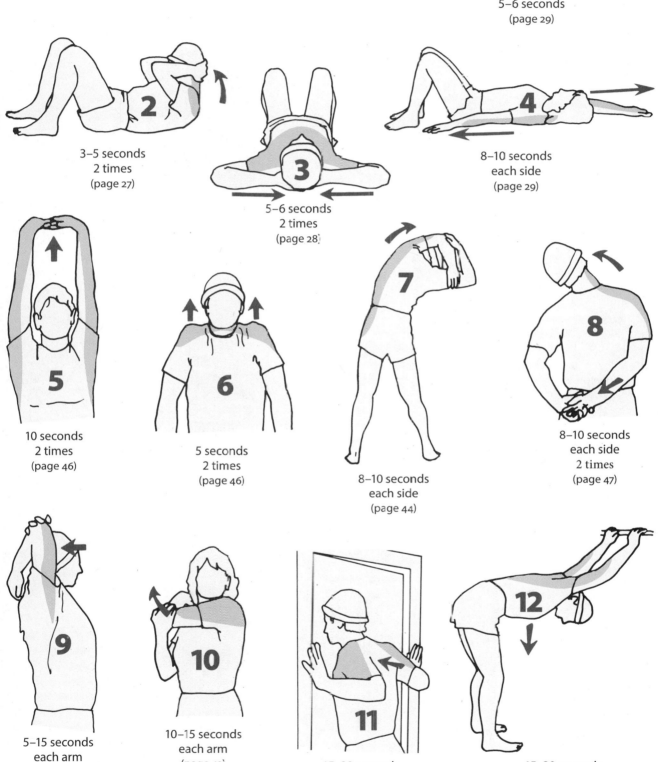

5–6 seconds
(page 29)

3–5 seconds
2 times
(page 27)

5–6 seconds
2 times
(page 28)

8–10 seconds
each side
(page 29)

10 seconds
2 times
(page 46)

5 seconds
2 times
(page 46)

8–10 seconds
each side
(page 44)

8–10 seconds
each side
2 times
(page 47)

5–15 seconds
each arm
2 times
(page 44)

10–15 seconds
each arm
(page 43)

15–20 seconds
(page 47)

15–20 seconds
(page 81)

STRETCHES FOR LOWER BACK TENSION

APPROXIMATELY 6 MINUTES

These stretches are designed for the relief of muscular low back pain and are also good for relieving tension in the upper back, shoulders, and neck. For best results do them every night just before going to sleep. Hold only stretch tensions that feel good to you. *Do not overstretch.*

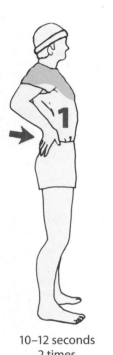

10–12 seconds
2 times
(page 46)

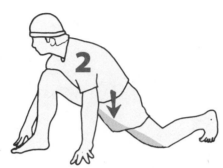

10–15 seconds
each leg
(page 51)

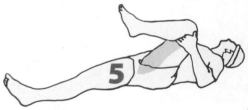

5–15 seconds
2 times
(page 33)

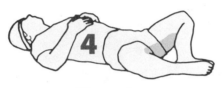

30 seconds
(page 26)

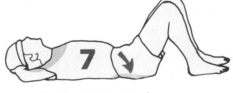

20–30 seconds
each leg
(page 63)

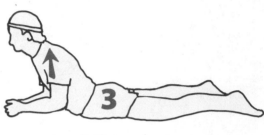

Contract 5–8 seconds,
then relax
2 times
(page 29)

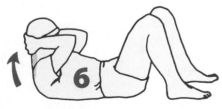

Hold for 3–5 seconds,
then relax
2 times
(page 27)

Rock gently back and forth
15–20 times
(page 26)

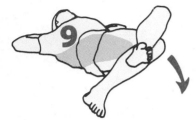

10–30 seconds
each leg
(page 27)

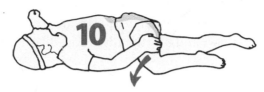

10–15 seconds
each leg
(page 32)

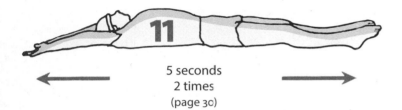

5 seconds
2 times
(page 30)

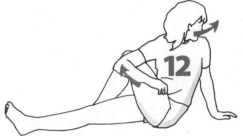

5–15 seconds
each side
(page 60)

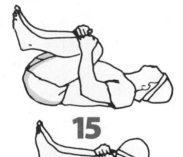

20 seconds
(page 58)

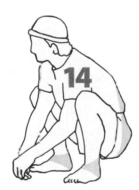

10–15 seconds
(page 65)

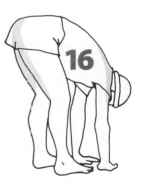

5–10 seconds
(page 55)

10–15 seconds
2 times
(page 63)

APPROXIMATELY 7 MINUTES

Stretch comfortably after a light warm-up of walking in place or riding a stationary bike for 2–3 minutes. Remember to stretch with control as you gradually limber up. Relax and breathe rhythmically.

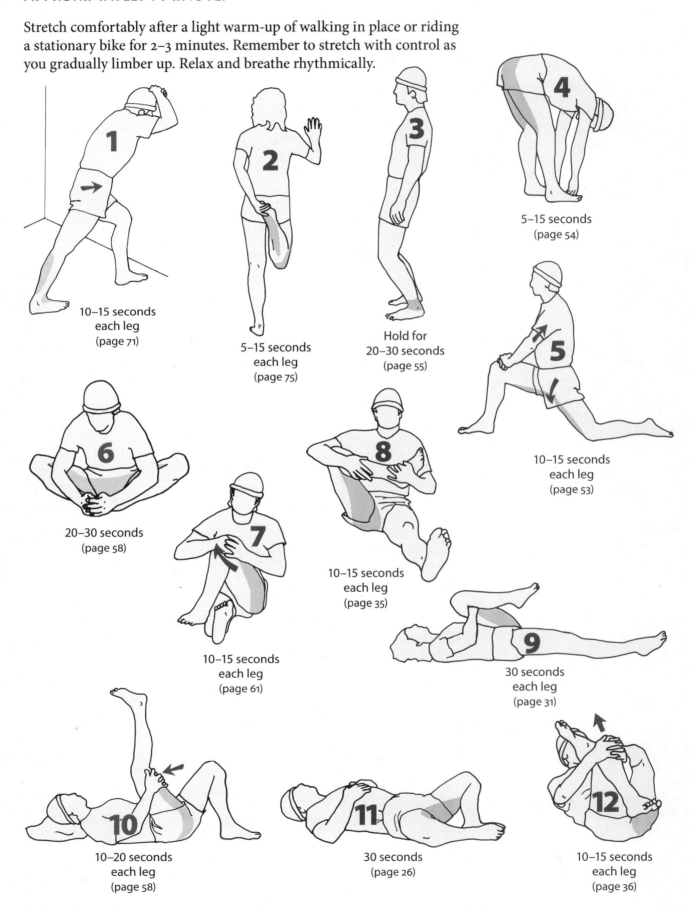

1 10–15 seconds
each leg
(page 71)

2 5–15 seconds
each leg
(page 75)

3 Hold for
20–30 seconds
(page 55)

4 5–15 seconds
(page 54)

5 10–15 seconds
each leg
(page 53)

6 20–30 seconds
(page 58)

7 10–15 seconds
each leg
(page 61)

8 10–15 seconds
each leg
(page 35)

9 30 seconds
each leg
(page 31)

10 10–20 seconds
each leg
(page 58)

11 30 seconds
(page 26)

12 10–15 seconds
each leg
(page 36)

SPONTANEOUS STRETCHES

You can stretch at odd times of the day. Reading a paper, talking on the phone, waiting for a bus . . . these are times for easy, relaxed stretching. Be creative; think of stretches to do during normally wasted time.

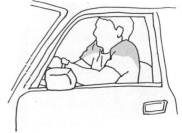

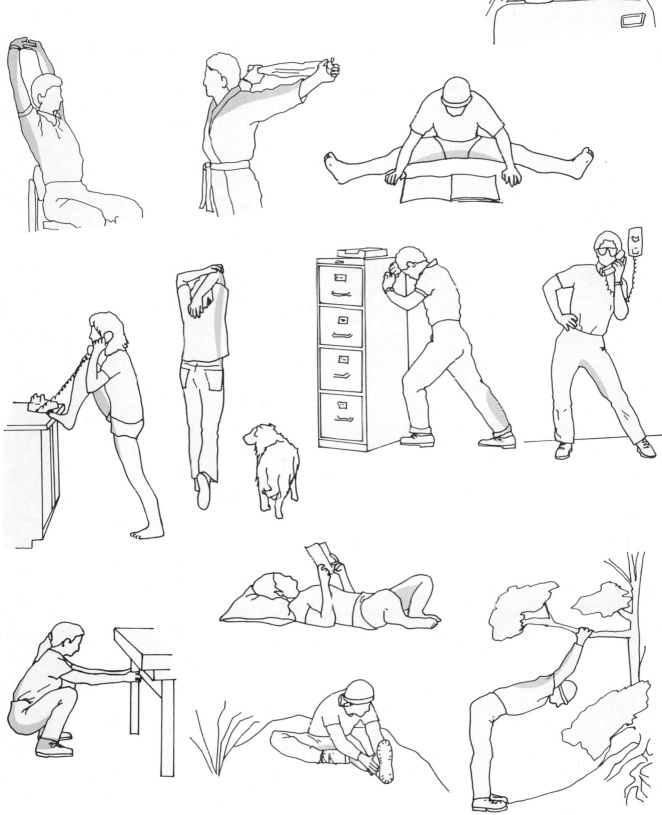

BLUE-COLLAR STRETCHES

APPROXIMATELY 6 MINUTES

Before you do any physical work — especially lifting — do some stretches. Stretching gives your muscles a signal they are about to be used, and a few minutes of stretching before starting work will make you feel better and help avoid injuries.

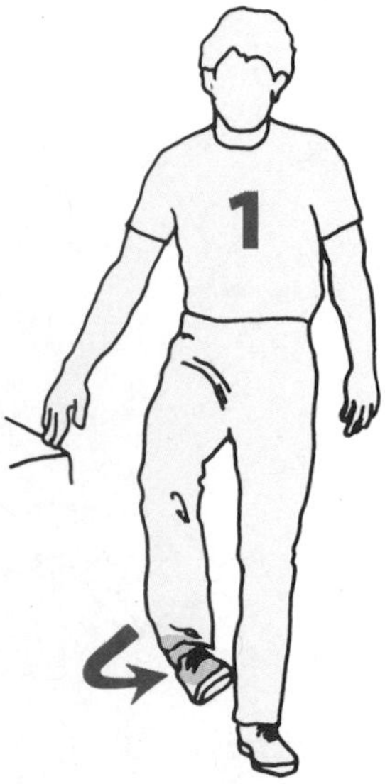

3

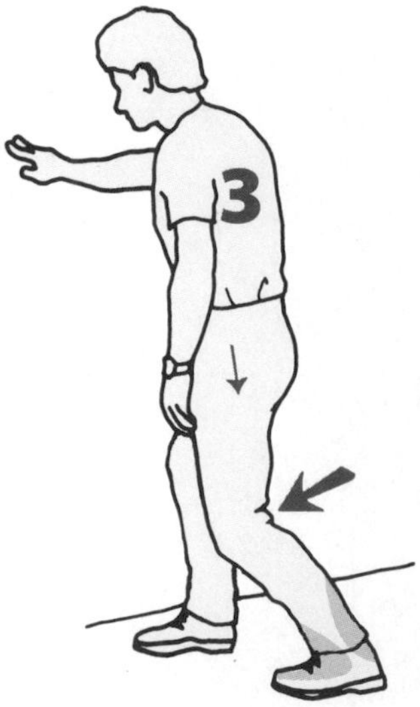

5–10 seconds
each leg
(page 71)

1

10–20 times
each foot
(page 71)

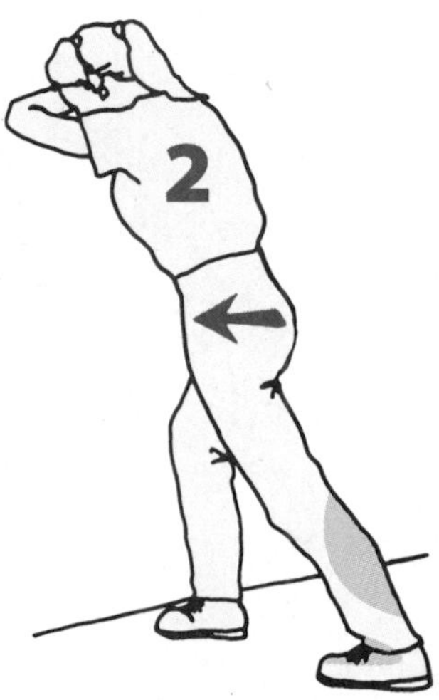

2

10–15 seconds
each leg
(page 71)

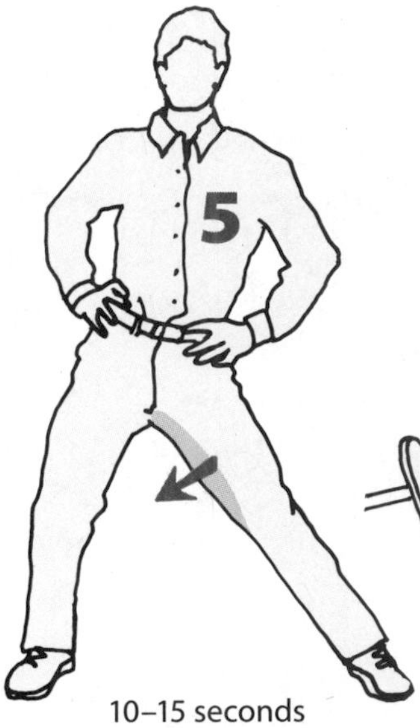

5

10–15 seconds
each leg
(page 73)

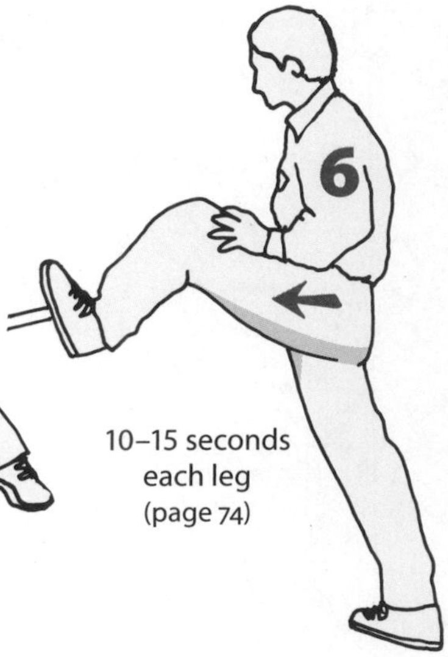

6

10–15 seconds
each leg
(page 74)

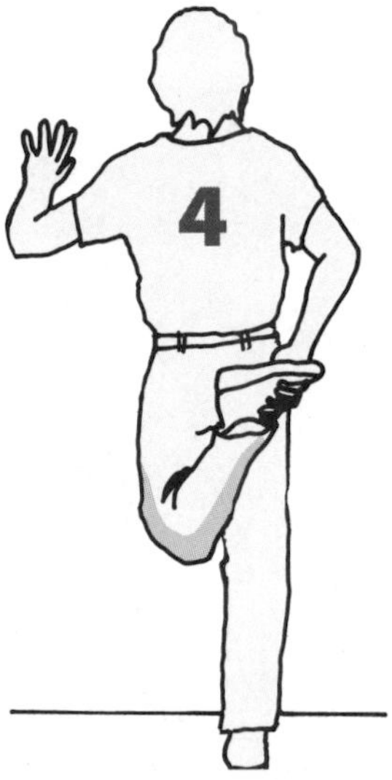

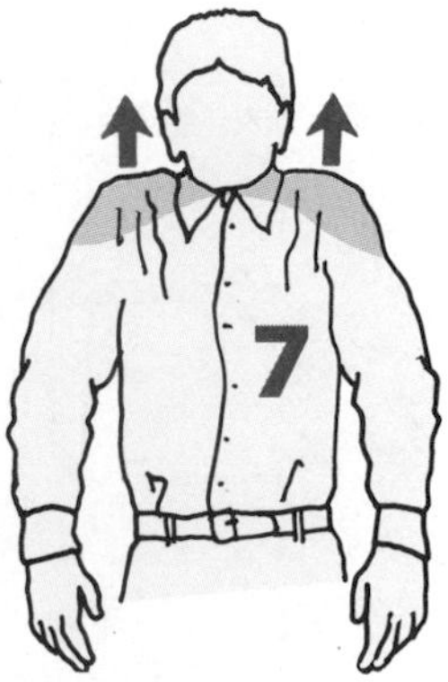

4

10 seconds
each leg
(page 75)

7

3–5 seconds
2 times
(page 46)

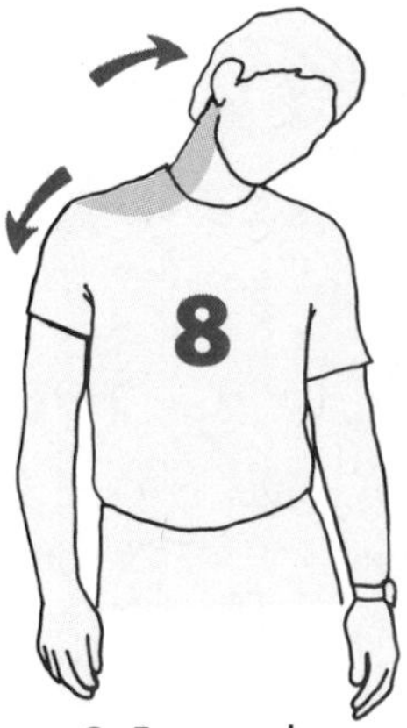

8

3–5 seconds
each side
(page 46)

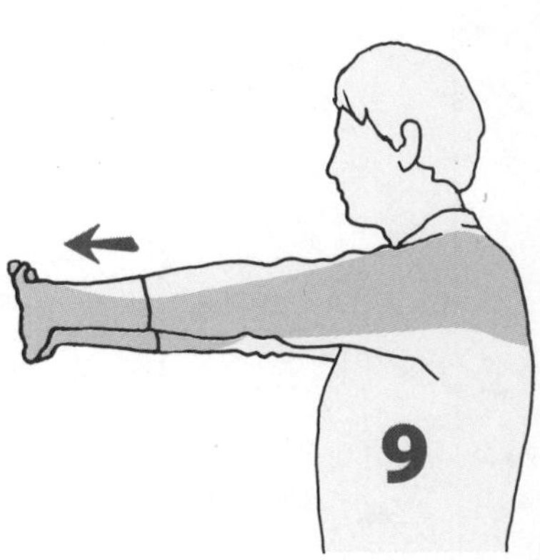

9

10 seconds
(page 45)

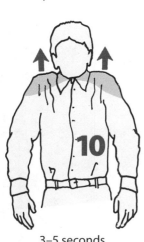

3–5 seconds
(page 46)

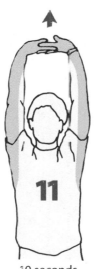

10 seconds
(page 46)

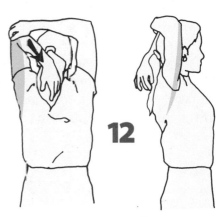

10 seconds
each arm
(page 44)

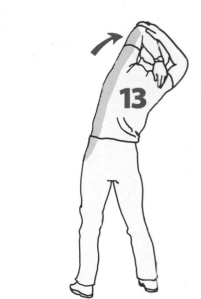

8–10 seconds
each side
(page 44)

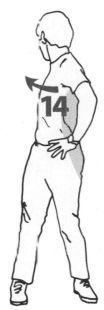

8–10 seconds
each side
(page 81)

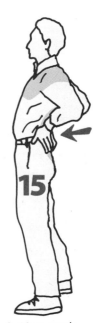

8–10 seconds
2 times
(page 46)

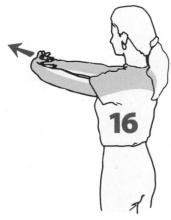

10 seconds
(page 45)

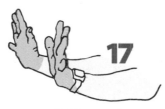

8–10 seconds
2 times
(page 88)

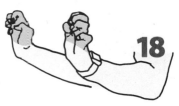

5–8 seconds
2 times
(page 88)

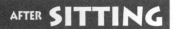

APPROXIMATELY 4 MINUTES

This is a series of stretches to do after sitting for a long time. The sitting position causes the blood to pool in the lower legs and feet, the hamstring muscles to tighten up, and the back and neck muscles to become stiff and tight. These stretches will improve your circulation and loosen up those areas that are tense from a prolonged period of sitting.

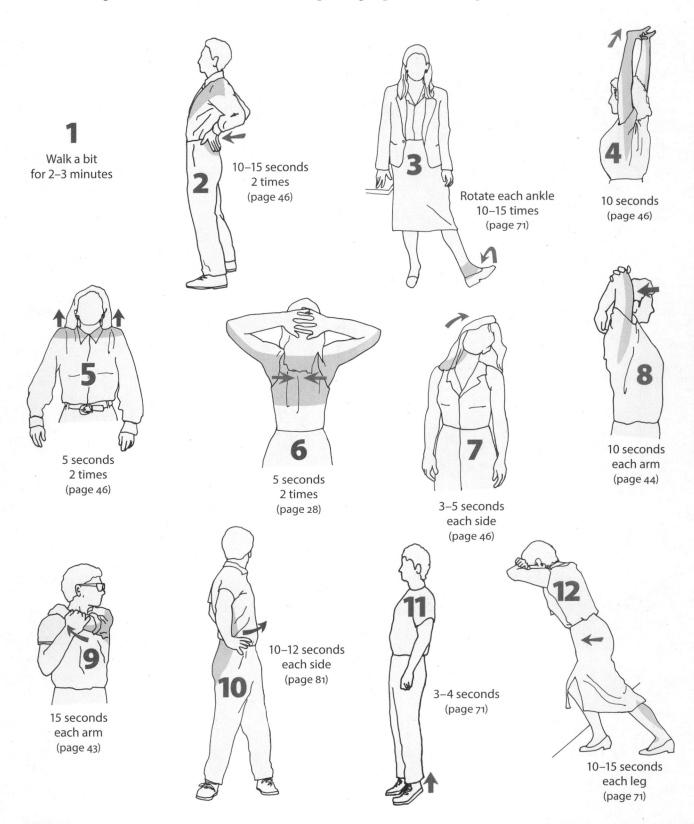

1
Walk a bit
for 2–3 minutes

2
10–15 seconds
2 times
(page 46)

3
Rotate each ankle
10–15 times
(page 71)

4
10 seconds
(page 46)

5
5 seconds
2 times
(page 46)

6
5 seconds
2 times
(page 28)

7
3–5 seconds
each side
(page 46)

8
10 seconds
each arm
(page 44)

9
15 seconds
each arm
(page 43)

10
10–12 seconds
each side
(page 81)

11
3–4 seconds
(page 71)

12
10–15 seconds
each leg
(page 71)

Stretching © 2010 by Bob and Jean Anderson. Shelter Publications, Inc.

BEFORE & AFTER GARDENING

APPROXIMATELY 4 MINUTES

Before you do any work in the garden, do a few minutes of easy stretching. This will help get your body ready to work efficiently without the usual tightness and stiffness that results from this kind of work. Stretch to reduce muscle tension and make work easier.

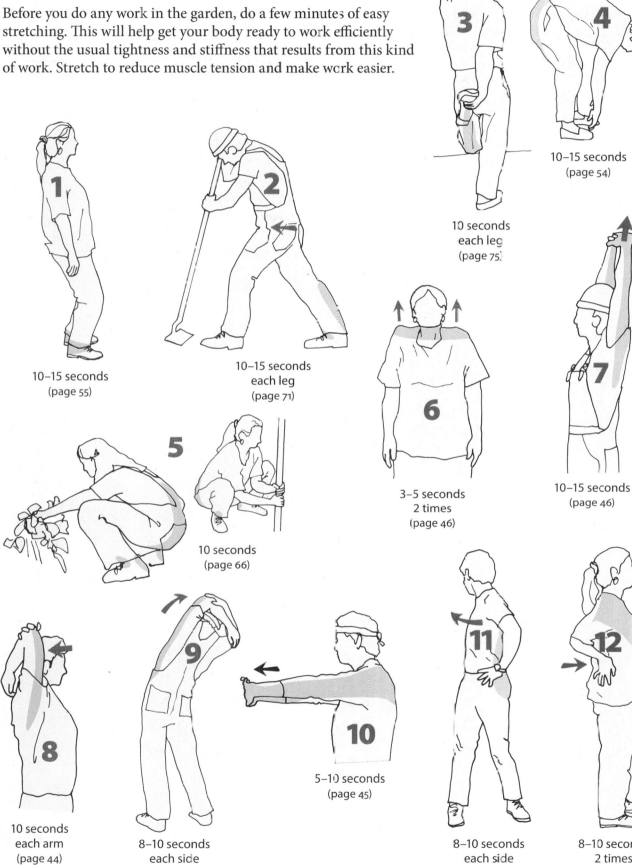

1
10–15 seconds
(page 55)

2
10–15 seconds
each leg
(page 71)

3
10 seconds
each leg
(page 75)

4
10–15 seconds
(page 54)

5
10 seconds
(page 66)

6
3–5 seconds
2 times
(page 46)

7
10–15 seconds
(page 46)

8
10 seconds
each arm
(page 44)

9
8–10 seconds
each side
(page 44)

10
5–10 seconds
(page 45)

11
8–10 seconds
each side
(page 81)

12
8–10 seconds
2 times
(page 46)

APPROXIMATELY 7 MINUTES

It is never too late to start stretching. In fact, the older we get, the more important it becomes to stretch on a regular basis.

With age and inactivity, the body gradually loses its range of motion; muscles can lose their elasticity and become weak and tight. But the body has an amazing capacity for the recovery of lost flexibility and strength if a regular program of fitness is followed.

The basic method of stretching is the same regardless of differences in age and flexibility. *Stretching properly means that you do not go beyond your comfortable limits.* You don't have to try to copy the drawings in this book. Learn to stretch your body without pushing too far; stretch by how you feel. It will take time to loosen up tight muscle groups that have been that way for years, but it can be done with patience and regularity. If you have any doubts about what you should be doing, consult your physician *before you start*.

Here is a series of stretches to help restore and maintain flexibility.

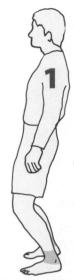

10–30 seconds
(page 55)

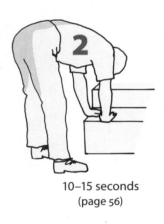

10–15 seconds
(page 56)

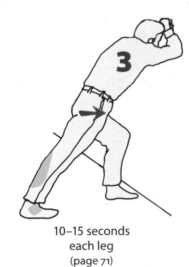

10–15 seconds
each leg
(page 71)

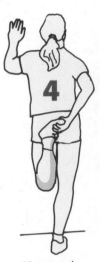

10 seconds
each leg
(page 75)

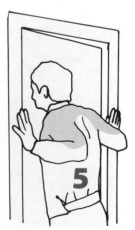

15–20 seconds
(page 47)

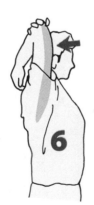

8–10 seconds
each arm
(page 44)

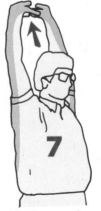

10–15 seconds
(page 46)

120 Routines

Stretching © 2010 by Bob and Jean Anderson. Shelter Publications, Inc.

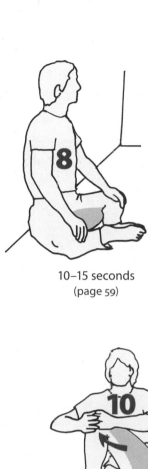

10–15 seconds
(page 59)

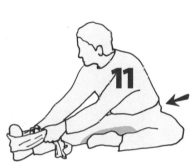

9 →

10–20 seconds
(page 58)

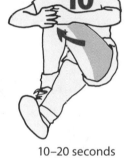

10–20 seconds
each leg
(page 61)

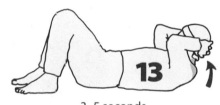

10–15 seconds
each leg
(page 40)

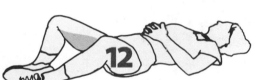

20–30 seconds
(page 26)

3–5 seconds
2 times
(page 27)

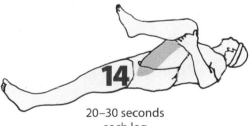

20–30 seconds
each leg
(page 63)

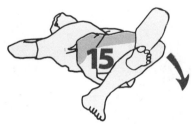

10–15 seconds
each side
(page 27)

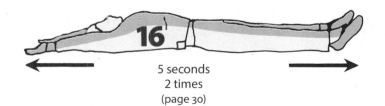

5 seconds
2 times
(page 30)

Stretching © 2010 by Bob and Jean Anderson. Shelter Publications, Inc

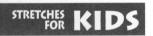

APPROXIMATELY 5 MINUTES

It's never too early to start stretching! Show your kids how to do these stretches (or show these to your kids' teachers, so they can get the whole class stretching). Explain to them that stretching is not a contest, and that they should stretch slowly, concentrating on the areas being stretched.

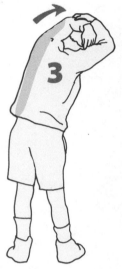

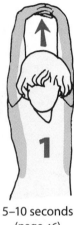

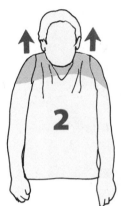

5–10 seconds
(page 46)

3–5 seconds
2 times
(page 46)

5–10 seconds
each side
(page 44)

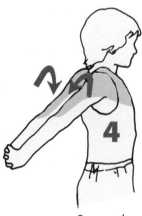

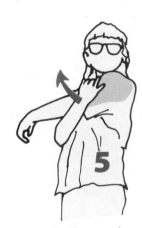

5 seconds
2 times
(page 47)

5–10 seconds
each arm
(page 43)

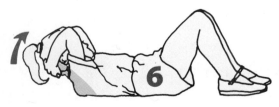

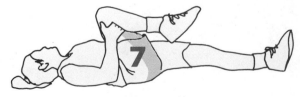

3 seconds
2 times
(page 27)

10 seconds
each leg
(page 63)

Stretching © 2010 by Bob and Jean Anderson. Shelter Publications, Inc.

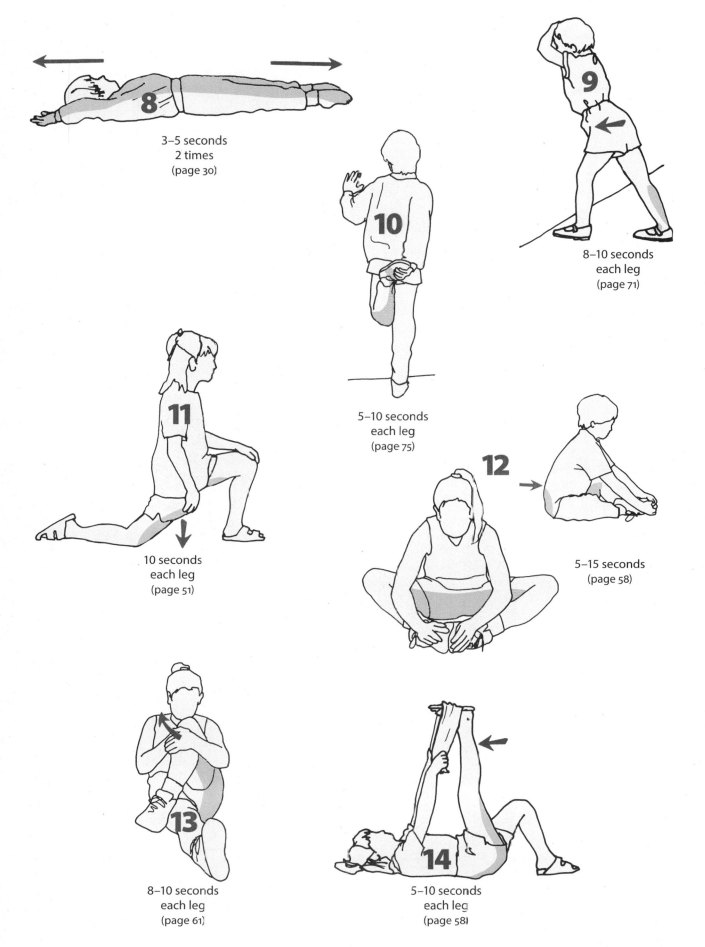

8

3–5 seconds
2 times
(page 30)

9

8–10 seconds
each leg
(page 71)

10

5–10 seconds
each leg
(page 75)

11

10 seconds
each leg
(page 51)

12

5–15 seconds
(page 58)

13

8–10 seconds
each leg
(page 61)

14

5–10 seconds
each leg
(page 58)

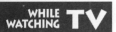

Many people think they don't have enough time to stretch, yet watch several hours of television a night. Well, you can stretch as you watch TV. This will not interfere with your viewing and you will be accomplishing something during otherwise sedentary times.

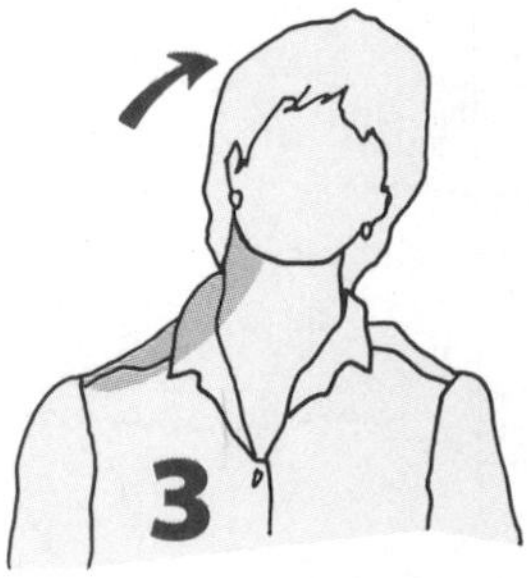

3
3–5 seconds
each side
(page 46)

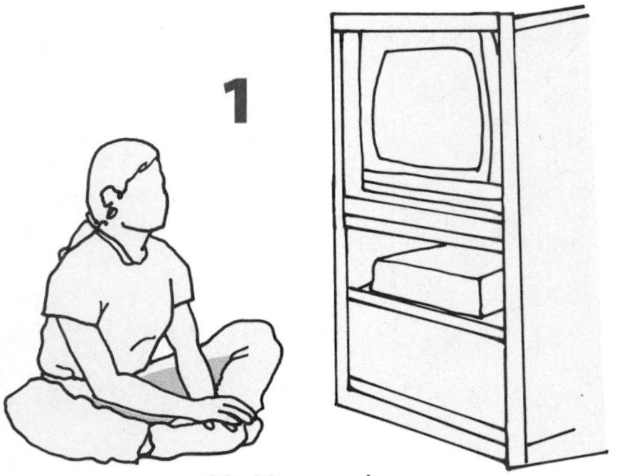

1
20–30 seconds
(page 58)

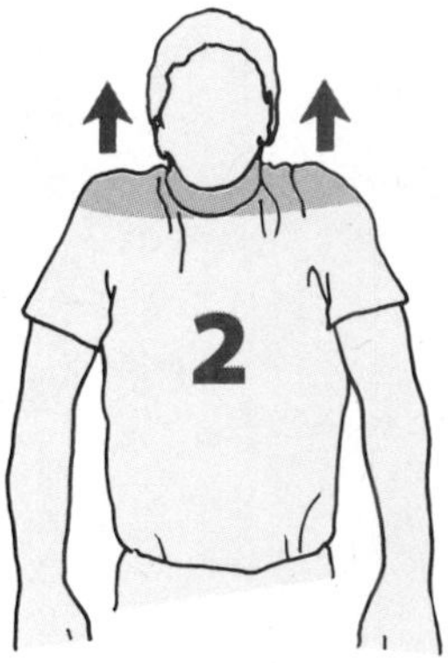

2
3–5 seconds
3 times
(page 46)

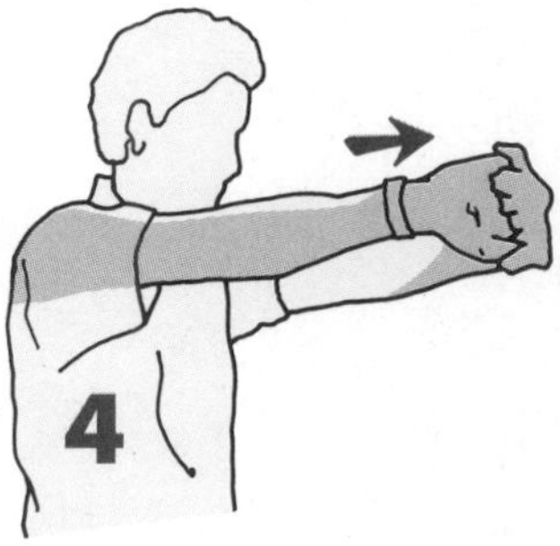

4
15 seconds
(page 45)

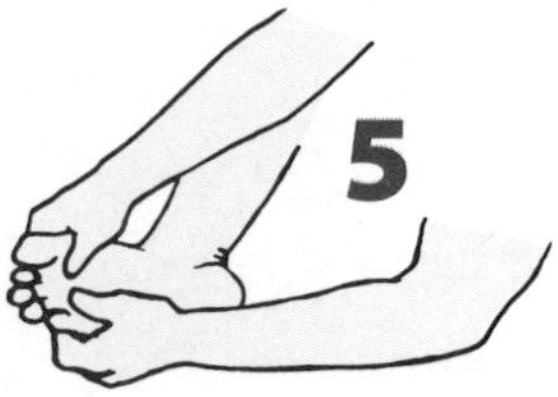

5
30–60 seconds
each foot
(page 34)

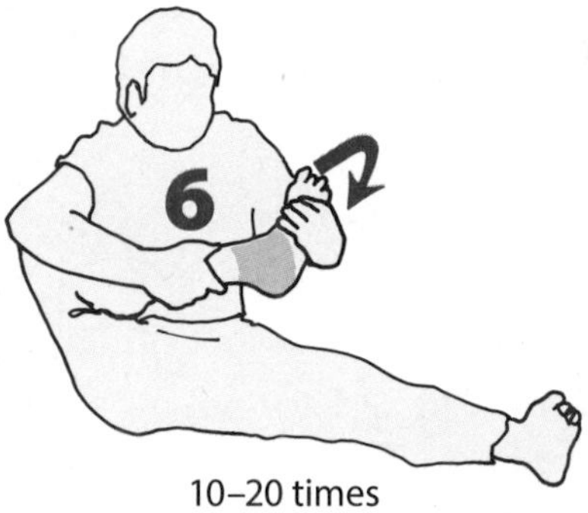

6
10–20 times
each foot
(page 34)

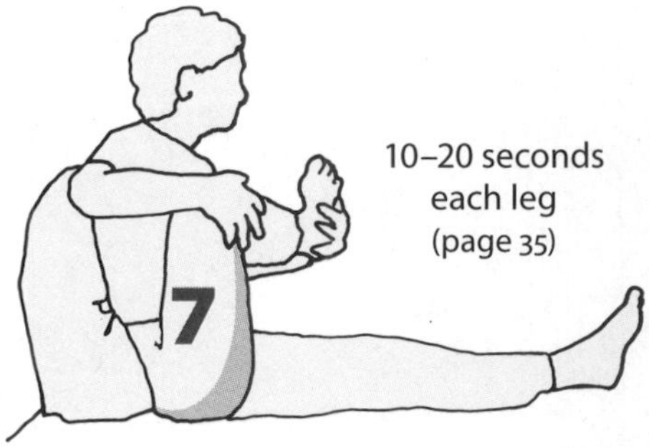

7
10–20 seconds
each leg
(page 35)

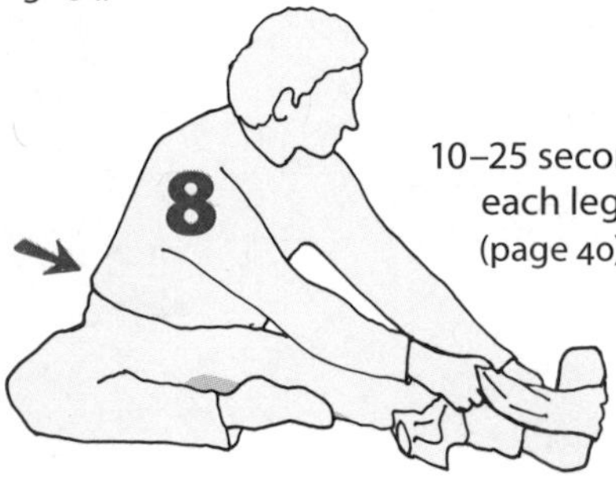

8
10–25 seconds
each leg
(page 40)

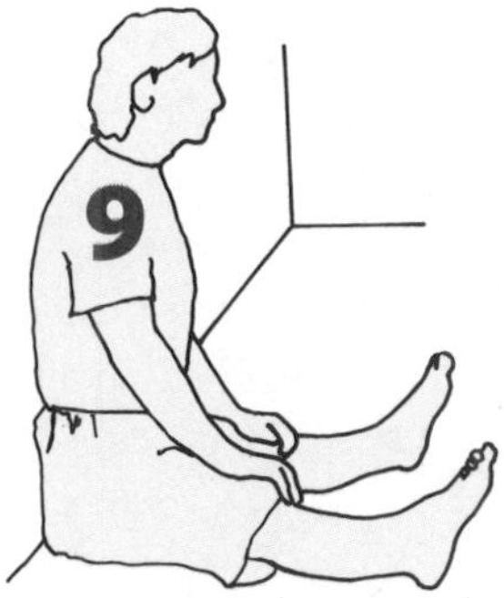

9
10–30 seconds
(page 98)

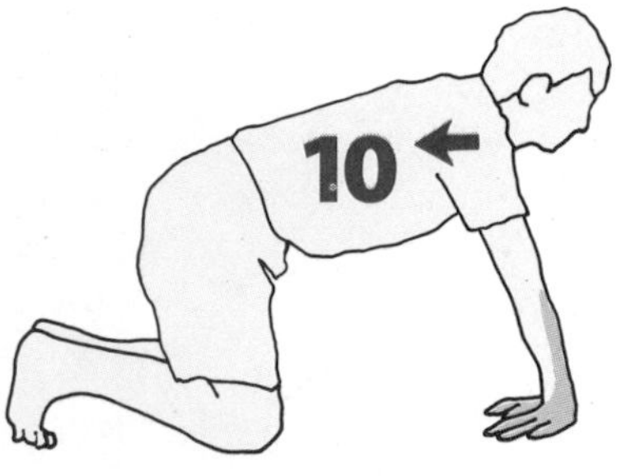

10
10–20 seconds
(page 42)

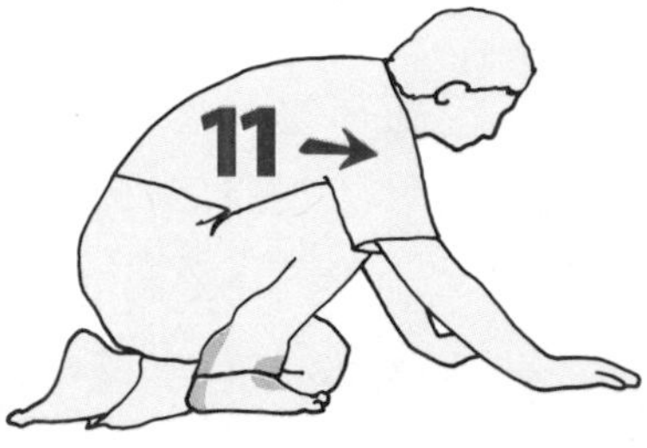

11
5–10 seconds
each leg
(page 50)

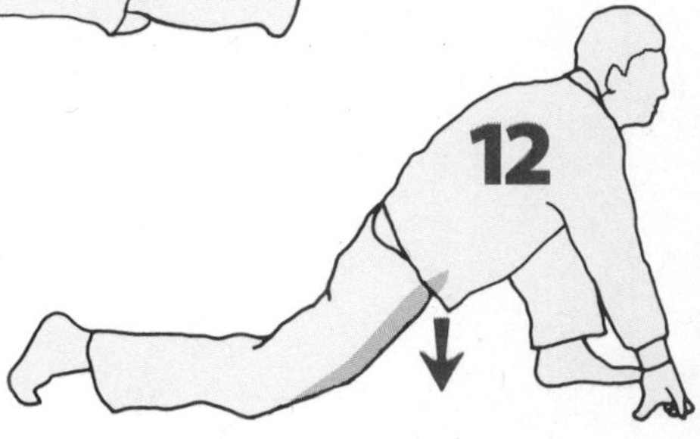

12
10–20 seconds
each leg
(page 51)

Stretching © 2010 by Bob and Jean Anderson. Shelter Publications, Inc.

WALKING

APPROXIMATELY 5 MINUTES

These stretches will make the movements of walking feel free and easy. Warm up by walking several minutes before stretching.

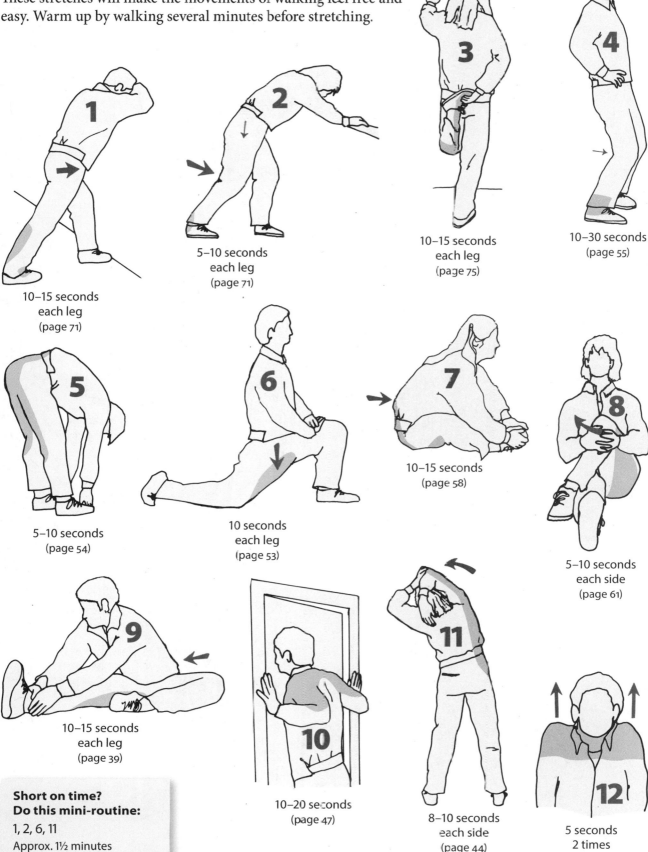

1 10–15 seconds each leg (page 71)

2 5–10 seconds each leg (page 71)

3 10–15 seconds each leg (page 75)

4 10–30 seconds (page 55)

5 5–10 seconds (page 54)

6 10 seconds each leg (page 53)

7 10–15 seconds (page 58)

8 5–10 seconds each side (page 61)

9 10–15 seconds each leg (page 39)

10 10–20 seconds (page 47)

11 8–10 seconds each side (page 44)

12 5 seconds 2 times (page 46)

**Short on time?
Do this mini-routine:**
1, 2, 6, 11
Approx. 1½ minutes

TRAVELER'S STRETCHES

APPROXIMATELY 2 MINUTES

Stretch at various times throughout your journey to help
your body feel less stiff and tight.

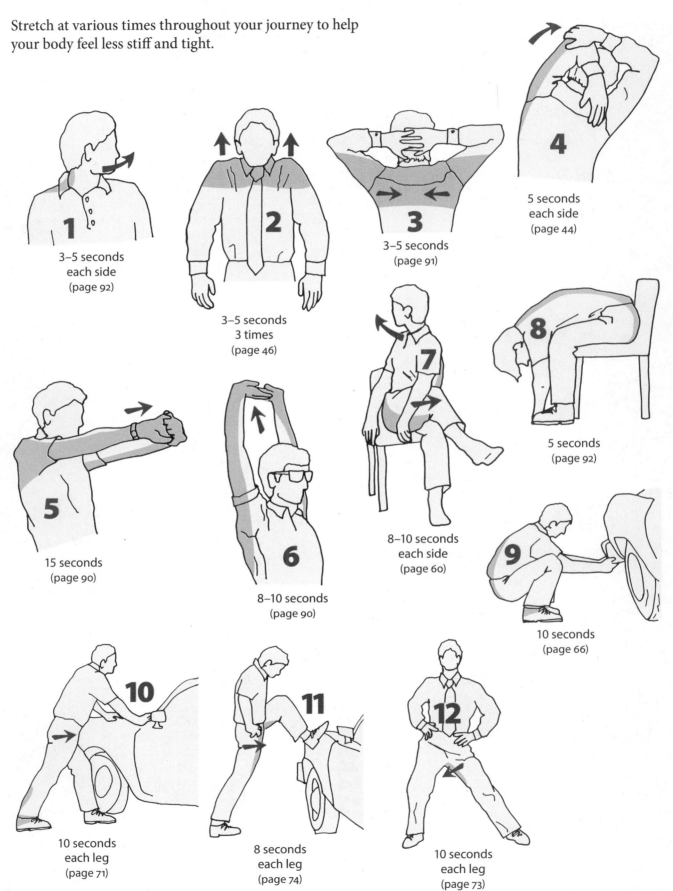

1 3–5 seconds
each side
(page 92)

2 3–5 seconds
3 times
(page 46)

3 3–5 seconds
(page 91)

4 5 seconds
each side
(page 44)

5 15 seconds
(page 90)

6 8–10 seconds
(page 90)

7 8–10 seconds
each side
(page 60)

8 5 seconds
(page 92)

9 10 seconds
(page 66)

10 10 seconds
each leg
(page 71)

11 8 seconds
each leg
(page 74)

12 10 seconds
each leg
(page 73)

AIRPLANE STRETCHES

Photocopy this page and take it along on your next flight. Stretching on the plane will relieve stress and stiffness and allow you to arrive in a more relaxed state. Don't be surprised if your fellow passengers follow your example and start stretching too. Especially good to do just before you land.

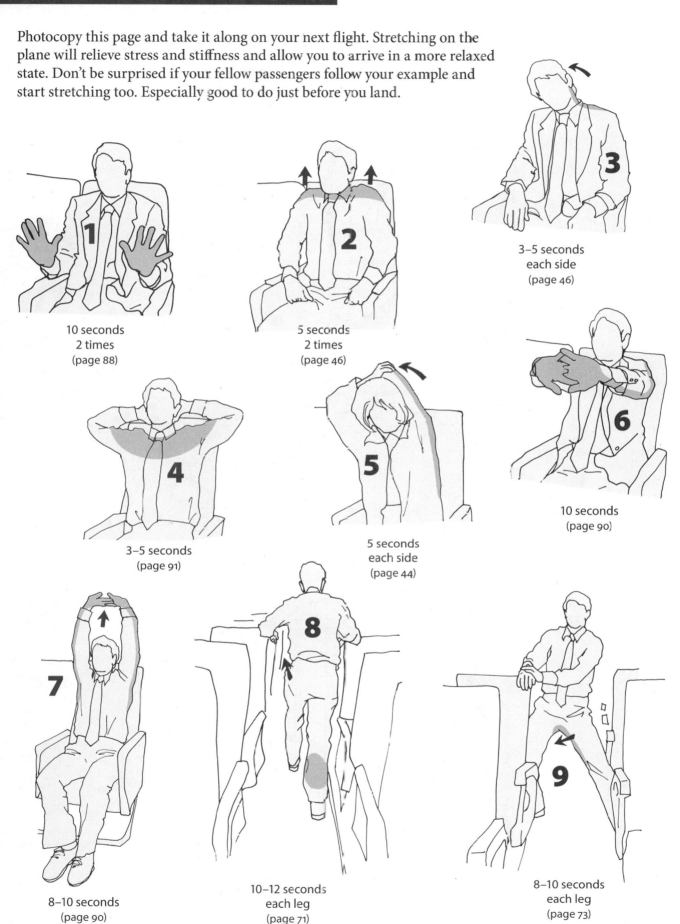

3
3–5 seconds
each side
(page 46)

1
10 seconds
2 times
(page 88)

2
5 seconds
2 times
(page 46)

4
3–5 seconds
(page 91)

5
5 seconds
each side
(page 44)

6
10 seconds
(page 90)

7
8–10 seconds
(page 90)

8
10–12 seconds
each leg
(page 71)

9
8–10 seconds
each leg
(page 73)

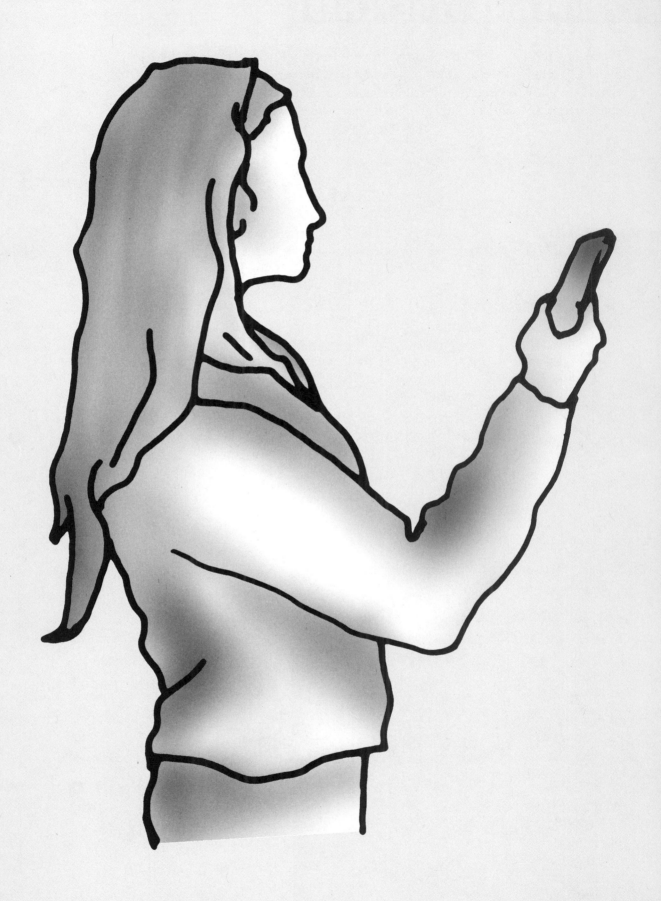

STRETCHING IN THE AGE OF COMPUTERS AND SMARTPHONES

Computers

Ten years ago, we updated this book to address the problems coming from sedentary office work, especially from too much time spent at a computer.

People were staying in the same position for long periods of time while working on computers. Even typewriters that were in usage earlier required some movement: putting in paper, turning the roller knob, working the carriage release lever. Computers eliminated these functions.

Phones

What's new?

The last ten years have seen a tremendous increase in smartphone usage, and this has caused problems, especially poor posture from looking downward most of the time.

In this section of the book, we'll outline the main problems that come from spending a lot of time on a computer and/or phone each day, and present simple stretches and tips that will improve your posture, make you feel better, and minimize pain.

DESK (COMPUTER) FITNESS

Sitting for hours at a time is a relatively recent phenomenon in human history. These days, most people working on computers sit for too long without a break, and problems are multiplying.

Computer Injuries

Fast, light-touch keyboards that allow high-speed typing have resulted in an epidemic of injuries to the hands, arms, and shoulders. Slowly, the thousands of repeated keystrokes and long periods of gripping and dragging a mouse damage the body. This happens even more quickly due to improper keyboarding technique and/or body positions that stress the tendons and nerves in the hand, wrist, arms, shoulders, and neck.

Typical problems

- **Repetitive strain injuries** — RSIs — (such as carpal tunnel syndrome and tendinitis) are typically caused by repetitive hand movements.
- **Back pain:** Sitting for long periods compresses your spine. If your posture is bad, gravity accentuates the problem.
- **Stiff muscles:** Not moving for long periods can cause neck and shoulder pain.
- **Tight joints:** Inactivity can cause joints to tighten, which makes moving more difficult or even painful.
- **Poor circulation:** When you sit very still, blood settles in the lower legs and feet and does not circulate well. There can be tingling, coldness, or numbness in the hands, and back pain.

What If You Have Such Symptoms?

We all have occasional aches and pains that go away in a day or two. But if you have recurring problems from using the computer, run, do not walk, to your doctor or health care provider. An early diagnosis can limit damage. Don't ignore the pain; you may sustain a serious injury. There are no quick fixes. No wrist splint, arm rest, split keyboard, spinal adjustment, etc. is going to get you right back to work at full speed. Even carpal

tunnel sufferers who have wrist release surgery can be back in pain if they don't make long-term changes in their techniques and work habits. Healing does happen but it may take months, not days.

Ergonomics Modern-day office ergonomics is the science of providing furniture, tools, and equipment that improve the comfort, safety, and health of office workers. Some basic principles:

- **Keyboard** should be set at a height so that forearms, wrists, and hands are aligned when keyboarding, and parallel to the floor, or bent slightly down from elbow to hand — the hands are never bent back.

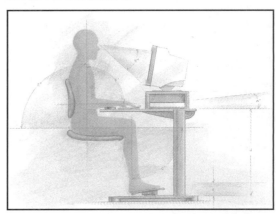

Preferably the stand or desk on which the keyboard sits is adjustable. There are many ergonomic keyboards available, some of them quite unusual.

- **Mouse pad** should be at a height where your arm, wrist, and hand are aligned and in "neutral." It's good if the stand or desk the mouse pad sits on is also adjustable.
- **Wrists**, while you are actually typing, should not rest on anything, and should not be bent up, down, or to the side, but should be in a straight line with your forearm, as viewed from above. Your arms should move your hands around, and instead of resting your wrists, stretch to hit keys with your fingers.
- **Chair** should be adjustable and comfortable. Set it so that your thighs are either parallel to the floor or at a slight downward angle from the hips to the knees. Sit straight, not slouching, and not straining forward to reach the keys. Stay relaxed.

Further Tips

- **Sit *and* stand.** Movement is important. Try adjusting the height or angle of your chair after a few hours, or stand after sitting for a period. In fact, the least stressful working position is one where the individual can "sit *and* stand" rather than "sit *or* stand." Many people now use standup mats or "anti-fatigue mats" that provide support and cushioning while standing.

- **Don't pound the keys.** Use a light touch.

- **Use two hands** to perform double-key operations such as **Command-P, Ctrl-C** or **Alt-F,** instead of twisting one hand to do them.

- **Hold the mouse lightly.** Don't grip it hard or squeeze it. Place it where you don't have to reach up or over very far to use it (close to the keyboard is best).

- **Use the tap-to-click setting for your trackpad.** Then you don't have to hold your thumb down to click or drag, and it puts less strain on your thumb and wrist.

- **Keep your arms and hands warm.** Cold muscles and tendons are at much greater risk for overuse injuries, and many offices are overly air-conditioned. Fingerless gloves help a lot.

- **Rest.** When you stop typing for a while, rest your hands in your lap and/or on their sides instead of leaving them on the keyboard.

- **Stretch.** Stretch frequently throughout the day *(see pages 132–135).*

- **Elevate your feet.** Elevating your feet daily for 5–10 minutes can help circulation. A very healthy habit.

- **Move.** Get up and move whenever you can. If possible, walk to talk to a near-by colleague instead of using the phone. Try using the stairs (at least for some floors) instead of the elevator.

- **Take breaks.** Some experts suggest a 10-second break every 3 minutes, others suggest a 1-minute break every 15 minutes, a 5-minute break every half hour, or a 15-minute break every 2 hours, etc. You can stretch and/or move around during these breaks.

- **Use a TheraCane®.** This is an excellent body tool to work out upper body tightness and tension. *(See page 235.)*

- **Breathing** Deep diaphragmatic breathing every hour helps you to reduce stress, create calmness and mental focus. If you are not sure you are using your diaphragm when breathing. *(See page 227, the Breath Builder, a tool to improve your diaphragmatic breath.)*

What Can Stretching Do?

- If you aren't injured, use the stretches on pages 132–135. Stretch regularly a few times a day and it may help you minimize repetitive strain injuries.

- If you are injured, take this book to your doctor or health care provider and ask which of the stretching programs you can follow. Point out that the stretching prescriptions on pages 228–229 can be used to customize a series of stretches for your particular condition.

- On the following four pages are stretching programs specifically designed for people who work at computers.

STRETCHES FOR KEYBOARD OPERATORS

APPROXIMATELY 1¼ MINUTES

Many people do not understand this, but working on a keyboard all day, day after day, is physically demanding. Repetitive strain injuries (RSIs) from mouse and keyboard use have risen dramatically. The routine below is specifically designed for keyboard operators and their potential (or actual) problems.

- If you are injured, see a doctor (preferably one with RSI experience) for advice on which stretches will help you recover. *(See the Stretching Prescriptions on pp. 228–229.)*

- If you are not injured now, do these stretches throughout the day as preventive medicine. (Stretch while making "saves," for example.)

- *See pp. 130–131, for more on RSI problems.*

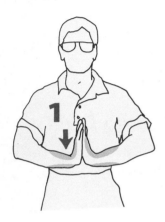

8 seconds
(page 89)

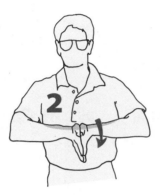

8 seconds
(page 89)

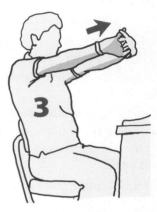

10 seconds 2
times
(page 90)

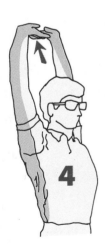

10–15 seconds
(page 46)

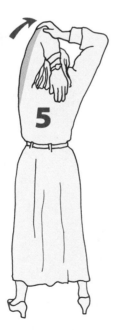

10 seconds
each arm
(page 44)

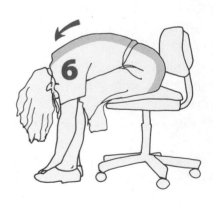

10 seconds
(page 92)

Move

It's important to move: take a 1-minute break every 10–15 minutes, or a 5-minute break every half hour; get up and move around.

Stretching © 2010 by Bob and Jean Anderson. Shelter Publications, Inc.

ONLINE STRETCHES

APPROXIMATELY 1 MINUTE

No matter how fast your connection, you're always waiting for something to load while online. (This will probably never change, for even as connections get faster and faster, files get larger and larger.) These stretches are for your upper body, especially neck, shoulders, and wrists.

- Whenever you are reading online, and not using the keyboard or mouse, you can do upper body stretches using both arms.
- After you follow this program a few times, you'll know these stretches by heart; thereafter do them frequently while online.

> If there isn't time to do them all at one time, break the routine into short combinations:
> 1, 2, 3 or 4, 5, 6 or 7, 8.

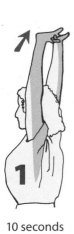

10 seconds
(page 46)

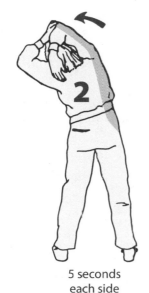

5 seconds
each side
(page 44)

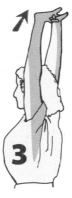

5 seconds
each side
(page 46)

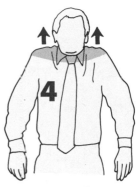

5 seconds
each side
(page 46)

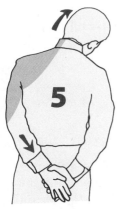

5 seconds
each side
(page 47)

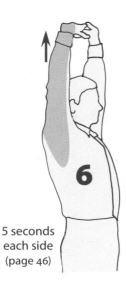

5 seconds
each side
(page 46)

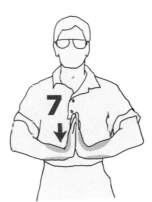

8 seconds
(page 89)

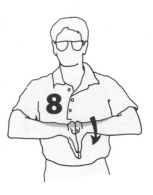

8 seconds
(page 89)

STRETCHES FOR GRAPHIC ARTISTS

APPROXIMATELY 1½ MINUTES

Concentrated effort on visual images puts a strain on your body as well as your eyes. Using a stylus with a drawing tablet can cause finger and wrist problems. Take frequent breaks to do these stretches, or do them while you're waiting for the computer to process information.

- Look at the stretching prescriptions on pages 228 to 229 for some other ideas.
- You can also do some exercises or move around.

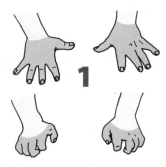

10 seconds each
position
(page 88)

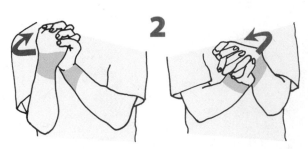

10 times
clockwise & counterclockwise (page 88)

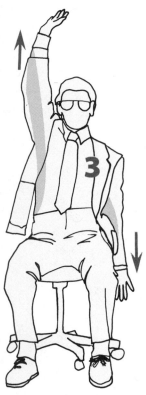

10 seconds each
side (page 84)

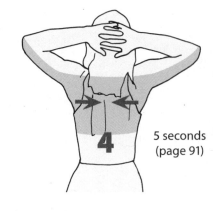

5 seconds
(page 91)

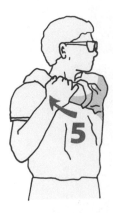

10 seconds each
arm (page 91)

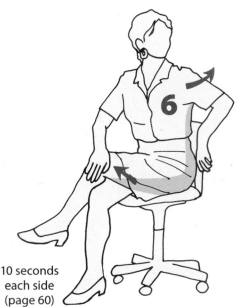

10 seconds
each side
(page 60)

Visual fitness

Every once in a while, look out the window or at a distant object. This different focus from close-up work relieves eye strain.

STRESSED-OUT STRETCHES

APPROXIMATELY 1½ MINUTES

- Had a tough day?
- Computer giving you problems?
- Going to an important meeting?
- Need to relax?

There are inevitable times during the day when the body signals it's had an overdose of stress. Don't let tension build up and ruin your good work. Pace yourself throughout the day. Take frequent stretch breaks!

- Breathe deeply.

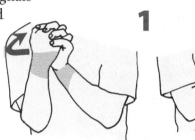

10 seconds
each position
(page 88)

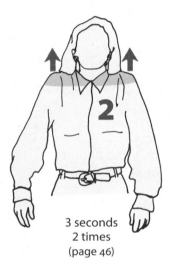

3 seconds
2 times
(page 46)

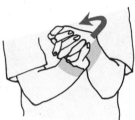

10 seconds 2 times
(page 90)

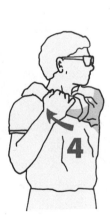

15 seconds each
arm (page 91)

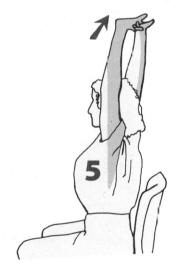

10 seconds (page 46)

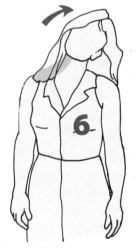

5 seconds each side
(page 46)

PHONE HEALTH PROBLEMS

Google research indicates there were between 3–4 billion smartphone users worldwide in 2019, and that number is growing.

According to RescueTime, an app for iOS and Android phones, people in 2019 spent an average of 3–4 hours every day on their smartphones, with 20% of users spending 4½ hours.

It sneaked up on us. Smartphones are life-changing devices, so useful and compelling that we've overlooked a major downside: bad posture! Which leads to back problems, among other things.

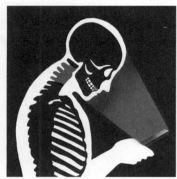

If you look at teenagers, they're invariably looking at their phones, heads bent forward, posture off-balance. Young people get off to a bad start in life when they unwittingly develop bad posture from bending over and staring at a small screen for hours on end. Unwittingly, because it's a gradual process, like the frog placed in a pot of slowly-warming water.

The same goes for adults. The next time you're in the streets, or are in a market, or on public transit, notice how people are bent over, looking at their phones.

(This isn't due entirely to phones: we hunch over when reading, driving, even walking. The head is almost always out of balance.)

The repetitive use of fingers (or thumbs) can contribute to repetitive stress injuries such as tendinitis or carpal tunnel syndrome.

Symptoms of tech neck (or text neck) are not just a stiff neck, but pain between shoulder blades, and sometimes headaches. Worse, over time, tendons and joints can become damaged and slouching permanent.

Poor posture while sitting, standing, walking, or looking at your phone can lead to more than upper body pain and stiffness; poor posture affects other parts of the spine, such as the middle and low back. Once sustained, these types of injuries are difficult to treat. Tendons are not muscles that tighten and contract, so tendon damage is hard to repair.

We encourage you to do some web research on the subject. Start by googling "tech neck"; there's a ton of information out there. We also encourage you to seek advice from a health care professional if you are having problems.

Tech Neck

Tech neck is a phrase describing neck (and shoulder) soreness that results from tucking your head down over your chin (sometimes called "hunchback slouch") while looking down at a phone screen. This causes the muscles in the back of your neck to contract in order to hold the head up.

An adult head weighs 10 to 11 pounds. As the angle of leaning forward increases, there's increasing stress on your spine. A 15-degree forward tilt is said to put a strain on your neck of 27 pounds (10 pounds from weight of the head, 17 pounds from imbalance).

Looking down at smart phones for long periods of time can cause the bones in the neck to mold into a curved position.

Text Neck

Text neck refers to the problems that come from *texting* on a phone.

The dangers of texting while driving are obvious, but there's also danger in texting while walking; there's been an increase in pedestrian accidents from people texting while walking. Some cities have even considered making texting while walking illegal.

Texting requires more concentration than talking and/or using voice recognition. (You can talk on a phone without staring at it.)

In these few pages, we'll show you some very simple things you can do to counteract the negative physical effects of using a smartphone.

Posture Check – Standing

How's your posture right now? Are you standing balanced evenly on both feet, or are you standing predominantly on one foot? Is your head forward, causing rounded shoulders and tension in your neck, shoulders, and upper and lower back? How about your jaw? Is it being held tight because you are clenching your teeth, creating tension throughout your upper body? Are your hands relaxed, or are they being held tight, in an uncomfortable position?

Here are some ideas to help you get back in balance and reduce unwanted muscle tension and tightness:

- **Focus on your legs and feet.** Try standing with your feet pointed straight ahead, almost shoulder-width apart. Now make sure your legs are straight, but knees not locked backwards. Make sure you're standing evenly on both feet with your weight equally distributed between your two feet. This helps keep your center of gravity directed downward. This is more of a position of power and relaxation than the position of weakness and instability that goes with standing with your weight on mostly one foot.

- **Next focus on your upper body and head.** While standing in a more balanced stance, lift your chest slightly upward while your head is lifted back above your shoulders. Your chin should be level to the floor/ground and you should be looking forward, not downward. Think: "Stand tall." Check your jaw to be sure it's relaxed. If not, simply say this to yourself: "Jaw relax," and unclench your teeth, letting your jaw relax slightly.

- *Focus on your shoulders.* Next, bring the top of your shoulders up toward your ears. Hold for 1–3 seconds. Repeat 3–5 times. Inhale as you bring your shoulders up; exhale as you bring them down. Say to yourself: "Shoulders hang, shoulders down."

- *Hands* If they are tight and tense, let them relax. Shake them out as on page 89. Think: "Hands relax."

- *Breathe* Learn to take at least 10 full diaphragmatic breaths every hour to help reduce stress.

- *Practice realigning yourself throughout the day.* This can reduce the pain and discomfort of poor posture.

During the day, do quick posture checks. If your shoulders are tight and tense, do some shoulder shrugs. If your jaw is relaxed, it will reduce the tension and tightness in your face and upper body. If you are standing out of balance, realign your legs and feet so that your weight is evenly distributed.

Three important things to practice:

1. Bring your phone up to eye level, rather than looking down.

2. Look down with your eyes, not your head.

3. Take a three minute break for every 15 to 20 minutes you talk on the phone.

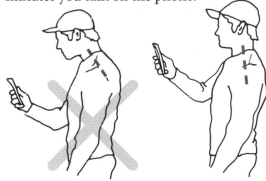

Your head controls your body.

Reducing Phone Stress

Google reports that "…mobile devices loaded with social media, email and news apps" are creating "…a constant sense of obligation, generating unintended personal stress." What can you do?

Turn off all notifications except for the ones you want to receive.

Delete apps or websites if they cause anxiety or stress. (Apps/websites like YouTube, Facebook, Twitter, WhatsApp, WeChat, TikTok, Instagram, etc. lure people into lots of time spent.)

Take breaks. Try a 24-hour "digital Sabbath." Many people who do this find an unexpected sense of peacefulness and calm without the digital leash and return to their devices refreshed.

There are books on how to "break up with your phone," that show you how to "…break up, then make up." The idea isn't to give up your phone, but to get a handle on usage, on hours spent.

Stretch! See *Phone Stretches* on the next two pages.

Phone Stickers

Here is an analog tool for your phone. It's not an app. It's a little printed reminder you can photocopy and tape on the back of your phone. There are two versions, for different size phones. (Packing or shipping tape works very well here.)

If you want to stretch, no need to start up an app. Just turn your phone over and do a few stretches.

It also reminds you to hold your phone at eye level.

> Photocopy one of these and tape to the back of your phone.
> OR
> Go to *shltr.net/phone-sticker* to download a color version.

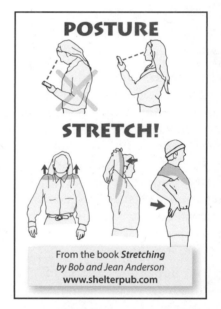

POSTURE

STRETCH!

From the book *Stretching* by Bob and Jean Anderson
www.shelterpub.com

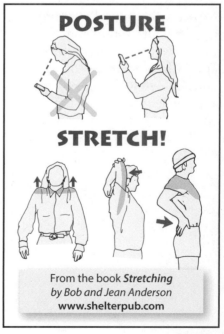

POSTURE

STRETCH!

From the book *Stretching* by Bob and Jean Anderson
www.shelterpub.com

APPROXIMATELY 1 MINUTE

- Do these whenever you need a break, or feel stiff.
- You needn't do all of these.
- Even one stretch can make a difference.
- Breathe.
- Stretch by the *feel*. If you do this, you'll develop body awareness: getting in touch with different parts of your body.

- Take a walk. Do something to get your blood circulating.
- After you finish the stretches, bring your phone up to eye level. Practice this often, and you'll develop a better habit.

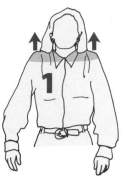

5 seconds 2 times
(page 46)

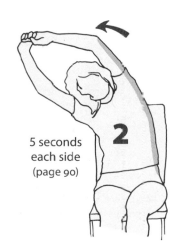

5 seconds
each side
(page 90)

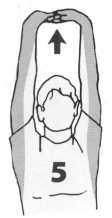

5 seconds each side
(page 46)

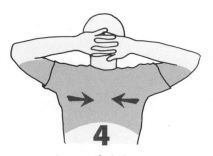

5 seconds 2 times
(page 28)

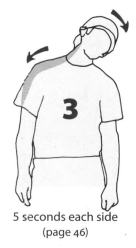

10 seconds 2 times
(page 46)

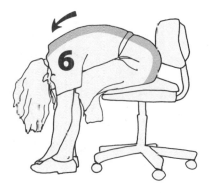

5 seconds
(page 92)

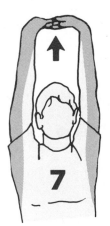

10 seconds 2 times
(page 46)

Stretching © 2010 by Bob and Jean Anderson. Shelter Publications, Inc.

PHONE STRETCHES (STANDING)

APPROXIMATELY 1½ MINUTES

- Stretch until you feel a bit of tension in your muscles.
- Hold it until you relax a bit.
- Then push gently a little farther.
- Concentrate on how your muscles and tendons feel.
- The "no gain no pain" principle does not apply to stretching.
- Breathe slowly and rhythmically.
- Practice bringing your phone up to eye level.

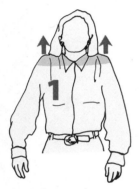

5 seconds
3 times
(page 46)

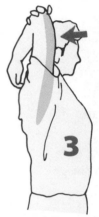

5–10 seconds each side
(page 92)

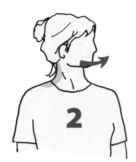

5 seconds each side
(page 44)

10–20 seconds (page 47)

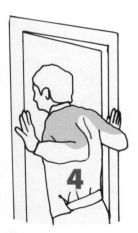

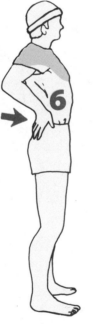

5–10 seconds each arm
(page 47)

10–12 seconds 2 times
(page 46)

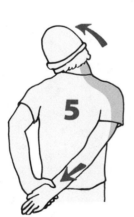

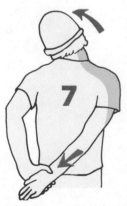

5–10 seconds each arm
(page 47)

THE IMPORTANCE OF EXERCISE

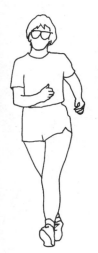

Stretching and good posture are not the only ways to counteract problems from smartphone usage, or "tech neck." Exercise increases your heart rate, sends blood to muscles, lubricates joints, and flushes out toxins that are causing pain.

Planning Plan to make exercise a part of your daily life, not just something you do at the end of the day — if you have time. Getting fit doesn't happen without planning, so you need a realistic plan for exercise to become an integral part of your life.

Make it a priority. Doing this will shape your future. Physical activity will become a priority centered around enjoyment, accomplishment, and improvement.

Be consistent. It takes longer to get into shape than it does to get out of shape. If you go a few days without exercise, don't worry; just don't go weeks or months without regular activity.

Stick with your routine. Getting fit doesn't happen by chance or without effort. It happens over time, with patience and a reasonable plan.

Learn an activity. Walking, hiking, running, cycling, swimming, weight training, etc. *Look at the list of activities on page 143.* You can google proper techniques/training for any activity you are interested in.

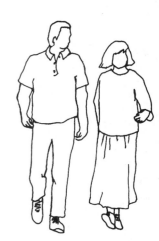

Take it easy. Don't overdo it when you begin. Start with a little activity, then *gradually* build it up over the year.

Rest is a very important part of getting the most out of exercise. Build rest days into your weekly plan. Rest helps prevent injuries, makes you stronger, and revitalizes the mind.

Staying hydrated improves physical and mental function, increases endurance, and helps the functioning of vital internal organs (heart, lungs, kidneys, etc.). Staying hydrated makes exercise easier and more enjoyable.

Elevate your feet every day.

Massage Get a massage as often as possible. *(See the massage body tools on pp. 228-229.)*

Staying in shape all year round will allow you to be prepared to do other activities such as vacuuming, washing the car, snow shoveling, gardening, cleaning house. Being in shape (staying strong, agile, and flexible) by regularly exercising and stretching will make it possible to do those activities more aerobically and safely.

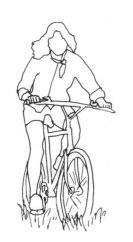
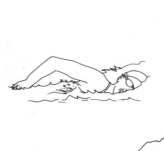
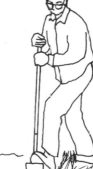

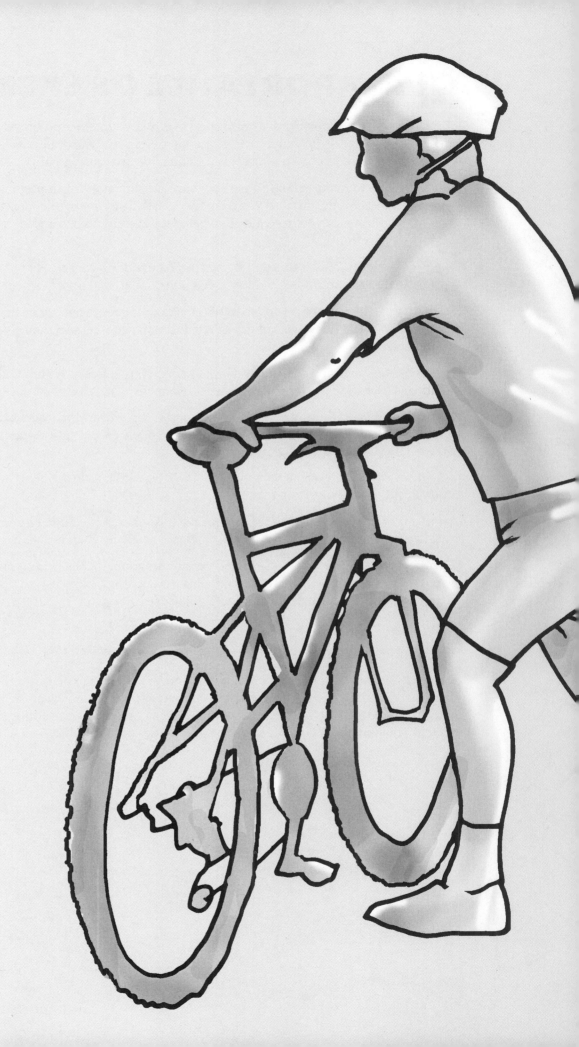

STRETCHING ROUTINES
Sports and Activities

In this section are stretching routines for sports and activities, arranged in alphabetical order.

Each time you do a stretch for the first time, read the *specific* instructions for that stretch. (See the page reference under each stretch.) After you follow the instructions a few times, you'll know how to do each stretch correctly. From then on, simply look at the drawings.

Warming up: For the more vigorous sports (running, football, etc.), I recommend that you do a short warm-up before stretching (jogging for 3–5 minutes with an exaggerated arm swing, for example). See p. 14, *Warming Up and Cooling Down*.

To teachers and coaches: These routines can serve as guidelines. You can add or subtract stretches to meet specific needs and time allotments.

Note: Be sure to read *How To Stretch* on pp. 12–13 before you do these routines.

AEROBIC EXERCISE

APPROXIMATELY 6 MINUTES

Do a mild warm-up of 2–3 minutes before stretching.

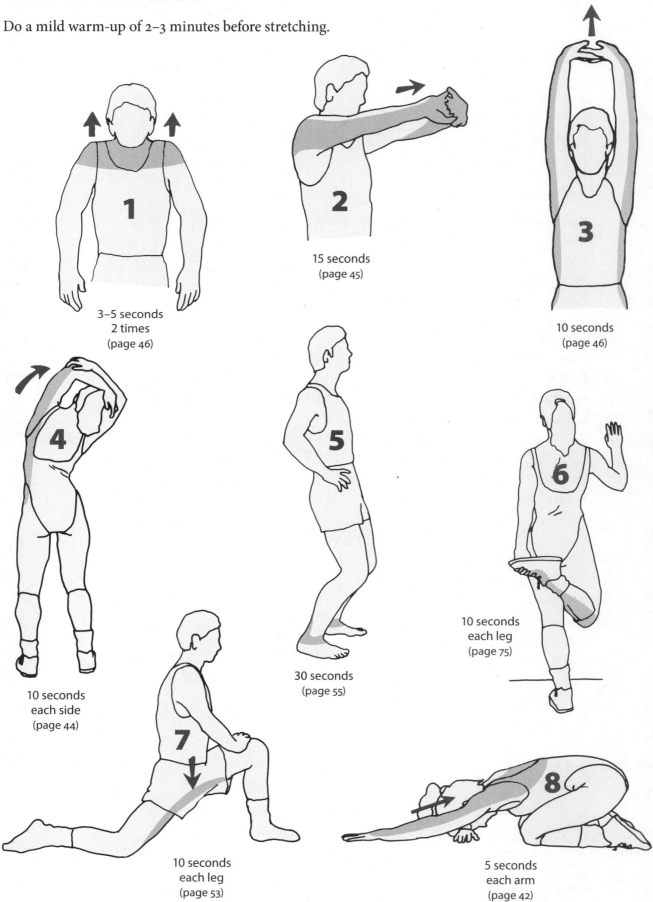

1
3–5 seconds
2 times
(page 46)

2
15 seconds
(page 45)

3
10 seconds
(page 46)

4
10 seconds
each side
(page 44)

5
30 seconds
(page 55)

6
10 seconds
each leg
(page 75)

7
10 seconds
each leg
(page 53)

8
5 seconds
each arm
(page 42)

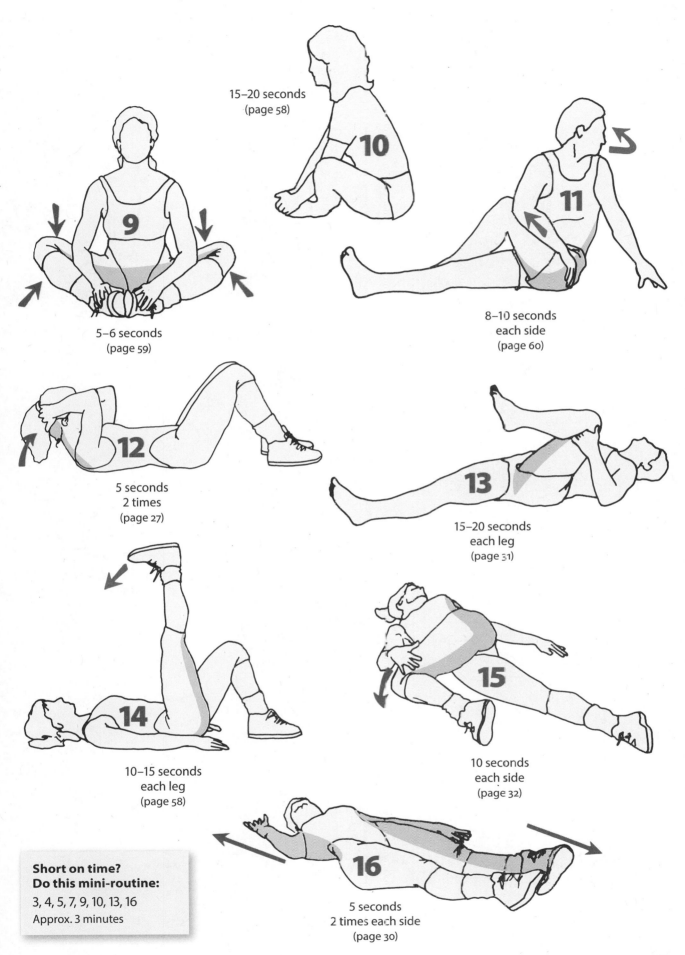

15–20 seconds
(page 58)

5–6 seconds
(page 59)

8–10 seconds
each side
(page 60)

5 seconds
2 times
(page 27)

15–20 seconds
each leg
(page 31)

10–15 seconds
each leg
(page 58)

10 seconds
each side
(page 32)

Short on time?
Do this mini-routine:
3, 4, 5, 7, 9, 10, 13, 16
Approx. 3 minutes

5 seconds
2 times each side
(page 30)

BADMINTON

APPROXIMATELY 6 MINUTES

Warm up with 2–3 minutes of walking before stretching.

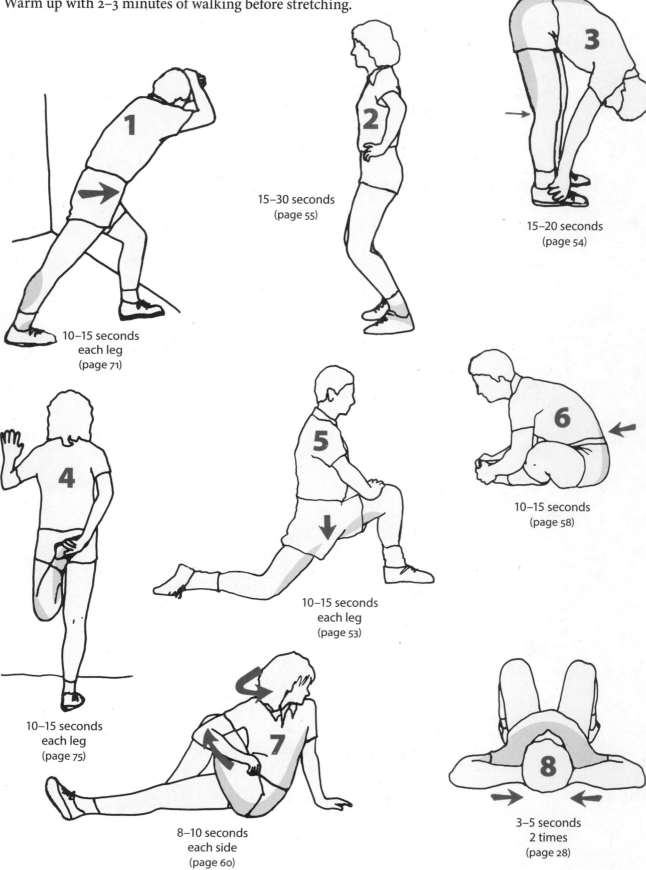

10–15 seconds
each leg
(page 71)

15–30 seconds
(page 55)

15–20 seconds
(page 54)

10–15 seconds
each leg
(page 75)

10–15 seconds
each leg
(page 53)

10–15 seconds
(page 58)

8–10 seconds
each side
(page 60)

3–5 seconds
2 times
(page 28)

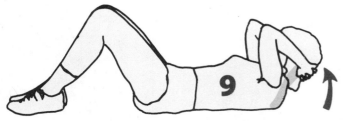

3–5 seconds
2 times
(page 27)

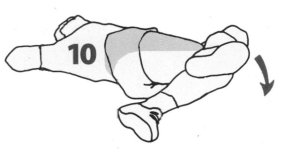

10-15 seconds
each side
(page 27)

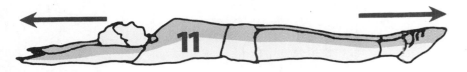

5 seconds
2 times
(page 30)

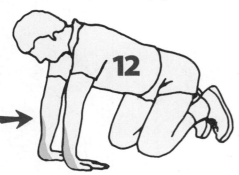

10–15 seconds
(page 42)

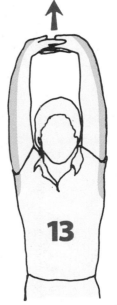

10–15 seconds
(page 46)

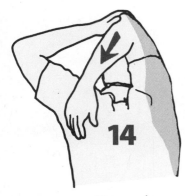

10 seconds
each arm
(page 44)

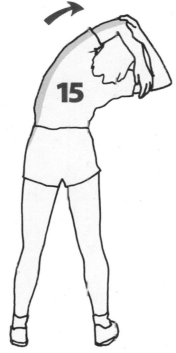

8–10 seconds
each side
(page 44)

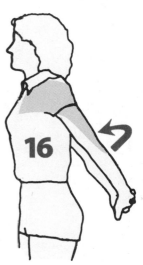

10–15 seconds
2 times
(page 47)

**Short on time?
Do this mini-routine:**
1, 2, 5, 13, 14, 15, 16
Approx. 3 minutes

BASEBALL/SOFTBALL

APPROXIMATELY 8 MINUTES

Jog around the baseball field once before stretching.

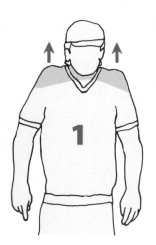

5 seconds
2–3 times
(page 46)

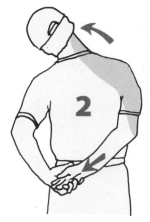

8–10 seconds
each arm
(page 47)

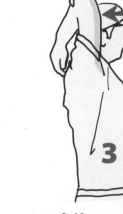

8–10 seconds
each arm
(page 44)

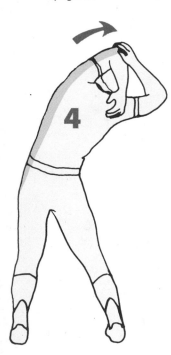

10 seconds
each side
(page 44)

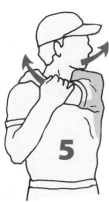

15 seconds
each arm
(page 43)

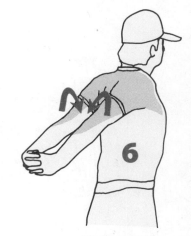

10–15 seconds
each arm
2 times
(page 47)

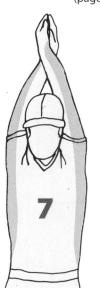

10–20 seconds
(page 43)

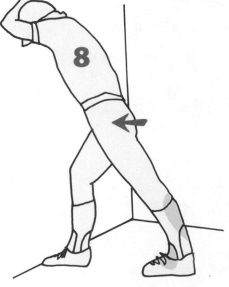

10–15 seconds
each leg
(page 71)

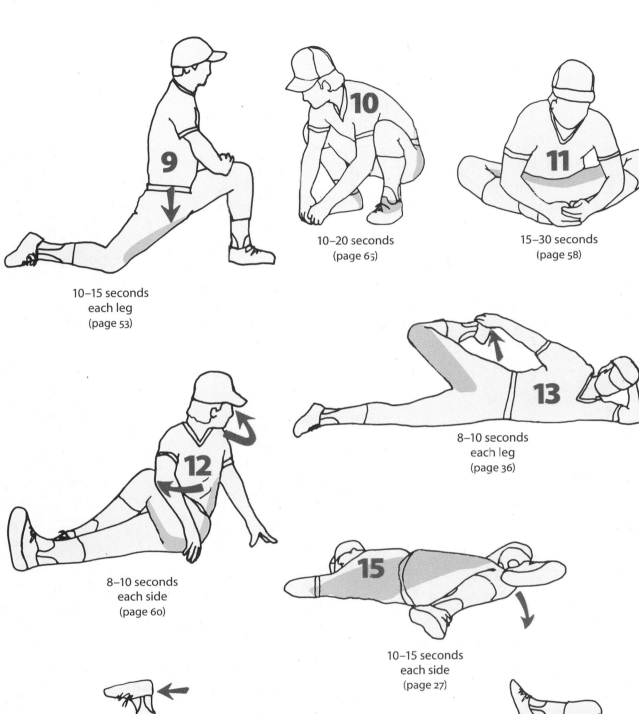

9

10–15 seconds
each leg
(page 53)

10

10–20 seconds
(page 65)

11

15–30 seconds
(page 58)

13

8–10 seconds
each leg
(page 36)

12

8–10 seconds
each side
(page 60)

15

10–15 seconds
each side
(page 27)

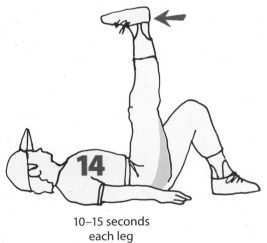

14

10–15 seconds
each leg
(page 58)

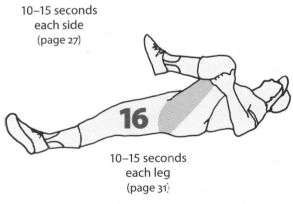

16

10–15 seconds
each leg
(page 31)

Short on time?
Do this mini-routine:
1, 3, 5, 9, 11, 12, 14, 16
Approx. 4 m nutes

BASKETBALL

Warm up by jogging for 3–5 minutes before stretching.

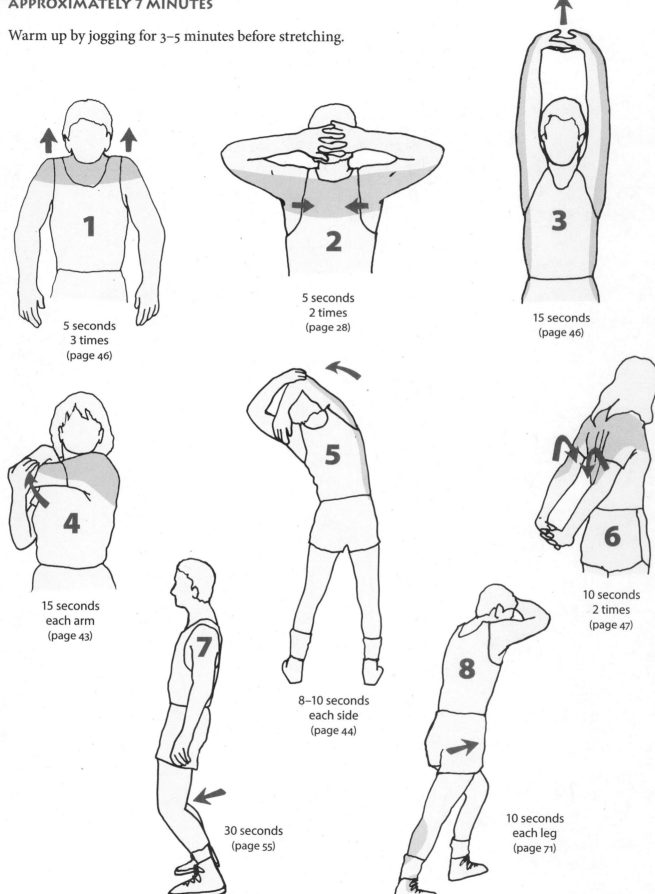

5 seconds
3 times
(page 46)

5 seconds
2 times
(page 28)

15 seconds
(page 46)

15 seconds
each arm
(page 43)

8–10 seconds
each side
(page 44)

10 seconds
2 times
(page 47)

30 seconds
(page 55)

10 seconds
each leg
(page 71)

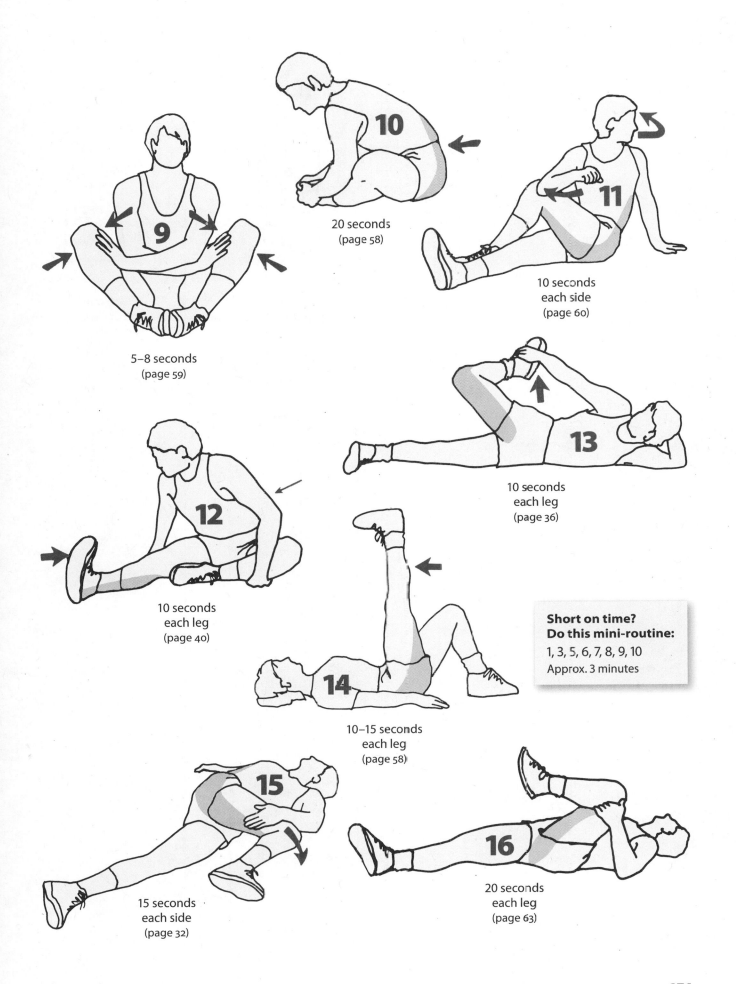

9

5–8 seconds
(page 59)

10

20 seconds
(page 58)

11

10 seconds
each side
(page 60)

12

10 seconds
each leg
(page 40)

13

10 seconds
each leg
(page 36)

14

10–15 seconds
each leg
(page 58)

15

15 seconds
each side
(page 32)

16

20 seconds
each leg
(page 63)

Short on time?
Do this mini-routine:
1, 3, 5, 6, 7, 8, 9, 10
Approx. 3 minutes

BOWLING

APPROXIMATELY 6 MINUTES

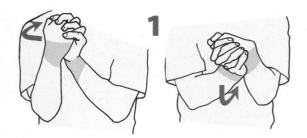

1

Rotate 10 times
each direction
(page 88)

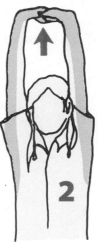

2

15 seconds
(page 46)

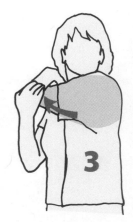

3

15 seconds
each arm
(page 43)

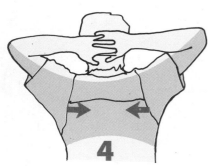

4

5 seconds
2 times
(page 91)

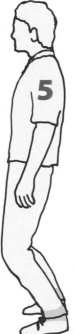

5

15–20 seconds
(page 55)

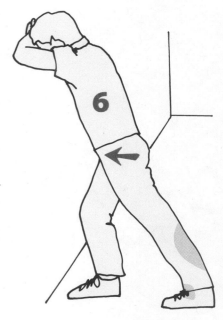

6

10–15 seconds
each leg
(page 71)

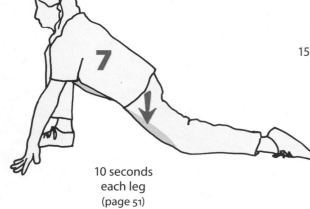

7

10 seconds
each leg
(page 51)

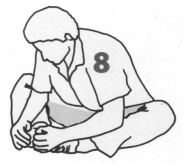

8

10 seconds
(page 58)

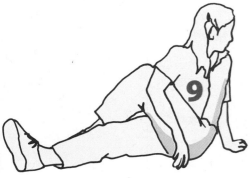

8–10 seconds
each side
(page 60)

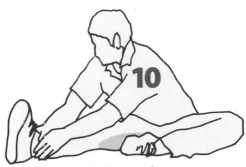

10–15 seconds
each leg
(page 39)

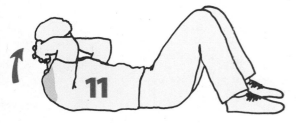

3 seconds
2 times
(page 27)

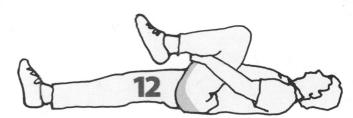

15–20 seconds
each leg
(page 31)

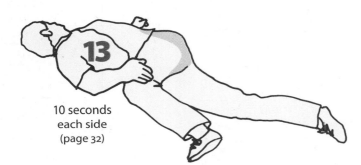

10 seconds
each side
(page 32)

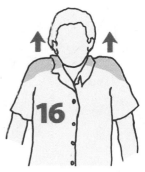

5 seconds
3 times
(page 46)

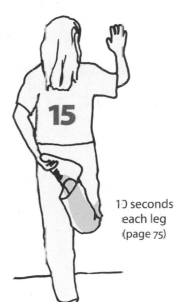

10 seconds
(page 58)

1) seconds
each leg
(page 75)

Short on time?
Do this mini-routine:
1, 2, 4, 5, 6, 7, 15
Approx. 2½ minutes

CYCLING

APPROXIMATELY 8 MINUTES

Walk for several minutes before stretching.

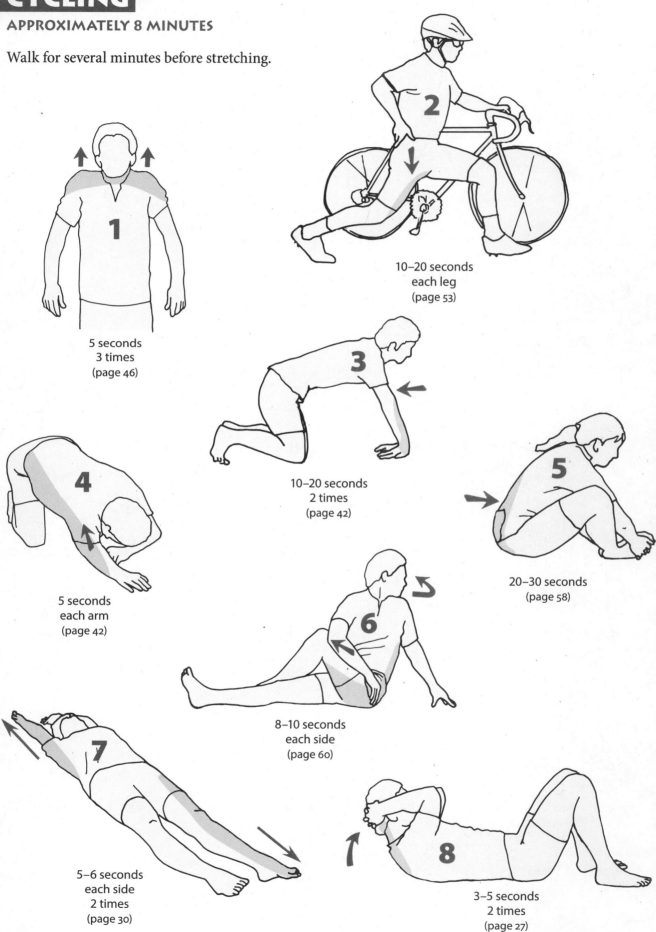

5 seconds
3 times
(page 46)

10–20 seconds
each leg
(page 53)

10–20 seconds
2 times
(page 42)

5 seconds
each arm
(page 42)

20–30 seconds
(page 58)

8–10 seconds
each side
(page 60)

5–6 seconds
each side
2 times
(page 30)

3–5 seconds
2 times
(page 27)

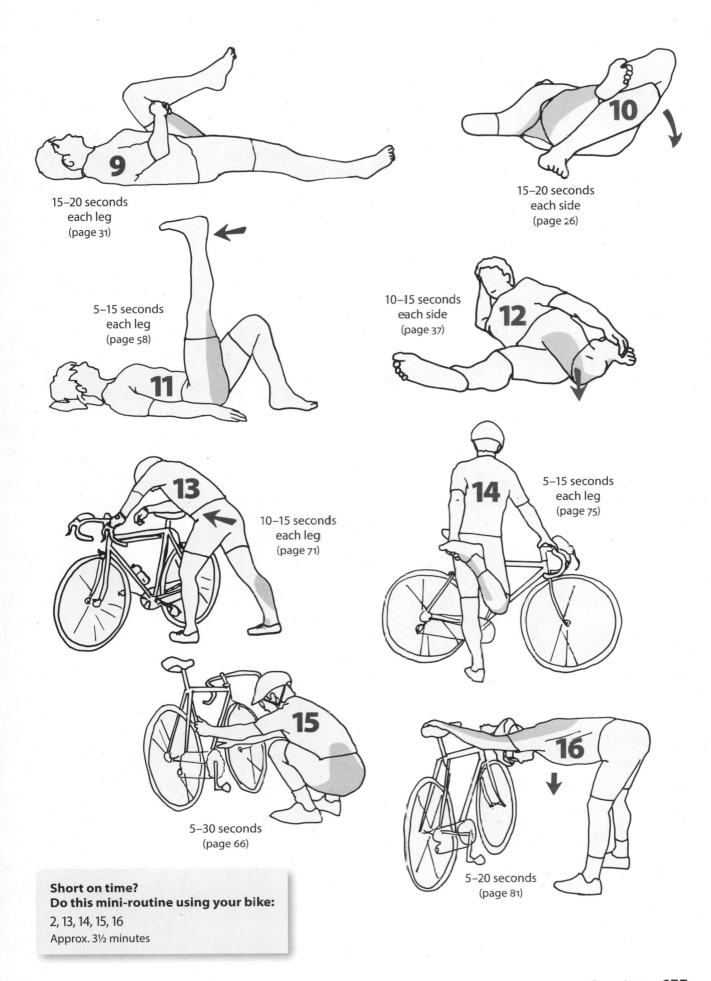

9

15–20 seconds
each leg
(page 31)

10

15–20 seconds
each side
(page 26)

11

5–15 seconds
each leg
(page 58)

12

10–15 seconds
each side
(page 37)

13

10–15 seconds
each leg
(page 71)

14

5–15 seconds
each leg
(page 75)

15

5–30 seconds
(page 66)

16

5–20 seconds
(page 81)

Short on time?
Do this mini-routine using your bike:
2, 13, 14, 15, 16
Approx. 3½ minutes

Stretching © 2010 by Bob and Jean Anderson. Shelter Publicaticns, Inc.

EQUESTRIAN SPORTS

APPROXIMATELY 5 MINUTES

Walk for 2–3 minutes before stretching.

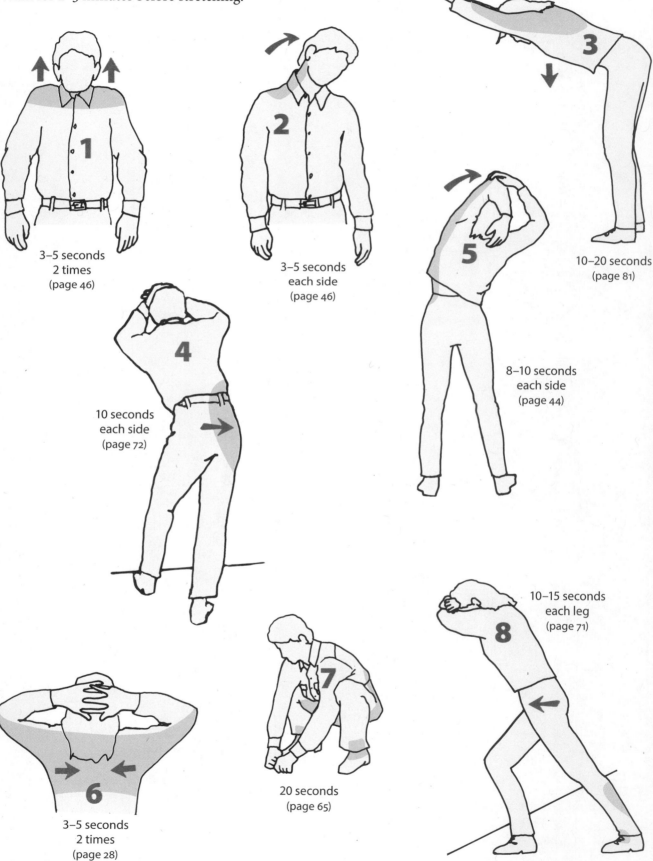

3–5 seconds
2 times
(page 46)

3–5 seconds
each side
(page 46)

10–20 seconds
(page 81)

10 seconds
each side
(page 72)

8–10 seconds
each side
(page 44)

10–15 seconds
each leg
(page 71)

20 seconds
(page 65)

3–5 seconds
2 times
(page 28)

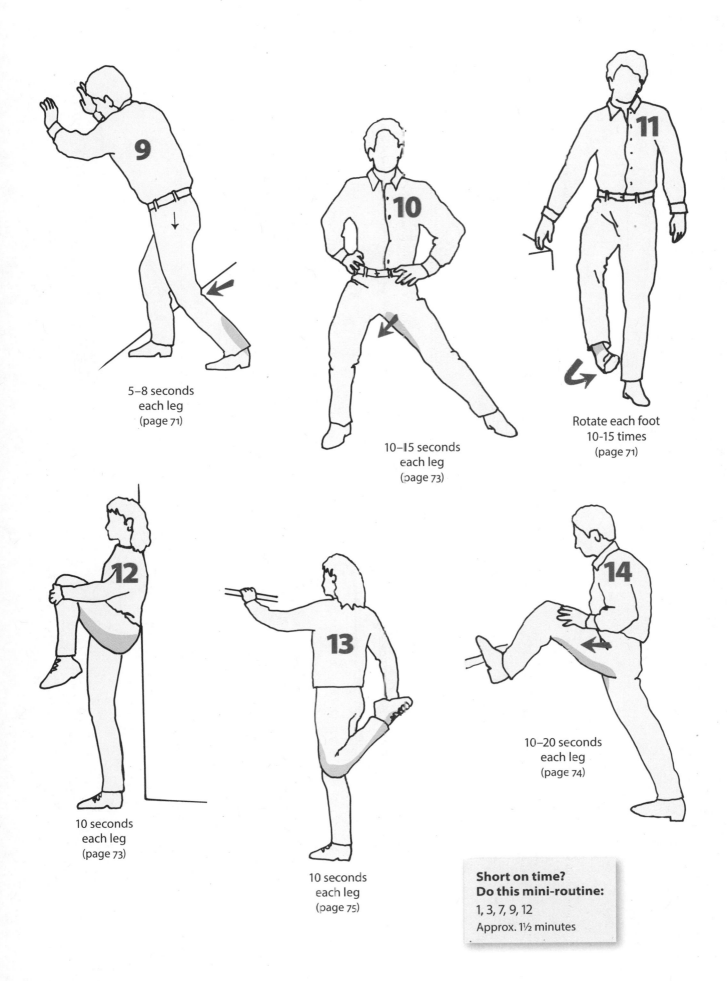

9

5–8 seconds
each leg
(page 71)

10

10–15 seconds
each leg
(page 73)

11

Rotate each foot
10-15 times
(page 71)

12

10 seconds
each leg
(page 73)

13

10 seconds
each leg
(page 75)

14

10–20 seconds
each leg
(page 74)

Short on time?
Do this mini-routine:
1, 3, 7, 9, 12
Approx. 1½ minutes

FIGURE SKATING

APPROXIMATELY 8 MINUTES

Warm up for 4–5 minutes before stretching.

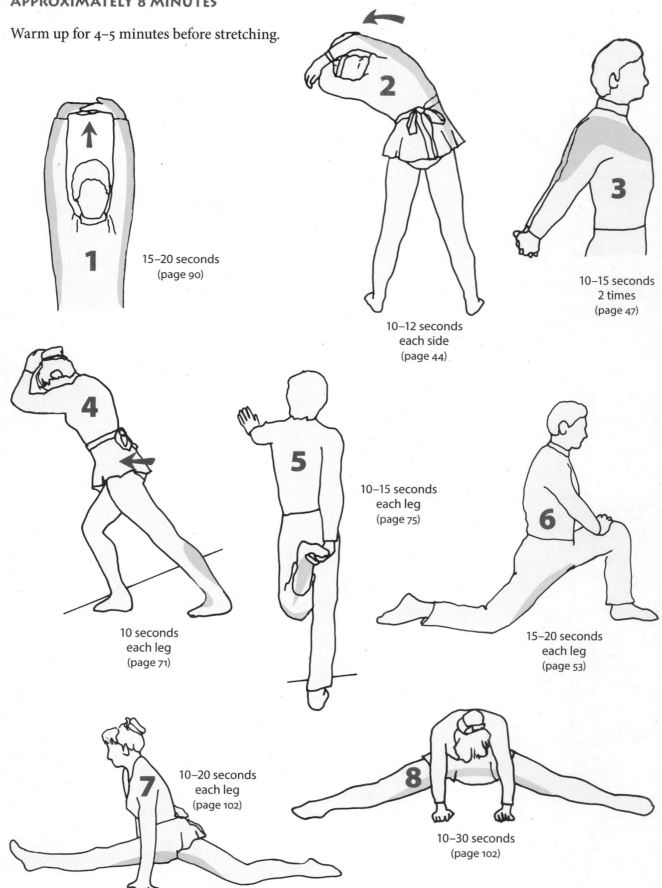

1 15–20 seconds
(page 90)

2 10–12 seconds
each side
(page 44)

3 10–15 seconds
2 times
(page 47)

4 10 seconds
each leg
(page 71)

5 10–15 seconds
each leg
(page 75)

6 15–20 seconds
each leg
(page 53)

7 10–20 seconds
each leg
(page 102)

8 10–30 seconds
(page 102)

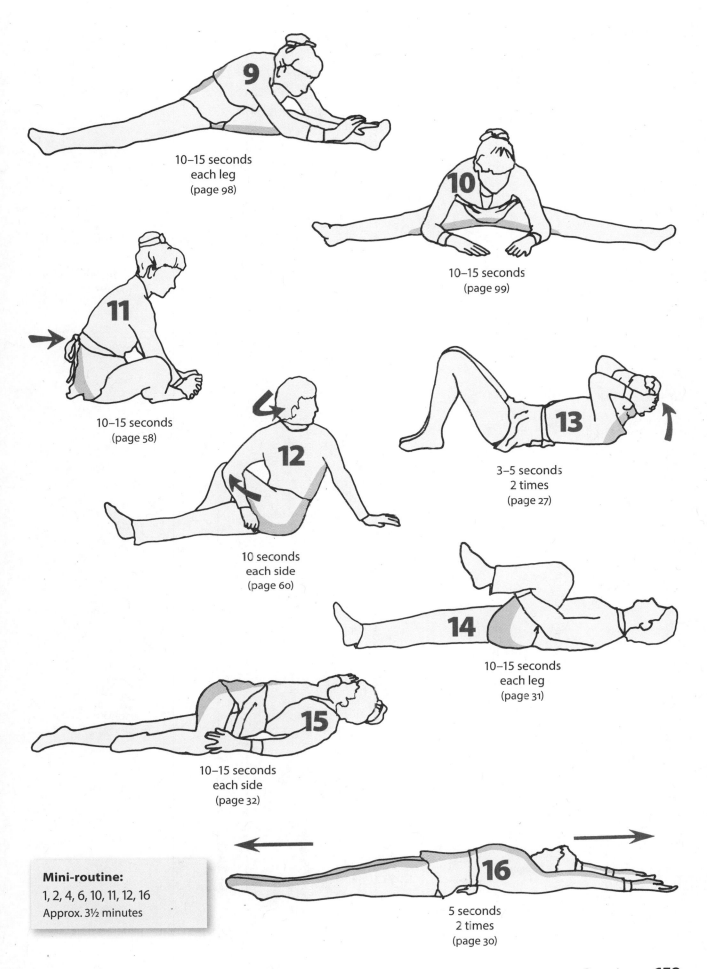

9

10–15 seconds
each leg
(page 98)

10

10–15 seconds
(page 99)

11

10–15 seconds
(page 58)

12

10 seconds
each side
(page 60)

13

3–5 seconds
2 times
(page 27)

14

10–15 seconds
each leg
(page 31)

15

10–15 seconds
each side
(page 32)

16

5 seconds
2 times
(page 30)

Mini-routine:
1, 2, 4, 6, 10, 11, 12, 16
Approx. 3½ minutes

FOOTBALL

APPROXIMATELY 6 MINUTES

Jog around the football field before stretching.

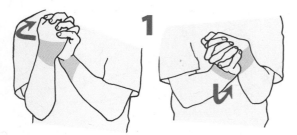

Rotate 10–15 times
each direction
(page 88)

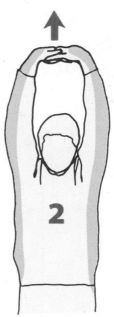

10 seconds
2 times
(page 46)

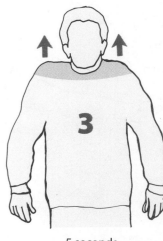

5 seconds
2 times
(page 46)

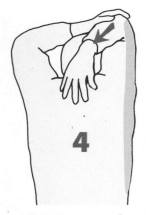

10–15 seconds
each arm
(page 44)

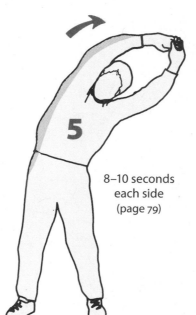

8–10 seconds
each side
(page 79)

30 seconds
(page 55)

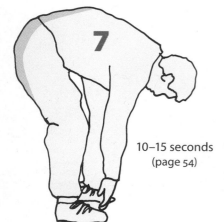

10–15 seconds
(page 54)

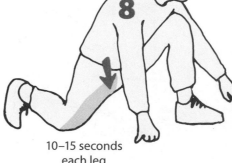

10–15 seconds
each leg
(page 51)

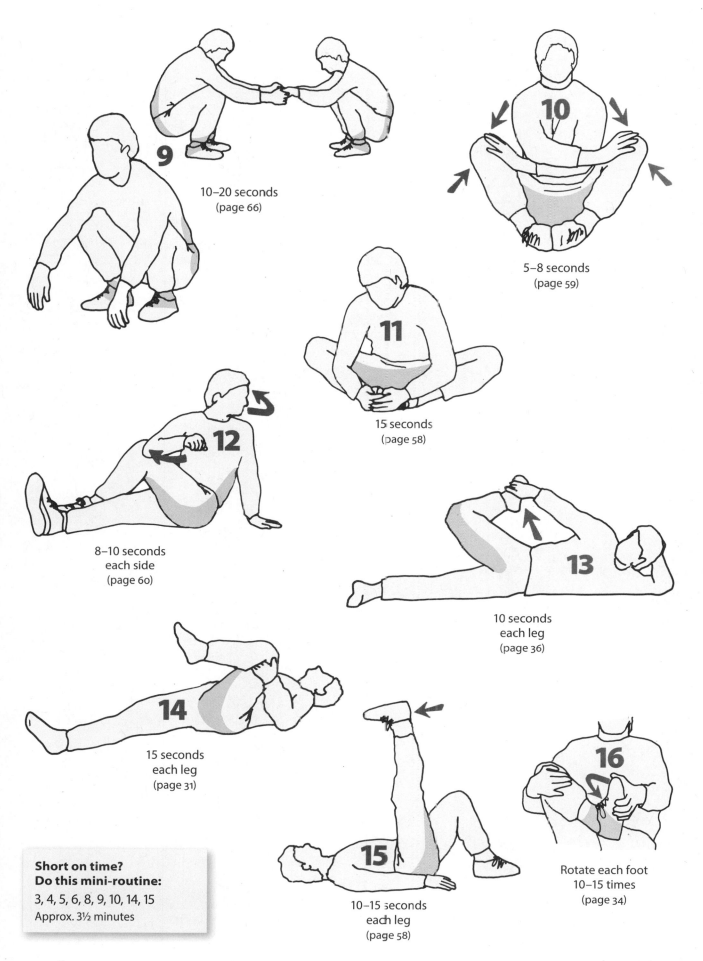

9
10–20 seconds
(page 66)

10
5–8 seconds
(page 59)

11
15 seconds
(page 58)

12
8–10 seconds
each side
(page 60)

13
10 seconds
each leg
(page 36)

14
15 seconds
each leg
(page 31)

15
10–15 seconds
each leg
(page 58)

16
Rotate each foot
10–15 times
(page 34)

Short on time?
Do this mini-routine:
3, 4, 5, 6, 8, 9, 10, 14, 15
Approx. 3½ minutes

GOLF

APPROXIMATELY 6 MINUTES

Walk for several minutes before stretching.

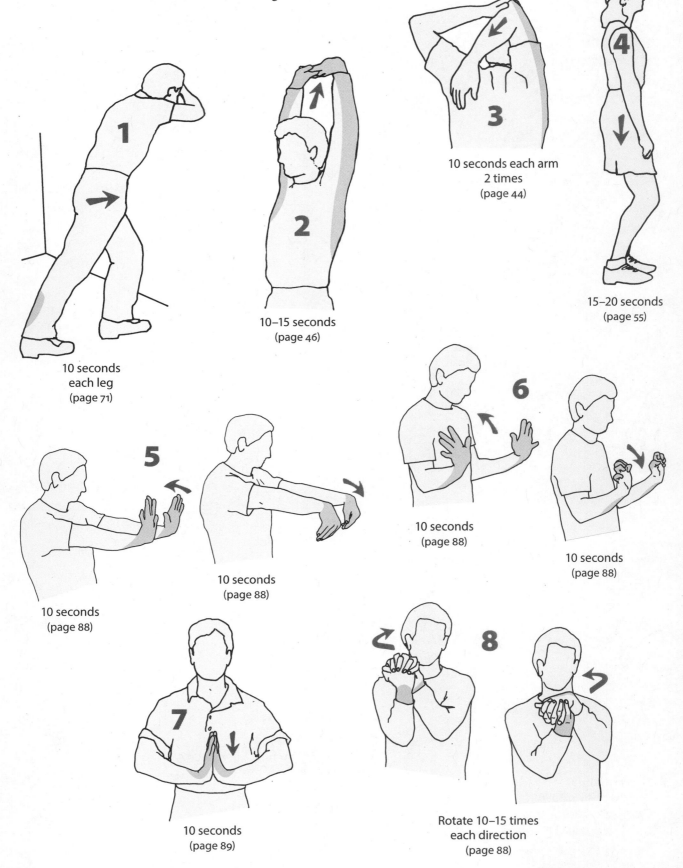

1 10 seconds each leg (page 71)

2 10–15 seconds (page 46)

3 10 seconds each arm 2 times (page 44)

4 15–20 seconds (page 55)

5 10 seconds (page 88)

10 seconds (page 88)

6 10 seconds (page 88)

10 seconds (page 88)

7 10 seconds (page 89)

8 Rotate 10–15 times each direction (page 88)

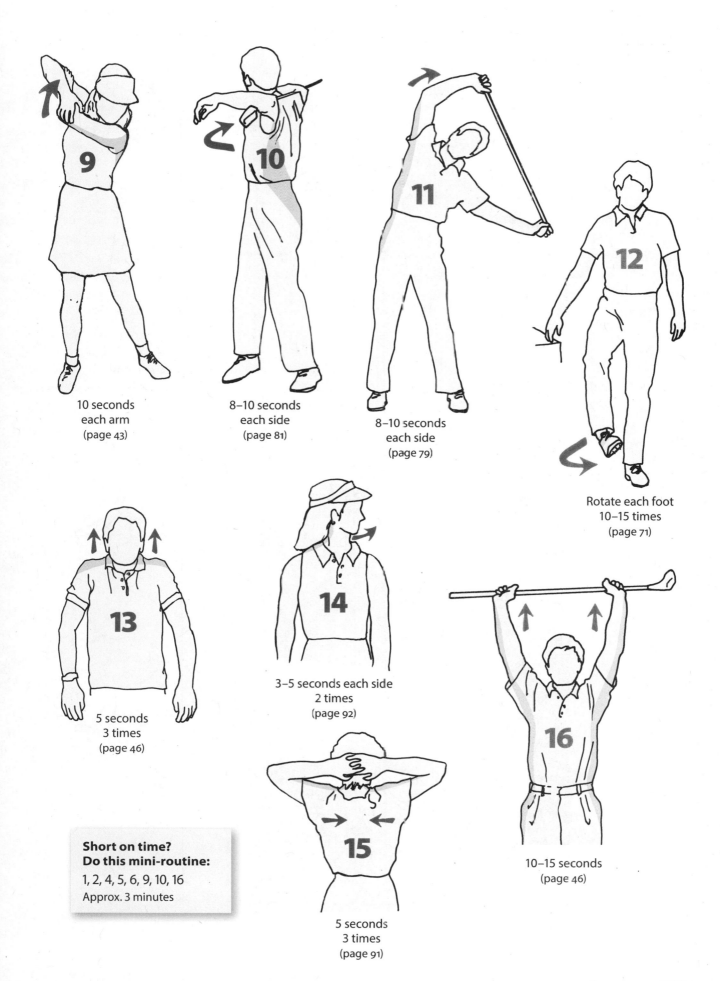

9
10 seconds
each arm
(page 43)

10
8–10 seconds
each side
(page 81)

11
8–10 seconds
each side
(page 79)

12
Rotate each foot
10–15 times
(page 71)

13
5 seconds
3 times
(page 46)

14
3–5 seconds each side
2 times
(page 92)

15
5 seconds
3 times
(page 91)

16
10–15 seconds
(page 46)

Short on time?
Do this mini-routine:
1, 2, 4, 5, 6, 9, 10, 16
Approx. 3 minutes

GYMNASTICS

APPROXIMATELY 8 MINUTES

Warm up for 4–5 minutes by walking or jogging before stretching.

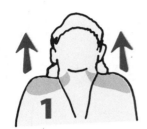

1

5 seconds
3 times
(page 46)

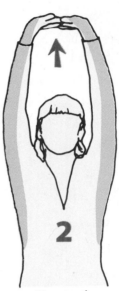

2

15 seconds
(page 46)

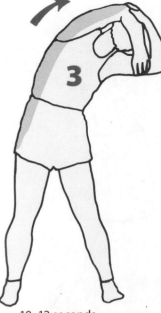

3

10–12 seconds
each side
(page 44)

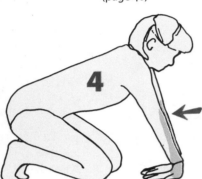

4

10–15 seconds
2 times
(page 42)

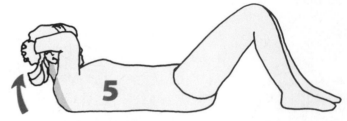

5

3–5 seconds
2 times
(page 27)

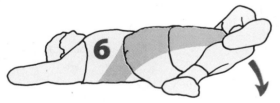

6

10–20 seconds
each side
(page 27)

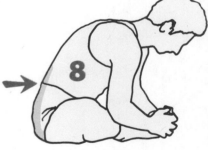

8

30 seconds
(page 65)

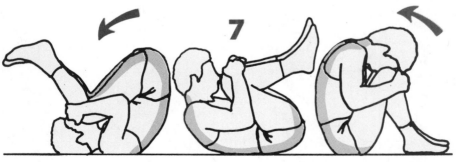

7

Gently roll
6–12 times
(page 63)

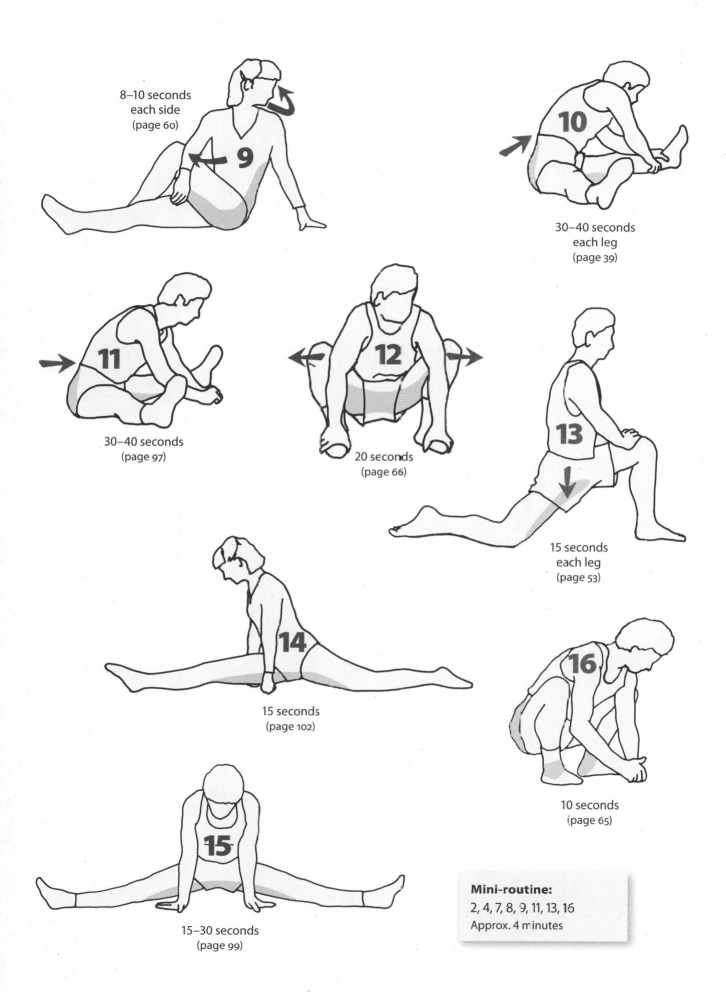

8–10 seconds
each side
(page 60)

9

10

30–40 seconds
each leg
(page 39)

11

30–40 seconds
(page 97)

12

20 seconds
(page 66)

13

15 seconds
each leg
(page 53)

14

15 seconds
(page 102)

16

10 seconds
(page 65)

15

15–30 seconds
(page 99)

Mini-routine:
2, 4, 7, 8, 9, 11, 13, 16
Approx. 4 minutes

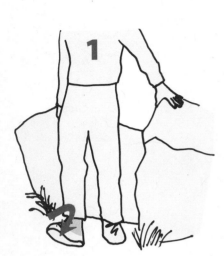

Rotate each foot
10–15 times
(page 71)

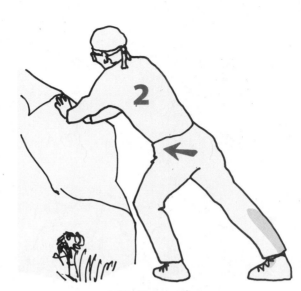

10–15 seconds
each leg
(page 71)

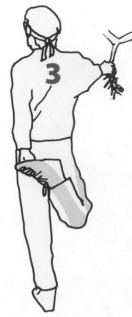

10–15 seconds
each leg
(page 75)

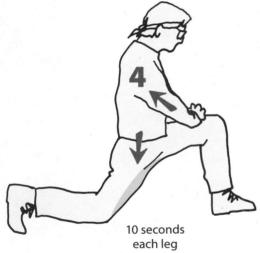

10 seconds
each leg
(page 53)

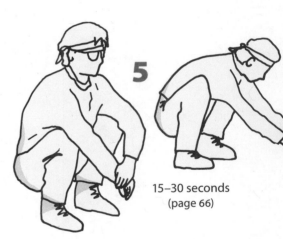

15–30 seconds
(page 66)

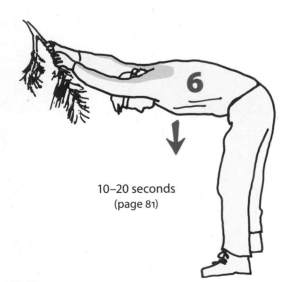

10–20 seconds
(page 81)

8–10 seconds
each arm
(page 44)

3–5 seconds
several times
(page 46)

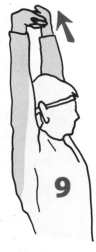

15 seconds
(page 46)

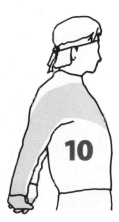

10–15 seconds
(page 47)

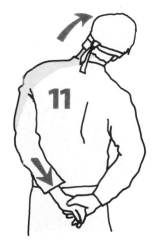

8–10 seconds
each side
(page 47)

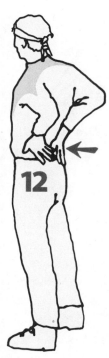

10 seconds
2 times
(page 46)

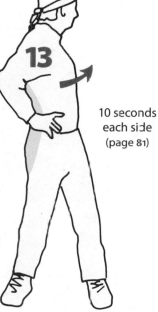
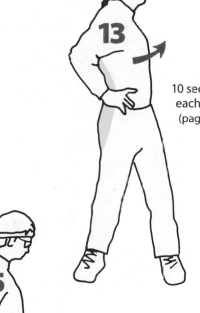

10 seconds
each side
(page 81)

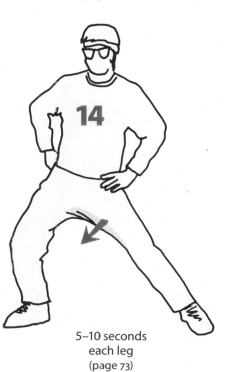

5–10 seconds
each leg
(page 73)

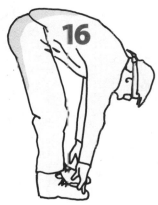

15–30 seconds
(page 55)

10–15 seconds
(page 54)

Short on time?
Do this mini-routine:
2, 4, 6, 8, 12, 13, 15
Approx. 3 minutes

ICE HOCKEY

APPROXIMATELY 8 MINUTES

Warm up by walking or riding a stationary bike for 2–4 minutes before stretching.

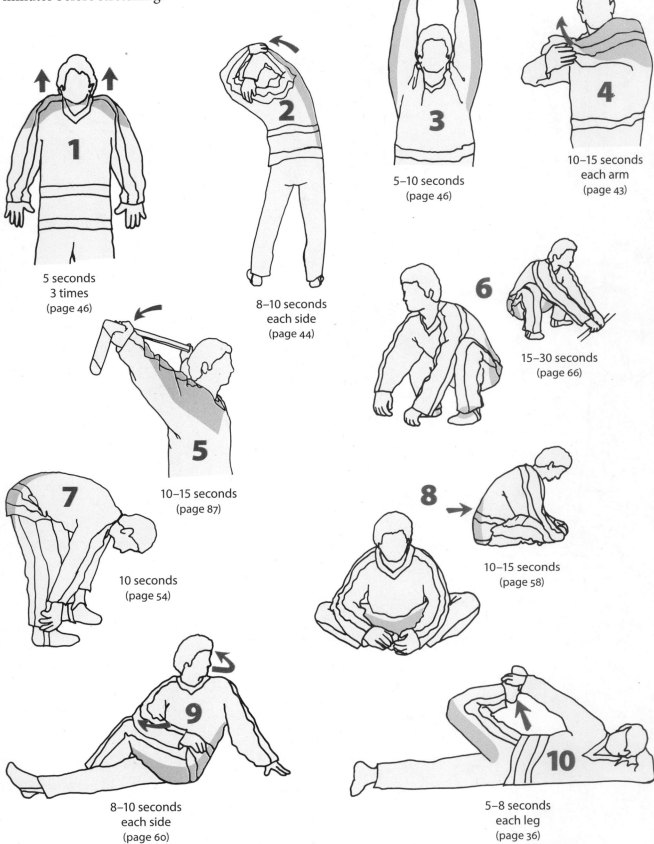

1
5 seconds
3 times
(page 46)

2
8–10 seconds
each side
(page 44)

3
5–10 seconds
(page 46)

4
10–15 seconds
each arm
(page 43)

5
10–15 seconds
(page 87)

6
15–30 seconds
(page 66)

7
10 seconds
(page 54)

8
10–15 seconds
(page 58)

9
8–10 seconds
each side
(page 60)

10
5–8 seconds
each leg
(page 36)

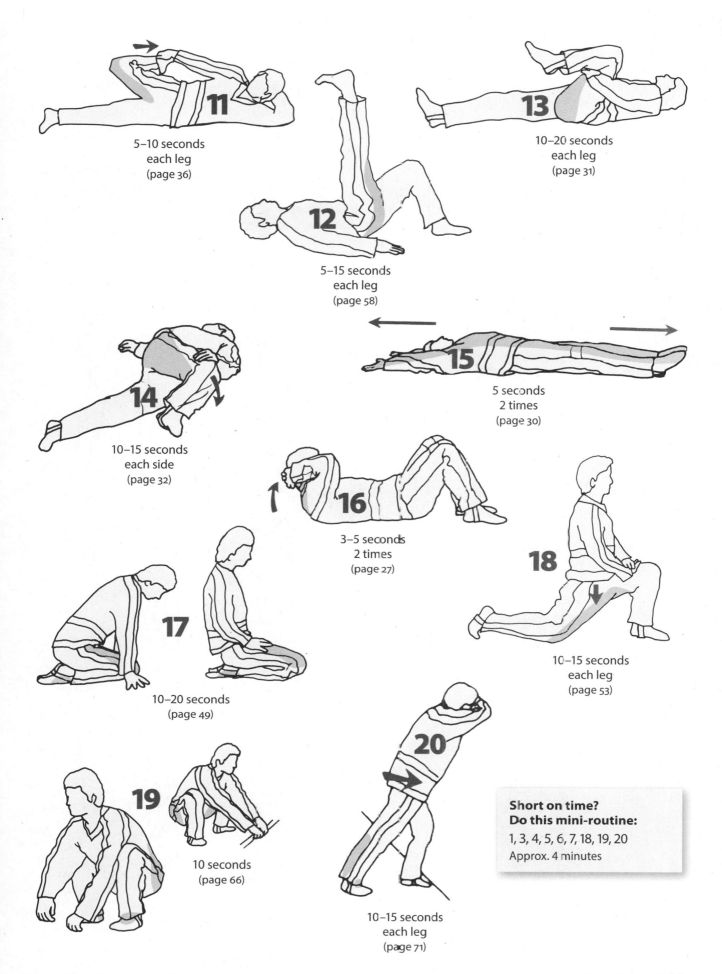

11

5–10 seconds
each leg
(page 36)

12

5–15 seconds
each leg
(page 58)

13

10–20 seconds
each leg
(page 31)

14

10–15 seconds
each side
(page 32)

15

5 seconds
2 times
(page 30)

16

3–5 seconds
2 times
(page 27)

17

10–20 seconds
(page 49)

18

10–15 seconds
each leg
(page 53)

19

10 seconds
(page 66)

20

10–15 seconds
each leg
(page 71)

**Short on time?
Do this mini-routine:**

1, 3, 4, 5, 6, 7, 18, 19, 20
Approx. 4 minutes

INLINE SKATING

APPROXIMATELY 6 MINUTES

Walk for several minutes before stretching.

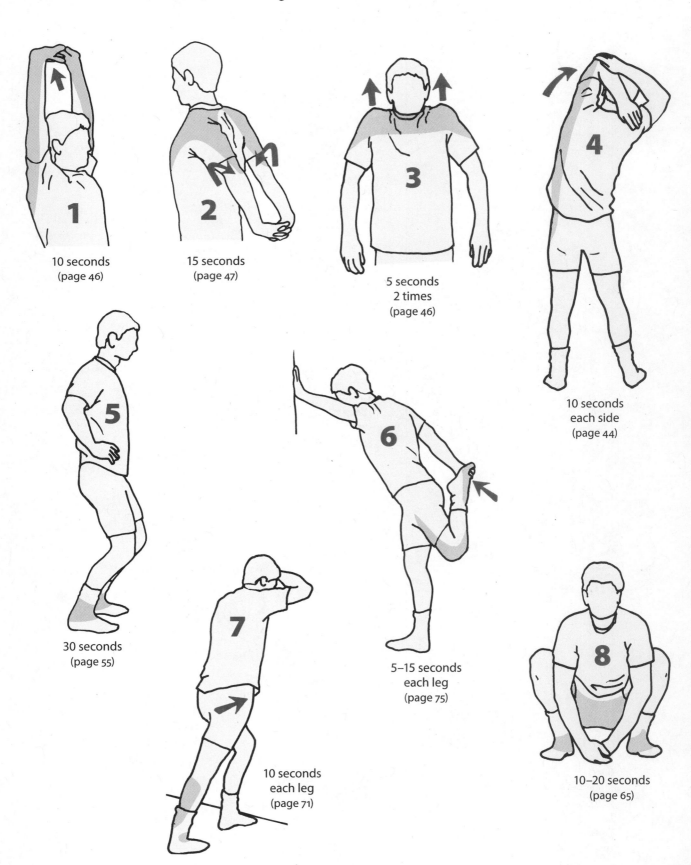

1
10 seconds
(page 46)

2
15 seconds
(page 47)

3
5 seconds
2 times
(page 46)

4
10 seconds
each side
(page 44)

5
30 seconds
(page 55)

6
5–15 seconds
each leg
(page 75)

7
10 seconds
each leg
(page 71)

8
10–20 seconds
(page 65)

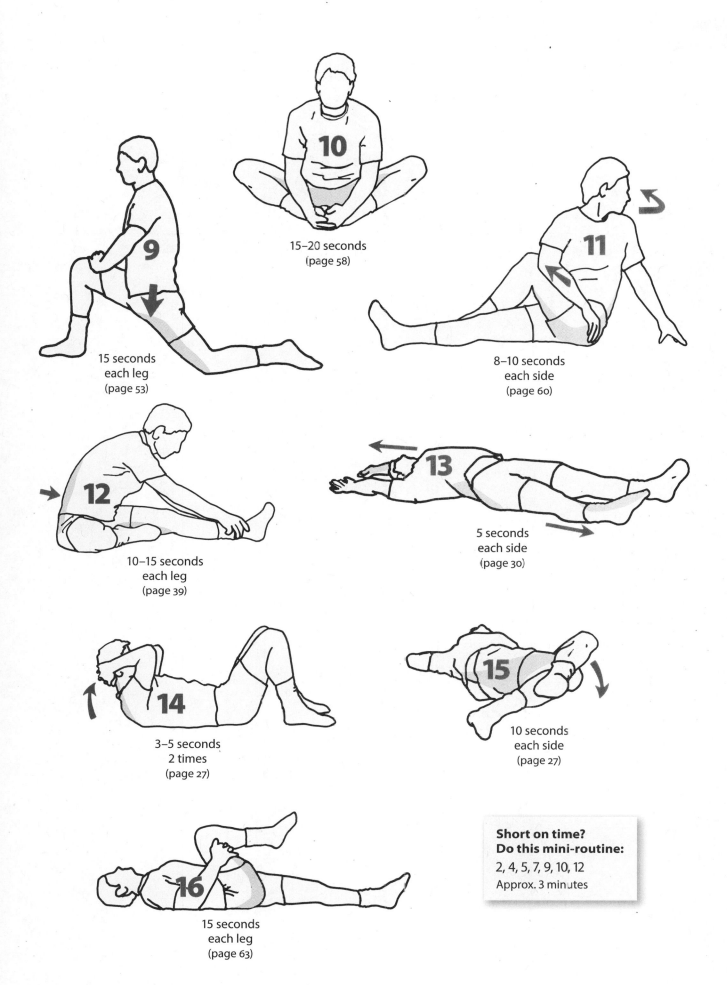

9
15 seconds
each leg
(page 53)

10
15–20 seconds
(page 58)

11
8–10 seconds
each side
(page 60)

12
10–15 seconds
each leg
(page 39)

13
5 seconds
each side
(page 30)

14
3–5 seconds
2 times
(page 27)

15
10 seconds
each side
(page 27)

16
15 seconds
each leg
(page 63)

Short on time?
Do this mini-routine:
2, 4, 5, 7, 9, 10, 12
Approx. 3 minutes

KAYAKING

APPROXIMATELY 7 MINUTES

Walk for several minutes before stretching.

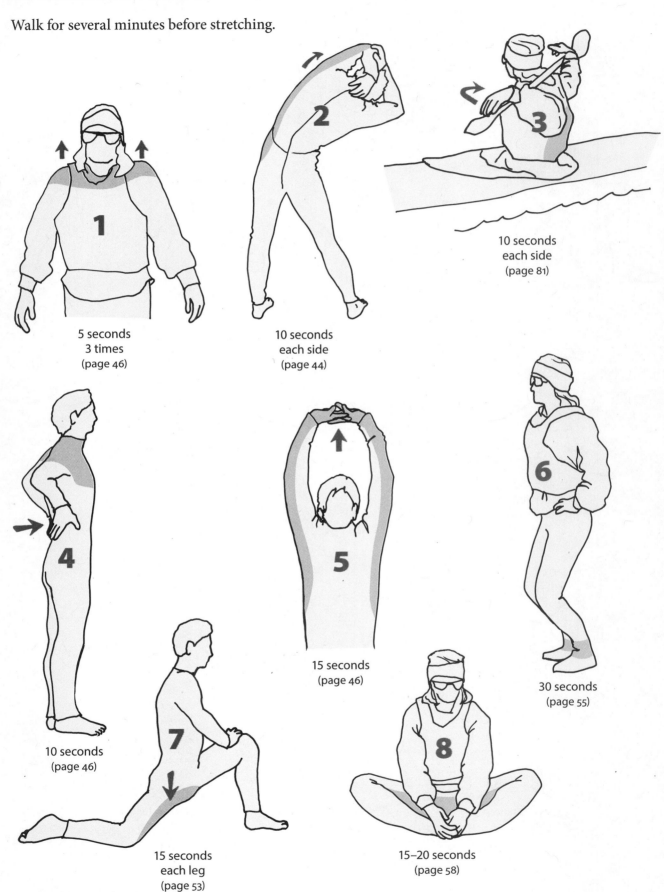

1
5 seconds
3 times
(page 46)

2
10 seconds
each side
(page 44)

3
10 seconds
each side
(page 81)

4
10 seconds
(page 46)

5
15 seconds
(page 46)

6
30 seconds
(page 55)

7
15 seconds
each leg
(page 53)

8
15–20 seconds
(page 58)

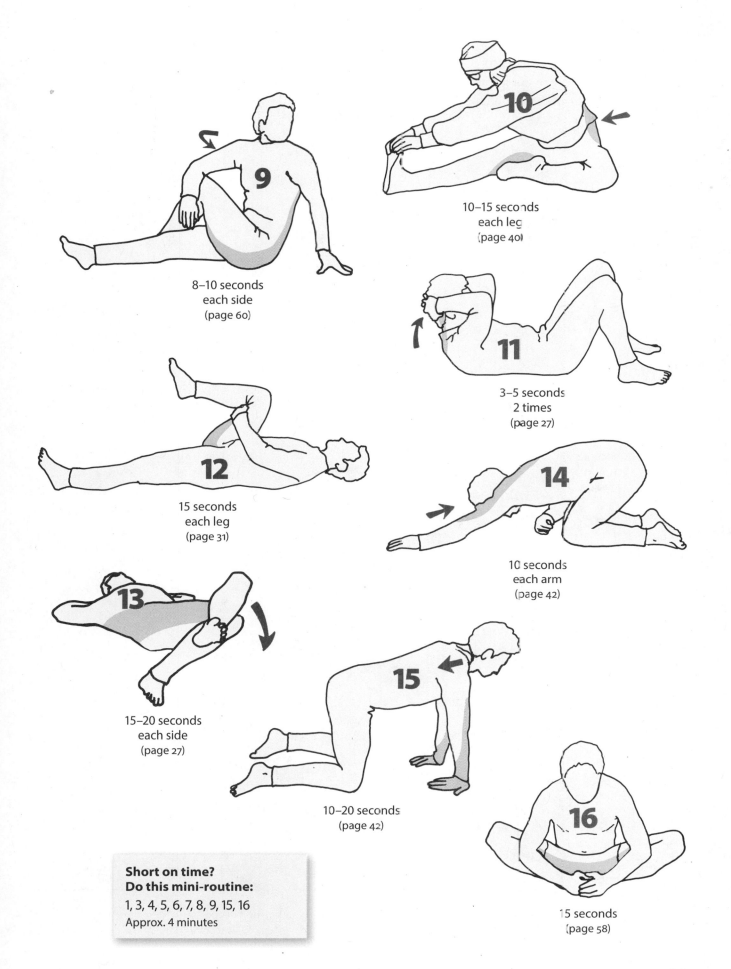

9

8–10 seconds
each side
(page 60)

10

10–15 seconds
each leg
(page 40)

11

3–5 seconds
2 times
(page 27)

12

15 seconds
each leg
(page 31)

14

10 seconds
each arm
(page 42)

13

15–20 seconds
each side
(page 27)

15

10–20 seconds
(page 42)

16

15 seconds
(page 58)

Short on time?
Do this mini-routine:
1, 3, 4, 5, 6, 7, 8, 9, 15, 16
Approx. 4 minutes

MARTIAL ARTS
APPROXIMATELY 7 MINUTES

Note: These stretches are not intended to replace your traditional routine, but can be used for improvement of overall flexibility. They should be preceded by a good warm-up.

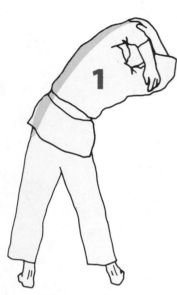

8–10 seconds
each side
(page 44)

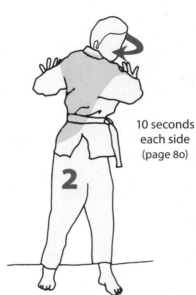

10 seconds
each side
(page 80)

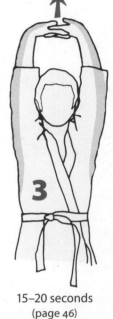

15–20 seconds
(page 46)

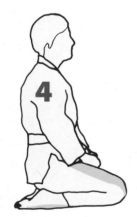

20–30 seconds
(page 49)

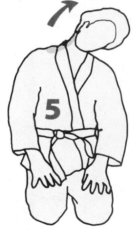

3–5 seconds
each side
(page 46)

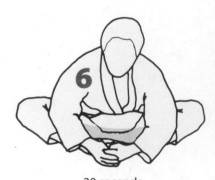

30 seconds
(page 58)

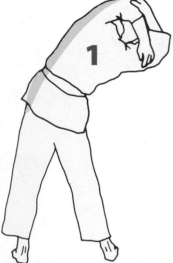

10 seconds
each side
(page 60)

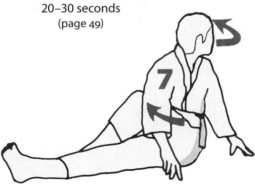

Roll back and forth
10–12 times
(page 63)

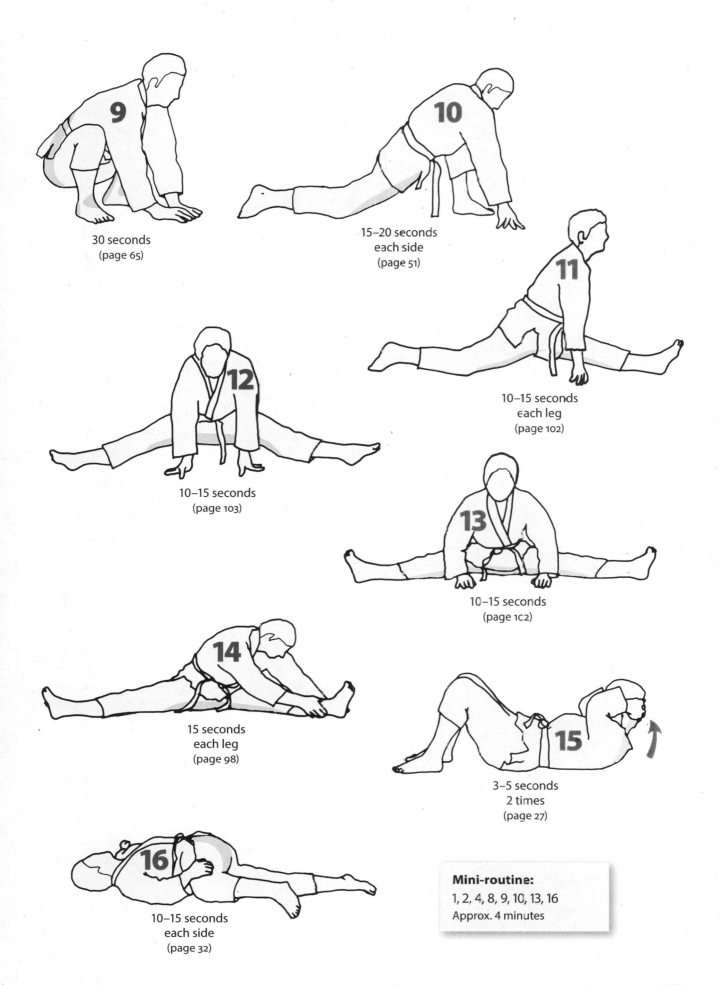

9
30 seconds
(page 65)

10
15–20 seconds
each side
(page 51)

11
10–15 seconds
each leg
(page 102)

12
10–15 seconds
(page 103)

13
10–15 seconds
(page 1c2)

14
15 seconds
each leg
(page 98)

15
3–5 seconds
2 times
(page 27)

16
10–15 seconds
each side
(page 32)

Mini-routine:
1, 2, 4, 8, 9, 10, 13, 16
Approx. 4 minutes

MOTOCROSS

APPROXIMATELY 6 MINUTES

Walk around for several minutes before stretching.

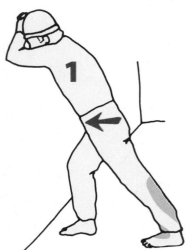

1

10–15 seconds
each leg
(page 71)

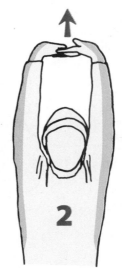

2

15 seconds
(page 46)

3

10 seconds
(page 47)

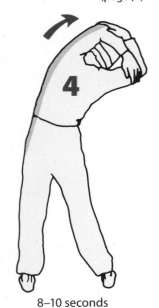

4

8–10 seconds
each side
(page 44)

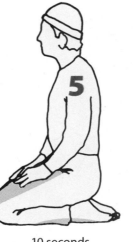

5

10 seconds
(page 49)

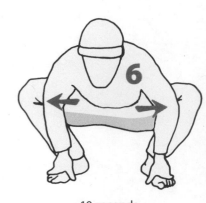

6

10 seconds
(page 66)

7

15 seconds
each leg
(page 52)

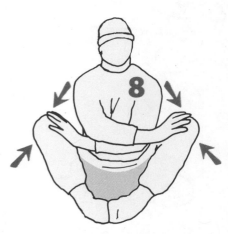

8

5–6 seconds
(page 59)

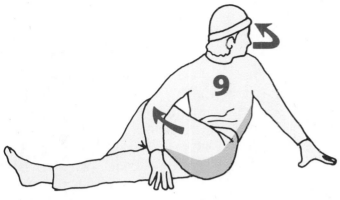

8–10 seconds
each side
(page 60)

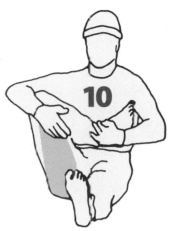

15 seconds
each leg
(page 35)

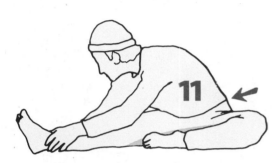

10–15 seconds
each leg
(page 39)

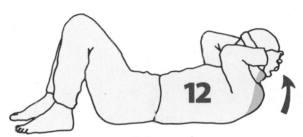

3–5 seconds
2 times
(page 27)

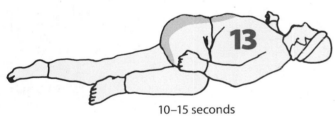

10–15 seconds
each side
(page 32)

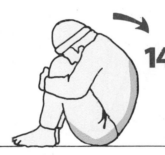

Roll back and forth
8–10 times
(page 63)

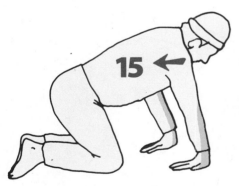

10–15 seconds
(page 42)

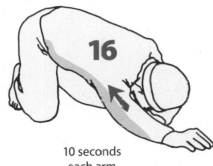

10 seconds
each arm
(page 42)

Short on time?
Do this mini-routine:
1, 2, 3, 6, 7, 11, 15, 16
Approx. 3 minutes

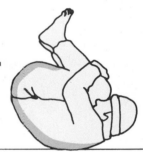

MOUNTAIN BIKING

APPROXIMATELY 6 MINUTES

Warm up by riding or walking for 3–5 minutes before stretching.

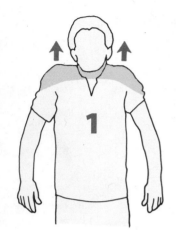

1

5 seconds
2 times
(page 46)

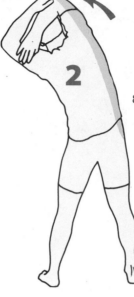

2

8–10 seconds
each side
(page 44)

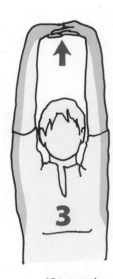

3

15 seconds
(page 46)

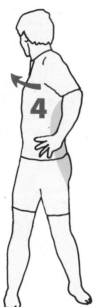

4

10 seconds
each side
(page 81)

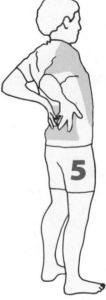

5

10–15 seconds
(page 46)

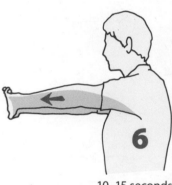

6

10–15 seconds
(page 45)

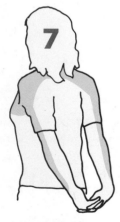

7

10–15 seconds
(page 47)

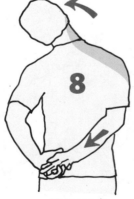

8

10 seconds
each arm
(page 47)

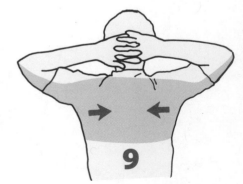

9

5 seconds
2 times
(page 91)

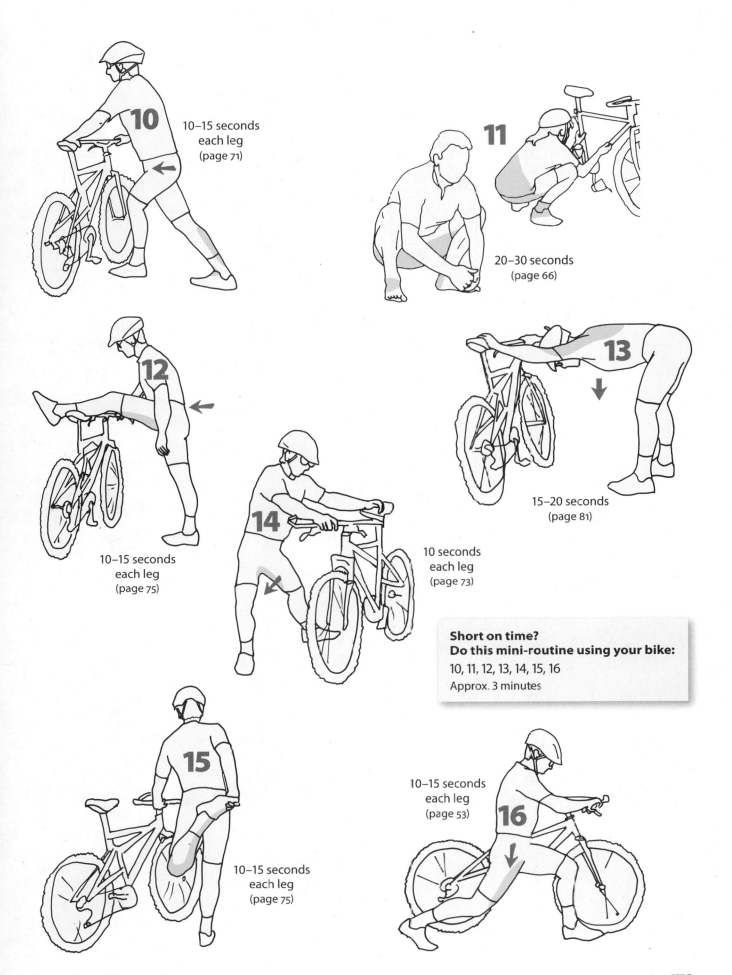

10 10–15 seconds
each leg
(page 71)

11 20–30 seconds
(page 66)

12 10–15 seconds
each leg
(page 75)

13 15–20 seconds
(page 81)

14 10 seconds
each leg
(page 73)

Short on time?
Do this mini-routine using your bike:
10, 11, 12, 13, 14, 15, 16
Approx. 3 minutes

15 10–15 seconds
each leg
(page 75)

16 10–15 seconds
each leg
(page 53)

APPROXIMATELY 7 MINUTES

Warm up for 2-4 minutes before stretching.

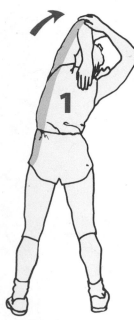

1

8–10 seconds
each side
(page 44)

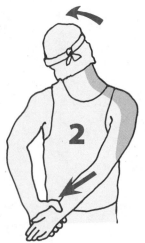

2

10 seconds
each arm
(page 47)

3

5 seconds
2 times
(page 46)

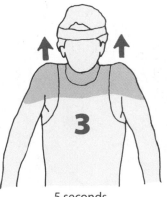

4

15 seconds
(page 46)

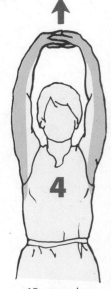

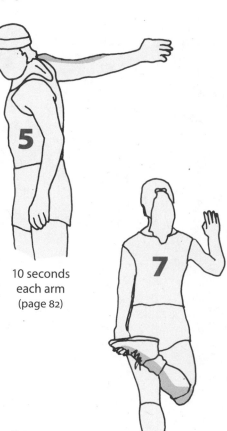

5

10 seconds
each arm
(page 82)

6

10 seconds
each leg
(page 71)

7

10–15 seconds
each leg
(page 75)

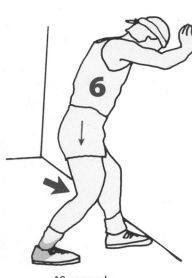

8

10–15 seconds
each leg
(page 71)

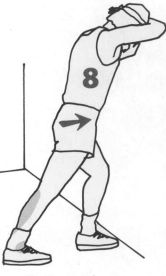

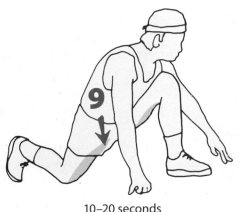

10–20 seconds
each leg
(page 51)

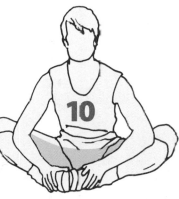

15–20 seconds
(page 58)

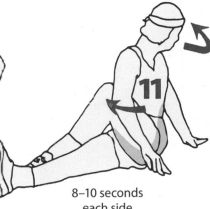

8–10 seconds
each side
(page 60)

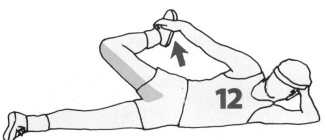

10 seconds
each leg
(page 36)

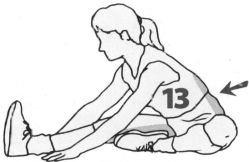

10–15 seconds
each leg
(page 39)

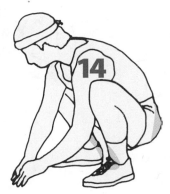

10–20 seconds
(page 65)

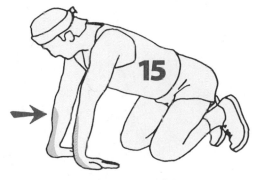

10–15 seconds
(page 42)

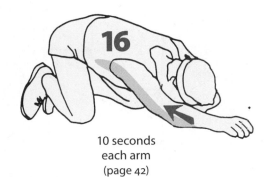

10 seconds
each arm
(page 42)

Short on time?
Do this mini-routine:
1, 2, 5, 7, 8, 9, 10, 11
Approx. 4 minutes

ROCK CLIMBING

APPROXIMATELY 6 MINUTES

Walk for several minutes before stretching.

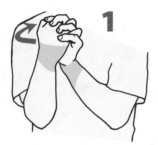

1

Rotate wrists
10 times clockwise
and counterclockwise
(page 88)

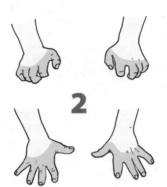

2

10 seconds each position
2 times
(page 88)

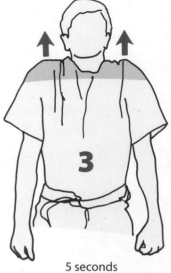

3

5 seconds
3 times
(page 46)

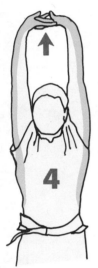

4

15 seconds
(page 46)

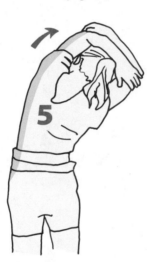

5

10 seconds
each side
(page 44)

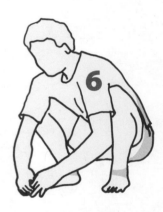

6

15–30 seconds
(page 65)

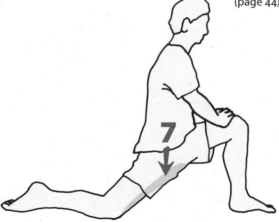

7

15 seconds
each leg
(page 53)

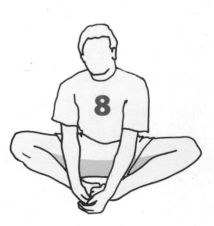

8

15–30 seconds
(page 58)

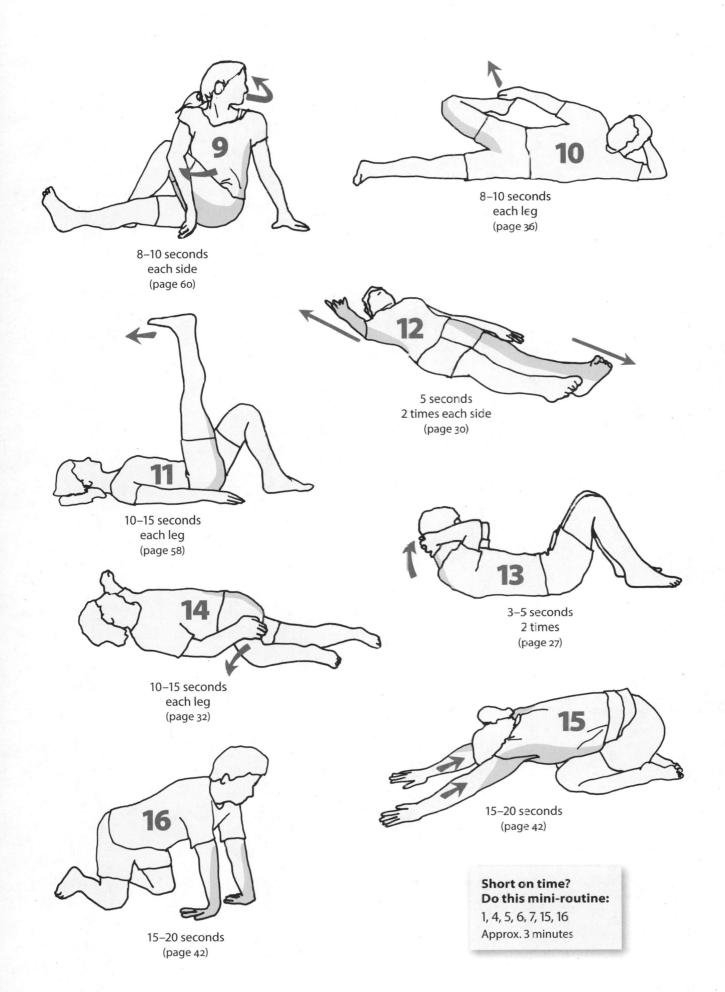

9

8–10 seconds
each side
(page 60)

10

8–10 seconds
each leg
(page 36)

12

5 seconds
2 times each side
(page 30)

11

10–15 seconds
each leg
(page 58)

13

3–5 seconds
2 times
(page 27)

14

10–15 seconds
each leg
(page 32)

15

15–20 seconds
(page 42)

16

15–20 seconds
(page 42)

Short on time?
Do this mini-routine:
1, 4, 5, 6, 7, 15, 16
Approx. 3 minutes

RODEO

APPROXIMATELY 5 MINUTES

Walk for several minutes before stretching.

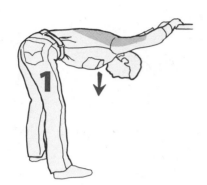

1

15–20 seconds
(page 81)

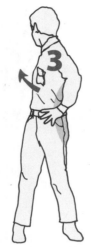

2

8–10 seconds
each side
(page 44)

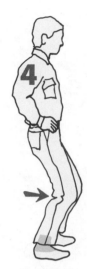

3

10 seconds
each side
(page 81)

4

20 seconds
(page 55)

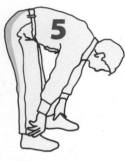

5

15 seconds
(page 54)

6

10 seconds
each leg
(page 75)

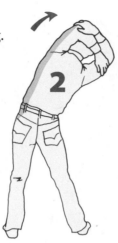

7

10 seconds
each leg
(page 75)

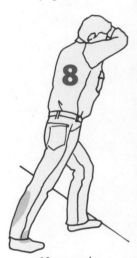

8

10 seconds
each leg
(page 71)

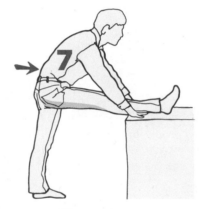

9

10 seconds
each leg
(page 52)

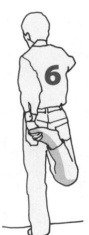

10

15 seconds
(page 42)

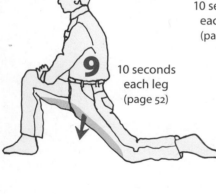

11

20 seconds
(page 65)

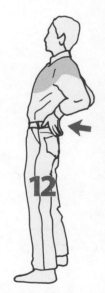

12

10 seconds
(page 46)

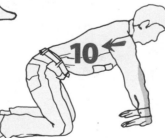

**Short on time?
Do this mini-routine:**
1, 2, 6, 8, 9, 12
Approx. 3 minutes

ROWING

APPROXIMATELY 6 MINUTES

Warm up by moving for 3–5 minutes before stretching.

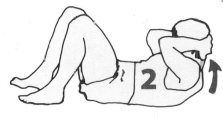

Contract 3–5 seconds
then relax 2 times
(page 27)

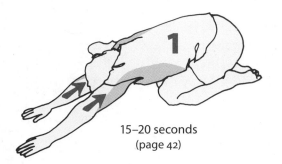

15–20 seconds
(page 42)

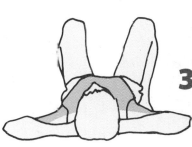

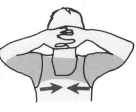

5 seconds
2 times
(page 28)

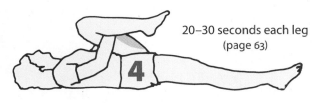

20–30 seconds each leg
(page 63)

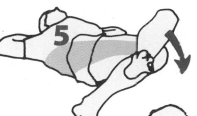

15–30 seconds
each leg
(page 27)

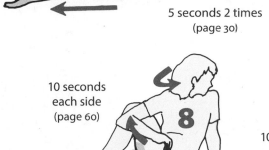

5 seconds 2 times
(page 30)

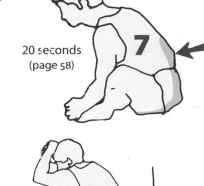

20 seconds
(page 58)

10 seconds
each side
(page 60)

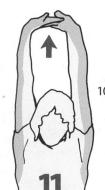

10–15 seconds
each leg
(page 53)

10–15 seconds
each leg
(page 71)

10–15 seconds
(page 46)

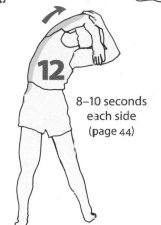

8–10 seconds
each side
(page 44)

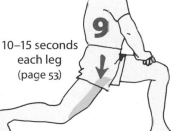

**Short on time?
Do this mini-routine:**

1, 7, 9, 10, 11, 12

Approx. 3 minutes

APPROXIMATELY 4 MINUTES

Warm up by jogging for 3–5 minutes before stretching.

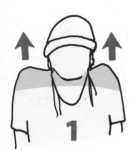

3–5 seconds
2 times
(page 46)

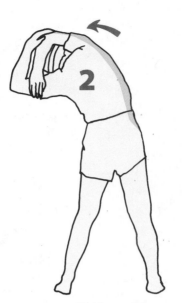

8–10 seconds
each side
(page 44)

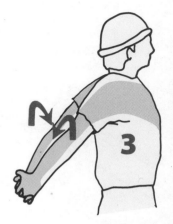

5–10 seconds
(page 47)

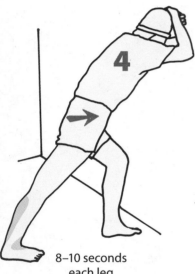

8–10 seconds
each leg
(page 71)

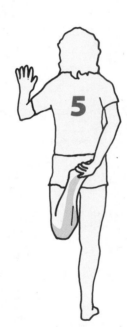

10–15 seconds
each leg
(page 75)

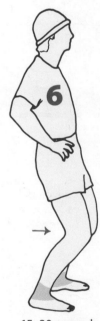

15–30 seconds
(page 55)

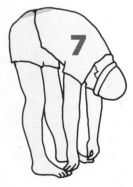

5–10 seconds
(page 54)

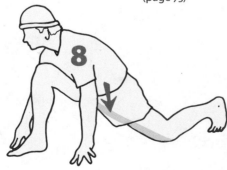

15 seconds
each leg
(page 51)

Short on time?
After a mild warm-up of 2–3
minutes, do this mini-routine:
3, 4, 5, 8
Approx. 1½ minutes

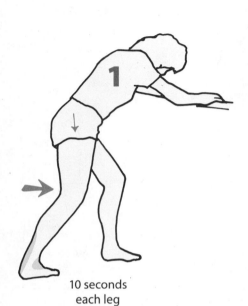

1

10 seconds
each leg
(page 71)

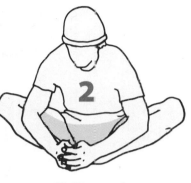

2

10–15 seconds
(page 58)

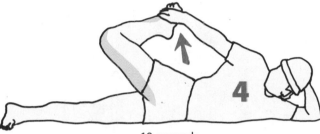

3

15 seconds
each leg
(page 61)

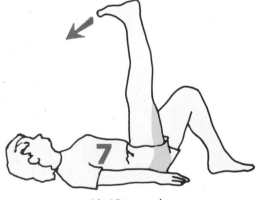

4

10 seconds
each leg
(page 36)

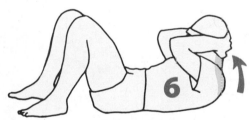

5

15 seconds
each leg
(page 31)

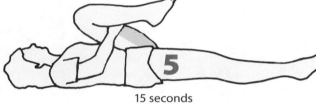

6

3–5 seconds
2 times
(page 27)

7

10–15 seconds
each leg
(page 58)

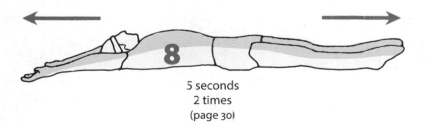

8

5 seconds
2 times
(page 30)

Short on time?
Do this mini-routine:
1, 5, 6, 8
Approx. 1½ minutes

SKIING (CROSS-COUNTRY)

APPROXIMATELY 3 MINUTES

Warm up by walking for several minutes with a big arm swing before stretching.

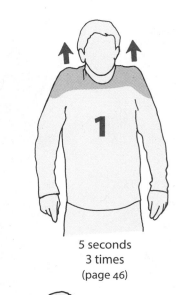

1

5 seconds
3 times
(page 46)

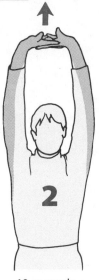

2

10 seconds
(page 46)

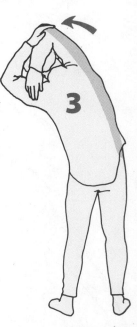

3

10 seconds
each side
(page 44)

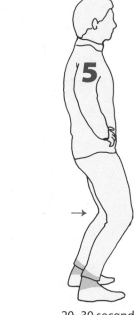

4

10 seconds
each side
(page 81)

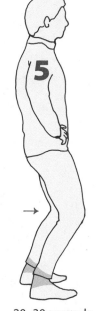

5

20–30 seconds
(page 55)

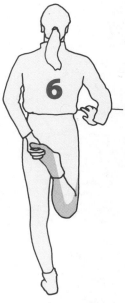

6

10–15 seconds
each leg
(page 75)

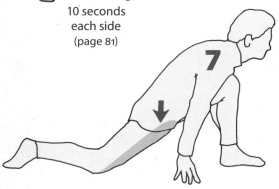

7

10–15 seconds
each leg
(page 51)

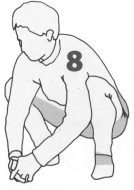

8

15–20 seconds
(page 65)

Short on time?
Do this mini-routine:
3, 4, 7, 8
Approx. 1½ minutes

APPROXIMATELY 4 MINUTES

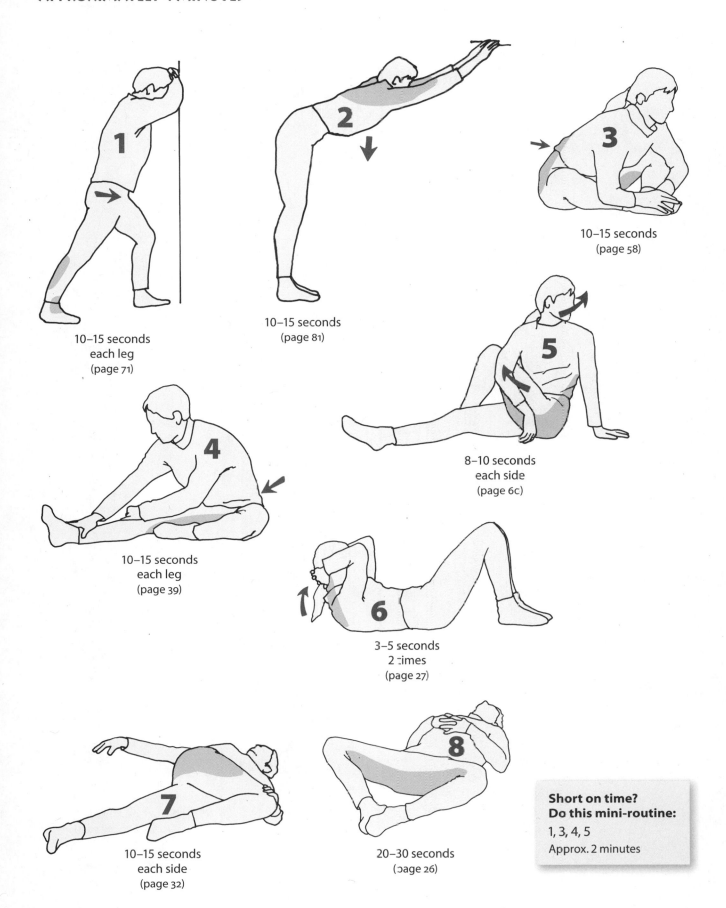

10–15 seconds
each leg
(page 71)

10–15 seconds
(page 81)

10–15 seconds
(page 58)

10–15 seconds
each leg
(page 39)

8–10 seconds
each side
(page 6c)

3–5 seconds
2 times
(page 27)

10–15 seconds
each side
(page 32)

20–30 seconds
(page 26)

Short on time?
Do this mini-routine:

1, 3, 4, 5
Approx. 2 minutes

SKIING (DOWNHILL)
APPROXIMATELY 3 MINUTES

Walk for 2–3 minutes.

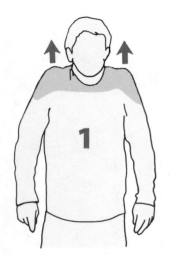

1

5 seconds
2 times
(page 46)

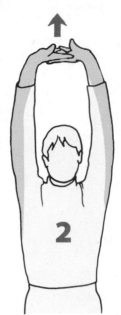

2

10 seconds
(page 46)

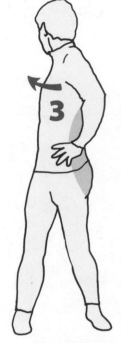

3

10 seconds
each side
(page 81)

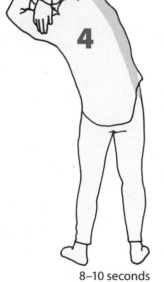

4

8–10 seconds
each side
(page 44)

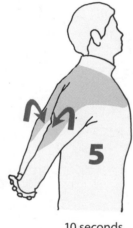

5

10 seconds
(page 47)

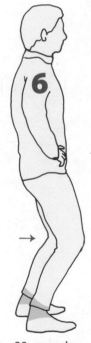

6

30 seconds
(page 55)

7

10–15 seconds
each leg
(page 75)

8

15 seconds
each leg
(page 51)

Short on time?
Do this mini-routine:
2, 3, 6, 8
Approx. 1½ minutes

1

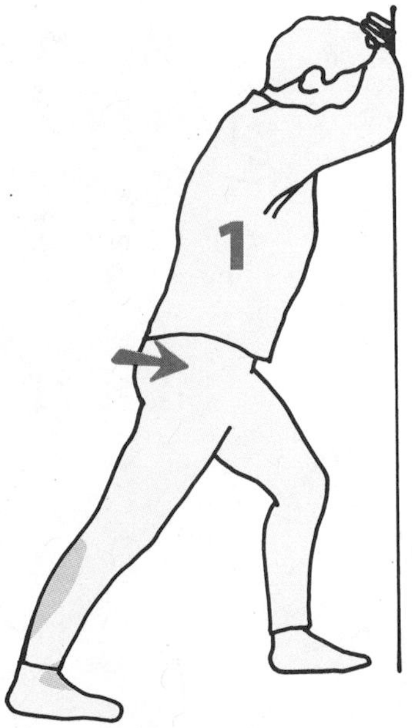

10–15 seconds
each leg
(page 71)

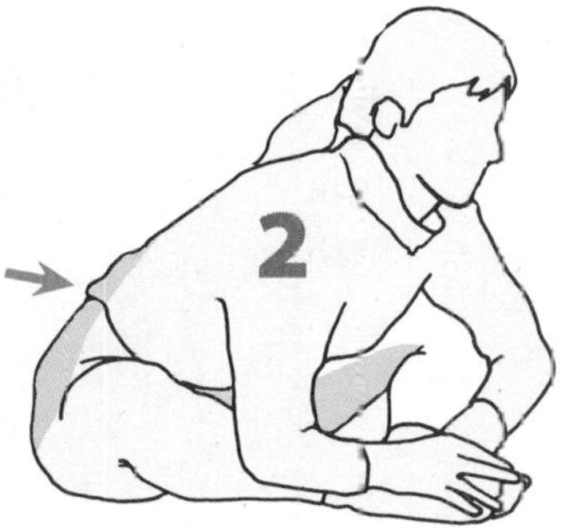

2

15–20 seconds
(page 58)

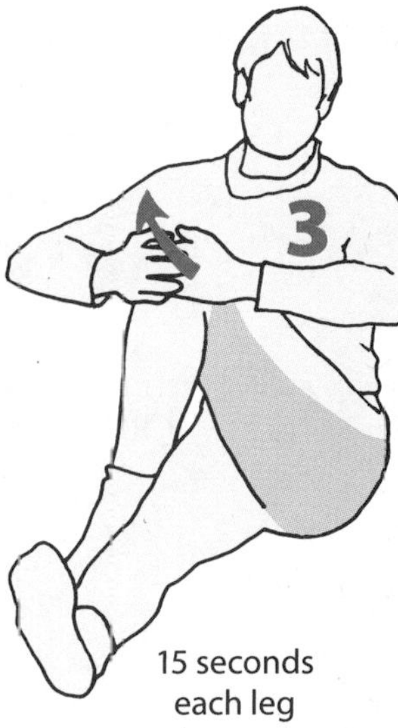

3

15 seconds
each leg
(page 61)

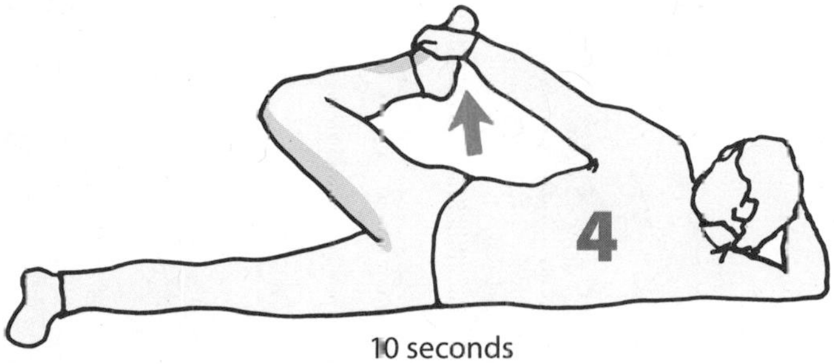

4

10 seconds
each leg
(page 36)

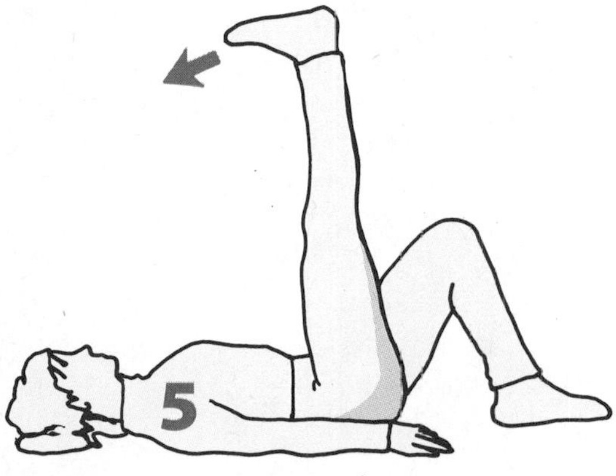

5

10 seconds
each leg
(page 58)

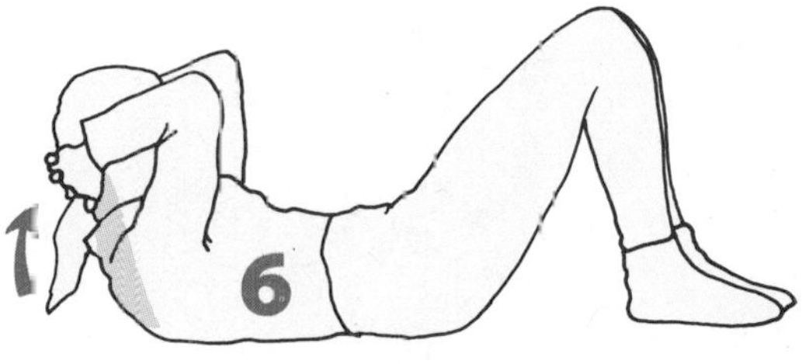

6

3–5 seconds
2 times
(page 27)

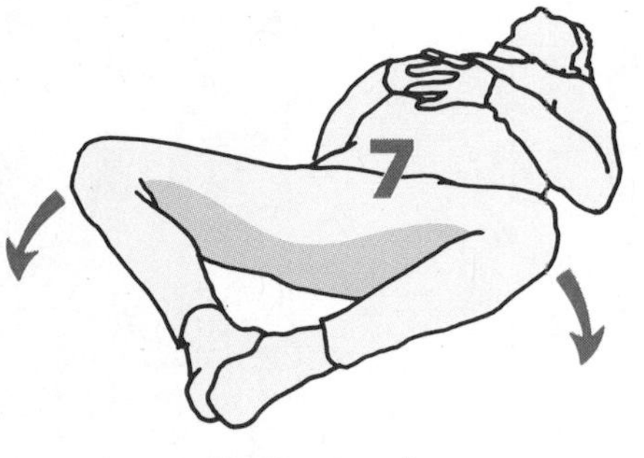

7

15–20 seconds
(page 26)

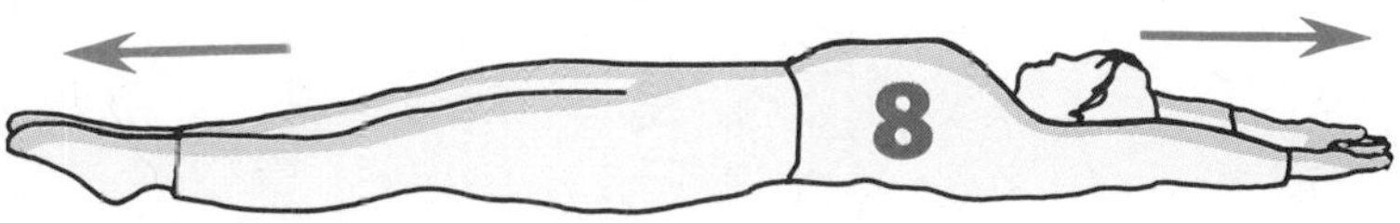

8

5 seconds
2 times
(page 30)

**Short on time?
Do this mini-routine:**

1, 5, 6, 8
Approx. 1½ minutes

SNOWBOARDING

APPROXIMATELY 5 MINUTES

Walk for several minutes before stretching.

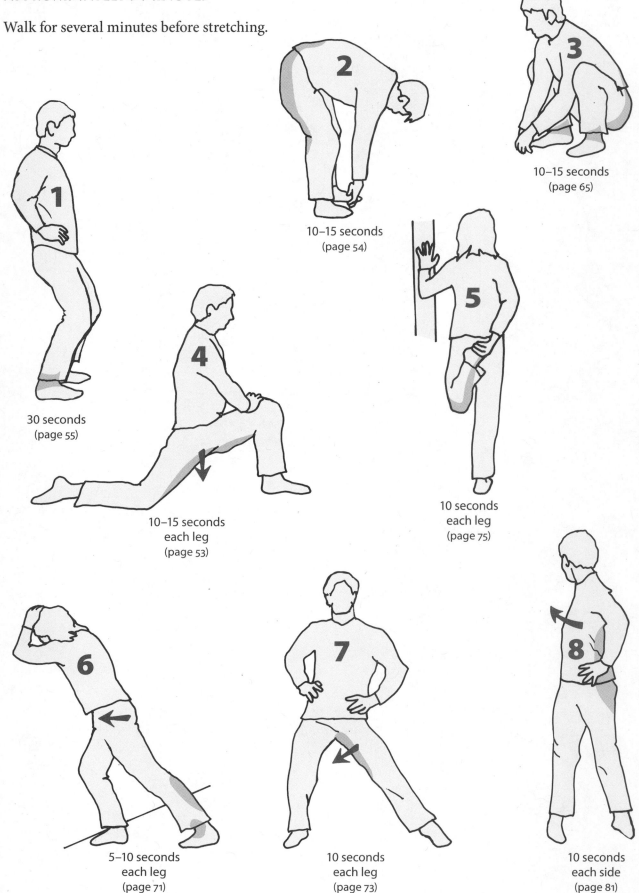

1

30 seconds
(page 55)

2

10–15 seconds
(page 54)

3

10–15 seconds
(page 65)

4

10–15 seconds
each leg
(page 53)

5

10 seconds
each leg
(page 75)

6

5–10 seconds
each leg
(page 71)

7

10 seconds
each leg
(page 73)

8

10 seconds
each side
(page 81)

Stretching © 2010 by Bob and Jean Anderson. Shelter Publications, Inc.

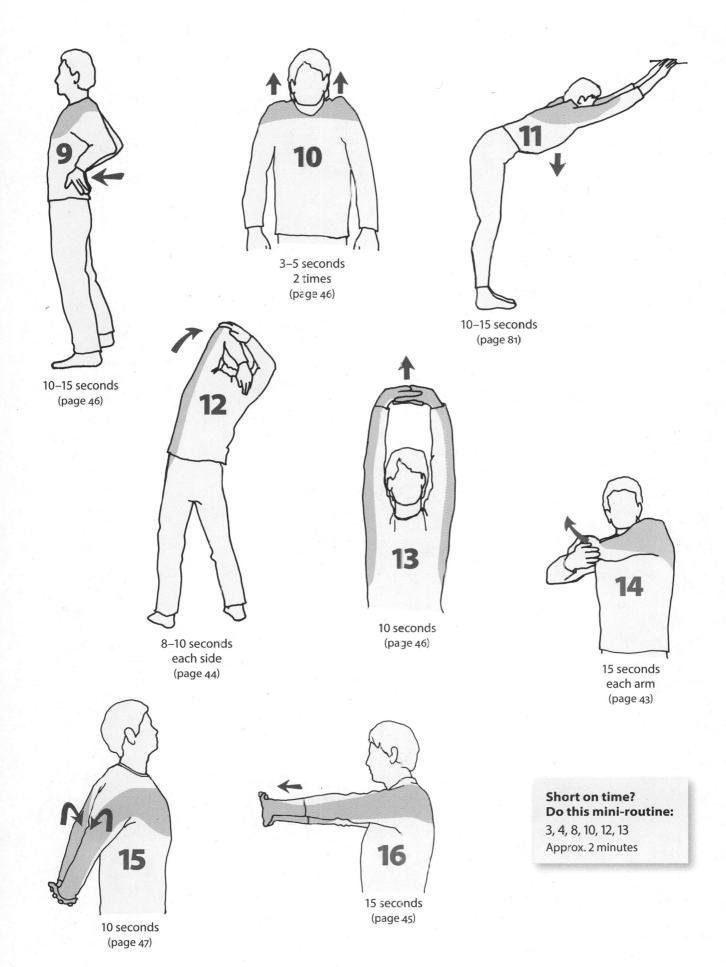

9

10−15 seconds
(page 46)

10

3−5 seconds
2 times
(page 46)

11

10−15 seconds
(page 81)

12

8−10 seconds
each side
(page 44)

13

10 seconds
(page 46)

14

15 seconds
each arm
(page 43)

15

10 seconds
(page 47)

16

15 seconds
(page 45)

Short on time?
Do this mini-routine:

3, 4, 8, 10, 12, 13
Approx. 2 minutes

APPROXIMATELY 3 MINUTES

Jog around the soccer field before stretching.

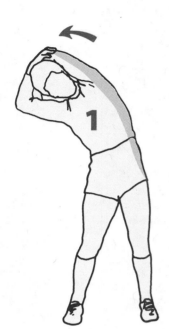

8–10 seconds
each side
(page 44)

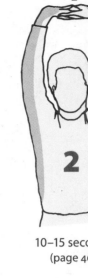

10–15 seconds
(page 46)

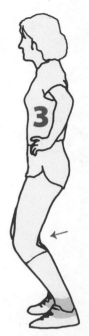

20–30 seconds
(page 55)

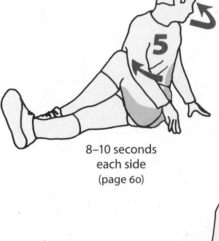

8–10 seconds
each side
(page 60)

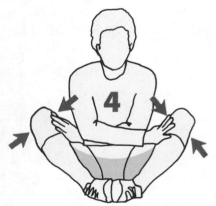

5–8 seconds
(page 59)

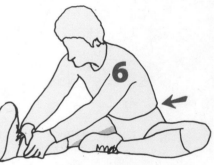

10–15 seconds
each leg
(page 39)

10–15 seconds
(page 65)

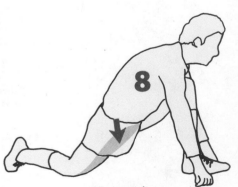

15 seconds
each leg
(page 52)

Short on time?
After a mild warm-up of 2–3
minutes, do this mini-routine:

1, 2, 3, 4, 8
Approx. 2 minutes

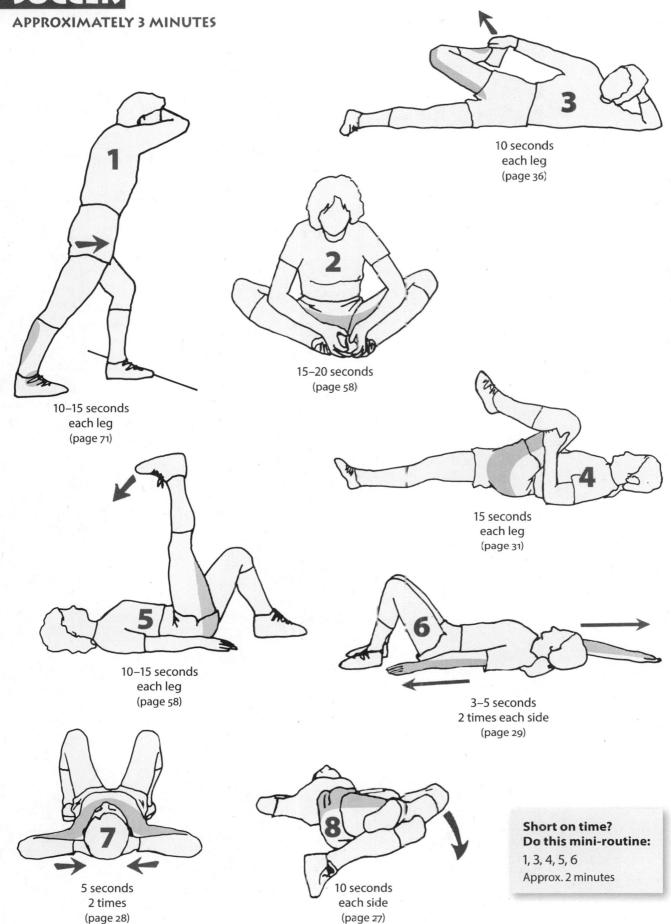

1

10–15 seconds
each leg
(page 71)

2

15–20 seconds
(page 58)

3

10 seconds
each leg
(page 36)

4

15 seconds
each leg
(page 31)

5

10–15 seconds
each leg
(page 58)

6

3–5 seconds
2 times each side
(page 29)

7

5 seconds
2 times
(page 28)

8

10 seconds
each side
(page 27)

**Short on time?
Do this mini-routine:**

1, 3, 4, 5, 6
Approx. 2 minutes

SURFING
APPROXIMATELY 6 MINUTES

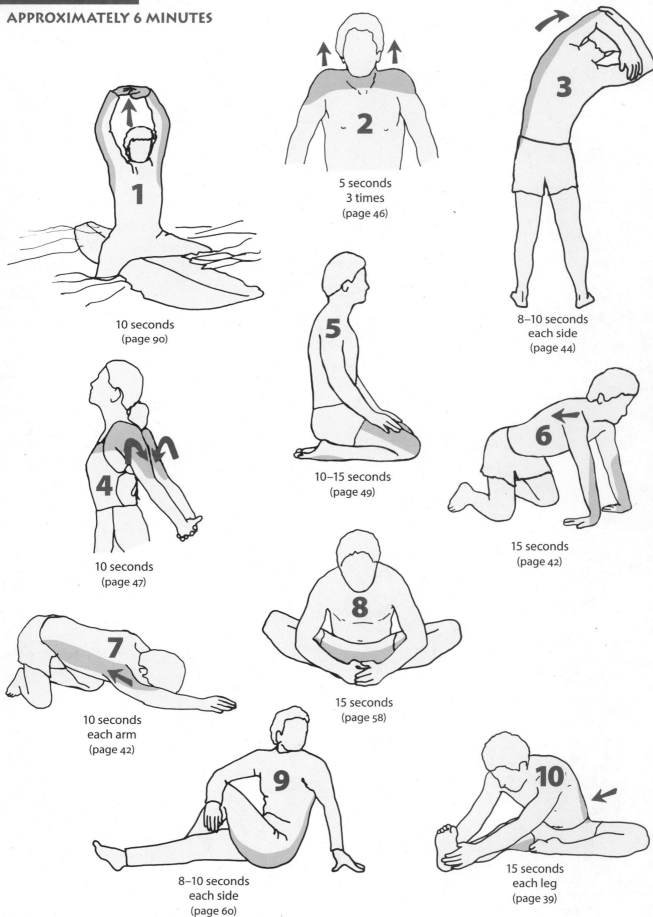

10 seconds
(page 90)

5 seconds
3 times
(page 46)

8–10 seconds
each side
(page 44)

10 seconds
(page 47)

10–15 seconds
(page 49)

15 seconds
(page 42)

10 seconds
each arm
(page 42)

15 seconds
(page 58)

15 seconds
each leg
(page 39)

8–10 seconds
each side
(page 60)

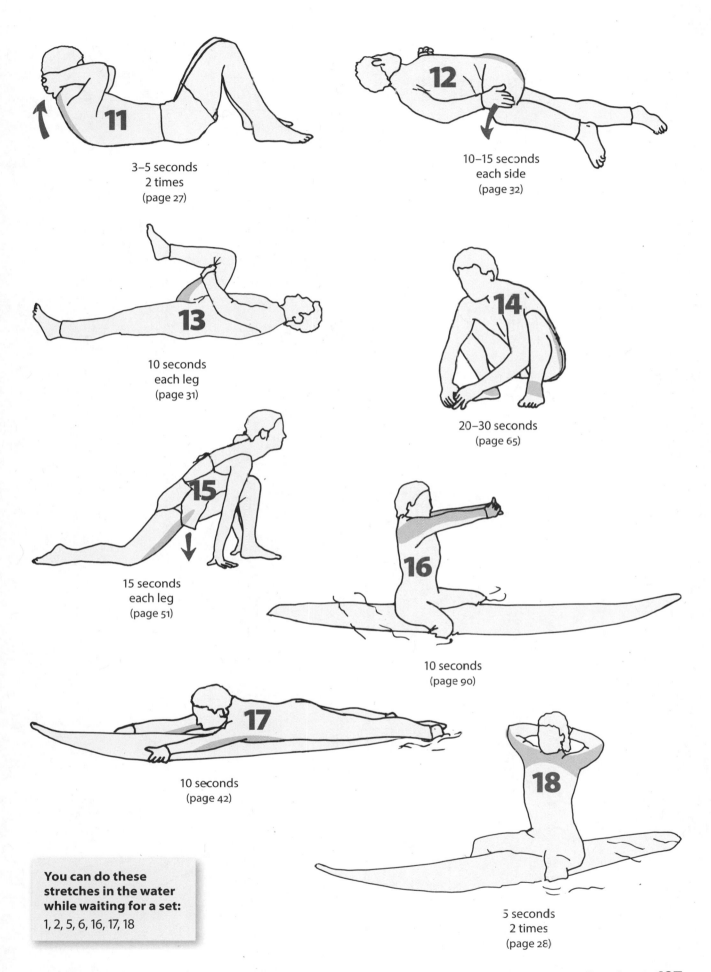

11

3–5 seconds
2 times
(page 27)

12

10–15 seconds
each side
(page 32)

13

10 seconds
each leg
(page 31)

14

20–30 seconds
(page 65)

15

15 seconds
each leg
(page 51)

16

10 seconds
(page 90)

17

10 seconds
(page 42)

18

5 seconds
2 times
(page 28)

You can do these
stretches in the water
while waiting for a set:
1, 2, 5, 6, 16, 17, 18

SWIMMING

APPROXIMATELY 5 MINUTES

Walk with a big arm swing for 2–3 minutes before stretching.

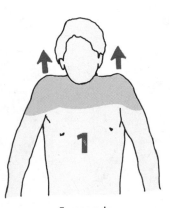

1

5 seconds
3 times
(page 46)

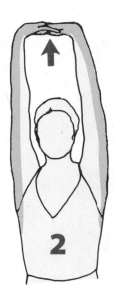

2

10–15 seconds
(page 46)

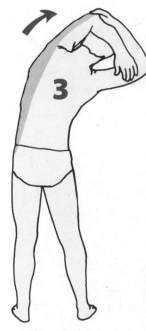

3

10 seconds
each side
(page 44)

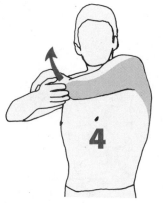

4

15 seconds
each arm
(page 43)

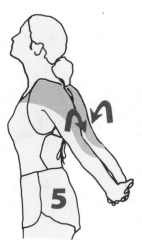

5

15 seconds
(page 47)

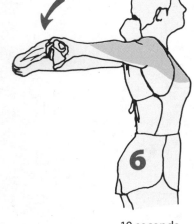

6

10 seconds
(page 87)

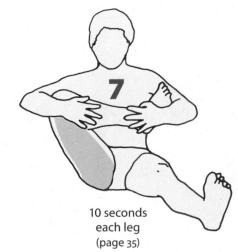

7

10 seconds
each leg
(page 35)

8

15 seconds
(page 58)

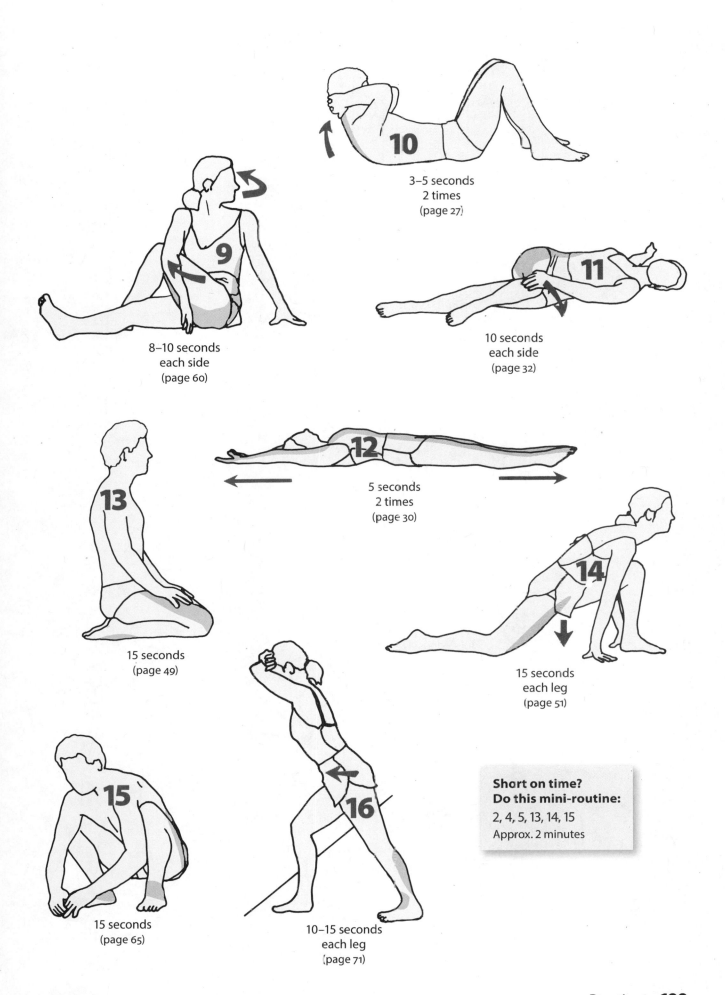

3–5 seconds
2 times
(page 27)

8–10 seconds
each side
(page 60)

10 seconds
each side
(page 32)

5 seconds
2 times
(page 30)

15 seconds
(page 49)

15 seconds
each leg
(page 51)

15 seconds
(page 65)

10–15 seconds
each leg
(page 71)

**Short on time?
Do this mini-routine:**
2, 4, 5, 13, 14, 15
Approx. 2 minutes

TABLE TENNIS

APPROXIMATELY 5 MINUTES

Walk for several minutes before stretching.

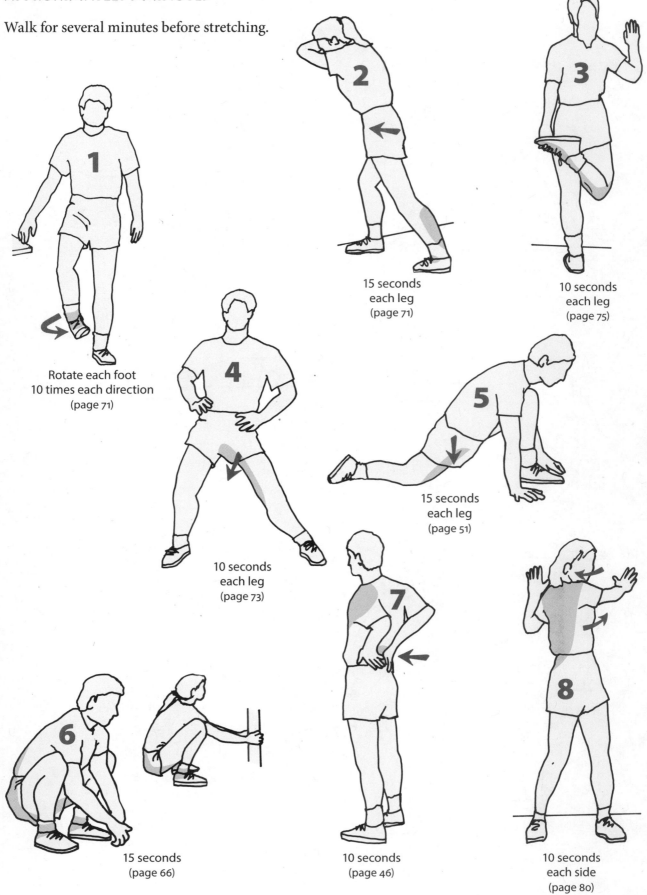

1

Rotate each foot
10 times each direction
(page 71)

2

15 seconds
each leg
(page 71)

3

10 seconds
each leg
(page 75)

4

10 seconds
each leg
(page 73)

5

15 seconds
each leg
(page 51)

6

15 seconds
(page 66)

7

10 seconds
(page 46)

8

10 seconds
each side
(page 80)

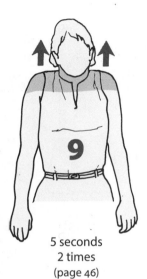

5 seconds
2 times
(page 46)

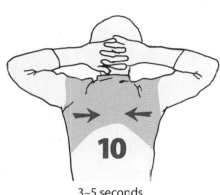

3–5 seconds
2 times
(page 91)

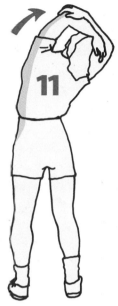

8–10 seconds
each side
(page 44)

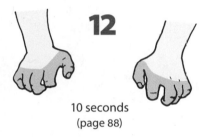

10 seconds
(page 88)

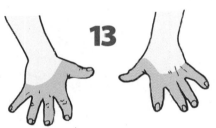

10 seconds
(page 88)

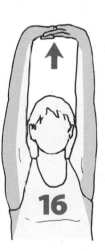

5–10 seconds
(page 46)

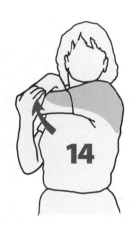

10–15 seconds
each arm
(page 43)

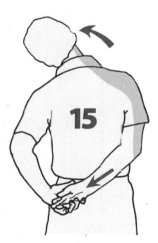

10 seconds
each arm
(page 47)

Short on time?
Do this mini-routine:
2, 3, 5, 8, 10, 11, 15
Approx. 1½ minutes

TENNIS

APPROXIMATELY 5 MINUTES

Walk or jog for several minutes before stretching.

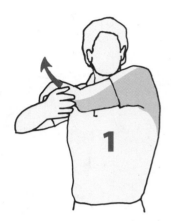

1

10 seconds
each arm
(page 43)

2

5 seconds
2 times
(page 46)

3

8–10 seconds
each side
(page 44)

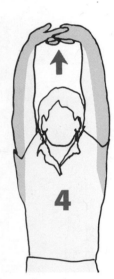

4

8–10 seconds
(page 46)

5

10 seconds
each side
(page 80)

6

10 seconds
each leg
(page 71)

7

10 seconds
each leg
(page 75)

8

15–20 seconds
(page 55)

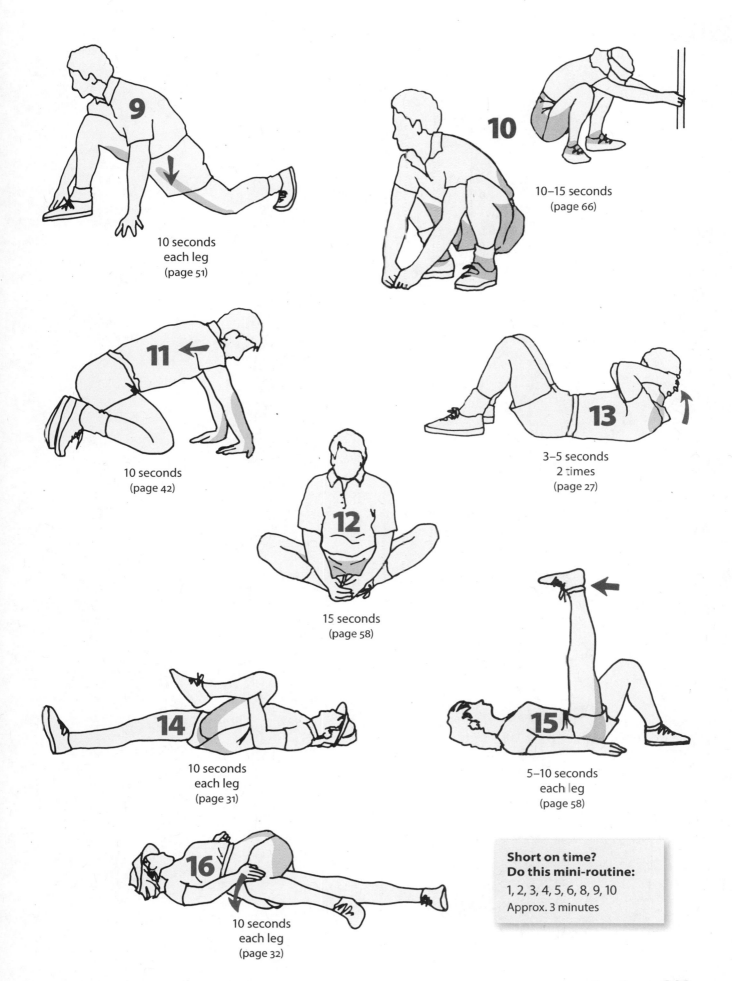

9

10 seconds
each leg
(page 51)

10

10–15 seconds
(page 66)

11

10 seconds
(page 42)

12

15 seconds
(page 58)

13

3–5 seconds
2 times
(page 27)

14

10 seconds
each leg
(page 31)

15

5–10 seconds
each leg
(page 58)

16

10 seconds
each leg
(page 32)

**Short on time?
Do this mini-routine:**

1, 2, 3, 4, 5, 6, 8, 9, 10
Approx. 3 minutes

TREKKING POLES

APPROXIMATELY 6 MINUTES

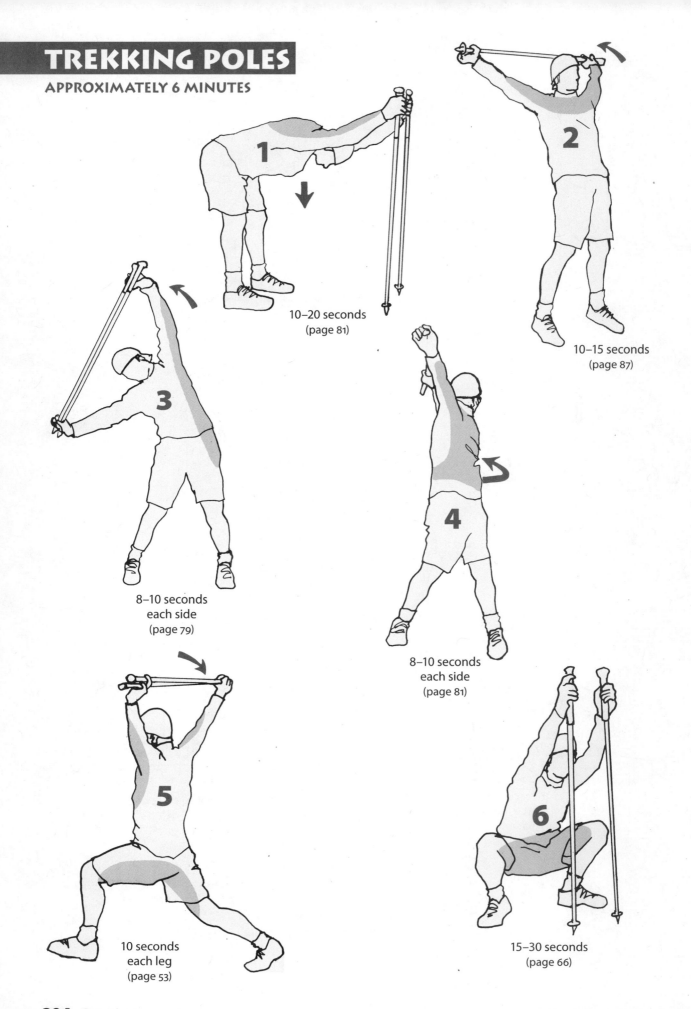

1 10–20 seconds
(page 81)

2 10–15 seconds
(page 87)

3 8–10 seconds
each side
(page 79)

4 8–10 seconds
each side
(page 81)

5 10 seconds
each leg
(page 53)

6 15–30 seconds
(page 66)

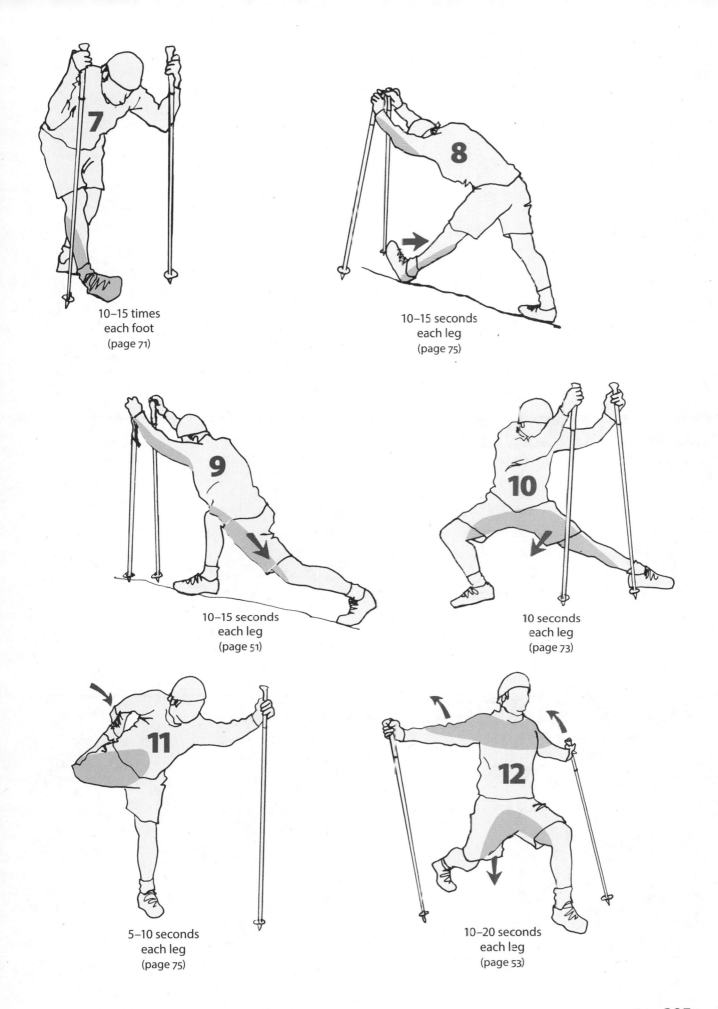

7

10–15 times
each foot
(page 71)

8

10–15 seconds
each leg
(page 75)

9

10–15 seconds
each leg
(page 51)

10

10 seconds
each leg
(page 73)

11

5–10 seconds
each leg
(page 75)

12

10–20 seconds
each leg
(page 53)

TRIATHLON (SWIMMING)

APPROXIMATELY 2½ MINUTES

Walk for several minutes before stretching.

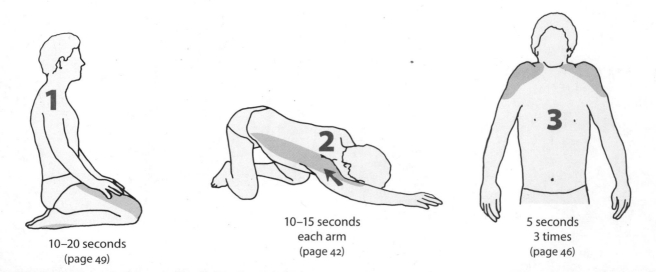

10–20 seconds
(page 49)

10–15 seconds
each arm
(page 42)

5 seconds
3 times
(page 46)

BEFORE & AFTER # TRIATHLON (CYCLING)

APPROXIMATELY 2 MINUTES

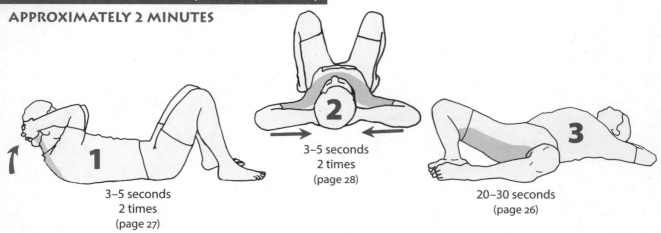

3–5 seconds
2 times
(page 27)

3–5 seconds
2 times
(page 28)

20–30 seconds
(page 26)

BEFORE & AFTER # TRIATHLON (RUNNING)

APPROXIMATELY 2 MINUTES

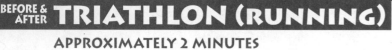

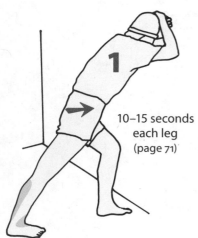

10–15 seconds
each leg
(page 71)

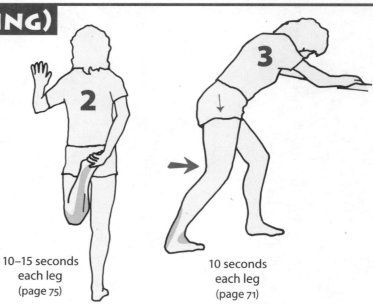

10–15 seconds
each leg
(page 75)

10 seconds
each leg
(page 71)

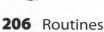

Stretching © 2010 by Bob and Jean Anderson. Shelter Publications, Inc.

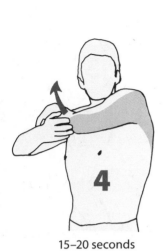

15–20 seconds
each arm
(page 43)

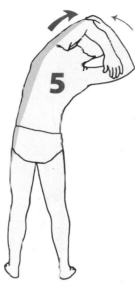

8–10 seconds
each side
(page 44)

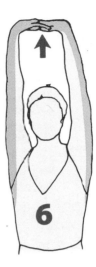

15–20 seconds
(page 46)

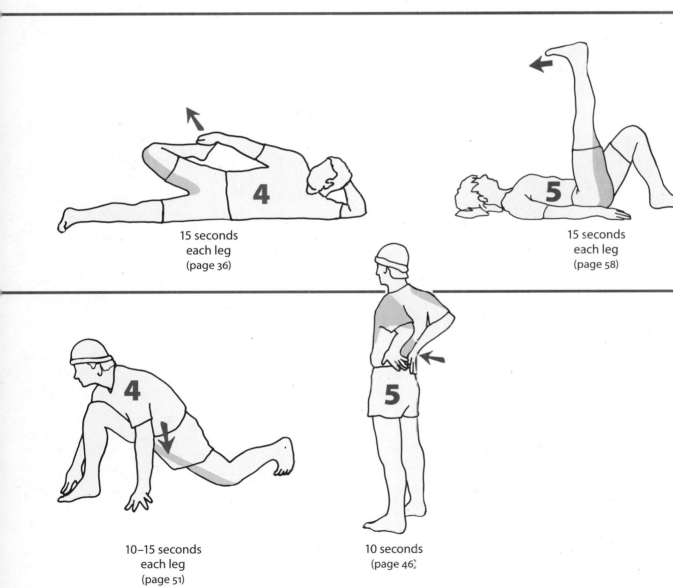

15 seconds
each leg
(page 36)

15 seconds
each leg
(page 58)

10–15 seconds
each leg
(page 51)

10 seconds
(page 46)

Stretching © 2010 by Bob and Jean Anderson. Shelter Publications, Inc.

VOLLEYBALL

APPROXIMATELY 6 MINUTES

Walk or jog for 2–3 minutes before stretching.

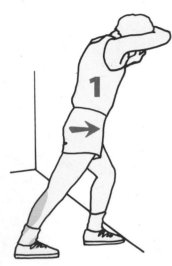

5–10 seconds
each leg
(page 71)

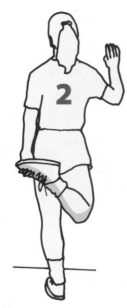

10 seconds
each leg
(page 75)

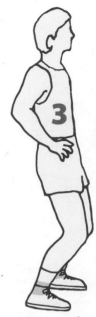

30 seconds
(page 55)

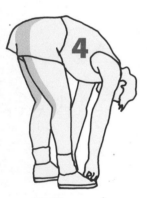

10–15 seconds
(page 54)

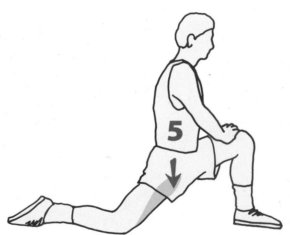

10–15 seconds
each leg
(page 53)

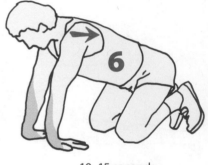

10–15 seconds
(page 42)

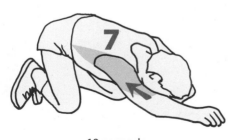

10 seconds
each arm
(page 42)

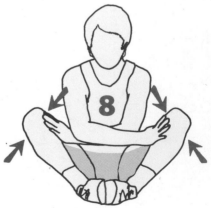

5–8 seconds
(page 59)

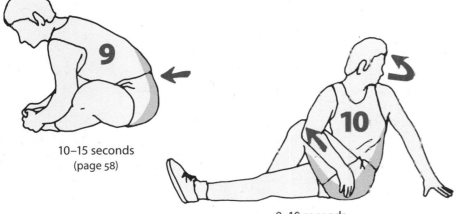

10–15 seconds
(page 58)

8–10 seconds
each side
(page 60)

20 seconds
(page 66)

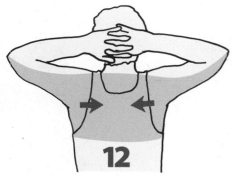

5 seconds
2 times
(page 91)

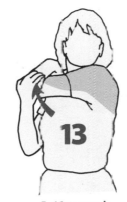

5–10 seconds
each arm
(page 43)

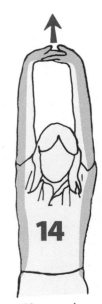

10 seconds
(page 46)

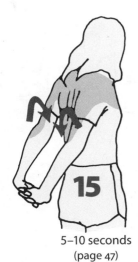

5–10 seconds
(page 47)

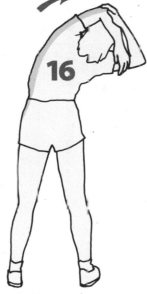

8–10 seconds
each side
(page 44)

Short on time?
Do this mini-routine:
1, 2, 3, 5, 13, 14, 15, 16
Approx. 3 minutes

WEIGHT TRAINING

APPROXIMATELY 7 MINUTES

Warm up by using a stationary bike or treadmill, etc., for 3–5 minutes before stretching.

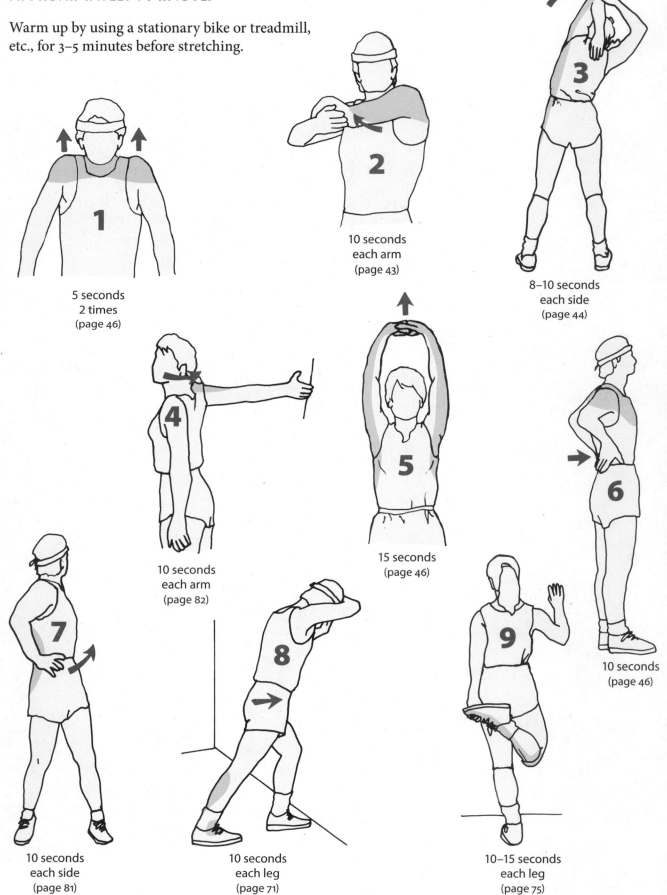

1
5 seconds
2 times
(page 46)

2
10 seconds
each arm
(page 43)

3
8–10 seconds
each side
(page 44)

4
10 seconds
each arm
(page 82)

5
15 seconds
(page 46)

6
10 seconds
(page 46)

7
10 seconds
each side
(page 81)

8
10 seconds
each leg
(page 71)

9
10–15 seconds
each leg
(page 75)

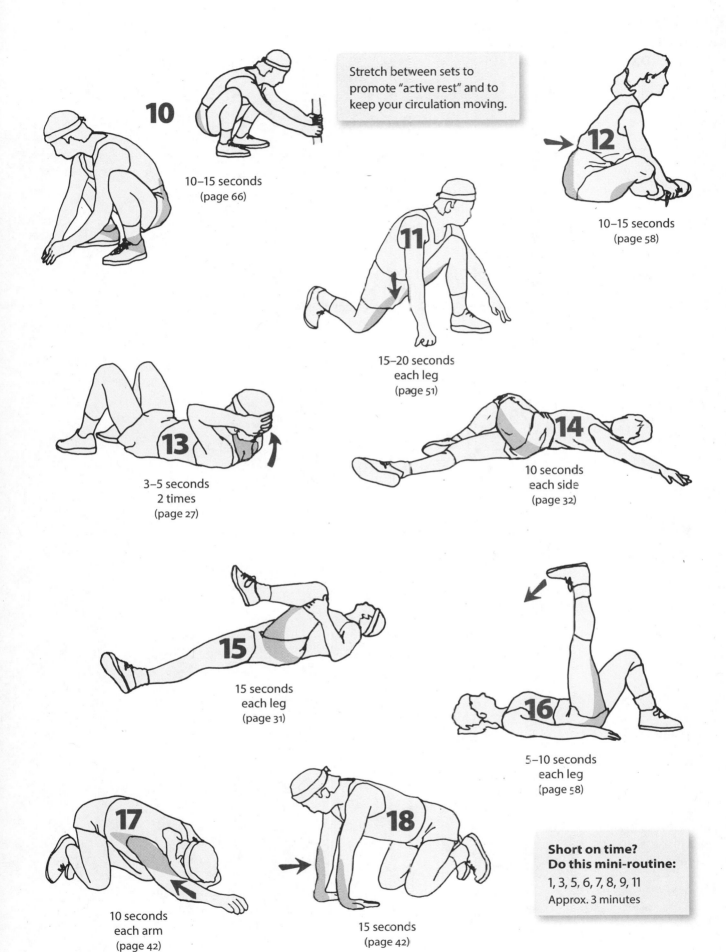

10

10–15 seconds
(page 66)

Stretch between sets to promote "active rest" and to keep your circulation moving.

11

15–20 seconds
each leg
(page 51)

12

10–15 seconds
(page 58)

13

3–5 seconds
2 times
(page 27)

14

10 seconds
each side
(page 32)

15

15 seconds
each leg
(page 31)

16

5–10 seconds
each leg
(page 58)

17

10 seconds
each arm
(page 42)

18

15 seconds
(page 42)

**Short on time?
Do this mini-routine:**
1, 3, 5, 6, 7, 8, 9, 11
Approx. 3 minutes

WINDSURFING

APPROXIMATELY 6 MINUTES

Walk for several minutes before stretching.

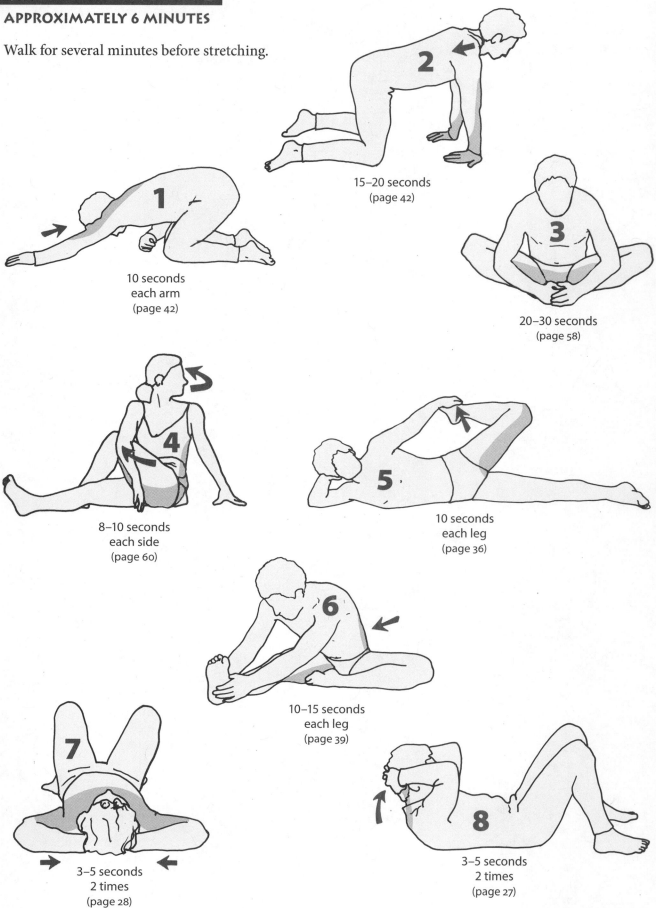

1
10 seconds
each arm
(page 42)

2
15–20 seconds
(page 42)

3
20–30 seconds
(page 58)

4
8–10 seconds
each side
(page 60)

5
10 seconds
each leg
(page 36)

6
10–15 seconds
each leg
(page 39)

7
3–5 seconds
2 times
(page 28)

8
3–5 seconds
2 times
(page 27)

Stretching © 2010 by Bob and Jean Anderson. Shelter Publications, Inc.

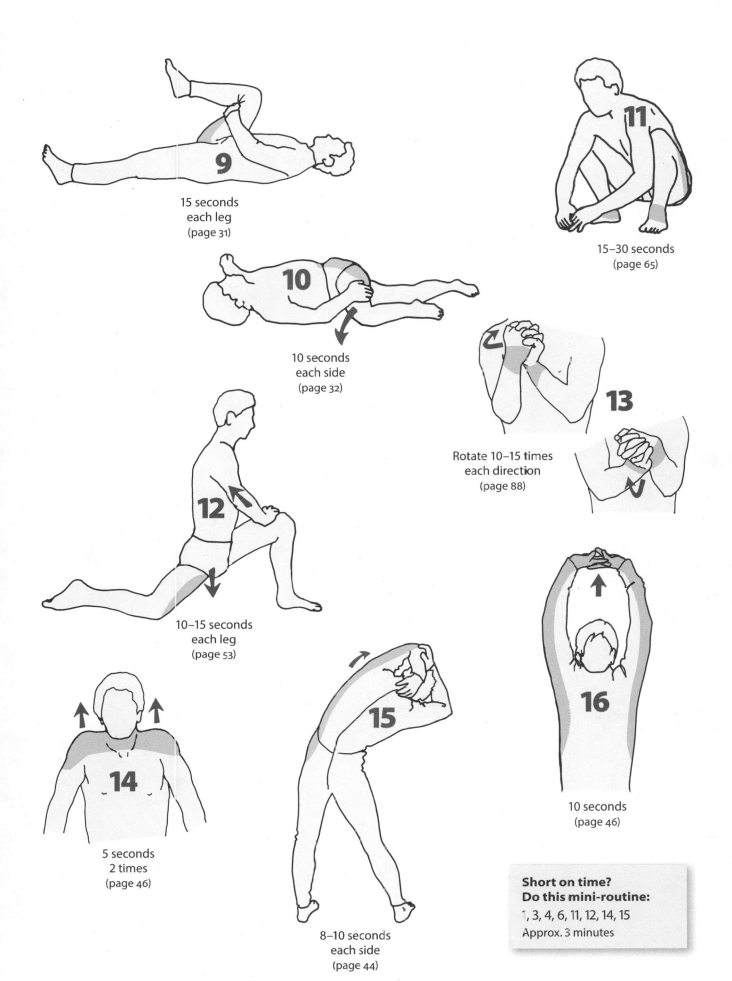

9

15 seconds
each leg
(page 31)

11

15–30 seconds
(page 65)

10

10 seconds
each side
(page 32)

13

Rotate 10–15 times
each direction
(page 88)

12

10–15 seconds
each leg
(page 53)

16

10 seconds
(page 46)

14

5 seconds
2 times
(page 46)

15

8–10 seconds
each side
(page 44)

Short on time?
Do this mini-routine:

1, 3, 4, 6, 11, 12, 14, 15

Approx. 3 minutes

WRESTLING
APPROXIMATELY 6 MINUTES

Jog for 2–3 minutes before stretching.

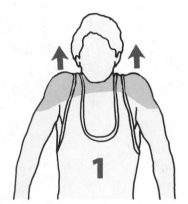

1
5 seconds
3 times
(page 46)

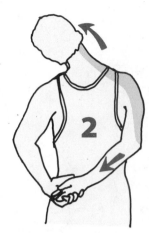

2
10 seconds
each arm
(page 47)

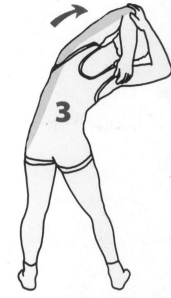

3
8–10 seconds
each side
(page 44)

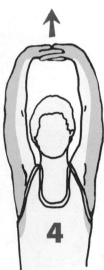

4
15 seconds
(page 46)

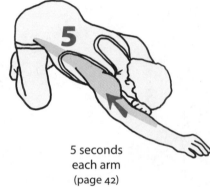

5
5 seconds
each arm
(page 42)

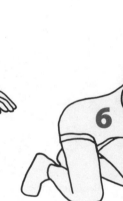

6
20 seconds
(page 42)

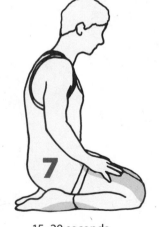

7
15–20 seconds
(page 49)

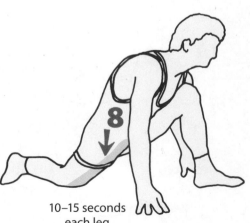

8
10–15 seconds
each leg
(page 51)

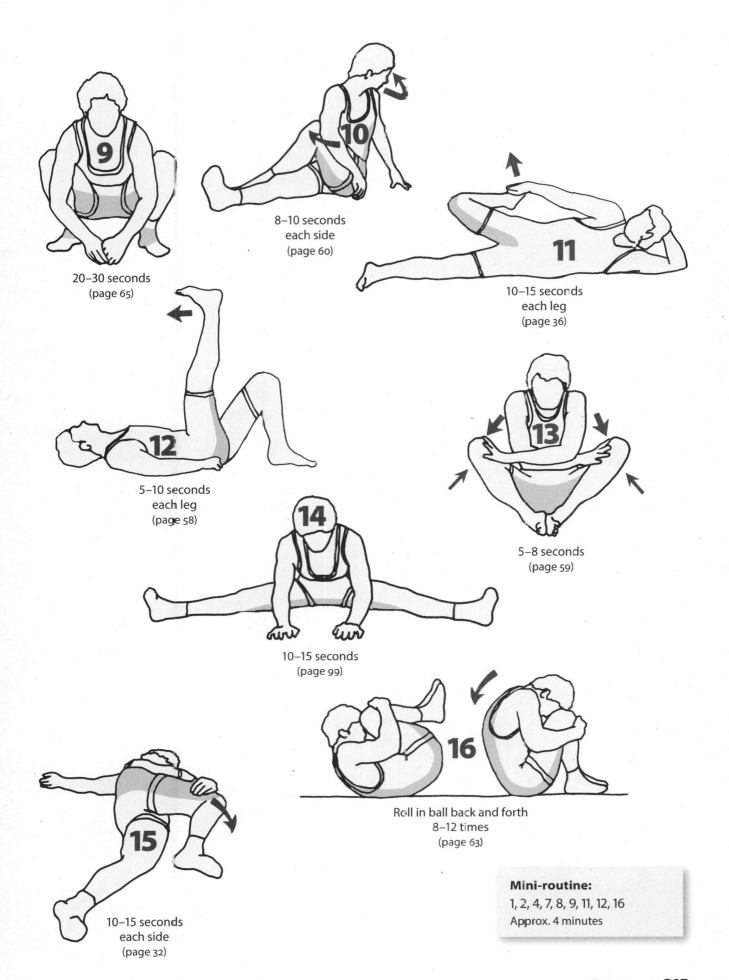

9
20–30 seconds
(page 65)

10
8–10 seconds
each side
(page 60)

11
10–15 seconds
each leg
(page 36)

12
5–10 seconds
each leg
(page 58)

13
5–8 seconds
(page 59)

14
10–15 seconds
(page 99)

15
10–15 seconds
each side
(page 32)

16
Roll in ball back and forth
8–12 times
(page 63)

Mini-routine:
1, 2, 4, 7, 8, 9, 11, 12, 16
Approx. 4 minutes

To Teachers and Coaches

For student athletes training has always stressed discipline, constantly pushing to new limits, and building maximum strength and power. As teachers and coaches, you are interested, of course, in team performance. But your most important goal is to educate the individuals under your supervision.

The best way to teach stretching is by your own example. When you yourself do the stretches and enjoy them, you will communicate this with enthusiasm. You will generate the same kind of attitude in your students.

In recent years, some attention has been given to stretching for injury prevention, but even here, there has been too much emphasis on maximum flexibility. *Stretching is entirely individual.* Let your students know that it is not a contest. There should be no comparisons made between students, because each is different. The emphasis should be on the feeling of the stretch, not on how far one can go. Stressing flexibility at the beginning will only lead to overstretching, a negative attitude, and possible injuries. If you notice someone who is tight or inflexible, don't single that person out; emphasize the proper stretches for that person alone, away from the group.

As a teacher/coach/guide, emphasize that stretching should be done with care and common sense. You do not have to set standards or push limits. Do not overwork or force your students to do too much. They will soon discover what feels right to them. They will improve naturally—and enjoy it.

It is important for students to understand that each and every one of them is an individual, with his or her own limits and a certain potential. All they can do is their best, nothing more.

The greatest gift you can give your students is to prepare them for the future. Teach them the value of regular exercise, of stretching daily, and of eating sensibly. Impress upon them that everyone can be fit, regardless of strength or athletic ability. Instill in your students an enthusiasm for movement and health that will last a lifetime.

APPENDIX

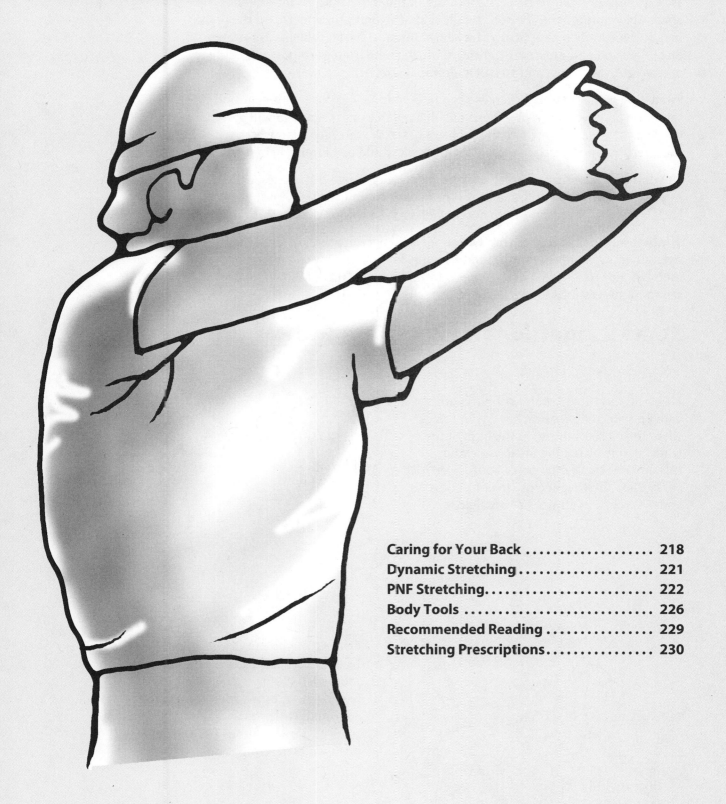

CARING FOR YOUR BACK

More than 50 percent of all Americans will suffer from some sort of back problem some time during their lives. Some problems may be congenital, such as sway back or *scoliosis* (lateral curvature of the spine). Others may be the result of an automobile accident, a fall, or sports injury (in which case the pain may subside, only to reappear years later). But most back problems are simply due to tension and muscular tightness, which come from poor posture, being overweight, inactivity, and lack of abdominal strength.

Stretching and abdominal exercises can help your back if done with common sense. If you have a back problem, consult a reliable physician who will give you tests to see exactly where the problem lies. Ask your physician which of the stretches and exercises shown in this book would be of most help to you.

Anyone with a history of lower back problems should avoid stretches, called hyperextensions, that arch the back. They create too much stress on the lower back, and for this reason I have not included any such stretches in this book.

The best way to take care of your back is to use proper methods of stretching, strengthening, standing, sitting, and sleeping. For it is what we do moment to moment, day to day, that determines our total health. In the following pages are some suggestions for back care. *(Also see pp. 26–33.)*

Some Suggestions for Back Care and Posture

Never lift anything (heavy *or* light) with your legs straight. Always bend your knees when lifting something, so the bulk of the work is done by the big muscles of your legs, not the small muscles of your lower back. Keep the weight close to your body and your back as straight as possible.

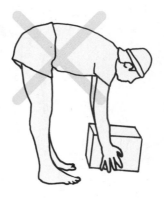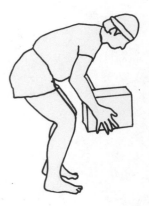

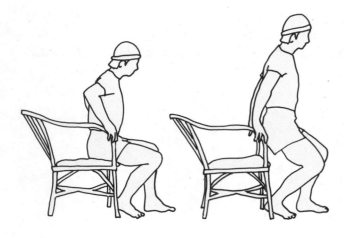

Getting in and out of chairs can be a hazard to your back. Always have one foot in front of the other when rising from a chair. Move your bottom to the edge and, with your back vertical and chin in, use your thigh muscles and arms to push yourself straight up.

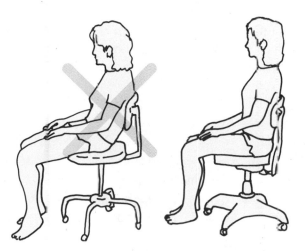

If your shoulders are rounded and your head tends to droop forward, bring yourself into new alignment. This position, when practiced regularly, will lessen back tension and keep the body fresh with energy. Pull your chin in slightly (not down, not up), with the back of your head being pulled straight up. Think of your shoulders being down.

Breathe with the idea that you want the middle of your back to expand outward. Tighten your abdominal muscles as you flatten your lower back into the chair. Do this while driving or sitting to take pressure off the lower back. Practice this often and you will naturally train your muscles to hold this more alive alignment without conscious effort.

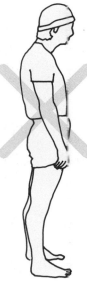

Do not stand with your knees locked. This tilts your hips forward and puts the pressure of standing directly on your lower back: a position of weakness. Let the quadriceps support the body in a position of strength. Your body will be more aligned through the hips and lower back with knees slightly bent.

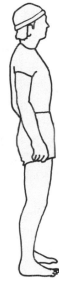

When standing, your knees should be slightly bent (½ inch), with feet pointed straight ahead. Keeping the knees slightly bent prevents the hips from rotating forward. Use the big muscles in the front of the upper legs (*quadriceps*) to control your posture when standing.

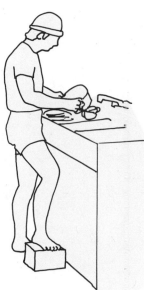

If you stand in one place for a period of time, as when doing the dishes, prop one foot up on a box or short stool. This will relieve some of the back tension that comes from prolonged standing.

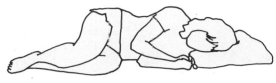

A good, firm sleeping surface helps in back care. If possible, sleep on one side or the other. Sleeping on your stomach can cause tightness in the lower back. If you sleep on your back, a pillow under your knees will keep your lower back flat and minimize tension.

When you are aware that your posture is bad, automatically adjust into a more upright, energetic position. Good posture is developed through the constant awareness of how you sit, stand, walk, and sleep.

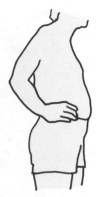

Many tight and so-called bad backs can be caused by excessive weight around the middle. Without the support of strong abdominal muscles, this extra weight will gradually cause a forward pelvic tilt, causing pain and tension in the lower back.

1. Develop the abdominal muscles by regularly doing abdominal curls. Exercise within your limits. It takes time and regularity. But if you don't get into it, the condition will only worsen.

2. Develop the muscles of the chest and arms by doing knee push-ups. These push-ups isolate the muscles in the upper body without straining the lower back. Start an easy three-set routine such as 10–8–6, or whatever — just get started!

3. Stretch the muscles in the front of each hip as shown on p. 51, and stretch the muscles of the lower back *(pp. 26–33 and 63–67)*. By strengthening the abdominal area and stretching the hip and back areas, you can gradually undo the forward pelvic tilt that is, in so many cases, the main cause of back problems.

4. Slowly let the size of your stomach shrink by not overeating.

5. Learn how to walk before you jog, and jog before you run. If you walk a mile a day (at one time) every day, without increasing your calorie intake, you will lose ten pounds of fat in one year.

A unique book on self-care for low-back pain:

Treat You Own Back, by Robin McKenzie, published by OPTP <www.OPTP.com>, 2006.

Dynamic Stretching

What's all this you hear these days about "dynamic stretching?" There have been recent media articles claiming that "dynamic stretching" is the preferred method for athletes, that static stretching is no longer useful before competition, and in fact, may even be harmful. First, some definitions:

- *Dynamic* stretching is defined as "…actively moving a joint through the range of motion required for a sport."
- *Static* stretching refers to holding a stretch with no movement.
- Stretching, as in this book, refers to a two-phase stretch with movement.*

What's going on here? It may have started with a well-publicized study in the 1994 Honolulu Marathon in which runners who stretched had more injuries than those who didn't. First, how did the control group stretch? If incorrectly (as many competitors do — pushing too far, or bouncing), it could well have increased injuries. And why conclude that stretching *caused* the injuries? (Curiously, these results applied only to white males, not women or Asians.)

Some sports trainers say athletes should not practice static stretching *before* competition (although many of them recommend it *after* the event). Here's what I recommend:

For athletes: After a warm-up, some gentle stretches will prepare you for dynamic stretches, drills, and further warming up. Mild stretches give your muscle a signal they are about to be used. And, static stretching (two-phase) after the event is highly beneficial.

For the general population (ordinary people, not competitive athletes): I believe two-phase stretching is as effective and useful as ever. Over 3½ million people (worldwide) have bought and used *Stretching* (the great majority of them not competitive athletes). We've received favorable feedback for over 30 years. Stretching makes people *feel* better.

And what about yoga? Hundreds of millions of people throughout the world practice yoga, which is actually static stretching. Would they be practicing yoga if it wasn't beneficial?

Curiously, if you check out dynamic stretches, many of them are really drills. Arm swings, leg swings, side bends, toe touches. Nothing new here; these movements have been used for years by athletes in warm-ups; they just weren't called "dynamic stretching."

Some of the new dynamic stretches look good to me, including those that take a regular stretch and add motion, mimicking sports-specific movements. You can see a video of these online at: *http://bit.ly/ja7n*. If I were a competitive athlete, I'd look into dynamic stretching, and — listen to my coach or trainer. But I'd keep static stretches in my toolbox.

To say that dynamic stretching replaces static stretching is short-sighted. One doesn't replace the other, any more than Nautilus machines replaced free weights (or television replaced radio). They each have their place. The millions of people throughout the world who have used *Stretching* will continue to use and benefit from the book. Competitive athletes and their coaches will continue evolving warming-up and stretching techniques, finding the best combination for optimum performance and avoidance of injury.

Stretching for ordinary people (such as office workers or computer users) is about feeling your body, paying attention to stiffness and flexibility. Tune into your body, never push things to the point of pain, never bounce, or do extreme stretches. Focus on how each stretch feels. Be sensitive to your body. You don't need a Ph.D. to tell you how you feel, any more than you "…need a weatherman to know which way the wind blows." Try some stretches (*for example, pp 15–21*) and you be the judge.

*My type of stretching isn't strictly "static." It consists of a two-phase stretch: the *easy stretch,* where you relax into the stretch, is followed by the *developmental stretch,* where you move it a little farther — always paying close attention to how your body feels.

PNF Stretching

PNF is the abbreviation for "proprioceptive neuromuscular facilitation," a physical therapy developed after World War II to help rehabilitate soldiers suffering from neurological disorders. By the '60s and '70s, physical therapists and sports trainers began using PNF techniques to increase flexibility and range of motion for healthy people, including athletes. In ensuing years, PNF practices have gained popularity with trainers and athletes seeking to optimize sports performance.

Though this book is primarily about two-phase, static stretching, I have also included some basic PNF stretches. PNF is most often used by athletes and by individuals who have less-than-normal range of motion or who have lost normal range of motion. The PNF stretches in this book can be done without a partner or assisting device. They are easy to learn and use. These stretches are mainly the *contract-relax-stretch technique* and the *antagonist contract-relax technique*. Following are descriptions and examples of these two types of PNF stretches.

Contract-Relax-Stretch Technique

Here the muscle is passively taken through a range of motion that produces a mild (not painful) stretch tension, then contracted (as forceful as a closed fist) for 4–5 seconds, then relaxed momentarily, and then taken once again into a mild static stretch for 5–15 seconds. This process may be repeated several times. Each time you can expect a slight increase in tension-free flexibility.

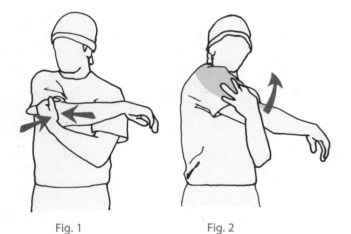

Fig. 1   Fig. 2

Isometric contraction — a muscular contraction in which you increase muscle tension, but the muscles do not lengthen and the joints do not move.

Important: Because of the moderate isometric contraction required in PNF, individuals with heart disease or high blood pressure should be cautioned in the use of PNF. (My approach to isometric contractions is to exert much less than maximal effort.)

Pull your elbow across your chest until a mild (not painful) stretch is felt, then move your elbow away from your body against the resistance of your opposite hand. Now hold a sustained (50–60 percent) isometric contraction for 4–5 seconds (*fig. 1*). (Do not hold your breath; breathe during contraction of the muscle you will be stretching next.) Relax momentarily and then use your hand and arm to pull your elbow further back across your chest until a mild stretch tension is again felt in the muscles just contracted (*fig. 2*). Hold a mild (moderate) stretch for 5–15 seconds. Repeat several times.

Antagonist Contract-Relax Technique

The second PNF technique uses the principle of contracting and relaxing opposing muscles, such as with the quadriceps (front thigh) and the hamstrings (back of thigh). In this PNF technique, you contract your quadriceps to relax your hamstrings, then stretch your hamstrings, as in figure 1 or 4. This action facilitates the hamstrings' relaxation through the reciprocal inhibition reflex. (Sounds complicated but is easy to do.) When you contract your quadriceps, as in figure 3, your hamstrings will relax.

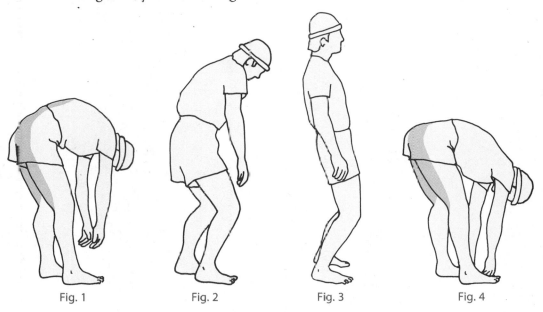

| Fig. 1 | Fig. 2 | Fig. 3 | Fig. 4 |

Try it out. Start in a standing position and slowly bend forward from the hips (keeping knees slightly flexed), until you reach a comfortable stretch (*fig. 1*). At this time note how far you are able to go. Return to a standing position, keeping your knees slightly flexed as you do so (*fig. 2*).

Now assume a flexed-knee position, with feet flat and pointed straight ahead (*fig. 3*). Hold for 15–20 seconds. This position contracts your quadriceps and relaxes your hamstrings, which should make it easier to stretch your hamstrings in the next position. Stand up straight and without bouncing go into the first stretch (*fig.1*). Hold for 5–15 seconds or so. You will probably be able to stretch farther now than you could the first time with the same amount of effort. Repeat figures 3 and 1 several times and expect slight-to-moderate flexibility gains (*fig. 4*).

These two examples should help you to understand and be able to use some basic PNF stretches. The PNF stretches are scattered throughout the book; being mixed in with the sustained (static) stretches. I think the combination of sustained (static) stretches and PNF stretches works quite well.

> **Caution:** Do not overdo the PNF stretches. Stay relaxed and don't strain during mild contractions. Keep breathing! Be comfortable in your approach. Straining and overdoing only leads to not doing!

On the next two pages is a summary of PNF stretches that appear in various places throughout the book.

PNF STRETCHES

Here are some PNF stretches, as described in the preceding two pages. Try them out to see if the technique works for you (helps you get more flexible). Once you get the idea, you can use the technique on any stretch. Contract-relax-stretch, contract-relax-stretch, etc.

Repeat each of these series several times. Hold each contraction 4–5 seconds, each stretch 5–15 seconds.

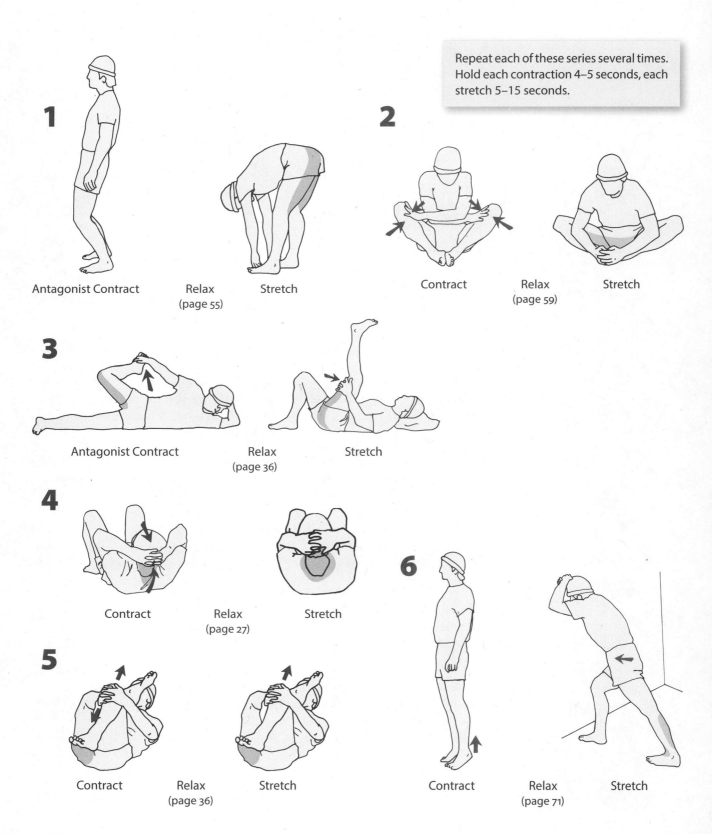

1
Antagonist Contract   Relax (page 55)   Stretch

2
Contract   Relax (page 59)   Stretch

3
Antagonist Contract   Relax (page 36)   Stretch

4
Contract   Relax (page 27)   Stretch

5
Contract   Relax (page 36)   Stretch

6
Contract   Relax (page 71)   Stretch

7

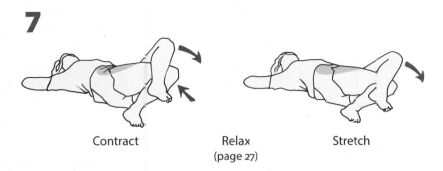

Contract   Relax   Stretch
                  (page 27)

Don't push it! No pain! *Feel* the stretch.
Listen to your body.

8

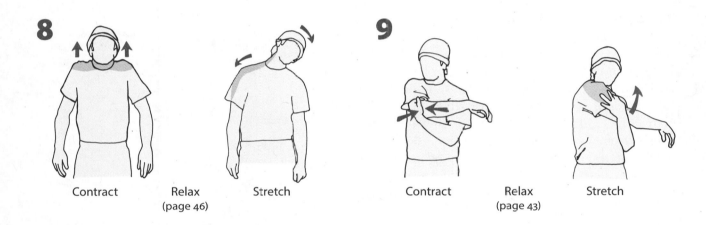

Contract   Relax   Stretch
              (page 46)

9

Contract   Relax   Stretch
              (page 43)

10

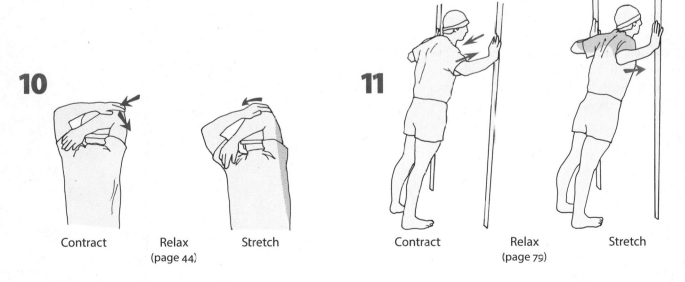

Contract   Relax   Stretch
              (page 44)

11

Contract   Relax   Stretch
              (page 79)

BODY TOOLS

Body tools are self-help devices that allow you to do body work (massage, acupressure) in a very precise way without a partner. I started using various body tools in the early '90s and found them really helpful. I also discovered that they worked exceptionally well when combined with regular stretching. So I introduced them to the participants at the camps I attended and clinics I gave and the response was excellent.

People like the fact that the tools are easy to use and that they are helpful with trigger points (knotted muscle tissue) and tension. They allow you to work on your body in completely different ways. You can easily access trigger points and sore spots. Tight muscle tissue can be loosened in just a few minutes with most of these tools. They make bodywork easy to do and pain reduction a reality.

Here are some tools that I use regularly and recommend.

TheraCane®

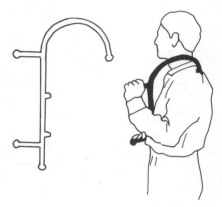

An acupressure tool that loosens tight, painful muscular areas. You use leverage and a slight downward pull to create the desired pressure wherever you want (mild pressure is recommended). Especially designed for the back of the neck, excellent for the mid-back (between shoulder blades), upper back, sides of neck, and shoulders. In fact, it can be used all over the body and even as a stretching aid. This tool has been extremely popular in many pain clinics throughout the United States. It's a great tool that many people find useful.

The Stick®

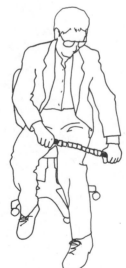

A non-motorized massage device used by serious athletes to loosen "barrier trigger points" (knotted-up muscles). The flexible core with revolving spindles easily molds to various body contours. This tool is wonderful for the legs, especially the calves, and can be used on all major muscle groups. You can use it through clothing or directly on the skin. The Stick provides instant myofascial release by relaxing healthy muscle fibers and promoting good circulation. Adequate blood supply allows muscles to feel better, work harder, last longer, and recover faster. Using this tool gets the muscles ready for activity, helps disperse lactic acid after a hard workout, helps prevent injuries, and hastens recovery time if injured.

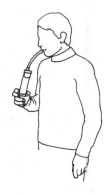

Breath Builder®

This device was originally designed for musicians to develop breath control; however it is excellent for anyone who wishes to develop restorative deep breathing. You blow into a tube and the pressure of your breath keeps a ping-pong ball afloat in the cylinder. It forces you to use your diaphragm muscles and to breathe correctly, with the goal of increasing your lung capacity. Taking more air into your lungs replenishes your bloodstream with oxygen and revitalizes every cell in your body (think of it!). The ball is a visual aid and tells you exactly what your diaphragm is doing by how high the ball floats in the cylinder. Comes with detailed instructions.

The Trigger Wheel®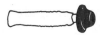

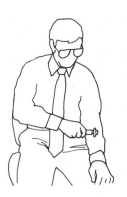

A 2″ nylon wheel on a 4″ handle for deep massage. The Trigger Wheel works on trigger points (knotted muscles) and can be used directly on skin or through light clothing. It works the way a tire rolls back and forth on pavement. Very effective in reaching specific sore spots, such as small areas in the neck, hands, wrists, arms, legs, and feet. You can carry it with you and use it spontaneously throughout the day to keep pain at a minimum.

The Foot Massage®

A 2″ × 9″ roller with raised knobs for foot massage, and rubber rings to protect the floor. A super tool for tired feet. The studded knobs give you pinpoint access to the bottom of the foot. Used to stimulate nerve endings, reduce discomfort, and improve circulation. Use on the job if you sit a lot.

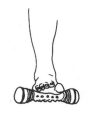

See pp. 234–235 for information on ordering any of these tools.

STRETCHING PRESCRIPTIONS

Here is a summary of the stretches in this book that can be used by health care professionals when prescribing individual fitness and rehabilitation programs. Circle the stretches that are appropriate for the individual.

Relaxing Stretches for Your Back • 26–33

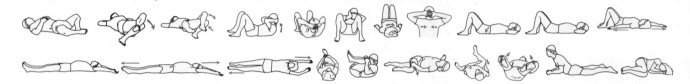

Stretches for the Legs, Feet, and Ankles • 34–41

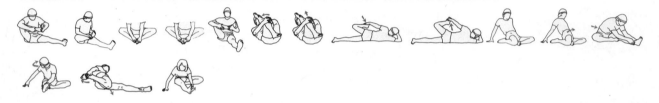

Stretches for the Back, Shoulders, and Arms • 42–48

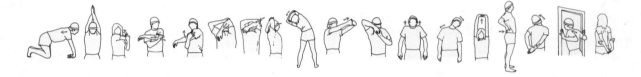

A Series of Stretches for the Legs • 49–53

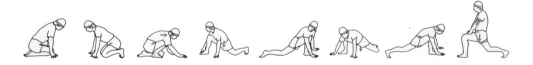

Stretches for the Lower Back, Hips, Groin, and Hamstrings • 54–61

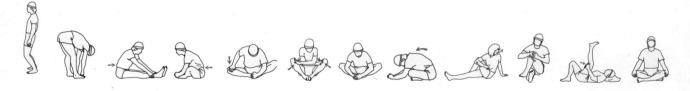

Stretches for the Back, Hips, and Legs • 63–67

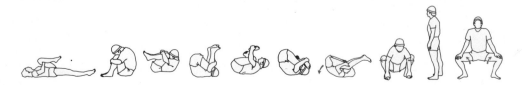

Elevating Your Feet • 68–70

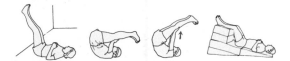

Standing Stretches for the Legs and Hips • 71–77

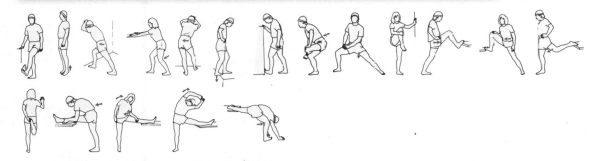

Standing Stretches for the Upper Body • 79–84

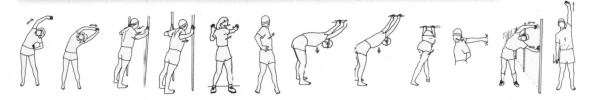

Chin Bar 85	Upper Body with Towel 86–87	Stretches for the Hands, Wrists, and Forearms • 88–89

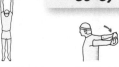

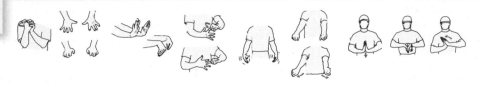

Sitting Stretches • 90–93

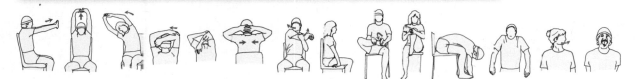

Leg and Groin Stretches with Feet Elevated • 94–96

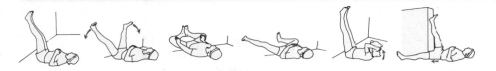

Stretching the Groin and Hips with Legs Apart • 97–100

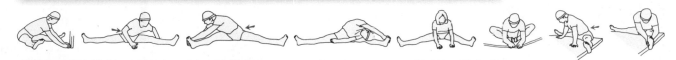

Learning the Splits • 101–102

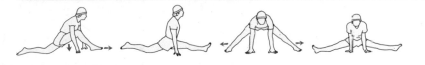

229

INDEX

RECOMMENDED READING

8 Steps to a Pain-Free Back: Remember When It Didn't Hurt. Esther Gokhale, L.Ac.. Pando Press, Stanford, CA. 2008.

A revolutionary new book on improving posture and treating back pain. A wonderful approach.

The Alexander Technique: How to Use Your Body without Stress. Wilfred Barlow and Nikolaas Tinbergen. Inner Traditions, Int'l, Richester, Va. 1991.

An updated edition of the classic guide to F. M. Alexander's technique for successful body dynamics.

Awareness through Movement. Moshe Feldenkrais. Harper, San Francisco. 1991.

Illustrated, easy-to-use exercises to improve posture, vision, motivation, and self-awareness.

The Courage to Start: A Guide to Running for Your Life. John "The Penguin" Bingham. Simon & Schuster, New York. 1999.

An inspiring look at the struggles of a man in his 40s learning to run. Funny, witty, and compassionate. Great inspiration for anyone who wants to start running.

Galloway's Book on Running. Jeff Galloway. Shelter Publications, Bolinas, Calif. 2020.

This classic has helped many thousands of runners get started and train sensibly. It continues to be a best seller.

Getting Back in Shape. Bob Anderson, Ed Burke and Bill Pearl. Shelter Publications, Bolinas, Calif. 2007.

How to get back into shape. 30 programs, each with the 3 components of fitness: stretching, weight training, and moving exercises. A simple, visual approach to life-long fitness.

Getting Stronger: Weight Training for Sports. Bill Pearl. Shelter Publications, Bolinas, Calif. 2005.

Over half a million copies in print, this is 3 books in one: weight training for sports; bodybuilding; and general conditioning. The most complete book on weight training ever produced.

Healing Moves: How to Cure, Relieve and Prevent Common Ailments with Exercise. Carol Krucoff and Mitchell Krucoff, M.D. Healthy Learning, N.Y. 2009.

A timely book by an award-winning health columnist and a renowned cardiologist on the importance of vigorous exercise for general good health. Exercise relieves stress, keeps weight down, improves sleep and helps the body resist illness. There are exercise programs for general health and fitness, as well as exercise prescriptions for specific illnesses and health problems.

Myofascial Pain and Dysfunction, The Trigger Point Manual, Vol 1, Upper Half of Body; Vol 2, The Lower Extremities. Williams and Wilkins, Media, N.Y. 1999.

A classic. Beautifully illustrated. In-depth descriptions and solutions to myofascial pain and dysfunction through trigger point therapy. A reference book that is a pleasure to read and learn from.

Orthopaedic Sports Medicine: Principles and Practices. Jesse C. DeLee, M.D. and David Drez, Jr., M.D. W. B. Saunders Company, Philadelphia. 2009.

Experts in orthopaedic sports medicine share their experiences in dealing with sports injuries. The contributors give an excellent review of their topic, followed by their recommendations for treatment and recovery. These are not books for casual reading; the 2 volumes are over $350.

Running Within: A Guide to Mastering the Body-Mind-Spirit Connection for Ultimate Training and Racing. Jerry Lynch and Warren A. Scott. Human Kinetics, Champaign, Ill. 1999.

Dr. Lynch brings us to the forefront of sports psychology. Here are mental tools for running farther and faster, as well as for integrating body, mind, and spirit.

8 Weeks to Optimum Health. Andrew Weil, M.D. Ballntine Books, N.Y. 2007.

Dr. Weil believes in the body's natural abilities to heal. His changes are not radical but rather a series of simple, small steps to optimum health: taking supplements, adjusting eating habits, eliminating toxins from the diet, and an exercise program based on walking and improving breathing patterns.

Super Power Breathing: For Super Energy, High Health & Longevity. Paul C. Bragg and Patricia N. D. Bragg, Ph.D. Health Science, Goleta, Calif. 2008.

Excellent book on using your lungs to improve your health and increase your resistance to disease. A classic.

Touch for Health: A Practical Guide to Natural Health Using Acupressure Touch and Massage. John F. Thie. Devorss & Company, Marina del Rey, Calif. 2005.

How to utilize acupressure effectively, how to use kinesiology to test you body's need for foods, how to guide your own physical well-being. A complete system for home health.

Stretching in the Office. Bob Anderson and Jean Anderson. Shelter Publications, Bolinas, Calif. 2002.

Stretches and exercises for people who work in offices or at computers. Routines that will relieve stress and tension and keep the body tuned. Keep in your desk drawer.

MORE ON STRETCHING
FROM BOB AND JEAN ANDERSON

Over the past 40 years, Bob and Jean have developed a variety of their own stretching and fitness products, all designed to help people stay flexible and fit. In addition, Bob has discovered a number of body tools and workout products that are distributed by Stretching, Inc.

Stretching DVD

A 57-minute DVD organized in six comfortably paced sections: a brief introduction, stretches for the neck and back, then legs and hips, then feet, and finally, the arms and shoulders. The tape and DVD conclude with a 14-minute stretching routine for all body parts that can be used for everyday fitness or for sports. Suitable for people of all ages and interests. (*The DVD is in spoken English and Spanish; also available in VHS.*)

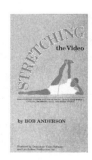

Stretching Charts

These large wall charts are great for learning how to stretch. They not only remind you to stretch (by being so visible), but guide you through a series of stretches (without having to look at the book). They come in both plain paper and laminated, and cover most of the routines in pp. 105–108 in this book.

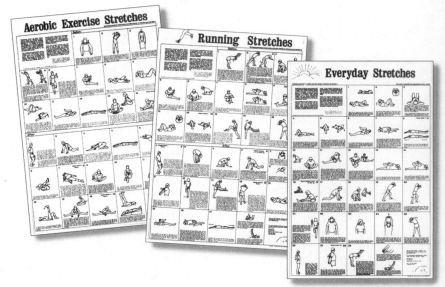

Stretching Chart Pads

These are miniature versions of the wall charts. They measure 8½ by 11 inches and come in pads of 40 identical sheets. As with the wall charts, full instructions are below each stretch. Used frequently by medical professionals, trainers, body workers, and coaches for their clients or team members.

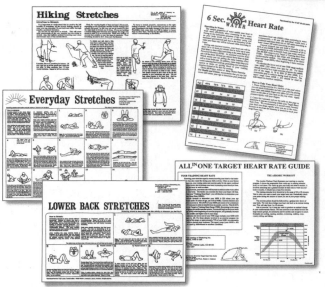

Stretch & Strengthen

This is a spiral-bound book for people in wheelchairs, the disabled, and the elderly. It contains stretching exercises and muscle-strengthening exercises performed with a circular resistive cord with tubular handles. Valuable for rehabilitation and for people with disabilities who want to increase their strength and flexibility.

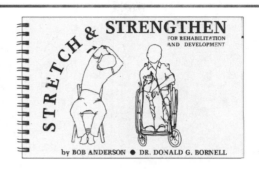

Body Tools

Body tools can be used in conjunction with stretching to help reduce muscular tension and pain. *(See pp. 226–227.)*

Shown here are: TheraCane® • The Foot Massage® Trigger Wheel® • Breath Builder® • The Stick®.

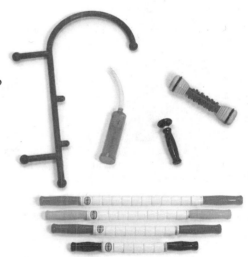

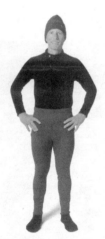
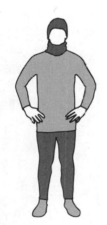

Maxit® Workout Gear

Functional sportswear for the person who wants warmth and dryness (97 percent wind-resistant) and breathability without layering. This blend of spun polyolefin (a new generation of polypropylene) and Lycra® is comfortable and durable. The clothing includes neckgators, balaclavas, sweatbands, headbands, undershirts, tights, shirts, socks. Great for all cold climate activities.

Call 1-800-333-1307 for a free catalog or visit Stretching's website at **www.stretching.com**

MORE FITNESS BOOKS FROM SHELTER PUBLICATIONS

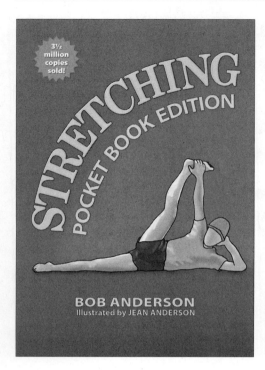

Stretching – Pocket Book Edition
Bob Anderson
Illustrated by Jean Anderson
$14.95   5" × 7¼"
ISBN: 978-0-936070-64-1

• The complete book in small size
• Take it with you when you travel.
• Stretches to do on airplanes, in hotel rooms, on the road

Revised!

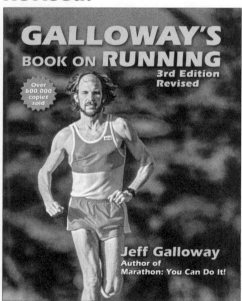

You can do it!

Two running books from Olympic runner Jeff Galloway, originator of the run walk run® method of training

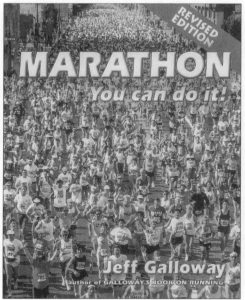

Galloway's Book on Running, 3rd Edition
Jeff Galloway
$21.95   7¼" × 9"
ISBN: 978-0-936070-85-8

• Now includes Jeff's run walk run® training method
• Over 600,000 copies sold

Marathon – You Can Do It!
Revised Edition
Jeff Galloway
$18.95   7¼" × 9"
ISBN: 978-0-936070-25-4

• In the past 35 years, Jeff has coached tens of thousands of people to run their first marathon
• Over 100,000 copies sold

LARGE FITNESS POSTERS FROM SHELTER
LAMINATED, WITH BRASS EYELETS

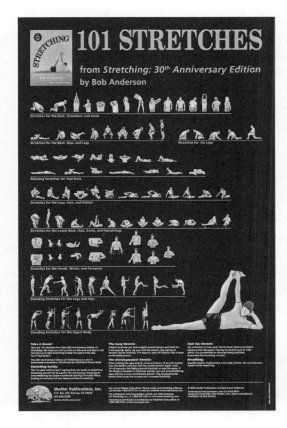

101 Stretches Poster

$19.95   21" × 32"

A large, beautiful four-color poster with 101 stretches, organized by body parts

From *Stretching,* by Bob and Jean Anderson

- Heavy 5-mil lamination, with two brass eyelets for secure hanging
- Hang on a wall as a reminder to stretch once in a while during the day.

Special: 30% discount for both posters
www.shelterpub.com

Free shipping on all retail sales within U.S.A.

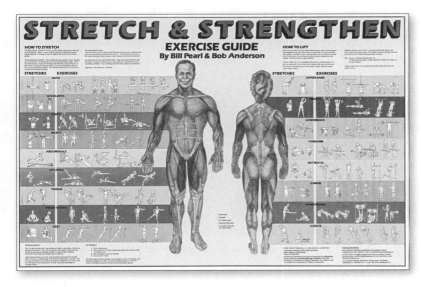

Stretch & Strengthen Poster

$19.95   23" × 36"

A four-color poster with stretches and weight training exercises

- From stretching guru Bob Anderson and bodybuilding legend Bill Pearl
- Body parts are color-coded, along with stretches and exercises for that body part
- Heavy 5-mil lamination, with two brass eyelets for secure hanging

Shelter Publications
P.O. Box 279
Bolinas, CA 94924
415-868-0280
800-307-0131 (orders)
www.shelterpub.com

ABOUT THE AUTHORS

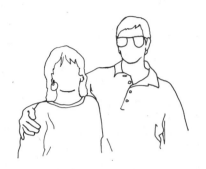

Bob Anderson is the world's most popular stretching authority. For over 40 years, Bob has taught millions of people his simple approach to stretching.

Bob and his wife Jean first published a homemade version of *Stretching* in a garage in southern California in 1975. The drawings were done by Jean, based on photos she took of Bob doing the stretches. This book was modified and published by Shelter Publications in 1980 for general bookstore distribution and is now known by lay people as well as medical professionals as the most user-friendly book on the subject. To date, it has sold over 3¾ million copies worldwide and has been translated into 23 languages.

Bob is fit and healthy these days, but it wasn't always so. In 1968, he was overweight (190 pounds — at 5′9″) and out of shape. He began a personal fitness program that got him down to 135 pounds. Yet one day, while in a physical conditioning class in college, he found he couldn't reach much past his knees in a straight-legged sitting position. So Bob started stretching. He found he soon felt better and that stretching made his running and cycling easier.

The American fitness boom was just starting, and the millions of people who started working out were discovering the importance of flexibility in their fitness programs. After several years of exercising and stretching with Jean and a small group of friends, Bob gradually developed a method of stretching that could be taught to anyone. Soon he was teaching his technique to others.

He began with professional sports teams: the Denver Broncos, the California (now Anaheim) Angels, the Los Angeles Dodgers, the Los Angeles Lakers, and the New York Jets. He also worked with college teams at Nebraska, UC Berkeley, Washington State, and Southern Methodist University, as well as other amateur and Olympic athletes in a variety of sports. He traveled around the country for years, teaching stretching to people at sports medicine clinics, athletic clubs, and running camps.

In the 1980s, Bob was a serious mountain runner and road biker. For ten years in a row he ran the Catalina Island Marathon in southern California, the 18-mile Imogene Pass run in Telluride, Colorado (which goes up over a 13,000-foot-high ridge), and the Pike's Peak Marathon. These days Bob spends most of his workout time on a mountain bike and hiking in the mountains above his house in Colorado, often going for 2–4 hour bike rides in the mountains, with occasional trips to Nevada. Though Bob works out a lot, he knows that training like this is not necessary for the average person to be fit. Through his travels, lectures, and workshops, he's kept in constant touch with people in all degrees of physical condition.

Jean Anderson has a B.A. in art from California State University at Long Beach. She began running and cycling (and stretching) with Bob in 1970. She developed a system of shooting photos of Bob doing the stretches, then making clear ink drawings of each stretch position. Jean was photographer, illustrator, typesetter, and editor of the first homemade edition of *Stretching*. These days she oversees Stretching Inc.'s mail-order business, and hikes and cycles to stay in shape.

CREDITS

Editor
Lloyd Kahn

Contributing Editor
Robert Lewandowski

Production Manager
Rick Gordon

Design
Rick Gordon, Jean Anderson, Lloyd Kahn

Cover Design
David Wills

Art Director
David Wills

Indexing
Frances Bowles

Proofreading
Robert Grenier

Models
Bob Anderson
Jean Anderson
Tiffany Anderson
Shari Boesel
Paul Comish
Kim Cooper
Debra Gentile
Karen Johnston
Bob Kahn
Evan Kahn
Will Kahn
Mari Lillestol
Jim Melo
Justine Melo
Victoria Pollard
Christina Reski
Dave Roche
JoAnne Sercl
Kelsey Sercl
Shane Sercl
Mary Ann Shipstad
Shawntel Staab
Peggy Sterling
Joyce Werth

Production Hardware
Apple Mac computers, Agfa Arcus II
scanner, GCC Elite XL 20/600 laser printer,
Epson Stylus Photo Pro 4800 printer

Production Software
Adobe InDesign, Adobe Photoshop,
Nisus Writer Pro, Microsoft Word

Typefaces
Minion Pro, Myriad Pro, Lithos Pro

Printing
Marquis Book Printing, Montmagny, Quebec,
Canada

Paper
57 lb. Rolland Enviro100 Schoolbook 100%
post-consumer recycled paper

Press
W8 ZMR web press zero make ready

Special thanks to the following people, who
helped with this book in one way or another:

Joan Creed
Drake Jordan
Evan Kahn
Lesley Kahn
Mari Lillestol
Brian Roberts
Tess Rubinstein
Mary Sangster
George Young
The folks at Publishers Group West